CLINICAL
NEUROSURGERY

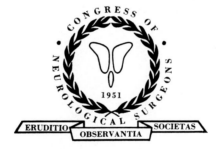

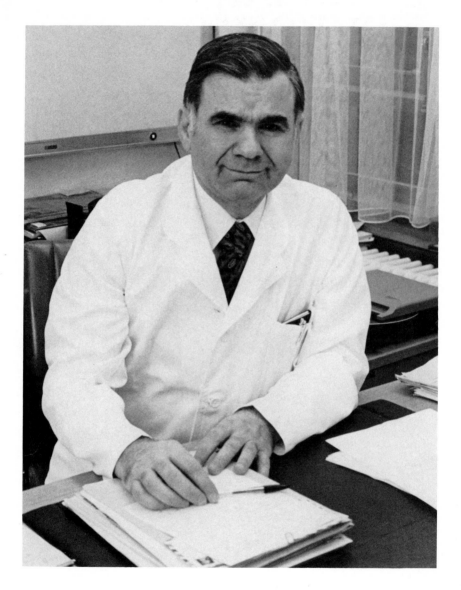

M. Gazi Yaşargil, M.D.

CLINICAL NEUROSURGERY

Proceedings

OF THE

CONGRESS OF NEUROLOGICAL SURGEONS

New Orleans, Louisiana

1986

WILLIAMS & WILKINS
Baltimore • Hong Kong • London • Los Angeles • Sydney

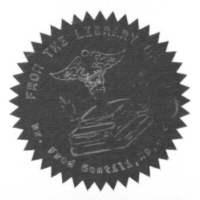

Printed in the United States of America

Library of Congress
Catalog Card Number
S4-12666
ISBN 0-683-02029-3

The Library of Congress cataloged this serial as follows:
Congress of Neurological Surgeons.
    Clinical neurosurgery. v. 1–1953–
Baltimore, Williams & Wilkins.
      v. ill. 24 cm.
    Annual.
    "Proceedings of the Congress of Neurological Surgeons."
    Issues for 1954–70 include the Membership roster of the Congress
of Neurological Surgeons.
    Each vol. honors an individual scientist and presents a biograph-
ical sketch, bibliography, and some of his original papers.
    Indexes:
      Vols. 1–19, 1953–72, in v. 19

    ISSN 0069-4827 = Clinical neurosurgery.
    1. Nervous system.—Surgery.   I. Congress of Neurological Sur-
geons. Proceedings. II. Congress of Neurological Surgeons. Membership roster. III. Title.
    [DNLM: W1 CL732]
RD593.A1C63   617.48   54-12666
                                           MARC-S

87 88 89 90 91
10 9 8 7 6 5 4 3 2 1

Preface

This volume constitutes the Proceedings of the 36th Annual Meeting of the Congress of Neurological Surgeons held in New Orleans, Louisiana, from September 14 to September 19, 1986. Joseph C. Maroon, M.D. (CNS President), Joseph M. McWhorter, M.D. (General Chairman), and Arthur L. Day, M.D. (Chairman, Scientific Sessions) organized an outstanding scientific program upon which this volume is based.

Dr. M. Gazi Yaşargil was the Honored Guest of the Congress. In three chapters, he reflects upon his surgical philosophy, his development as a surgeon, and the future of microneurosurgery. He succinctly describes his principles of microsurgery and illustrates their application in the treatment of "inaccessible" tumors.

The main theme of the scientific program was the "Future of Neurosurgery." The 30 chapters in the general text provide "cutting edge" insights into the surgical treatment of cerebral ischemia, cerebral aneurysm, spinal instability, spinal arteriovenous malformation, orbital tumors, base of skull tumors, and ventricular tumors. The future impact of acquired immunodeficiency syndrome (AIDS) upon neurosurgery is discussed in frank detail. Five chapters are devoted to the potential role of magnetic resonance imaging, ultrasound imaging, and electrical monitoring in the diagnosis and treatment of spinal disorders. Controversies in the medical and surgical management of head and spine trauma are debated by a group of internationally recognized experts. The contents of this volume confirm both the exciting future and continuing challenge of neurosurgery.

I would like to express my appreciation to the members of the Editorial Board for their superb effort in putting together this volume. My secretary, Ms. Marianne Lorini, is also to be congratulated for her help in this endeavor. A special thanks is expressed to Ms. Carol-Lynn Brown, Williams & Wilkins, for her guidance and support.

JOHN R. LITTLE, M.D.
Editor

Editorial Board

JANET W. BAY, M.D.	WALTER J. LEVY, M.D.
ARTHUR L. DAY, M.D.	HAROLD L. REKATE, M.D.
MICHAEL J. EBERSOLD, M.D.	JON H. ROBERTSON, M.D.
STEVEN L. GIANNOTTA, M.D.	WARREN R. SELMAN, M.D.
STEPHEN J. HAINES. M.D.	JAMES H. WOOD, M.D.

v

Honored Guests

1952—Professor Herbert Olivecrona, Stockholm, Sweden
1953—Sir Geoffrey Jefferson, Manchester, England
1954—Dr. Kenneth G. McKenzie, Toronto, Canada
1955—Dr. Carl W. Rand, Los Angeles, California
1956—Dr. Wilder G. Penfield, Montreal, Canada
1957—Dr. Francis C. Grant, Philadelphia, Pennsylvania
1958—Dr. A. Earl Walker, Baltimore, Maryland
1959—Dr. William J. German, New Haven, Connecticut
1960—Dr. Paul C. Bucy, Chicago, Illinois
1961—Professor Eduard A. V. Busch, Copenhagen, Denmark
1962—Dr. Bronson S. Ray, New York, New York
1963—Dr. James L. Poppen, Boston, Massachusetts
1964—Dr. Edgar A. Kahn, Ann Arbor, Michigan
1965—Dr. James C. White, Boston, Massachusetts
1966—Dr. Hugo A. Krayenbühl, Zurich, Switzerland
1967—Dr. W. James Gardner, Cleveland, Ohio
1968—Professor Norman M. Dott, Edinburgh, Scotland
1969—Dr. Wallace B. Hamby, Cleveland, Ohio
1970—Dr. Barnes Woodhall, Durham, North Carolina
1971—Dr. Elisha S. Gurdjian, Detroit, Michigan
1972—Dr. Francis Murphey, Memphis, Tennessee
1973—Dr. Henry G. Schwartz, St. Louis, Missouri
1974—Dr. Guy L. Odom, Durham, North Carolina
1975—Dr. William H. Sweet, Boston, Massachusetts
1976—Dr. Lyle A. French, Minneapolis, Minnesota
1977—Dr. Charles G. Drake, London, Ontario, Canada
1979—Dr. Frank H. Mayfield, Cincinnati, Ohio
1980—Dr. Eben Alexander, Jr., Winston-Salem, North Carolina
1981—Dr. J. Garber Galbraith, Birmingham, Alabama
1982—Dr. Keiji Sano, Tokyo, Japan
1983—Dr. C. Miller Fisher, Boston, Massachusetts
1985—Dr. Hugo V. Rizzoli, Washington D.C.
     Dr. Walter E. Dandy (posthumously), Baltimore, Maryland
1985—Dr. Sidney Goldring, St. Louis, Missouri
1986—Dr. M. Gazi Yaşargil, Zurich, Switzerland

Officers of the Congress
of
Neurological Surgeons
1986

JOSEPH C. MAROON, M.D.
President

DONALD O. QUEST, M.D.
President-Elect

FREMONT P. WIRTH, M.D.   MICHAEL SALCMAN, M.D.
Vice-President   *Secretary*

HAL HANKINSON, M.D.
Treasurer

EXECUTIVE COMMITTEE

ROBERT A. RATCHESON, M.D.   PAUL CROISSANT, M.D.
MARTIN B. CAMINS, M.D.   EDWARD R. LAWS, JR., M.D.
ARTHUR L. DAY, M.D.   LAWRENCE PITTS, M.D.
STEVEN GIANNOTTA, M.D.   J. CHARLES RICH, M.D.
ROBERTO C. HEROS, M.D.   CHRISTOPHER SHIELDS, M.D.
JOE M. MCWHORTER, M.D.   JOHN M. TEW, JR., M.D.
THOMAS SAUL, M.D.

JOE M. MCWHORTER, M.D., *Chairman, Annual Meeting Committee*
ARTHUR L. DAY, M.D., *Chairman, Scientific Program Committee*

Contributors

ADNAN ABLA, M.D., Allegheny General Hospital, Pittsburgh, Pennsylvania

MICHAEL L. J. APUZZO, M.D., Professor, Department of Neurological Surgery, University of Southern California, School of Medicine, Los Angeles, California

DONALD P. BECKER, M.D., Professor and Chairman, Division of Neurological Surgery, University of California Los Angeles, Los Angeles, California

ANDREW R. BLIGHT, PH.D., New York University, New York, New York

DALE E. BREDESEN, M.D., University of California San Francisco, San Francisco, California

WILLIAM F. CHANDLER, M.D., Associate Professor, Division of Neurosurgery, University of Michigan, Ann Arbor, Michigan

MARSHALL CHEUNG, PH.D., University of California Los Angeles, Los Angeles, California

GUY L. CLIFTON, M.D., Associate Professor, Division of Neurosurgery, Medical College of Virginia, Richmond, Virginia

JOHN P. CONOMY, M.D., Chairman, Department of Neurology, Cleveland Clinic Foundation, Cleveland, Ohio

PAUL R. COOPER, M.D., Associate Professor, Division of Neurosurgery, New York University Medical Center, New York, New York

GEORGE F. CRAVENS, M.D., Division of Neurosurgery, Louisiana State University, New Orleans, Louisiana

JOSEPH J. CRISCO, III, M.S., Department of Orthopedics and Rehabilitation, Yale University, New Haven, Connecticut

H. ALAN CROCKARD, F.R.C.S., Department of Surgical Neurology, The National Hospitals of Nervous Diseases, Queen Square, London, England

VINCENT DECRESCITO, PH.D., New York University, New York, New York

PAUL D. DERNBACH, M.D., Department of Neurosurgery, Cleveland Clinic Foundation, Cleveland, Ohio

GEORGE J. DOHRMANN, M.D., PH.D., Associate Professor, Division of Neurosurgery, University of Chicago, Chicago, Illinois

R. M. PEARDON DONAGHY, M.D., Emeritus Professor, Division of Neurosurgery, University of Vermont, Burlington, Vermont

JOHN L. DOPPMAN, M.D., Department of Radiology, National Institutes of Health, Bethesda, Maryland

PAUL S. DWAN, M.D., Division of Neurosurgery, University of California Los Angeles, Los Angeles, California

HOWARD M. EISENBERG, M.D., Professor and Chairman, Division of Neurosurgery, University of Texas, Galveston, Texas

EUGENE S. FLAMM, M.D., Professor, Division of Neurosurgery, New York University, New York, New York

NICOLE C. FODE, R.N., M.S., Department of Neurological Surgery, Mayo Clinic, Rochester, Minnesota

EDMUND FRANK, M.D., Kaiser Permanente, Medical Care Program, Clackamas, Oregon

WILLIAM A. FRIEDMAN, M.D., Assistant Professor, Division of Neurological Surgery, University of Florida, Gainesville, Florida

GEORGE GADE, M.D., University of California Los Angeles, Los Angeles, California

STEVEN L. GIANNOTTA, M.D., Associate Professor, Division of Neurological Surgery, University of Southern California, Los Angeles, California

JOHN A. GRUNER, PH.D., New York University, New York, New York

MARK N. HADLEY, M.D., Division of Neurological Surgery, Barrow Neurological Institute, Phoenix, Arizona

HAROLD J. HOFFMAN, M.D., F.R.C.S.(C) Professor, Division of Neurosurgery, University of Toronto, Toronto, Ontario, Canada

ANTHONY F. JABRE, M.D., Universitatsspital Zurich, Zurich, Switzerland

CLIFFORD R. JACK, JR., M.D., Department of Neurological Surgery, Mayo Clinic, Rochester, Minnesota

JOHN S. KENNERDELL, M.D., Professor, Division of Ophthalmology and Neurology, Eye and Ear Hospital, Pittsburgh, Pennsylvania

HARVEY S. LEVIN, PH.D., University of Texas, Galveston, Texas

ROBERT M. LEVY, M.D., PH.D., University of California San Francisco, San Francisco, California

WALTER J. LEVY, JR., M.D., Division of Neurosurgery, University of Missouri, Columbia, Missouri

JOHN R. LITTLE, M.D., Chairman, Department of Neurosurgery, Cleveland Clinic Foundation, Cleveland, Ohio

JEAN-PIERRE MACH, M.D., PH.D., Associate Professor, Ludwig Institute for Cancer Research, Epalinges, Switzerland

JOSEPH C. MAROON, M.D., Chairman, Department of Neurosurgery, Allegheny General Hospital, Pittsburgh, Pennsylvania

LAWRENCE F. MARSHALL, M.D., Division of Neurological Surgery, University of California Medical Center, San Diego, California

EDWARD H. OLDFIELD, M.D., Department of Surgical Neurology, National Institutes of Health, Bethesda, Maryland

MANOHAR M. PANJABI, PH.D., Department of Orthopedics and Rehabilitation, Yale University, New Haven, Connecticut

LAWRENCE H. PITTS, M.D., Associate Professor, Division of Neurosurgery, University of California, San Francisco, California

JACK L. PULEC, M.D., Clinical Professor, Division of Otorhinolaryngology, University of Southern California, Los Angeles, California

MARK L. ROSENBLUM, M.D., Division of Neurosurgery, University of California San Francisco, San Francisco, California

PETER ROTH, Medical Illustrator, Universitatsspital Zurich, Zurich, Switzerland

JONATHAN M. RUBIN, M.D., PH.D., Associate Professor of Radiology, University of Michigan, Ann Arbor, Michigan

CLARENCE T. SASAKI, M.D., Section of Otolaryngology, Yale University, New Haven, Connecticut

THOMAS G. SAUL, M.D., Associate Professor, Division of Neurosurgery, University of Cincinnati, Cincinnati, Ohio

VOLKER K. H. SONNTAG, M.D., Division of Neurological Surgery, Barrow Neurological Institute, Phoenix, Arizona

DONALD H. STEWART, JR., M.D., Syracuse, New York

THORALF M. SUNDT, JR., M.D., Professor and Chairman, Department of Neurological Surgery, Mayo Clinic, Rochester, Minnesota

GEORGE W. SYPERT, M.D., Professor, Division of Neurosurgery, University of Florida, Gainesville, Florida

LEE L. THIBODEAU, M.D., Section of Neurosurgery, Yale University, New Haven, Connecticut

NICOLAS DE TRIBOLET, M.D., Professor and Chairman, Neurosurgical Service, Centre Hospitalier Universitaire Vandois, Lausanne, Switzerland

MEREDITH A. WEINSTEIN, M.D., Department of Diagnostic Radiology, Cleveland Clinic Foundation, Cleveland, Ohio

BRYCE K. A. WEIR, M.D., Professor and Chairman, Department of Surgery, University of Alberta, Edmonton, Alberta, Canada

AUGUSTUS A. WHITE, III, M.D., Department of Orthopaedic Surgery, Harvard Medical School, Boston, Massachusetts

M. G. YAŞARGIL, M.D., Universitatsspital Zurich, Neurochirurgische Klinik, Zurich, Switzerland

WISE YOUNG, M.D., PH.D., Division of Neurosurgery, New York University, New York

Biography of M. Gazi Yaşargil, M.D.

Mahmut Gazi Yasargil was born July 6, 1925, in Lice, a village in eastern Turkey, approximately 200 miles west of the Turko-Iranian border, and 100 miles north of Syria. At the time of Gazi's birth, the population of Lice was 5,000 to 6,000 and the infant mortality rate was about 165 per 1,000 live births. Children were then regarded, particularly among the well educated, as precious assets, to be guarded, guided, loved, and protected. This was certainly true of the two Yasargil sons and daughter. While the family was still young, a move was made to Ankara, partly because of its excellent educational institutions. A tribute to the family's judgment is made by the fact that all three children are quite successful, and two are professors in some branch of medicine in Switzerland today.

Gazi attended Ankara public schools from 1931 to 1943, when he graduated from the Gymnasium. The children were all strongly influenced by their father, who doted on things academic and encouraged the children to work, and to learn from every possible experience. Friends and neighbors of similar background often came to the Yasargil house and carried on spirited discussions on many subjects, including medicine and neurology. At an early age, Gazi became familiar with the terminology of medicine in general and of neurology in particular, as one of Gazi's father's friends was a neurologist.

In 1944, Gazi entered medical school at Frederick Schiller University in Jena, Germany. However, classes were disrupted in 1945 because of World War II and young Gazi transferred to medical school at Basel, Switzerland, where he obtained his medical degree in 1950. Here he was greatly influenced by Professor Muller, a psychiatrist, and his senior thesis was written on the effects of drugs on delirium tremens. This kept Gazi in contact with the principles of cerebral anatomy and physiology, but the concepts of psychiatry were not precise enough for him. His mathematical mind yearned for a problem that he could solve, for a truth which became evident.

In the meantime, Gazi met Professor Hugo Krayenbühl, who headed neurosurgery at the University of Zurich. Young Doctor Yasargil was much impressed by this learned scholar and surgeon, and by the logic and precision of the nervous system. One could localize pathology from a painstaking history of the symptoms and their development, and gain a knowledge of nervous system anatomy and function. Thus, careful examination revealed the location of pathology, while the behavior and pattern of the development of symptoms could reveal the nature of the process. Moreover, if one studied the various tracts of the nervous system, one could determine where along the pathway the process had progressed, and if it were localized or disseminated. It now remained to seek new techniques for examinations that could refine the location of the lesion and perhaps give a clue to its nature.

Gazi joined Dr. Krayenbühl in neurological surgery on January 4, 1953. His admiration for the Chief increased, as many facets of care, evaluation, investigation, and theory were revealed to him. Near this same time, a new technique, stereotactic surgery, made its debut. Deep brain lesions were approached without direct vision, by advancing a slender instrument along a set of coordinates, until one reached the site of the problem. Gazi expressed an interest in stereotactic surgery, and he was dispatched to Germany to learn the technique. He found, however, that it was ideal for destroying a given area or a sharply localized lesion, but was not of great value in the repair or reconstruction of tissues.

This was somewhat of a disquieting revelation to Gazi, as his interest at that time was focused on vascular lesions such as aneurysms and arteriovenous malformations. Arteriography, the x-ray technique developed by Lima and Moniz in Portugal, was of greater interest to Gazi, as it actually allowed one to see blood vessels and their exact location. One could now tell whether a vessel required occlusion or repair. For the first time, one could study the angiograms and devise a more precise and physiologically sound operation for ligation or coating of various lesions.

After overcoming the irritating effects of the contrast agents used in arteriography, experience with vascular lesions grew, revealing many problems. One actually needed to count the vessels entering a malformation or aneurysm, and to note the borders of the vessels, so one could recognize them during surgery. The vessels thus identified were often small and their exploration might lead to disruption and bleeding.

New methodology, however, was developing that held some promise. The technique of microsurgery allowed the surgeon to see, by using a dissecting microscope, the lesion in magnified form. The surgery of such fine structures was being studied in the United States, and Gazi was interested. After conveying his interest to Dr. Krayenbühl, an arrangement was made with the Microvascular Laboratory at the University of Vermont, in Burlington, for Dr. Yasargil to join the research staff, where he worked from October 25, 1965 to January 4, 1967. Gazi entered the work wholeheartedly, beginning on the fundamentals, as he wished to miss nothing. In 6 weeks, he finished the exercises customarily performed by a student in 3 months, and was ready for that for which he had come—experience in the handling of the living, functional cortical vessels. This included the direct opening, closing, patching, and surface grafting of the cortical vessels. In essence, Gazi repeated the whole extensive experience that had first been tried on extremities and intra-abdominal vessels. However, the vessels Gazi worked with were only 0.5 to 2.0 mm in size!

This remarkable surgeon did not complain about working on the simple problems or that he was ready for the complex. Instead, he studied the available literature and only when he had mastered that knowledge did he plan the research beyond that point. Thus, Gazi gradually decreased the problems to be studied. After just improving the technique of coagulating the small cortical branches that had to be sacrificed, he worked hard and long on preserving every salvageable branch.

A method was sought to allow a vessel (superficial temporal complex) to be grafted into the cortical branch (middle cerebral complex) of the brain. A study of grafts, patch grafts, and replacement grafts had previously been performed with unacceptable failure rates. Gazi conceived of the idea of using the superficial temporal artery as a direct connection into a middle cerebral branch that did not entail the removal of a segment of the superficial temporal artery, and hence did not require a double suture line. The superficial temporal vessel was simply sectioned far enough out to allow it to be sutured to the middle cerebral branch by a single end-to-side anastomosis. This technique provided a greatly improved patency rate and the results were reported in 1967.

Neurosurgeons are familiar with these techniques and with the recent Bypass Study. Under the rules of the study, the procedure was shown not to be helpful in altering mortality and morbidity rates. To give meaning to our data, a study of the physics and physiology of the nervous system blood supply should now be planned.

Perhaps Gazi's greatest contribution to neurosurgery has been his deep and thoughtful study of the subarachnoid spaces. We have all known that careful intracranial operations have low mortality and morbidity rates, provided the brain and its vessels are not injured. What Gazi has done is to demonstrate that many, if not most, intracranial procedures can be done in the subarachnoid space with an intact pia and arachnoid. The problem is that the depths of the wound are sometimes great, the light is poor, and one cannot always be certain where the arachnoid leaves off and the vascular surface remains. Great familiarity with the tissue is needed, and having been there, 10, 20, or 100 times before, is of great importance. Using this knowledge, he has achieved exceedingly low mortality and morbidity rates.

Certainly neurosurgery owes a tremendous debt to the fertile, busy mind of this experienced pioneer. We shall not often see its like. I am grateful to Gazi for what he has taught me. We should all be grateful for what he has taught any of us willing to listen. Mostly we should be grateful on behalf of the thousands of our patients for his demonstration that, with devotion and personal sacrifice, modern neurosurgical procedures can safely be performed.

Yes, the village of Lice is famous for two things: it is the birthplace of Mahmut Gazi Yasargil, and, too, it is the site of a great earthquake. We do not have incontrovertible evidence as to what was cause and what was effect.

R. M. PEARDON DONAGHY, M.D.
BURLINGTON, VERMONT

Bibliography of M. Gazi Yaşargil, M.D.

1. YAŞARGIL, M. G. Zur Pathogenese und Therapie des Delirium tremens und des pathologischen Rauschzustandes, Dissertation. Basel, Orell Füssli Verlag, 1950.
2. YAŞARGIL, M. G. Erfahrungen über die Behandlung des chronischen Alkoholismus mit den Methoden des sogenannten bedingten Reflexes. In: *Beihhefte zur Alkoholfrage in der Schweiz*, Heft 23. Basel, Benno Schwabe Verlag, 1952.
3. YAŞARGIL, M. G. Zur Pathogenese und Therapie des Delirium tremens und des pathologischen Rauschzustandes. Schweiz. Arch. Neurol. Neurochir. Psychiatr., *68:* 342–370, 1952.
4. YAŞARGIL, M. G. Vertebralisangiographie. Schweiz. Arch. Neurol. Neurochir. Psychiatr., *76:* 398–399, 1954.
5. KRAYENBÜHL, H., and YAŞARGIL, M. G. Eine seltene subtentorielle Tumorkombination: Clivus-Meningeom und Acusticus-Neurinom. Acta Neurochir., *5:* 92–101, 1956.
6. KRAYENBÜHL, H., and YAŞARGIL, M. G. Die vaskulären Erkrankungen im Gebiete der A. vertebralis und A. basialis. Stuttgart, Georg Thieme Verlag, 1957.
7. KRAYENBÜHL, H., and YAŞARGIL, M. G. Der subtentorielle Kollateralkreislauf im angiographischen Bild: Einer pathologische Beitrag zur Klinik der vaskulären bulbopontinen Syndrome. Dtsch. Z. Nervenheilkd., *177:* 103–116, 1957.
8. KRAYENBÜHL, H., and YAŞARGIL, M. G. Klinischer und pathologisch-anatomischer Beitrag zur Sturge-Weber-Krabbe'schen Krankheit. Dermatologica, *115:* 555–571, 1957.
9. YAŞARGIL, M. G. Die Röntgendiagnostik des Exophthalmus unilateralis: Eine Studie anhard von 110 Fällen. Ophthalmologica, *133:* 212–214, 1957.
10. YAŞARGIL, M. G. Die Röntgendiagnostik des Exophthalmus unilateralis. *Bibl. Ophthalmol.*, Basel, S. Karger, 1957.
11. YAŞARGIL, M. G. Vertebralisangiographie. In: *Röntgendiagnostik, Ergebnisse 1952–56*, edited by Schinz, Glanner, and Uehlinger, pp. 282–306. Stuttgart, Georg Thiemé Verlag, 1957.
12. KRAYENBÜHL, H., and YAŞARGIL, M. G. Das Hirnaneurysma. Docum Geigy (Chir.), 4: 143, 1958.
13. KRAYENBÜHL, H., and YAŞARGIL, M. G. Das Kleinhirnhämangiom. Schweiz. Med. Wochenschr., *88:* 99–104, 1958.
14. KRAYENBÜHL, H., and YAŞARGIL, M. G. Der zerebrale kollaterale Blutkreislauf im angiographischen Bild. Acta Neurochir., *6:* 30–80, 1958.

15. YAŞARGIL, M. G. Leberfunktion und Lebertherapie bei endogen Psychosen. Psychiatr. Neurol., *135:* 401–419, 1958.

16. KRAYENBÜHL, H., and YAŞARGIL, M. G. L'anévrysme de l'artère communicante antérieure. Paris, Masson, 1959, pp. 41–70 and 91–107.

17. MÜLLER, C., and YAŞARGIL, M. G. Zur Psychiatrie der stereotaktischen Hirnoperationen bei extrapyramidaler Erkrankungen. Schweiz. Arch. Neurol. Neurochir. Psychiatr. *84:* 136–154, 1959.

18. YAŞARGIL, M. G., and KRAYENBÜHL, H. Le traitement chirurgical de la maladie de Parkinson. Med. Hyg., *17:* 147–149, 1959.

19. YAŞARGIL, M. G., WYSS, O., and KRAYENBÜHL, H. Beitrag zur Behandlung extrapyramidaler Erkrankungen mittels gezielter Hirnoperationen. Bericht uber 75 eigene Fälle. Schweiz. Med. Wochenschr., *89:* 143–150, 1959.

20. KRAYENBÜHL, H., and YAŞARGIL, M. G. Bilateral thalamotomy in parkinsonism. Dig. Neurol. Psychiatr., *28:* 375, 1960.

21. KRAYENBÜHL, H., and YAŞARGIL, M. G. Bilateral thalamotomy in parkinsonism. J. Nerv. Ment. Dis., *130:* 538–541, 1960.

22. KRAYENBÜHL, H., and YAŞARGIL, M. G. Bilateral operations on the thalamus and pallidum for parkinsonism. J. Neurol. Psychiatr., *23:* 349–350, 1960.

23. KRAYENBÜHL, H., and YAŞARGIL, M. G. Le traitement chirurgical du parkinsonism. Riv. Romagna Med., *12:* 1–12, 1960.

24. YAŞARGIL, M. G. Stereotaktische Hirnoperation. *Panorama*, Sept. 1960.

25. KRAYENBÜHL, H., WYSS, O., and YAŞARGIL, M. G. Bilateral thalamotomy and pallidotomy as treatment for bilateral parkinsonism. J. Neurosurg., *18:* 429–444, 1961.

26. KRAYENBÜHL, H., and YAŞARGIL, M. G. Ergebnisse der stereotaktischen Operationen beim Parkinsonismus, inbesondere der doppelseitigen Eingriffe. Dtsch. Z. Nervenheilkd., *182:* 530–541, 1961.

27. KRAYENBÜHL, H., and YAŞARGIL, M. G. Die Angiographie der Thrombose der A. basialis. Schweiz. Med. Wochenschr., *91:* 1504–1507, 1961.

28. KRAYENBÜHL, H., and YAŞARGIL, M. G. Chirurgische Behandlung von Rückenmarksangiomen. *Panorama*, Sept. 1962, p. 10.

29. KRAYENBÜHL, H., and YAŞARGIL, M. G. Relief of intention tremor due to multiple sclerosis by stereotaxic thalamotomy. Confin. Neurol., *22:* 368–374, 1962.

30. KRAYENBÜHL, H., and YAŞARGIL, M. G. Röntgenologischer Beitrag zur Diagnose zerebraler Arachnoidalzysten der Temporalregion. Schweiz. Arch. Neurol. Neurochir. Psychiatr., *89:* 327–339, 1962.

31. OSACAR, E. M., YAŞARGIL, M. G., and KRAYENBÜHL, H. El trata-
mento quirurgico de la enfermedad de Parkinson. Acta Neurol.
LatinoAm., *8:* 128–162, 1962.

32. SENNING, A., WEBER, G., and YAŞARGIL, M. G. Zur operativen
Behandlung von Tumoren der Wirbelsäule. Schweiz. Med. Wochenschr., *92:* 1574–1576, 1962.

33. YAŞARGIL, M. G. Die Ergebnisse der stereotaktischen Operationen
bei Hyperkinesien. Schweiz. Med. Wochenschr., *92:* 1550–1555,
1962.

34. YAŞARGIL, M. G. Die Vertebralisangiographie: Ihre Bedeutung für
die Diagnostik der Tumoren. Acta Neurochir. [Suppl. 9] (Wien),
1962.

35. YAŞARGIL, M. G. Die Musiktherapie im Orient und Okzident.
Schweiz. Arch. Neurol. Neurochir. Psychiatr., *90:* 301–326, 1962.

36. KRAYENBÜHL, H., SIEGFRIED, J., and YAŞARGIL, M. G. Résultats
tardifs des opérations stéréotaxiques dans le traitement de la
maladie de Parkinson. Rev. Neurol., *108:* 485–494, 1963.

37. KRAYENBÜHL, H., and YAŞARGIL, M. G. Varicosis spinalis. Schweiz.
Arch. Neurol. Neurochir. Psychiatr., *92:* 74–92, 1963.

38. YAŞARGIL, M. G. Akute Lähmungen. Praxis, *52:* 190–193, 1963.

39. YAŞARGIL, M. G. Der Hirnschlag. Schweiz. Arch. Neurol. Neurochir. Psychiatr., *91:* 553–564, 1963.

40. KRAYENBÜHL, H., AKERT, K., HARTMANN, K., and YAŞARGIL, M.
G. Etude de la corrélation anatomo-clinique chez des malades
opérés de Parkinsonisme. Neurochirurgie, *10:* 397–412, 1964.

41. KRAYENBÜHL, H., and YAŞARGIL, M. G. Verschluss der A. cerebralis
media: Ergebnisse der Klinischen und Katamnestischen Untersuchungen. Schweiz. Arch. Neurol. Neurochir. Psychiatr., *94:*
287–304, 1964.

42. YAŞARGIL, M. G. Ergebnisse der angiographischen Untersuchungen
beim Exophthalmus. Presented at the 14th Biennial Congress of
the International College of Surgeons, Vienna, 1964, pp. 209–214.

43. HUBER, A., and YAŞARGIL, M. G. Orbitale angiographie. In: *Röntgendiagnostik*, Vol. 3, edited by G. Schinz. Stuttgart, Georg
Thieme Verlag, 1965 (English edition, 1969).

44. KRAYENBÜHL, H., SIEGFRIED, J., KOHENOF, M., and YAŞARGIL,
M. G. Is there a dominant thalamus? Confin. Neurol., *26:* 246–
249, 1965.

45. KRAYENBÜHL, H., and YAŞARGIL, M. G. Stereotaktische Geräte.
In: *Röntgendiagnostik*, Vol. 3, edited by G. Schinz, pp. 388–411.
Stuttgart, Georg Thieme Verlag, 1965 (English edition, 1969).

46. KRAYENBÜHL, H., YAŞARGIL, M. G., and DECKER, K. Kraniozere-

brale Erkrankugen. Pneumoenzephalographie und Angiographie. In: *Röntgendiagnostik*, Vol. 3, edited by G. Schinz. pp. 265–344. Stuttgart, Georg Thieme Verlag, 1965 (English edition, 1969).

47. KRAYENBÜHL, H., YAŞARGIL, M. G., and SIEGFRIED, J. Interventions stéréotaxiques pour hyperkinésies à développment infantile. Infanz. Anorm., *64:* 582–596, 1965.

48. KRAYENBÜHL, H., and YAŞARGIL, M. G. Zur Diagnose der subtentoriellen Hirntumoren. Schweiz. Arch. Neurol. Neurochir. Psychiatr., *96:* 337–355, 1965.

49. KRAYENBÜHL, H., and YAŞARGIL, M. G. Die Zerebrale Angiographie. Stuttgart, Georg Thieme Verlag, 1965 (Italian edition, 1967; English edition, 1968).

50. KRAYENBÜHL, H., and YAŞARGIL, M. G. Angiographie der Hirngefässe. In: *Röntgenodiagnostik*, edited by H. R. Schinz, pp. 314–342. Stuttgart, Georg Thieme Verlag, 1965 (English edition, 1968).

51. KRAYENBÜHL, H., and YAŞARGIL, M. G. Klinik und Behandlung des Torticollis spasticus. Schweiz. Arch. Neurol. Neurochir. Psychiatr., *96:* 356–365, 1965.

52. YAŞARGIL, M. G. Die Operative Behandlung des Morbus Parkinson. Dtsch. Med. Wochenschr., *90:* 1296–1297, 1965.

53. YAŞARGIL, M. G. L'importance des artères lenticulostriées dans les occlusions des artères cérébrales. In: *Symposium International sur la Circulation Cerebrale*, pp. 41–43. Paris, Edition Sandoz, 1965.

54. FILIPPA G, REGLI, F, and YAŞARGIL, M. G. Beitrag zur Diagnostik der inneren Hirnvenenthrombose. Dtsch. Med. Wochenschr., *91:* 1025–1034, 1966.

55. FILIPPA, G., REGLI, F., and YAŞARGIL, M. G. Zur Nosologie der inneren Hirnvenenthrombose. Anatomie und pathologische-anatomische Veränderungen. Dtsch. Med. Wochenschr., *91:* 1049–1054, 1966.

56. KRAYENBÜHL, H., and YAŞARGIL, M. G. Die angiodiagnostische Bedeutung der Aa. lenticulostriatae. Neurochirurgie, *9:* 1–11, 1966.

57. KRAYENBÜHL, H., and YAŞARGIL, M. G. Percutaneous vertebral angiography in 900 cases. Acta Radiol., *5:* 263–266, 1966.

58. KRAYENBÜHL, H., and YAŞARGIL, M. G. Trattamento chirurgico del morbo di Parkinson. Medica Tedesca, *2:* 133–134, 1966.

59. KRAYENBÜHL, H., YAŞARGIL, M. G., and SIEGFRIED, J. Le diagnostic de l'exophthalmie unilatérale en neurochirurgie. Notre expérience neuroradiologique, notamment avec la méthode de soustraction. Confin. Neurol., *28:* 224–227, 1966.

60. DONAGHY, R. M. P., and YAŞARGIL, M. G. (eds.): *Micro-Vascular Surgery.* Stuttgart, Georg Thieme Verlag, and St. Louis, C. V. Mosby, 1967.

61. KRAYENBÜHL, H., and YAŞARGIL, M. G. Die Anwendung des binokularen Mikroskopes in der Neurochirurgie. Wien Z. Nervenheilkd., *25:* 268–277, 1967.

62. KRAYENBÜHL, H., and YAŞARGIL, M. G. Les signes artériographiques les plus typiques permettant d'évoquer une néoformation des lobes cérébelleux. Ann. Radiol., *10:* 819–826, 1967.

63. YAŞARGIL, M. G. Entwicklung der Diagnose und der chirurgischen Behandlung cerebrovascularer Erkrankungen. Schweiz. Med. Wochenschr., *97:* 1734–1736, 1967.

64. YAŞARGIL, M. G. Experimental small vessel surgery in the dog including patching and grafting of cerebral vessels and the formation of functional extra-intracranial shunts. In: *Micro-Vascular Surgery,* edited by R. M. P. Donaghy and M. G. Yasargil. Stuttgart, Georg Thieme Verlag, and St. Louis, C. V. Mosby, 1967.

65. DONAGHY, R. M. P., and YAŞARGIL, M. G. Microangeional surgery and its techniques. Prog. Brain Res., *30:* 263–267, 1968.

66. FISCH, U., and YAŞARGIL, M. G. Der translabyrinthäre Zugang für die Akustikus-Neurinome. Med. Hygiene, *26:* 1190–1191, 1968.

67. FISCH, U., and YAŞARGIL, M. G. Transtemporale extrapyramidale Eingriffe am inneren Gehörgang. Pract. Oto-rhino-laryngol., *30:* 377–386, 1968.

68. KRAYENBÜHL, H., and YAŞARGIL, M. G. Die neuroradiologische Diagnose und Therapie der Hirngefässverschlüsse. Ther. Umsch., *25:* 462–469, 1968.

69. KRAYENBÜHL, H., and YAŞARGIL, M. G. Die Anwendung des Mikroskopes bei Operationen des Zentralnervensystems. Praxis, *57:* 214–217, 1968.

70. KRAYENBÜHL, H., and YAŞARGIL, M. G. Die neuroradiologische Diagnose und Therapie der zerebralen arteriovenosen Gefässmissbildungen. Ther. Umsch., *25:* 485–490, 1968.

71. KRAYENBÜHL, H., and YAŞARGIL, M. G. Das Operationsmikroskop in der Neurochirurgie. Sandorama, *Nov.:* 11–13, 1968.

72. KRAYENBÜHL, H., and YAŞARGIL, M. G. Die Anwendung des Operationsmikroskops in der Behandlung der vaskulärer zerebrospinalen Erkrankungen. Münch. Med. Wochenschr., *110:* 1931–1934, 1968.

73. KRAYENBÜHL, H., and YAŞARGIL, M. G. Die neuroradiologische Diagnose und Therapie der zerebralen sackförmigen Aneurysmen. Ther. Umsch., *25:* 480–485, 1968.

74. YAŞARGIL, M. G. Die Anwendung des Operationsmikroskops in der Neurochirurgie. Zeiss Inform., *70:* 129–131, 1968.

75. YAŞARGIL, M. G. Experimental and clinical microsurgery of cerebral vessels. IX Congresso Latinoamericano de Angiologia, Lima, Peru, October 4–9, 1968.

76. YAŞARGIL, M. G. Fragen aus der Praxis. Pneumoenzephalographie und Karotisangiographie ambulant. Dtsch. Med. Wochenschr., *38:* 1826, 1968.

77. YAŞARGIL, M. G. Klinische Erfahrungen bei konstruktiven mikrochirurgischen Eingriffen an Hirnarterien. Presented at the Fourth International Symposium of the Research Group on Cerebral Circulation, Salzburg, Austria, Sept. 25–29, 1968.

78. CROWELL, R., and YAŞARGIL, M. G. Experimental microvascular autografting. Technical note. J. Neurosurg., *31:* 101–104, 1969.

79. KRAYENBÜHL, H., and YAŞARGIL, M. G. The use of the binocular microscope in neurosurgery. In: *Microneurosurgery*, edited by R. Rand. St. Louis, C. V. Mosby, 1969.

80. KRAYENBÜHL, H., and YAŞARGIL, M. G. La Micro-chirurgie du cerveau. In: *Livre de la Santé.* Monte Carlo, Editions Auret, 1969.

81. KRAYENBÜHL, H., and YAŞARGIL, M. G. Cerebral venous and sinus thrombosis. Rev. Brasil Cardiovasc., *5:* 367–370, 1969.

82. KRAYENBÜHL, H., YAŞARGIL, M. G., and McCLINTOCK, H. G. Treatment of spinal cord malformations by surgical excision. J. Neurosurg., *30:* 427–435, 1969.

83. YAŞARGIL, M. G. Clinical experience in microsurgical operations of cerebral vessels. Rev. Brasil Cardiovasc., *5:* 1969.

84. YAŞARGIL, M. G. Experimental small vessel surgery in the dog. Rev. Brasil Cardiovasc., *5:* 1969.

85. YAŞARGIL, M. G. Die Subarachnoidale Blutung. Schweiz. Med. Wochenschr., *99:* 1629–1632, 1969.

86. YAŞARGIL, M. G. Die Vertebralisangiographie. Tagung der Deutschen Neuroradiologischen Arbetsgemeinschaft, Zurich, Switzerland, April 24–26, 1969.

87. YAŞARGIL, M. G. *Microsurgery Applied to Neurosurgery.* Stuttgart, Georg Thieme Verlag, 1969.

88. YAŞARGIL, M. G. Die Bedeutung der Mikrochirurgie in der Hirnchirurgie. Dtsch. Med. Wochenschr., *94:* 1496–1497, 1969.

89. YAŞARGIL, M. G. L'utilisation du microscope pour opérations dans les interventions sur le système nerveux central et plus particulièrement lors d'atteinte vasculaire. Med. Hyg., *870:* 530–533, 1969.

90. YAŞARGIL, M. G., and FISCH, U. Unsere Erfahrungen in der mikrochirurgischen Extirpation der Acusticusneurinome. Arch. Klin.

Exp. Ohren-Nasen-Kehlkopfheilkd., *194:* 243–248, 1969.

91. YAŞARGIL, M. G. [Possibilities and limitations of vascular surgery of the central nervous system.] Bull. Schweiz. Akad. Med. Wiss., *24:* 487–493, 1969.

92. GUERRISI, R., and YAŞARGIL, M. G. Studio sperimentale su aneurismi artificialimente creati con l'ausilio del microscopio, in ratti e conigli. Minerva Neurochir., *14:* 140–144, 1970.

93. KRAYENBÜHL, H., and YAŞARGIL, M. G. Diagnosis and therapy of intracranial aneurysms. Surg. Ann., *2:* 327–343, 1970.

94. KRAYENBÜHL, H., and YAŞARGIL, M. G. The use of the binocular microscope in neurosurgery. Adv. Ophthalmol., *22:* 62–65, 1970.

95. YAŞARGIL, M. G. Die Anwendung des Operationsmikroskopes in der Behandlung der Vaskulären Zerebrospinalen Erkrankungen. In: *Zerebrale arterielle Durchblutungsstörungen. Symposium der Deutschen Gesellschaft für Angiologie.* München, October 24 and 25, 1968, pp. 163–167. Stuttgart, F. K. Schattar Verlag, 1970.

96. YAŞARGIL, M. G. Bedeutung und Grenzen der mikrochirurgischen Technik bei Hirngefässkrankheiten. Actuelle Chir., *5:* 5–10, 1970.

97. YAŞARGIL, M. G. Der Kopfschmerz bei organischen, zerebrovaskulären Erkrankungen. In: *Cephalaea,* edited by A. G. Hommel, pp. 121–136. Zurich, Switzerland, Adliswil, 1970.

98. YAŞARGIL, M. G., KRAYENBÜHL, H., and JACOBSON, J. H. II. Microneurosurgical arterial reconstruction. Surgery, *76:* 221–233, 1970.

99. YAŞARGIL, M. G. Structure and reaction of cerebral arteries. In: *Research on the Cerebral Circulation,* edited by J. S. Meyer, M. Reivich, H. Lechner, and O. Eichhorn. Springfield, IL, Charles C Thomas, 1970, pp 275–278.

100. YAŞARGIL, M. G. Intracranial microsurgery. Clin. Neurosurg., *17:* 250–256, 1970.

101. YAŞARGIL, M. G. Surgery of vascular lesions of the spinal cord with the microsurgical technique. Clin. Neurosurg., *17:* 257–265, 1970.

102. YAŞARGIL, M. G. and KRAYENBÜHL, H. The use of the binocular microscope in neurosurgery. Bibl. Ophthalmol., *81:* 62–65, 1970.

103. YAŞARGIL, M. G. Strombahnwiederherstellende Operationen im intrakraniellen Gefässbereich. In *Zerebrale arterielle Durchblutungsstörungen.* Symposium der Deutsch Gesellschaft für Angiologie, München, October 24 and 25, 1968. Stuttgart, F. K. Schattauer, 1970.

104. PEERLESS, S. J., and YAŞARGIL, M. G. Adrenergic innervation of the cerebral blood vessels in the rabbit. J. Neurosurg., *35:* 148–154, 1971.

105. YAŞARGIL, M. G. Diagnosis and treatment of spinal cord arterio-

venous malformations. In: *Progress in Neurological Surgery*, Vol. 4, edited by H. Krayenbühl, P. E. Maspes, and W. H. Sweet, pp. 355–428. Basel, S. Karger, 1971.

106. YAŞARGIL, M. G. Orbito-Angiographie. 1 Welkongress über Ultraschall-diagnostik in der Medizin, Vienna, June 2–7, 1969. In: *Ultrasono Graphia Medica, II*, edited by J. Beck and K. Ossini. pp. 385–393, 1971.

107. FLAMM, E. S., YAŞARGIL, M. G., and RANSOHOFF, J. Alteration of experimental cerebral vasospasm by adrenergic blockade. J. Neurosurg., *37*: 294–301, 1972.

108. FLAMM, E. S., YAŞARGIL, M. G., and RANSOHOFF, J. Control of cerebral vasospasm by parenteral phenoxybenzamine. Stroke, *3*: 421–426, 1972.

109. KRAYENBÜHL, H., and YAŞARGIL, M. G. Das normale Hirngefässsystem im angiographischen Bild. In: *Der Hirnkreislauf*, edited by H. Gänshirt, pp. 161–200. Stuttgart, Georg Thieme Verlag, 1972.

110. KRAYENBÜHL, H., and YAŞARGIL, M. G. Klinik der Gefässmissbildungen und Gefässfisteln. In: *Der Hirnkreislauf*, edited by H. Gänshirt, pp. 465–510. Stuttgart, Georg Thieme Verlag, 1972.

111. KRAYENBÜHL, H., and YAŞARGIL, M. G. Radiological anatomy and topography of the cerebral veins. In: *Handbook of Clinical Neurology*, Vol. 1, pp. 102–117. Amsterdam, North Holland, 1972.

112. KRAYENBÜHL, H., YAŞARGIL, M. G., FLAMM, E. S., and TEW, J. M., JR. Microsurgical treatment of intracranial saccular aneurysms. J. Neurosurg., *37*: 678–686, 1972.

113. LANDOLT, A. M., YAŞARGIL, M. G., and KRAYENBÜHL, H. Disturbances of the serum electrolytes after surgery of intracranial arterial aneurysms. J. Neurosurg., *37*: 210–218, 1972.

114. PEERLESS, S. J., YAŞARGIL, M. G., and KENDALL, M. J. The adrenergic and cholinergic innervation of the cerebral blood vessels. In: *Proceedings of the 4th European Congress of Neurosurgery, Present Limits of Neurosurgery*, Prague, 1971, pp. 199–202. Prague, Avicenum Czechoslovak Medical Press, 1972.

115. YAŞARGIL, M. G. Intracranial microsurgery. Proc. R. Soc. Med., *65*: 15–16, 1972.

116. YAŞARGIL, M. G. Mikrotechnische Behandlung der Hirnarterien-Verschlüsse. Verh. Dtsch. Ges. Inn. Med., *78*: 487–492, 1972.

117. YAŞARGIL, M. G. Microsurgical approach to the cerebrovascular diseases. In: *Proceedings of the 4th European Congress of Neurosurgery, Present Limits of Neurosurgery*, Prague, 1971, pp. 357–361. Prague, Avicenum Czechoslovak Medical Press, 1972.

118. YAŞARGIL, M. G. Die klinischen Erfahrungen mit der Miktrotechnik. Schweiz. Arch. Neurol. Neurochir. Psychiatr., *111:* 493–504, 1972.

119. YAŞARGIL, M. G., and KRAYENBÜHL, H.. Radiological anatomy and topography of the cerebral arteries. In: *Handbook of Clinical Neurology,* Vol. I, edited by P. J. Vinken and G. W. Bruyn, pp. 65–101. Amsterdam, North Holland, 1972.

120. CROWELL, R. M., and YAŞARGIL, M. G. End-to-side anastomosis of superficial temporal artery to middle cerebral artery branch in the dog. Neurochirurgia, *16:* 73–77, 1973.

121. YAŞARGIL, M. G. Die Behandlung der intrakraniellen sackförmigen Aneurysmen. Ophthalmologica, *167:* 189–192, 1973.

122. YAŞARGIL, M. G. Subarachnoidale Blutung (Aneurysmen und Angiome). In: *Innere Medizin in Praxis und Klinik,* Vol. 2, H. Hornbostel, W. Kaufmann, and W. Siegenthaler, pp. 7/39–7/42. Stuttgart, Georg Thieme Verlag, 1973.

123. YAŞARGIL, M. G. Microsurgical experience in surgery of acoustic neurinomas (abstr.). In: *Advances in Neurosurgery,* p. 250. Berlin, Springer Verlag, 1973.

124. YAŞARGIL, M. G. Extra-intracranial arterial anastomosis for transient cerebral ischemic attacks. In: *Recent Progress in Neurological Surgery, Proceedings of the Symposia of the Fifth International Congress of Neurological Surgery,* Tokyo, Oct. 7–12, 1973, pp. 15–151. Amsterdam, Excerpta Medica, 1973.

125. YAŞARGIL, M. G., YONEKAWA, Y., ZUMSTEIN, B., and STAHL, H. J. Hydrocephalus following spontaneous hemorrhage. Clinical features and treatment. J. Neurosurg., *39:* 474–479, 1973.

126. YONEKAWA, Y., and YAŞARGIL, M. G. Practice of microvascular anastomosis. Jpn. Z., *1:* 345–351, 1973.

127. FOX, J. L., and YAŞARGIL, M. G. Fluorescein angiography in microvascular surgery: A study using the rodent artery. Stroke, *5:* 196–206, 1974.

128. FOX, J. L., and YAŞARGIL, M. G. The effect of DC electrical current on the rodent artery. Surg. Neurol., *2:* 13–16, 1974.

129. FOX, J. L., and YAŞARGIL, M. G. The experimental effect of direct electrical stimulation on intracranial arteries and the blood-brain barrier. J. Neurosurg., *41:* 582–589, 1974.

130. FOX, J. L., and YAŞARGIL, M. G. The role of the hydroxyl ion during vasodilation of arteries caused by DC negative electrical current. Surg. Neurol., *2:* 343–345, 1974.

131. YAŞARGIL, M. G. Mikrotechnische Behandlung der Hirnarterienverschlüsse. In: *Aktuelle Probleme der Akuten zerebralen Durch-*

blutsstorüngen, Diagnose und Therapie, edited by P. W. Duchosal and B. Krakenbühl, pp. 78–89. Bern, Hans Huber, 1974.

132. YAŞARGIL, M. G. Microtechnique applied to cerebrovascular diseases. In: *Reconstructive Surgery of Brain Arteries,* pp. 233–236. Balatonfüred, 1972, 1974.
133. YAŞARGIL, M. G., and CARTER, L. P. Saccular aneurysms of the distal anterior cerebral artery. J. Neurosurg., *40:* 218–223, 1974.
134. YAŞARGIL, M. G., and DAMUR, M. Thrombosis of the cerebral veins and dural sinuses. In: *Radiology of the Skull and Brain, Angiography,* Vol. 4, pp. 2375–2400. St. Louis, C. V. Mosby, 1974.
135. YAŞARGIL, M. G., and FOX, J. L. The microsurgical approach to acoustic neurinomas. Surg. Neurol., *2:* 393–398, 1974.
136. YAŞARGIL, M. G., YONEKAWA, Y., DENTON, I., PIROTH, P., and BENES, I. Experimental intracranial transplantation of autogenic omentum majus. J. Neurosurg., *40:* 213–217, 1974.
137. FOX, J., L., and YAŞARGIL, M. G. The relief of intracranial vasospasm: An experimental study with methylprednisolone and cortisol. Surg. Neurol., *3:* 214–218, 1975.
138. KRAYENBÜHL, H., and YAŞARGIL, M. G. Cranial chordomas. Prog. Neurol. Surg., *6:* 380–434, 1975.
139. KRAYENBÜHL, H., and YAŞARGIL, M. G. Chondromas. Prog. Neurol. Surg., *6:* 435–463, 1975.
140. YAŞARGIL, M. G., DeLONG, W. B., and GUARNASCHELLI, J. J. Complete microsurgical excision of cervical extramedullary and intramedullary vascular malformations. Surg. Neurol., *4:* 211–224, 1975.
141. YAŞARGIL, M. G. Die subarachnoidale Blutung, Subarachnoid Hemorrhage, Diagnosis and Therapy. Schweiz. Rundsch. Med. Praxis, *15:* 439–444, 1975.
142. YAŞARGIL, M. G., and FOX, J. L. The microsurgical approach to intracranial aneurysms. Surg. Neurol., *3:* 7–14, 1975.
143. YAŞARGIL, M. G., FOX, J. L., and RAY, M. W. The operative approach to aneurysms of the anterior communicating artery. Adv. Tech. Stand. Neurosurg., *2:* 113–170, 1975.
144. YAŞARGIL, M. G., and DePREUX, J. Microsurgical experiments in 12 cases of intramedullary hemangioblastomas. Neurochirurgie, *21:* 425–434, 1975.
145. SCHREIBER, A., WALKER, N., NISHIKAWA, M., and YAŞARGIL, M. G. [Microvascular studies on the knee joint.] Z. Orthop., *114:* 706–708, 1976.
146. VOIGT, K., and YAŞARGIL, M. G. Cerebral cavernous haemangiomas or cavernomas. Incidence, pathology, localization, diagnosis, clin-

ical features, and treatment. Review of the literature and report of an unusual case. Neurochirurgia, *19:* 59–68, 1976.

147. YAŞARGIL, M. G. Subokzipitale—transmeatale mikrotechnische Exstirpation des Akustikus-neurinomes. In: *Kopf- und Hals-Chirurgie*, edited by H.H. Naumann, pp. 545–587. Stuttgart, Georg Thieme Verlag, 1976.

148. YAŞARGIL, M. G. Development of a motorized microscope stand. In: *Clinical Microneurosurgery*, edited by W. T. Koos, F. W. Böck, and R. F. Spetzler. Stuttgart, Georg Thieme Verlag, 1976.

149. YAŞARGIL, M. G. Indural spinal arteriovenous malformations: Tumors of the spine and spinal cord. In: *Handbook of Clinical Neurology*, edited by P. J. Vinken and G. W. Bruyn, pp. 481–523. Amsterdam, North Holland, 1976.

150. YAŞARGIL, M. G., ANTIC, J., LACIGA, R., DE PREUX, J., FIDELER, R. W., and BOONE, S. C. The microsurgical removal of intramedullary spinal hemangioblastomas. Report of twelve cases and a review of the literature. Surg. Neurol., *6:* 141–148, 1976.

151. YASARGIL, M. G., ANTIC, J., LACIGA, R., JAIN, K. K., and BOONE, S. C. Arteriovenous malformations of the vein of Galen: Microsurgical treatment. Surg. Neurol., *6:* 195–200, 1976.

152. YAŞARGIL, M. G., ANTIC, J., LACIGA, R., JAIN, K. K., HODOSH, R. M., and SMITH, R. D. Microsurgical pterional approach to aneurysms of the basilar bifurcation. Surg. Neurol., *6:* 83–91, 1976.

153. YAŞARGIL, M. G., and CHATER, N. L. Surgical results of Professor Yasargil's series. In: *Microsurgical Anastomoses for Cerebral Ischemia*, edited by G. M. Austin, pp. 359–367. Springfield, IL, Charles C Thomas, 1976.

154. YAŞARGIL, M. G., JAIN, K. K., and LACIGA, R. Arteriovenous malformations of the splenium of the corpus callosum: Microsurgical treatment. Surg. Neurol., *5:* 5–14, 1976.

155. YAŞARGIL, M. G., JAIN, K. K., ANTIC, J., LACIGA, R., and KLETTER, G. Arteriovenous malformations of the anterior and the middle portions of the corpus callosum: Microsurgical treatment. Surg. Neurol., *5:* 67–80, 1976.

156. YAŞARGIL, M. G., KASDAGLIS, K., JAIN, K. K., and WEBER, H. P. Anatomical observations of the subarachnoid cisterns of the brain during surgery. J. Neurosurg., *44:* 298–302, 1976.

157. YAŞARGIL, M. G., and PERNECZKY, A. Operative Behandlung der intramedullaren spinalen Tumoren. In: *Spinale raumfordernde Prozesse*, edited by W. Schiefer and H. H. Wieck, pp. 299–312. Erlangen, Verlag Peri Med., 1976.

158. YAŞARGIL, M. G., and SMITH, R. D. Association of middle cerebral artery anomalies with saccular aneurysms and Moyamoya disease. Surg. Neurol., *6:* 39–43, 1976.

159. YAŞARGIL, M. G., and SO, S. C. Cerebellopontine angle meningioma presenting as subarachnoid hemorrhage. Surg. Neurol., *6:* 3–6, 1976.

160. YONEKAWA, Y., and YAŞARGIL, M. G. Extra-intracranial arterial anastomosis. Clinical and technical aspects, results. Adv. Tech. Stand. Neurosurg., *3:* 47–78, 1976.

161. FRIEDE, R. L., and YAŞARGIL, M. G. Suprasellar neoplasm with a granular cell component. J. Neuropathol. Exp. Neurol., *36:* 769–782, 1977.

162. FRIEDE, R. L., and YAŞARGIL, M. G. Supratentorial intracerebral epithelial (ependymal) cysts: Review, case reports, and fine structure. J. Neurol. Neurosurg. Psychiatry, *40:* 127–137, 1977.

163. NISHIKAWA, M., YAŞARGIL, M. G., YAGI, N., and FISCH, U. Experimental extracranial-intracranial anastomosis. Surg. Neurol., *8:* 249–253, 1977.

164. SCHREIBER, A., WALKER, N., NISHIKAWA, M., and YAŞARGIL, M. G. Experimental autologous transplantation of the knee joint: Contributions of microvascular surgery (a preliminary report). Ital. J. Orthop. Traumatol. *3:* 283–288, 1977.

165. YAŞARGIL, M. G. Microsurgical operation of herniated lumbar disc. In: *Advances in Neurosurgery,* edited by R. Wüllenweber, M. Brock, J. Hamer, M. Klinger, and O. Spoerri, p. 81. Berlin, Springer Verlag, 1977.

166. YAŞARGIL, M. G., GASSER, J. C., HODOSH, R. M., and RANKIN, T. V. Carotid-ophthalmic aneurysms. Direct microsurgical approach. Surg. Neurol., *8:* 155–165, 1977.

167. YAŞARGIL, M. G., and SMITH, R. D. Surgery on the carotid system in the treatment of hemorrhagic stroke. Adv. Neurol., *16:* 181–209, 1977.

168. YAŞARGIL, M. G., SMITH, R. D., and GASSER, J. C. Microsurgical approach to acoustic neurinomas. Adv. Tech. Stand. Neurosurg., *4:* 93–100, 1977.

169. YAŞARGIL, M. G., VISE, W. M., and BADER, D. C. Technical adjuncts in neurosurgery. Surg. Neurol., *8:* 331–336, 1977.

170. YAŞARGIL, M. G., and YONEKAWA, Y. Results of microsurgical extra-intracranial arterial bypass in the treatment of cerebral ischemia. Neurosurgery, *1:* 22–24, 1977.

171. YONEKAWA, Y., and YAŞARGIL, M. G. Brain revascularization by transplanted omentum: A possible treatment of cerebral ischemia. Neurosurgery, *1:* 256–259, 1977.

172. MEYERMANN, R., and YAŞARGIL, M. G. Ultrastructural studies of

cerebral aneurysms and angiomas gained operatively. Adv. Neurol., *20:* 557–567, 1978.

173. SCHUBIGER, O., and YAŞARGIL, M. G. Extracranial vertebral aneurysm with neurofibromatosis. Neuroradiology, *15:* 171–173, 1978.

174. WALKER, N., NISHIKAWA, M., SCHREIBER, A., and YAŞARGIL, M. G. Autogenous whole joint transplantation with microsurgical vascular anastomoses. Microsurgery, Bonn, October 4–7, pp. 288–292. Amsterdam, Excerpta Medica, 1978.

175. WALKER, N., NISHIKAWA, M., SCHREIBER, A., and YAŞARGIL, M. G. [How important is the blood supply in the etiology of arthrosis?] Z. Orthop., *116:* 434–435, 1978.

176. WEINSTEIN, P. R., CHATER, N. L., and YAŞARGIL, M. G. Microsurgical treatment of intracranial cerebrovascular occlusive disease. In: *Practice of Surgery: Neurosurgery.* Hagerstown, Md., Harper & Row, 1978.

177. YAŞARGIL, M. G. Subarachnoidale Blutung (Aneurysmen und Angiome). In: *Innere Medizin in Praxis und Klinik,* edited by H. Hornbostel, W. Kaufmann, and W. Siegenthaler, pp. 7.40–7.42. Stuttgart, Georg Thieme Verlag, 1978.

178. YAŞARGIL, M. G. Mikrochirurgie der Kleinhirnbrückenwinckel-Tumoren. In: *Kleinhirnbrückenwinckel-Tumoren, Diagnostik und Therapie,* edited by D. Plester, S. Wende, and N. Nakayoma, pp. 215–257. Berlin, Springer Verlag, 1978.

179. YAŞARGIL, M. G., BOEHM, W. B., and HO, R. E. Microsurgical treatment of cerebral aneurysms at the bifurcation of the internal carotid artery. Acta Neurochir., *41:* 61–72, 1978.

180. YAŞARGIL, M. G., FIEDELER, R. W., and RANKIN, T. P. Operative treatment of spinal angioblastomas. In: *Spinal Angiomas, Advances in Diagnosis and Therapy,* edited by H. W. Pis and R. Djindjian, pp. 171–188. Berlin, Springer Verlag, 1978.

181. YAŞARGIL, M. G., SMITH, R. D., and FIRTH J. L. Anterior communicating arterial aneurysms. In: *Operative Surgery: Neurosurgery,* pp. 233–251. London, Butterworth, 1978.

182. YAŞARGIL, M. G., SMITH, R. D., and FIRTH, J. L. The principles of microsurgery applied to aneurysm surgery. In: *Operative Surgery, Neurosurgery,* edited by C. Rob and R. Smith, pp. 225–232. London, Butterworth, 1978.

183. YAŞARGIL, M. G., SMITH, R. D., and GASSER, C. Microsurgery of the aneurysms of the internal carotid artery and its branches. Prog. Neurol. Surg., *9:* 58–121, 1978.

184. YAŞARGIL, M. G., YONAS, H., and GASSER, J. C. Anterior choroidal artery aneurysms: Their anatomy and surgical significance. Surg. Neurol., *9:* 129–138, 1978.

185. ZUMSTEIN, B., YONEKAWA, Y., and YAŞARGIL, M. G. Extra-intra-

cranial arterial anastomosis for cerebral ischemia: Technique and results in 90 cases. In: *International Conference on Atherosclerosis*, edited by L. A. Carlson *et al.*, pp. 257–263. New York, Raven Press, 1978.

186. HUBER, A., and YAŞARGIL, M. G. Möglichkeiten und Bedeutung der angiographischen Diagnostik in der Ophthalmologie. Ber. Dtsch. Ophthalmol. Ges., *76:* 21–37, 1979.

187. SCHREIBER, A., WALKER, N., NISHIKAWA, M., and YAŞARGIL, M. G. [Joint transplantation using microsurgical vascular technics.] Acta Orthop. Belg., *45:* 403–411, 1979.

188. SHIMIZU, Y., YAŞARGIL, M. G., and SMITH, R. D. Thrombogenesis in experimental microvascular anastomosis. J. Microsurg., *1:* 39–49, 1979.

189. WALKER, N., NISHIKAWA, N., SCHREIBER, A., and YAŞARGIL, M. G. Die Prognose der autologen Kniegelenktransplantation. Orthop. Praxis, *8:* 687–689, 1979.

190. ZUMSTEIN, B., and YAŞARGIL, M. G. [Cerebral microsurgical bypass anastomoses in extra and intracranial vascular occlusions.] Internist, *20:* 553–558, 1979.

191. YAŞARGIL, M. G., MORTARA, R. W., and CURCIC, M. Meningiomas of basal posterior cranial fossa. Adv. Tech. Stand. Neurosurg., *7:* 115, 1980.

192. ZUMSTEIN, B., and YAŞARGIL, M. G. [Improvement in brain circulation by microsurgical bypass anastomoses.] Bull. Schweiz. Akad. Med. Wiss., *36:* 209–222, 1980.

193. ZUMSTEIN, B., and YAŞARGIL, M. G. Verbesserung der Hirndurchblutung durch mikrochirurgische Bypass-Anastomosen. Der Kassenarzt, *20:* 4133–4144, 1980.

194. ZUMSTEIN, B., YAŞARGIL, M. G., CURCIC, M., and NAUTA, H. J. Experiences with the extra- to intracranial bypass in the surgical management of cerebral aneurysms (9 cases). Neurol. Res., *2:* 327–343, 1980.

195. ZUMSTEIN, B., YAŞARGIL, M. G., and KELLER, H. M. Prevention of cerebral ischemia by extra-intracranial microanastomosis. In: *Arteriographies Cerebrales Extracraniennes Asymptomatiques*, edited by R. Courbier, J. M. Jausseron, and M. Recci, pp. 334–344. Lyon, Documentation Médical Oberval, 1980.

196. MEYERMANN, R., and YAŞARGIL, M. G. Ultrastructural findings in the intima of vessels of cerebral angiomas gained operatively. In: *Cerebral Microcirculation and Metabolism*, edited by J. Cervos-Navarro and E. Fritschka, pp. 361–367. New York, Raven Press, 1981.

197. MEYERMANN, R., and YAŞARGIL, M. G. Ultrastructural studies of

cerebral berry aneurysms obtained operatively. Adv. Neurosurg., 9: 174–181, 1981.

198. WIESER, H. G., and YAŞARGIL, M. G. Die selektive Amygdalo-Hippokampektomie als chirurgische Behandlungsmethode der "mediobasal-limbschen" psychomotorischen Epilepsie. EEG EMG, 12: 56, 1981.

199. YOUNG, P. H., and YAŞARGIL, M. G. Use of small diameter synthetic grafts in carotid bypasses in rats. J. Microsurg., 3: 3–6, 1981.

200. ZUMSTEIN, B., and YAŞARGIL, M. G. [Improvement of cerebral blood circulation by microsurgical bypass-anastomoses (author's transl).] Schweiz. Rundsch. Med. Prax, 70: 1866–1873, 1981.

201. WALSER, H., YAŞARGIL, M. G., and CURCIC, M. Auditory brain stem responses in patients with posterior fossa tumors. Surg. Neurol., 18: 405–415, 1982.

202. WIESER, H. G., and YAŞARGIL, M. G. Selective amygdalohippocampectomy as a surgical treatment of mesiobasal limbic epilepsy. Surg. Neurol., 17: 445–457, 1982.

203. WIESER, H. G., and YAŞARGIL, M. G. "Selective amygdalo-hippocampectomy" as a surgical treatment of mesiobasal limbic epilepsy (author's transl). Neurochirurgia, 25: 39–50, 1982.

204. YAŞARGIL, M. G. Suboccipital transmeatal microsurgical excision of acoustic neuromas. In: Head and Neck Surgery, edited by H. H. Naumann, pp. 553–595. Stuttgart, Georg Thieme Verlag, 1982.

205. YAŞARGIL, M. G., and SMITH, R. D. Management of aneurysms of anterior circulation by intracranial procedures. In: Neurological Surgery, edited by J. R. Youmans, pp. 1663–1696. Philadelphia, W. B. Saunders, 1982.

206. YOUNG, P. H., and YAŞARGIL, M. G. Experimental carotid artery aneurysms in rats: A new model for microsurgical practice. J. Microsurg., 3: 135–146, 1982.

207. HAAS, H. L., WIESER, H. G., and YAŞARGIL, M. G. Aminopyridine and fiber potentials in rat and human hippocampal slices. Experientia, 39: 114–115, 1983.

208. HUBER, A., and YAŞARGIL, M. G. Ophthalmic artery aneurysms. Klin. Monatsbl. Augenheilkd., 182: 537–543, 1983.

209. NAUTA, H. J., DOLAN, E., and YAŞARGIL, M. G. Microsurgical anatomy of spinal subarachnoid space. Surg. Neurol., 19: 431–437, 1983.

210. VALAVANIS, A., WELLAUER, J., and YAŞARGIL, M. G. The radiological diagnosis of cerebral venous angiomas: Cerebral angiography and computed tomography. Neuroradiology, 24: 193–199, 1983.

211. SANDVOSS, G., SMITH, R. D., and YAŞARGIL, M. G. Experimental

microsurgical exposure of cranial nerves III, IV, and VI in the cat. Neurochirurgia, *27:* 129–132, 1984.

212. SGIER, F., and YAŞARGIL, M. G. Chronic subdural hematoma. Surgical treatment under microsurgical conditions. Schweiz. Rundsch. Med. Prax., *73:* 547–553, 1984.

213. YAŞARGIL, M. G. *Microneurosurgery,* Vols 1 and 2. Stuttgart, Georg Thieme Verlag, 1984.

214. YAŞARGIL, M. G., SYMON, L., and TEDDY, P. J. Arteriovenous malformations of the spinal cord. Adv. Tech. Stand. Neurosurg., *11:* 61–102, 1984.

215. SHOKRY, A., JANZER, R. C., VON HOCHSTETTER, A. R., YAŞARGIL, M. G., and HEDINGER, C. Primary intracranial germ-cell tumors. A clinicopathological study of 14 cases. J. Neurosurg., *62:* 826–830, 1985.

216. YAŞARGIL, M. G. Subarachnoidale Blutung (Aneurysme und Angiome). In: *Innere Medizin in Praxis und Klinik,* edited by H. Hornbostel, W. Kaufmann, and W. Siegenthaler, pp. 740–743. Stuttgart, Georg Thieme Verlag, 1985.

217. YAŞARGIL, M. G. Forward. In: *Cerebrovascular Surgery,* Vol. 4. Berlin, Springer Verlag, 1985.

218. YAŞARGIL, M. G., TEDDY, P. J., and ROTH, P. Selective amygdalohippocampectomy. Operative anatomy and surgical technique. Adv. Tech. Stand. Neurosurg., *12:* 93–123, 1985.

219. SANDVOSS, G., CERVOS-NAVARRO, J., and YAŞARGIL, M. G. Intracranial repair of the oculomotor nerve in cats. Neurochirurgia, *29:* 1–8, 1986.

Contents

——————————————— I ———————————————

CHAPTER 1

CHAPTER 2

CHAPTER 3

CHAPTER 4

CHAPTER 5

——————————————— II ———————————————

CEREBROVASCULAR SURGERY

CHAPTER 6

CHAPTER 7

CHAPTER 8

V

TRAUMA

I

1

Presidential Address: from *Aequanimitas* to Icarus

JOSEPH C. MAROON, M.D.

The theme of the 35th meeting of the Congress of Neurological Surgeons is New Frontiers in Neurosurgery. The scientific program is replete with learned discussions of the great advances in diagnostic imaging, laser technology, neurotransmitters, and innovative surgical procedures. Our honored guest, professor Gazi Yaşargil, has demonstrated, in a virtuoso fashion, the frontiers one may reach with *chiriurgie*, or work with our hands, under magnification.

Rather than discuss additional, technical frontiers, I feel it is a time for reflection and perspective. We have heard the inspiring, personal neurosurgical reflections of Dr. Yaşargil; the historically steeped and erudite discussion of the social transformation of American medicine by Dr. Paul Starr, which was further advanced by my good friend Dr. Donald Stewart. We have all looked at what has preceded in an attempt to understand the present and, perhaps, to glimpse the future.

I also have looked back, as well as within, to find a topic for my address to you. I considered what personal reflections of mine might have special meaning to most here. I found help in rereading the address delivered by Sir William Osler in 1899 to the students and faculty of The University of Pennsylvania upon his departure to the then fledgling Johns Hopkins University (6). He spoke to his friends of two qualities which, he said, might contribute to their success, or help them in times of failure.

With the Congress dedicated to the younger neurosurgeon who is usually struggling for success, but also encompassing the older neurosurgeon who has had much greater exposure to failure, I thought it propitious to explore these two Oslerian qualities as they pertain to the neurosurgeon's professional and personal life.

The qualities Osler described were imperturbability and *aequanimitas*. He defined imperturbability as "coolness" and presence of mind under all circumstances, calmness amid storm, and clearness of judgment in moments of grave peril. To describe the second quality he referred to that wisest of Roman rulers, Antoninus Pius. As Antoninus lay dying in his home in Etruria, he summed up his philosophy of life with the watchword "*aequanimitas*." It is a character trait so difficult to attain, yet necessary in success as well as in failure. *Aequanimitas* derives from the Latin words *aequus*, or "even," and *animus*, meaning "mind" or "spirit"; therefore meaning even in mind, temperament, and composure, or combined in modern parlance with imperturbability to mean "balance" or "equanimity."

I propose, with some trepidation, to direct your attention for a few minutes to this quality of balance, or *Aequanimitas*, the importance of it, the consequences of not possessing it (I'm an expert in that field!) and, perhaps, a suggestion for its attainment.

In my search to better understand "balance," Sir William's advice sent me further back in history and mythology to the Greek myth of Daedalus and his son, Icarus—the earliest example I could find dealing with the problems and consequences of not attaining balance or equanimity in one's life (5).

Imprisoned by King Minos of Crete in a labyrinthian prison with no roof, Daedalus and Icarus escaped by ingeniously constructing wings of feathers and wax and flying out. But before attaining flight, Daedalus cautioned Icarus, his young impetuous son, not to fly too low, lest the sea wet the feathers of his wings and make them too heavy to fly. Nor, Daedalus said, should Icarus fly too high, lest the sun melt the wax, scorch his wings and cause him to fall to the earth. Above all, Daedalus warned Icarus not to be diverted by the birds he would see soaring in the sky. He might thus experience the hubris of flight, forget his limitations, and surely fall and die.

We all know that in the exultation of the flight, Icarus failed to heed his father's advice. Feeling the great thrill of soaring, up, up he flew, up so near the sun that the wax binding his wings melted, and he plummeted into the sea, to be swallowed by the waves (Fig. 1.1).

I must confess, that the full significance of this story eluded me until I entered neurosurgical practice. Like Icarus, I was young and impetuous. Eager to test my wings and fly, I decided early on to operate upon a young mother of two with an enormous left internal carotid artery aneurysm. After hours of tedious dissection, I finally clipped what I thought was the neck of the aneurysm. Then I closed the wound and departed from the operating room. I soared like Icarus, congratulating myself on my deft hands, sharp eyes, and exquisite judgment. I allowed myself proud thoughts of how few others could perform such an operation with such expertise.

Thirty minutes later a call from the recovery room informed me of my patient's hemiplegic, aphasic, and subsequently comatose state. An angiogram showed a complete occlusion of the internal carotid artery

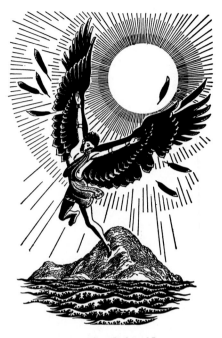

FIG. 1.1. The flight of Icarus.

because of a misplaced clip. My ensuing depression and despondency matched—in a negative way—my elation and, yes, my hubris, my over-inflated pride, of just a few minutes before. At that moment I painfully recalled the familiar proverb with its Icarian message: "Pride goeth before the fall and a haughty spirit before destruction" (7).

Despite this, and the subsequent scorching of my wings on many other operative occasions, it took me a long time to realize the wisdom of my colleague Bob Selker's statement that "complications are God's way of keeping surgeons humble." For several years I rode the surgeon's roller coaster. I soared to peaks with my surgical successes and plummeted into the valley of depression with my failures. Ah, balance. A balance of sorts came only when I realized that despite the skills and training required of us, the Golden Rule still applies. For surgeons, it is to do unto others with the same surgeon's skill, the same judgment and, above all, the same compassion with which we would want something done unto us. Furthermore, I found it helpful to remember the words of the barber-surgeon Ambrose Paré, in the 1500s: "We dress the wound," he said, and "God cures the patient." Complications and cures—they both come from God. Maybe it's better that way. It certainly leads to better balance.

As neurosurgeons, we are constantly inclined to test the frontiers of possibility: the giant basal meningioma, the cervical intramedullary tumor, and the giant aneurysm. In operating on all of these, there is the unmistakable strain of nonacceptance which is the primal mark of Icarus in our nature. The rewards of neurosurgical nonacceptance may be great—a cured patient or perhaps a new technique that could benefit many future patients. But the consequences may just as easily be disastrous, with paralysis or death from violating neuroanatomical laws akin to the violation of the laws of physics by Icarus.

We must constantly seek the balance between good judgment, experience, and our technical abilities. Good judgment comes from experience but, unfortunately, experience comes most often from poor judgment. Unlike Icarus, however, we are able to learn from our experiences and not drown in our mistakes if the Oslerian qualities of hard work, scholarship, and humility characterize our practice.

But *aequanimitas* in our profession is only part of the balance we must attain if we wish to be successful. For even if we succeed in getting our professional life under control, we have only just begun. We still have vital personal issues to confront—physical fitness, spirituality, and family—before we can achieve a truly balanced life. Unfortunately I was a very slow learner. It was only quite recently that I discovered the interrelated nature of these other aspects. Only then did a more complete understanding of the full meaning of equanimity—or balance—become apparent to me.

A recent experience I had with my children greatly helped with this understanding. Permit me to share it with you. One night I was reading a book entitled *I Dare You*, by William Danforth (3). The book not only challenges the reader to superior accomplishment, but also demonstrates that the only way to true success is through a balanced life. I showed it to my daughter Laura, not quite 11, and my son Michael, 15, with the hope of encouraging them into persevering during those most difficult years. The book requires each reader to consider the four major areas of personal commitment: professional (or educational), family/social, spiritual, and physical. Then a "picture" is drawn of one's life to determine how four-square it is (Fig. 1.2), with the length of each arm proportional to the degree of commitment. I asked Laura and Mike to draw their square.

They then said: "It's your turn." After comparing my "square" to theirs, it was obvious their responses (and lives) were in much better balance than mine. I also immediately recognized, with this simplistic approach, that many of the principles and ideals I had *wanted* to impart to my own children had, in me, become weakened or lost altogether as seen in my square.

Although unorthodox for an address such as this, I now request and

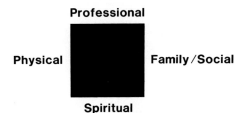

FIG. 1.2   The relationship of professional, educational, family/social, physical, and spiritual components as depicted in a "square."

challenge each of you with the same task. You received a piece of paper when you entered. Take 30 seconds now and draw your own square. Later, in the quiet moments you reserve for yourself, think about its configuration and the best way to balance it.

Now, one further request. Think just for a minute about your most valued possession—that thing without which, as Shakespeare wrote, "life would be bound in shallows and in misery" (11). I think many would agree it is good health. Yet when most of us look at our squares we see how little importance is placed on the physical side. So I believe that the challenge that each of us must face is to understand the relationship of *our* squares—our goals—to equanimity—to balance—especially to health—both mental and physical.

Let us now examine a typical neurosurgeon's square (Fig. 1.3). Then we'll look at each side and some of the consequences of over and underemphasis—or imbalance.

We shall begin with the professional. As many will agree, this component frequently is out of proportion to the other three sides. Yet, when professional interests replace the others, then, as night follows day, the family/social, spiritual, and physical sides all atrophy. Such imbalance may translate into tragedy—or in fact, several tragedies. Often, they create neurosurgical widows—women who know that they have husbands somewhere, but who also know that sighting them is best accomplished at airports between neurosurgical meetings (Fig. 1.4). An overemphasis on the professional also affects children, whose material affluence—coupled with parental neglect—make them susceptible to the temptations of drugs, alcohol, and delinquency. Perhaps worst of all, overvalued professional interest detaches the family from the spiritual moorings so necessary for daily life. Finally, the imbalance promotes the hypotonic corpus and adiposity somewhat characteristic of our profession.

Next take a closer look at the physical side of our square and consider the physiological consequences of neglect in this area. Specifically, let's look at the breakdown of physical equanimity—let's look at the dangers of stress.

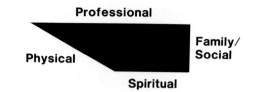
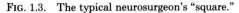

FIG. 1.3. The typical neurosurgeon's "square."

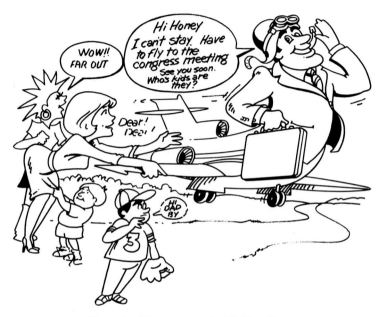

FIG. 1.4. The neurosurgical "widow."

One of the first modern physiologists to speak of equanimity—and stress—in health was Claude Bernard (1). In the late 1800s he stated; "It is the fixity of the *milieu interieur* which is the primary condition for a free and independent life. All the vital mechanisms of the body, varied as they are, have only one object: that of preserving balance and equilibrium." There can be little doubt that this was Bernard's greatest biological generalization. Fifty years later, and building on Bernard's observations, the American physiologist Walter Cannon suggested that the coordinated physiological processes—which maintains an organism's *milieu interieur*—should be called homeostasis—or physiological equanimity (2). Is this concept now beginning to sound familiar?

In the 1930s, Hans Selye went several physiologic steps further. He demonstrated that animals subjected to prolonged severe stress suffered from hypertrophy of the adrenal glands, atrophy of the thymus and lymph nodes, and the appearance of gastrointestinal ulcers (10). It was Selye who formulated the now classic "adaptation syndrome" which deals with the body's positive and negative reactions to stress.

In the last several years, scientists in such diverse fields as immunology, neuroendocrinology, neurochemistry, neuropharmacology, and the behavioral fields have all added observations related to the physiology of stress. Yet, for all their advances—and some are profound—they have all rediscovered what Galen stated in the second century A.D. He said that the emotional state of an individual can cause—and, in some cases— relieve disease. Specifically, Galen said that cancer struck far more frequently in melancholy rather than in sanguine persons—something we're just beginning to reconsider today (13).

The belief that disease was a consequence of psychic or spiritual imbalance governed medicine—both in theory and practice—in the Orient and the Occident until well after the 17th century rise of modern science with its mechanistic view of physiology. Yet, some of the old theories weren't so far fetched. It wasn't until the last 20 years, for example, that immune system alteration was documented in patients suffering from stress. It was observed, for example, that during the first few months of bereavement, widows and widowers were highly susceptible to disease and that people hospitalized for severe depression—usually resulting from psychic stress—often had a hampered immune system (9).

So, while we're looking for a balance, let us look at how the immune system normally functions. Then perhaps, we can determine the ways in which mental or physical imbalance may cause disease. As you know, our white blood cells constitute a highly effective army of defenders against those substances—living and inert—that are not part of the human body.

Normally when a virus, bacterium, or other foreign substance first enters the body, it is engulfed by a macrophage (Fig. 1.5). The macrophage then secretes lymphokines and interleukin-1 (IL-1), and they activate the T cells, which join the fight. The activated T cell then produces interleukin-2 (IL-2) which, in turn, stimulates other T cells to grow and divide. The Ts also secrete a lymphokine called B-cell growth factor (BCGF) which causes B cells to multiply and produce antibodies. Finally, the T cells produce a lymphokine called γ interferon (IF) with protean defensive capabilities. Of tremendous importance, we now know there are bidirectional circuits between the central nervous system and this phenomenal immunological system (Fig. 1.6). Lymphokines, thymosins, and certain complement proteins, called immunotransmitters, all appear to transfer information from the immune centers to the brain (4).

A major conceptual shift has thus occurred in neuroscience with the discovery that the linkage between the brain, the glands, and the immune

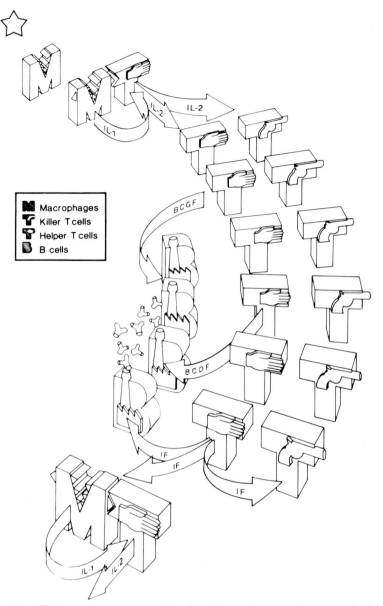

FIG. 1.5.   The immune response to infection. The mechanism of action of the immune system.

system is modulated by numerous chemicals, mostly peptides, in addition to classical neurotransmitters.

This all adds up to a wholly mechanistic substantiation of a self-correcting, functional circuit that ties the behavioral activity of the brain to the neuroendocrine and immunologic systems of the body—Bernard, Cannon, and Selye would be ecstatic! So, what does all this have to do with the physical side of our square?

Physical fitness and exercise now makes tremendous sense—and not just because we feel good doing it. We now know exercise stimulates the brain to release chemicals such as endorphins and enkephalins, which reduce anxiety and create a sense of well-being—naturally, without extraneous pharmacological influences, such as drugs.

Even more startling are studies which indicate that exercise affects macrophages and T cells and results in increased levels of interleukin-1 and interferon, both of which strengthen our immune system defenses (Fig. 1.7). In fact both substances are presently being used experimentally today in the treatment of cancer—a disease recognized 1900 years ago by Galen to be associated with excessive stress and depression which we now know suppress our immune system and peptides like interleukin-1 and interferon. So—it is not solely the good feeling one derives from running through green pastures, or swimming in still waters, although that feeling is both potent and palpable. No, we are also substantiating the premise that exercise in and of itself enhances our immunological system in a very positive way and additionally, as stated centuries ago in the 23rd Psalm, "restoreth our soul" (8).

I may have taken a circuitous path, but I have attempted to illustrate just one of the many ways a biological substratum underpins the aphorism, "As a man thinketh in his heart, so he shall be." We literally *are* what we think, as mediated through definable anatomic and neurochemical pathways (Fig. 1.6). Our character and our health—to a large extent—the sum of *all* of our thoughts. It's as simple as this: good thoughts and actions are unlikely to produce bad results. Bad thoughts and actions can never produce good results.

Yes, you say, but what are good thoughts? What is the *good* life? What guidelines do we have for right thinking and right living? What should our relationship be towards our families and friends? our patients? our society at large? Obviously, such questions extend beyond the scope of this address—and must be answered by each of us individually. But clearly, each of us must adopt for himself an acceptable way of life and a livable personal religion and spirituallty—the third arm of our square which we will now discuss.

One of the earliest spiritual guidelines designed to maintain equanimity in man and peace among men is found in the Old Testament—and then

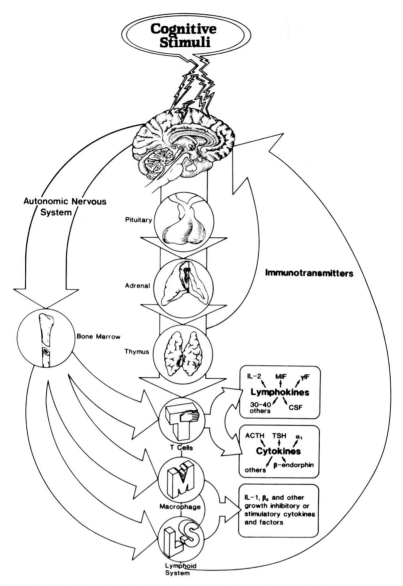

FIG. 1.6. The bidirectional relationship of the brain, the glands, the immune system, and the autonomic nervous system.

is reemphasized in the New Testament by St. Matthew and St. Mark (14, 15). "Thou shall love they neighbor as thyself." With certain variations this commandment can be found in the most diverse religions and philosophies. The so-called Golden Rule—"Do unto others as you would

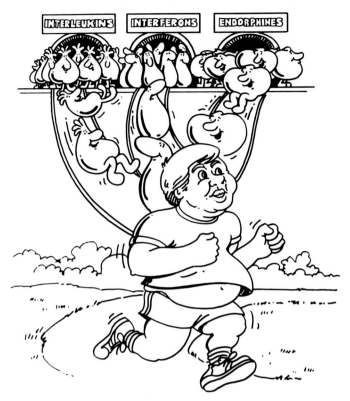

Fig. 1.7.   The beneficial effects of exercise.

have them do unto you"—is but a modification of the idea of loving our neighbors.

Perhaps that is why this commandment appears so often—and in so many places. Zoroaster taught it to the fire worshipers in Persia 3000 years ago. Confucius, Lao-Tse, and Buddha incorporated loving one's neighbor' into their doctrines. It appears, of course, in Judaism and Christianity. Above all, despite the variations in religions, the existence and importance of a higher authority is accepted by the adherents of every religious group.

Hans Selye contemplated spiritually, particularly as it applies to physicians (10). In discussing what is the aim of life, he concluded that it is our responsibility to incite love, goodwill, gratitude, respect, and all other positive feelings that render use useful, and, indeed, indispensable to our patients and neighbors. By so doing we express an "egotistic altruism" that is rewarded many times over by similar feelings from others towards ourselves. There is much wisdom in this philosophy.

Physicality and spirituality are irrevocably intertwined, and lead to equanimity—to balance.

The final arm of the square is the family. The family is so important that it is said that no other success can compensate for failure at home. Concomitantly, there is no greater stress—or distress—than that which arises from rancor or problems at home. The pain of a sick, injured, or retarded child or one on drugs, or the breakup of a marriage, those are among the most severely destabilizing forces to anyone's equilibrium. Family problems—and unfortunately they must come to all of us sooner or later— again summon the great need for spirituality, for a belief in a higher authority—to bring ease, to bring understanding, to bring coping, and even to bring survival.

Just as the family may be the source of tears and sorrow, it may also be the fount of our joys and laughter. Certainly we are delighted with our children's academic and athletic achievements, but perhaps the greatest joy comes from experiencing those intangibles of love and trust shared between parent and child, the purity of their uncluttered minds, and the unconditional love that is expressed in the everyday sharing of activities.

I lay no claims to being a paragon of excellence or an outstanding figure as a physician-father. I do know, however, that children are amazingly resilient and that even though wilted by lack of attention, time, and love, they quickly rebound to our caring with a blossoming that matches the freshness of flowers. We must carefully look at *their* developing squares and help them by our example to obtain balance in all four components. Our children are not so much vessels to be filled with money, cars, clothes and material goods, but rather are fires to be lit with love, caring, and support, and are kept burning by our presence physically and emotionally.

In this short time, I have attempted to illustrate what I believe to be the necessity of seeking a balance, or personal equanimity, in all aspects of our lives, of guarding against soaring too high with success, as did Icarus, or sinking so low with failure as to wetten our wings with the heaviness of depression which, in our profession, may at times seem ubiquitous. We must travel from Icarus to *aequanimitas* to the present.

Having discussed with you each arm of our square, we have seen the importance of some form of spirituality in all aspects of our lives. Differing slightly with William Danforth, I submit that a triangle might best depict the physicians' approach towards equilibrium—with spirituality permeating *all* aspects of our professional, family, and physical lives (Fig. 1.8).

Equilibrium—we all require it—for ourselves, our families, and our patients. We have discussed the bidirectional pathways between our brain and immune system and the profound mental and physical conse-

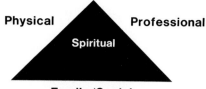

Physical   Professional

Spiritual

Family/Social

FIG. 1.8.   The relationship of spirituality to the physical, professional, and family/social aspects.

quences that many of us have experienced, of not maintaining such a state. Equilibrium—equal measure to all four sides of our square or our triangle. In the quietness of our own hearts: we must work to maintain our balance. To those less fortunate—like myself—who find ourselves at times out of balance, I would suggest—or perhaps urge—that we follow the admonition of St. Luke who, as quoted by Dr. Bruce Sorensen in his classic and sensitive Presidential Address, said: "Physician, heal thyself" (12).

REFERENCES

1. Bernard, C. *An Introduction to the Study of Experimental Medicine.* MacMillan and Company, New York, 1927.
2. Cannon, W. B. *The Wisdom of the Body.* W. W. Norton, New York, 1932.
3. Danforth, W. *I Dare You.* St. Louis, Missouri. Privately published and printed, December 1954.
4. Hall, N. R., McGillis, J. P., Spangello, B. L., and Goldstein, A. L. Evidence that thymosins and other biological response modifiers can function as neuroactive immunotransmitters. J. Immunol, *135:* 806–813, 1985.
5. Hazo, S. *The Feast of Icarus.* Pittsburgh, Palaemon Press, Limited, 1984.
6. Osler, W. *Aequanimitas,* pp. 1–13. McGraw-Hill, New York, 1906.
7. Proverbs 16:18. *Holy Bible,* New International Version, p. 840. Zondervan Bible Publishers, Grand Rapids, Mich., 1978.
8. Psalm 23:1-6. *Holy Bible.* New International Version, p. 687. Zondervan Bible Publishers, Grand Rapids, Mich., 1978.
9. Solomon, G. F. Emotions, stress and central nervous system and immunity. Ann. N.Y. Acad. Sci. *164:* 335–343, 1969.
10. Selye, H. *Stress without Distress.* J. B. Lippincott, Philadelphia, 1974.
11. Shakespeare, W. *Julius Caesar,* Act IV, Scene iii, line 217. Doubleday, New York.
12. Sorensen, B. *Physician Heal Thyself.* Clin. Neurosurg., *25:*1–8, 1978.
13. Stein, M., Keller, S. E., and Schleifer, S. J. Stress and immunomodulation: the role of depression and neuroendocrine function. J. Immunol., 827–832, 1985.
14. St. Mark, 12:31. *Holy Bible,* New International Version. Zondervan Bible Publishers, Grand Rapids, Mich., p. 1353, 1978.
15. St. Matthew, 19:19. *Holy Bible.* New International Version, p. 1316. Zondervan Bible Publishers, Grand Rapids, Mich., 1978.

2

Reflections of a Neurosurgeon

M. GAZI YAŞARGIL, M.D.

The reflection of information from the past and its anteflection into the defined time period is one dimension of the present, whereas the immeasurable individual time of a person is the other dimension of the present. The time-consciousness of man is imbedded in his given-time (*Moira, Nemesis*). The "being of time" opens itself only for man. This enables us to attempt to understand and accept the concepts of life and death.

Reflecting on history, we realize that three different chains of events are interwoven:

(*a*) All beings inherit a common cosmic history, which seems to be precisely disposed but difficult to decode.

(*b*) All living beings have a common genetical history which developed slowly, and its presentment began in ancient times. The first scientific speculation began 380 years ago with the introduction of the microscope by Van Leuwenhook and R. Hooke, who gave us the definiton of the "cell." Actual scientific research and presentation began with Darwin, 126 years ago.

(*c*) Only human beings have a civilization and cultural history. This began probably 500,000 years ago with the development of tools and then accelerated 30,000 years ago with the first scripts; 6,000 years ago with ideograms, pictograms, alphabets, numbers, and calendars; 2,500 years ago with dialectic dispute during the Hellenistic culture; 500 years ago with printed books (1452); and in our age, that is during the past 100 years, with instant transmission of communications (telephone, radio, television, and satellites).

The genetic information of billions of years is well filtrated and distilled despite its complex transmutations. We are just learning to read, interpret, and understand this fantastic alphabet which consists of 4 letters and 6 words but 1.3 million books (i.e., plants and animals).

16

Our cultural history, although relatively short, is entirely incomplete. Great parts remain undiscovered, are already destroyed, neglected, concealed, misinterpreted or misunderstood; or are, in general, not well studied and analyzed in an organized systematic manner. Every generation has its own particular approach to history and its own interpretation of facts.

The human brain develops ideas and concepts, which prepare us for anticipated actions. It creates philosophical, moral, and political ideologies not only for individuals but also for collective societies. Are the good ideologies, however, always the result of our rational thinking and the bad ones of irrational thinking? In his 18th century "*A Treatise of Human Nature*" David Hume warned us: "The moral laws are not the result of our ratio!"

We expect our "ratio" to indicate which path we should follow, for instance: "how to behave correctly" and "how to decide and perform correctly." Is our genetic conscience more reliable than the "cultural conscience"? If neuronal hurricanes occur in individual brains as well as in the "brain" of collective societies, then the expected actions of the conscience seem to be entirely paralyzed. Human beings, therefore, are still searching to find additional compasses.

In ancient times such imaginative compasses have been extrapolated to holy places and objects, as well as to persons and institutions. For several centuries during the Hellenistic and Roman cultures, Pythia was the holy person in the Apollo temple at Delphi, and her answers were always in the form of oracles. In the 6th century before Christ, Croesus, the Emperor of Lydia, sent a delegation to Delphi in order to ask how he should handle Cyrus and the Persians. Pythia oracled: "If you cross Halys, you will destroy an empire." We all know what happened. Croesus did cross the Halys, which culminated in his own defeat and the destruction of his own empire.

In every confrontation lurks a decision whether to "cross over a borderline." This is especially true in the case of decisions and planning for surgery. We, like Croesus, must be careful in our interpretations of the information which is available to us. Do we really know as much as we think we do, and can we really extrapolate our knowledge to correct action as we cross anatomical borders?

Before an operation the surgeon may calculate and predict the possible duration of a procedure; it should be over in 1, 2, or 3 hours. But what makes us feel uneasy? We are aware that we have to cross over a borderline, a borderline which exists between the readiness of the patient to accept the proposed intervention in his given-time and our decision to include the destiny of the patient with our own destiny and dexterity, which is our given-time.

Animals are naturally endowed with a horizontal head and body. Their head and extremities are fully developed as tools. They act instinctively and, therefore, usually correctly. The human body, however, stands perpendicular and attempts to balance the head between the horizontal and vertical coordinates within its given lifetime. The human brain also tries to form a balance between knowledge and ignorance, and to gain prospective perspectives to the horizontal which will reflect the past into the future, in order to create an active anticipatory present. It attempts to know what is the correct procedure here and now; what is right and what is wrong; and where to go!

Our extremities are in some way stagnated organs on an embryological level. The mouth, hands, and feet are not tools in the same sense that they are in the case of animals. Our "open-system" of the brain allows us to create tools, new ideas, and new concepts. This is not just the result of our process of adaptation for survival. Our open system continuously and actively participates in evolution, enhancing creative adaptation and improvement in the quality of survival. It also further actively participates in innovative creativeness, the initiative which is inherent in us.

As doctors of medicine and, more specifically, as surgeons, we have to combine our scientific knowledge and technical abilities with the art of medicine to acquire an accurate diagnosis and appropriate therapy for our patients. But what is knowledge? What is science? What is the art of medicine? If we compare the answers given today with the responses of the previous centuries there would be a great disparity, and yet each generation believes that it is correct, and is firm in its convictions. Obviously many things were neither correct nor final in previous times, nor are they so today. Nevertheless, we have made great advances in science in the past and will hopefully continue to do so in the future. Did we make advances also in the art of medicine? In daily confrontation of the destiny of our patients, their diseases, and the outcome of our surgical treatment, we may appear to know exactly what we are going to do, whereas in reality we are unsure of the line along which our reflections, logic, and emotions will lead us. We trust our knowledge, experience, imagination, and extrapolation to our direct scheduled actions. We hope that the tissue, organs, and overall system of the patient will accept our surgical manipulations and will respond, at least positively. These facts express a very real and special situation, namely, the following, that no less than the reluctant brain of a medical doctor is attempting to help another brain. Subsequently the following questions arise: What is the actual condition of this brain which is capable of reflecting and making decisions? Where are the roots of these critical judgments? Allow me to take you back almost 2400 years and to a place 6000 miles to the East.

Socrates, who has become a worldwide symbol of the moral, autonomous, and therefore self-conscious, self-responding person, was one of the greatest philosophers, but he called himself only "a midwife for the birth of critical thoughts." In his dialogues, he never gave a definitive answer to his questions, but in his analytic philosophy he left the search for answers to the questioning of his students. In reality, his line of thought or questioning is a level of reasoning which explores the reliability of the human brain and thus inquires into the reliability of human thought and decision.

Politics, faith, love, logic, ethics, and aesthetics are inseparable entities. The above form of self-questioning, as first initiated by Socrates, is a form of self-examination by the brain to try to understand these entities and thus to understand its own essential being. Through self-awareness and exercise of analytic judgment (What is real? What is good? What is beauty? What is courage? What is innocence? What is right?) the beginnings of critical reflection are initiated which play an important avant-garde role not only in art and philosophy, but also in all sciences and technologies.

The seeds of this dialectic, conceptualized way of thinking have been scattered from Athens to Mesopotamia to Central Asia to the South of Spain (Andalusia) and have finally settled into the fertile soil of the Occident. They have sprouted and blossomed over the past 900 years, without, surprisingly, the strands of continuity being interrupted.

We realize that the human being is distinctly unique. In a sense, man possesses a "neuronal compass" which has and can guide him to his intellectual destiny. He has evolved from a purely instinctual creature to a rational, reflective, and self-steering being. The architectural arrangement of the brain is of an old construction. A one billion-year-old brainstem, with a 500-million-year-old diencephalon and cerebellum, is coupled to a telencephalon which is 30 million years old. The holistic imagination is postulated to be a function of the cortex. It potentiates and modifies the drives of the limbic system. In many instances perhaps it is the limbic system and lower archaic systems which control the cortex. These reciprocal functions must always be in delicate balance. It is, therefore, necessary to exercise caution and careful judgment in order to avoid the rigidities and inflexibilities of both archaic instincts and learned dogmas. The validity of all sciences, philosophies, arts, and technologies is the liability which arises from open questioning and discussion. We must explain our process of reasoning both inwardly to ourselves and outwardly to others. This was the concern of Socrates and from his method of self scrutiny arose the concept of critical reflection. In open discussion will be achieved the harmony of topos, chronos, and logos (space, time, and logic).

Socrates was teaching us, with his analytic philosophy, the relativity of our feelings, beliefs, thoughts, and behavior. His conscience told him to follow his "logos," which cannot be translated merely as "logic" because it conveys a much wider significance. With his paradigm, *Socrates* opened a new period of cultural history which has continued until our century. The new cultural period began with *Einstein* in the early 1900s, who made us aware of the relativity of nature itself. But do we fully understand this opening onto a new threshold of our understanding that Einstein gave us?

Euclid, Galileo, Newton, and their contemporaries represent milestones in our cultural history. *Einstein* and his contemporaries succeeded in new breakthroughs. Our imagination, however, still adheres to *Euclid*'s 3-dimensional space-ideology, even though the physicists and mathematicians are presenting new theories of multidimensioned space and time. We have trouble imagining the 4th dimension, cannot comprehend the 5th or the 6th, yet we will understand that space and time are entirely different entities as understood up to the present time. Similarly, logos also has another dimension. It had been assumed, even as late as the 19th century, that what *Aristotle* said was the final word on logic. *Kant* asserted that logic, as developed by Aristotle, was, of all philosophical disciplines, a finished and complete subject, even down to its finest details. This view has been shown to be mistaken, as argued by *Russel* and *Whitehead*, who both used symbolic logic. They developed a new type of logic, which was much broader in scope than the Aristotelian logic; indeed, it contained classical logic as a very minor part.

The human being discovered long ago the relativity of the senses, but only later was he able to calculate and reason what exists beyond our small "perception-window," using mathematics and physics. Similarly, man realized long ago the relativity of our concepts, and we are now able to calculate and to prove what a *dynamic cosmos* exists beyond this static "concept-window." It has been a long and complicated journey from the analytic philosophy of *Socrates* to the logistic philosophy of *Russel, Whitehead, Wittgenstein,* and *Heidegger.*

Critical judgments are always counterbalanced by the scales of our conscience. The main constituents of our conscience have become more pronounced: *faith, love, politics, logics,* and *ethics* all have become more prominent. However, one other component of our conscience should be pronounced: critical aesthetics. The concept of critical aesthetics has been reduced nowadays to only a "judgment of beauty." It is more than this. It is a sense of perception. Beauty, goodness, and strength appear to be only positive attributes. If they are accepted alone without critical reflection, it becomes easy to be seduced into complacency. Ugliness may be beautiful; madness may be interesting; and weakness, faultiness, and timidity may be appealing. *Emmanuel Kant* and *Alexander Gottlieb Baumgarten* reminded us 200 years ago of the importance of critical aesthetics. Baumgarten even insisted that aesthetics be treated as a science. Although there have been an enormous number of philosophical tractates within the past 100 years concerning politics, logic, ethics, and aesthetics, there is surprisingly no book available dealing with ethics which includes aesthetics and vice versa. There are no reflections such as: What are the aesthetics of ethics and the ethics of aesthetics?

In addition to this, during discussions concerning critical aesthetics most associations deal with the five senses of sight, sound, touch, taste, and smell. The "vestibular sense" seems to have been excluded in relation to critical aesthetics. Not only does it control the balance during physical activities, but also it "balances" the processes of thought. Which sense regulates the velocity, rhythm, and relative proportions of thought to fulfill the requirements of mental harmony? The balance of our upright position is secured by small stones known as statoliths. The small weights (or stones) of the pharmacist are called scruples. Without scruples there will be no balance between aesthetical ethics and ethical aesthetics and, therefore, no balance in our critical reflection. We are asked by our conscience to take care of our scruples! Too many as well as too few may be wrong.

Faith, love, politics, logic, ethics, and aesthetics have been for ever inseparable forces in medicine. We have to approach our patients, who are trying to survive their illness and who are stranded sometimes in a delicate balance between life and death, with our critical judgment. The surgical patient must have the best anesthetics, and the surgeon must have the best aesthetics. This requires the surgeon to use not only the combination of his senses but also the critical reflection of his scientific knowledge, his ethical concern in his philosophical thoughts and religious belief, his artistic abilities, technical dexterity and, finally, fairness in the game with the nature.

SUGGESTED READINGS

Aristotle. *Nicomachear Ethics*, translated in German by F. Dirlmeier, Stuttgart, 1969.
Baumgartner A. G. *Aestetica*, 1750.
Einstein, A. *Spezielle Relativitätstheorie*, 1905.
Einstein, A. *Allgemeine Relativitätstheorie*, 1916.
Euclid. *Elements*, 300 B. C.
Galileo Galilei. *Discorsi*, 1638.
Heidegger, M. *Sein und Zeit*, 1927.
Hume, D. *A Treatise of Human Nature*, 1739/1740.
Kant, E. *Kritik der Urteilskraft*, 1790.
Newton, I. *Philisophiae Naturalis Principie Mathematica*, 1687.
Russel, B. Whitehead, A. N. *Principia Mathematica.* Cambridge, 1910/1913.
Socratres. *"Laches " of Platon: Sämtliche Werke*, vol 1. Rowohlt, 1957.
Whitehead, A. N. *Process and Reality*, 1927.
Wittgenstein, L. The tractus logico-philosophias, 1922. In: *Philosphical Investigation.* Blackwell, Oxford, 1965.

CHAPTER

3

Neurosurgical Horizons

M. GAZI YAŞARGIL, M.D., WILLIAM F. CHANDLER, M.D.,
ANTHONY F. JABRE, M.D., and PETER ROTH

THE DEVELOPMENT OF NEUROLOGICAL DIAGNOSIS AND INDICATIONS FOR SURGERY

With the advances in surgical and medical technology came the age of specialization. Cushing said that the birth of neurosurgery began with Sir Victor Horsley being named "Surgeon for the Paralyzed and Epileptic at the National Hospital in London" in 1886. It was Cushing who was the first to do exclusively neurosurgery. Not everyone agreed with this concept of specialization. There were still general surgeons who did a variety of neurosurgical procedures until the 1950s. Now that neurosurgery is clearly defined as a specialty, should there be further subspecialization? Should there be neurosurgeons who do exclusively aneurysms, acoustic neuromas, etc? What does the future hold?

We should remember that the roots of the now-sturdy tree of neurosurgery lie in several areas: neuroanesthesia, aseptic techniques, antibiotics, neuroanatomy, neurophysiology, laboratory investigations, neuroradiography, neuropharmacology and, finally, innovations in techniques in terms of apparatuses and surgical approaches. The ability to formulate a preoperative diagnosis and apply appropriate therapy for various neurological disease states has evolved over many decades to a degree that would have been beyond the comprehension of the early pioneers in neurosurgery. Before 1910 Cushing used only a careful history, meticulous examination, and his inherent knowledge to reach a tentative diagnosis. Electrophysiological evaluations such as electromyography (EMG), electroencephalography (EEG), electrocardiography (EKG), and electronystagmography (ENG) were available only after 1935. Radiologic evaluation began with simple skull and spine x-rays. Contrast studies began with placing air in the ventricular system, then advanced to putting iodide materials into the spinal fluid, and eventually evolved to introducing contrast materials into the vascular system. Angiography progressed to selective and superselective injections and recently developed portable digital subtraction angiography. The computer age brought about computerized tomography (CT) and magnetic resonance imaging (MRI).

Developments in nuclear medicine supplied the first images of brain tumors with radionuclide scans in 1950. They also demonstrated imaging of the cerebrospinal fluid (CSF) pathways with radioiodinated serum albumin (RISA) and other agents. Cerebral blood flow was determined with radioactive xenon, and positron emission tomographic (PET) scanning provided actual metabolic information about the brain. PET, along with single photon emission computed tomography (SPECT) and possibly magnetic resonance spectroscopy (MRS), is also providing dynamic functional information regarding brain physiology.

Advances in ultrasound technology have afforded us carotid artery imaging, transcranial blood flow measurements, and the monitoring of air embolism during neurosurgical procedures. Intraoperative real-time ultrasound imaging of the brain provides localization and characterization of tumors, abscesses, and vascular malformations.

The sequential developments in various areas of medicine have equipped the neurosurgeon with a vast armamentarium of diagnostic modalities and technical capabilities (1–3, 8–10, 15–17). It remains, however, the final decision of the neurosurgeon regarding the operability of the patient. A detailed discussion regarding the stepwise thought processes involved in the decision for or against surgery is beyond the intentions of this paper. Table 3.1 gives a hypothetical line of reasoning used to assess the indications and contraindications of surgery.

Although modern diagnostic and imaging devices provide an enormous amount of morphological information, it is still inadequate compared to the anatomical detail which is available and necessary for the microneurosurgeon. Preoperative imaging still cannot predict where the seventh and eighth cranial nerves lie in relation to an acoustic neuroma, nor can it always tell if a glioma in the suprasellar region arises from the optic nerves or the hypothalamus. Even though we may know the size, shape, extension, consistency, and vascularity of a mass preoperatively, we are still uncertain as to the precise diagnosis. We still find ourselves operating on what we are certain is a glioma, only to discover that the lesion is in fact an abscess, encephalitis, or infarct. What does the peritumoral hypodensity mean? Does it imply perifocal edema or metabolic change? For example, a meningioma with observed peritumoral hypodensity at surgery will have severe adherences between the tumor capsule and the pia-arachnoidal layers. In cases with no peritumoral hypodensity there are no adherences to be observed. Conversely, acoustic tumors usually have no peritumoral edema and are thus usually not adherent to surrounding tissue. However, rare cases which show surrounding low density

TABLE 3.1

Indications and Contraindications for Surgery

1. Initial assessment of patient's overall condition
2. Physical examination (neurological signs and symptoms)
3. Preliminary "working" diagnosis
4. Diagnostic studies (radiographic studies, laboratory investigations)
    A. Specific differential diagnosis (tumor, hemorrhage, infarctions, infection)
    B. Localization
    C. Relationship of lesion to surrounding tissue (gyri, sulci, fissures, cisterns, arteries, veins, sinus, nerves, mucosal sinuses)
    D. More specific diagnosis based on above information (type of tumor, hemorrhage, infarction, abscess, encephalitis)
5. Operability
    A. Assumption of histology of the lesion (malignant or benign)
    B. Overall medical condition of the patient (age, associated diseases)
    C. Technical challenge (proximity to vessels, nerves, sinuses)
    D. Eloquent areas
    E. Approachability (deep-seated lesion)
    F. Timing of operation
6. Neurosurgical team: neurosurgeon, neuroanesthetist, operating room personnel, recovery room personnel, intensive care personnel, consulting service personnel, physical and occupational therapists

areas are often extremely adherent and can be difficult to remove. Cases 1–4 (Figs. 3.1–3.4) demonstrate these concepts. The precise anatomical relations between parent arteries and aneurysms, and the precise construction of arteriovenous malformations, (AVMs) are recognized during surgery, not from preoperative angiograms. We must continue to work with our neuroradiologic collegues to motivate each other to develop more precise and meaningful diagnostic studies.

We are still very much "in the dark" regarding the prognosis of a variety of neurosurgical problems ranging from aneurysms to lumbar disc disease. We can do a technically perfect clipping of a recently ruptured aneurysm in a grade I patient, only to have the patient die 3 weeks later due to cerebral ischemia from vasospasm. Based on our present knowledge, these events are unpredictable; therefore, it is impossible for the surgeon to reach a completely rational approach in planning the timing of aneurysm surgery. Another seemingly unpredictable factor is the response and readaptation of the brain to a specific traumatic event. Included in this response are the reactions of the cerebral vasculature, the CSF, and the neurochemical and neurophysiological changes of the brain parenchyma. In the example of a ruptured aneurysm, the cerebrovascular reaction may be vasospasm; the CSF system may exhibit hydrocephalus; and the parenchymal reaction may result in irreparable loss of neurologic function. The question of how we affect the prognosis through

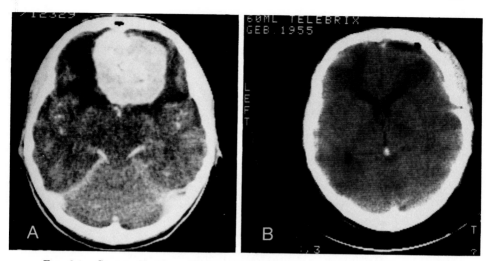

FIG. 3.1. Case 1. K. M., a 29-year-old female with a diagnosis of psycho-organic syndrome, suffered a grand mal seizure in 1984. A CT scan (A) showed a tuberculum sella lesion consistent with meningioma with bilateral hypodensity surrounding the lesion. Surgery was performed via a right pterional approach with complete removal. The tumor capsule was densely adherent to the surrounding arachnoid layer. The postoperative course was uneventful. Histology confirmed a meningotheliomatous meningioma. Follow-up CT scan 2 weeks after surgery (B) shows residual bilateral low density areas.

understanding and controlling these various responses remains unanswered.

We agree with the work of Mazziota and Phelps (14), who pointed out in 1986:

> The investigation of cerebral function has been one of the most difficult and challenging endeavors of the last century. However, even with the aid of neurophysiology, neuropsychology, and neuroradiology to furnish vastly improved understanding of cerebral function, there is still remarkably little knowledge about the local neurochemistry and neurophysiology of the human cerebral substructure. The available information has been gained from the extrapolation of animal studies to humans, a strategy that is limited in the study of human disease states. PET has provided previously unavailable insight into these local functional relationships.

The future clinical relevancy of these studies remains to be demonstrated and subsequently utilized.

Over the past 20 years there have been significant advances in the

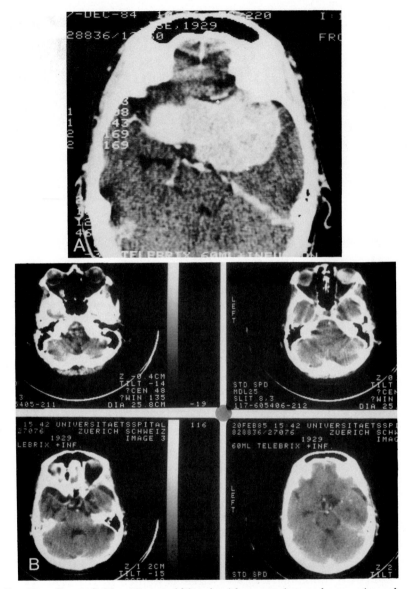

FIG. 3.2.   Case 2. G. M., a 55-year-old female with progressive psycho-organic syndrome.
A CT scan (A) showed a large meningioma of the tuberculum sella. No area of surrounding
hypodensity is visible. The tumor was removed through a right pterional approach with no
evidence of adherence between tumor and arachnoid layer. The histological diagnosis was
consistent with meningotheliomatous meningioma. Follow-up CT scan 2 months after
surgery is shown (B). Her postoperative course was uneventful.

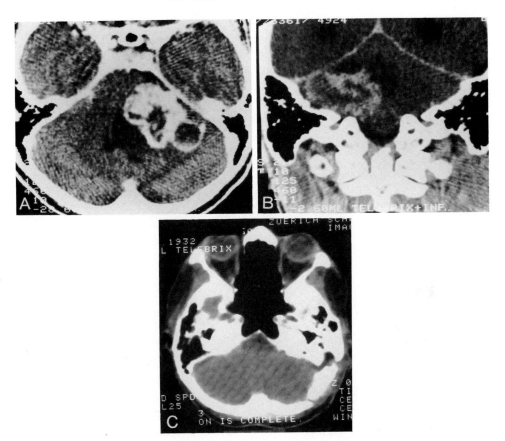

FIG. 3.3. Case 3. B. H., a 50-year-old female with hypacusis and hypesthesia in right-trigeminal distribution. A CT scan (A and B) showed a large cystic acoustic neurinoma with an area of hypodensity superomedially. Exploration confirmed enormous adhesions between tumor capsule and arachnoidal layer. Such peritumoral hypodensity is extremely rare in cases of acoustic neurinomas. The postoperative CT scan 2 weeks following surgery is shown (C). Her postoperative course was uneventful.

technical aspects of our neurosurgical procedures. We have established standards for classical neurosurgery and have more recently defined the microsurgical technique which will be further elaborated below. We have greatly improved the control of hemostasis with bipolar coagulation, surgical clips, and chemical hemostasis. Controlled suction has added a measure of safety, and ultrasonic suction (CUSA) has aided in precise resection. The laser is another technical advancement that is becoming well established in neurosurgery. Some of the newest technical advances include CT- or MR-guided stereotaxic biopsy, and implantation and stereotaxic radiosurgery as developed in Stockholm. Advances are being made with the flexible endoscope and with endovascular techniques. The current use of computer-guided laser surgery is perhaps a bit of the future already present. Table 3.2 reviews some of these technical advances.

The training of future neurosurgeons should include not only a study of classical neurosurgical methods, it should also include complete understanding of applied microtechniques. Students of neurosurgery should

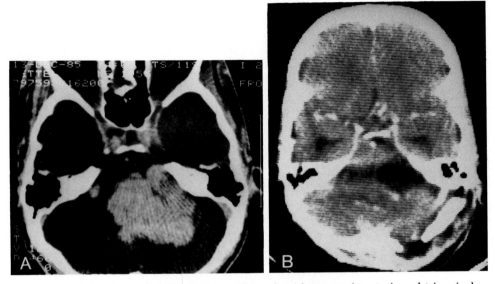

FIG. 3.4.   Case 4. W. H., a 31-year-old female with progressive ataxia and trigeminal dysesthesia associated with anacusis on the right side. CT scan (A) showed a large tumor but with no peritumoral low density changes. This is more commonly seen with acoustic neurinomas, as in this case. The follow-up CT scan (B) 10 days after surgery is shown. Her postoperative course was uneventful.

TABLE 3.2
Technical Advances

A. *Surgical Therapy*
   Classical neurosurgery
   Classical neurosurgery + microtechnique
   Surgical adjuncts: bipolar coagulation, clip, laser, chemical hemostasis, intermittent suction (CSF, blood), rotosuction, ultrasonic suction
B. *New, Revised, and Augmented Methods*
   Endoscopic (flexible)
   Endovascular (flexible)
   Stereotactic brachytherapy
   Stereotactic γ-radiation
   Stereotactic controlled laser surgery

have a thorough knowledge of and respect for the cisternal, sulcal, and fissural anatomy of the brain. The brain is a unique organ in that it is not round and encapsulated like other organs, but is comprised of extensive infoldings which can be used to the surgeon's and patient's advantage. Currently *every* region of the brain is surgically accessible with an acceptable risk to the patient. The surgical microscope remains the *key* to allowing this accessibility. Case reports 5 and 6 (Figs. 3.5 and 3.6) are presented to illustrate this point.

PROBLEMS WITH MICROSURGERY—THE MICROSCOPE

The surgical microscope was first introduced into the neurosurgical operating suite by Kurze (12) in 1957. However, the full merit of the microscope and its subsequent widespread application in neurological surgery had to await the development of microvascular procedures in the 1960s (4–7, 11, 13, 18). In addition, the combination of microtechnique and other new modalities (such as precise hemostasis with bipolar coagulation) vastly improved the safety of approaches to the brain, brainstem, and spinal cord.

The surgical microscope should be more appropriately called the surgical telescope, as in fact (despite what is generally believed) it provides a final magnification of only 2–10×. Actually most neurosurgeons use only 2–4× magnification for the majority of procedures. Therefore, the microscope's most useful function is not the enlargement of objects in the operative field but rather the stereoscopic, sharply focused vision it allows through a small gap. This is made possible by this optical device's ability to reduce the interpupillary distance of the surgeon's eyes (generally around 60 mm) to 16 mm, which is the distance between the two objective lenses. This permits the surgeon to work in a field four times smaller, as the light reflected from an image can enter the surgical microscope through an opening of only 16 mm and be perceived stereoscopically. This ability provided by the microscope combined with microtechnique provides greater accuracy and makes it possible for the surgeon to reach and treat deep lesions of the brain through small openings with minimal retraction.

The lack of free and effortless mobility inherent in the original surgical microscope imposed awkward and uncomfortable positions for the neurosurgeon during long and delicate procedures. Over the past 15 years, many attempts have been made to overcome this mechanical problem. Eventually the weight-counterbalanced microscope, coupled with an electromagnetic brake system at various joints, seemed to provide absolute stability with good (but still not optimal) mobility. The addition of a mouth switch allowed effortless movement of the microscope (as well as focusing capability) and left the surgeon's hands free for surgical manipulations.

The initially designed electromagnetic brake system was a passive system. This meant that in case the electric current was interrupted, with the microscope poorly balanced it could fall downward under its own weight, thereby endangering the patient beneath. In commercial development this was ultimately changed to an active brake system, which under similar circumstances would move the microscope upward, away from the operative field. Unfortunately, this seemingly useful modification resulted in a much heavier and more cumbersome microscope stand. Further improvements, such as the addition of computerized

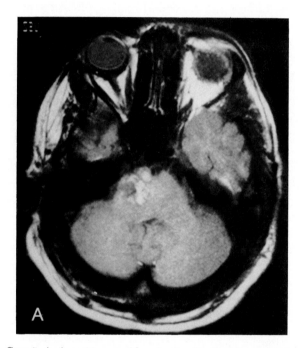

FIG. 3.5. Case 5. A. A., a 33-year-old male who developed a staggering gait and right-sided weakness 3 months prior to admission. In addition he was found to have nystagmus and ataxia. MRI (A) showed a left sided pontomesencephalic lesion. A vertebral angiogram (B) showed displacement of perforators of the P-1 segment but no pathological vascularization. MRI scan (C–E) shows multiple septated arms of high signal intensity in the T-2-weighted images suspicious for a cavernoma. Surgery was performed via a lateral supracerebellar approach with complete resection. Histology confirmed cavernoma. Postoperative MRI (F and G) shows postoperative tumor bed (T-2 image). His postoperative course was uneventful and he returned to full working capacity.

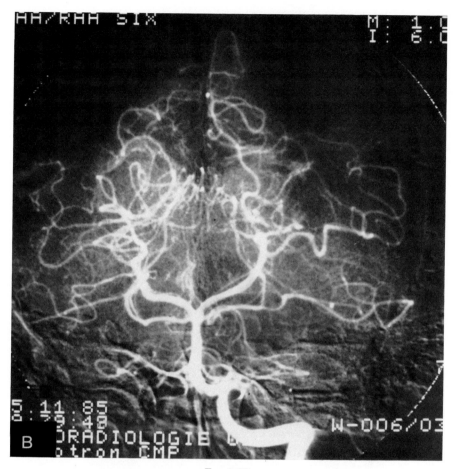

FIG. 3.5*B*

robotics to constantly keep the microscope balanced, may solve some of these difficulties.

FUTURE DEVELOPMENTS IN NEUROSURGERY?

Improving the working condition of the "telescopic" neurosurgeon is of primary importance. Looking through the narrow openings of the microscope's eyepieces and maintaining a relatively fixed posture of the head, neck, and body can be very tiring during a long and complex procedure and may affect the surgeon's technical performance. A high resolution stereoscopic color television monitor placed outside the operative field might provide more freedom and better mobility for the

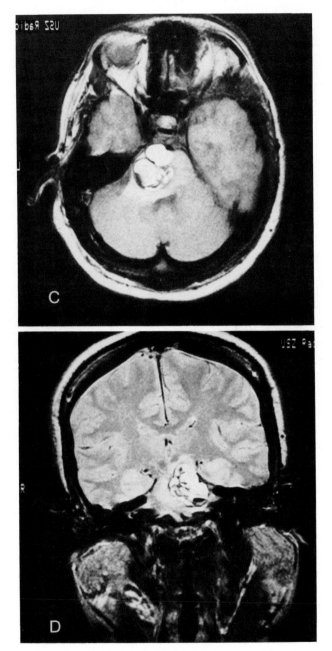

FIG. 3.5C and D

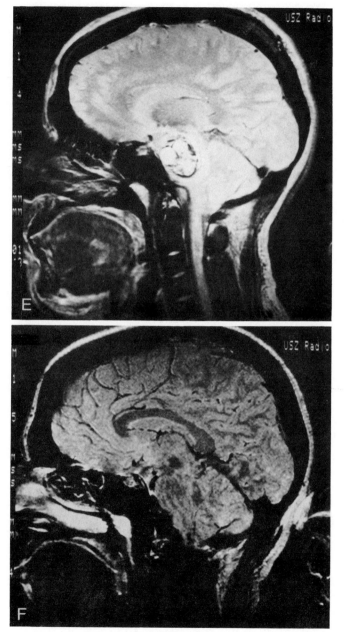

FIG. 3.5*E* and *F*

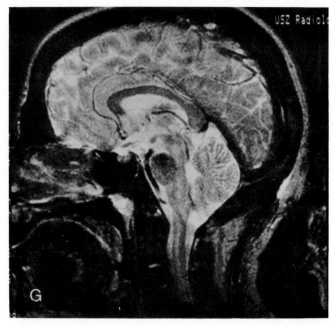

FIG. 3.5G

surgeon. Through this indirect surgical viewing (as is commonly done at endoscopy), it might even be possible to replace the operating microscope with a better optical system containing stereoscopic cameras. Becoming familiar with the techniques of indirect operating would seem to be merely a matter of practice and adjustment.

The minimal gap necessary to perform direct surgical manipulation is presently related to the distance required by the operating microscope for stereoscopic vision (about 16 mm) and to the surgeon's ability to maneuver microinstrumentation (such as a sucker and bipolar forceps). Further narrowing of the gap is necessary to improve the safety of our intrusions into the brain. This may be possible with the development of stereoscopic flexible endoscopy. This would permit both transcisternal and endovascular procedures with negligible brain manipulation. In addition, the combination of extra- and intravascular endoscopic approaches for difficult vascular lesions (such as basilar artery aneurysms) would provide a degree of precision not currently possible.

The planning of a surgical approach is perhaps the most challenging part of an operation. The data derived from ancillary studies such as angiography, CT, MRI, etc., is compiled and computed in the surgeon's imagination to create a 3-dimensional (3-D) image of the lesion as well as its adjacent structures. These normal structures may or may not be distorted or displaced. This subjective task may in many cases prove to be quite difficult, especially with deep lesions such as complex subcortical angiomas and tumors.

With modern technology it would seem possible to transfer the surgeon's 3-D concept of the pathology into a computerized 3-D replica of the lesion itself. The 2-dimensional information provided by anatomical studies (angiography, CT scanning, ultrasonography, MRI, etc.) could be conveyed to a computer capable of converting it into a 3-D format. This would depict the lesion in 3-D, surrounded by normal structures such as ventricles, deep nuclei, cranial nerves, vessels, etc. The computer could also be programmed to reconstruct the image in any orientation, thereby permitting approaches from any desired angle. The use of color graphics could further enhance structural details. In addition, during surgery this stereoscopic image could be projected into the operative field, providing the surgeon a continuous spatial configuration of the lesion within the brain (Fig. 3.7).

Furthermore, in situations that required the use of laser or CUSA, the position of the laser beam or CUSA tip could be computer monitored in relation to the precise 3-D boundaries of the lesion. Such controlled maneuverability would permit easier, safer, and more efficient operative approaches for many types of lesions.

The perfection of microtechnique requires endless hours of practice in the laboratory in conjunction with progressively complex clinical exposure. It is conceivable that a 3-D imaging system could also be used for instructional purposes. The computer could simulate a lesion such as an angioma or tumor with its anatomical surroundings on a stereoscopic monitor. The young neurosurgeon, using an electronic system, could attempt to dissect the mass under variable circumstances which could be preadjusted. The experience of the surgeon would dictate the speed of dissection, complexity of the lesion, etc., and expected difficulties encountered (such as bleeding from an arteriovenous malformation (AVM) could be simulated. Exposure of this kind would greatly improve the "telescopic" ability of young neurosurgeons before clinical exposure.

Despite our considerable advances in operative approaches to the brain, the imagination of the neurosurgeon must never cease to reach for even better means of providing more precise visualization of the lesion both before as well as during operation. The tools of the neurosurgeon must be constantly improved and advanced. Only by continual reassessment and development beyond our present boundaries can we hope to make our intrusions into the brain not just possible but safe for all our patients. The transition to new ideas is achieved by integrating the past and present knowledge with our imagination to form a bridge to new developments of the future.

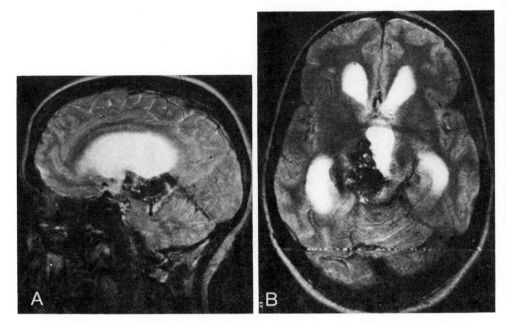

Fig. 3.6.   Case 6. C. M., a 20-year-old female student who suffered her first hemorrhage
at the age of 9. At 14 years of age her second hemorrhage resulted in right-sided severe
sensomotoric hemiparesis. An angiogram showed a deep localized mesencephalic arteriovenous malformation. The lesion was declared inoperable. The patient was treated with
proton beam irradiation in 1980 but suffered three subsequent hemorrhages. MRI scan in
July 1986 shows position of the AVM (*A* and *B*) and hydrocephalus (T-2). Vertebral
angiogram (*C* and *D*) shows the lesion with dilated vein of Galen and reflux venous drainage
through the parietooccipital veins and via the basilar vein to the cavernous sinus. The
postoperative vertebral angiogram (*E* and *F*) shows complete resection of the lesion, which
was performed within the transverse fissure with preservation of normal vasculature. The
postoperative CT scan is also shown (*G*).

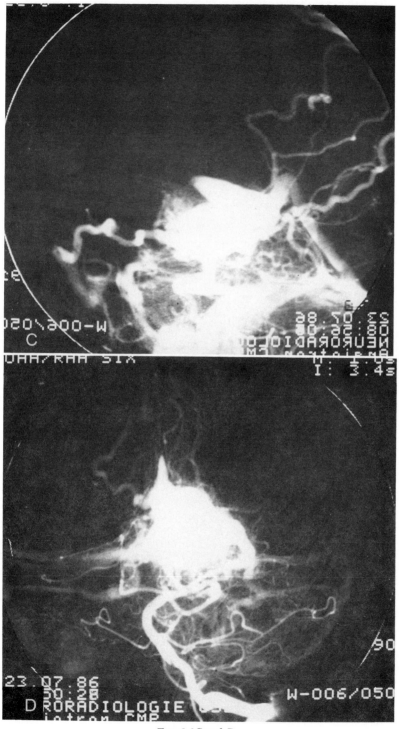

FIG. 3.6C and D

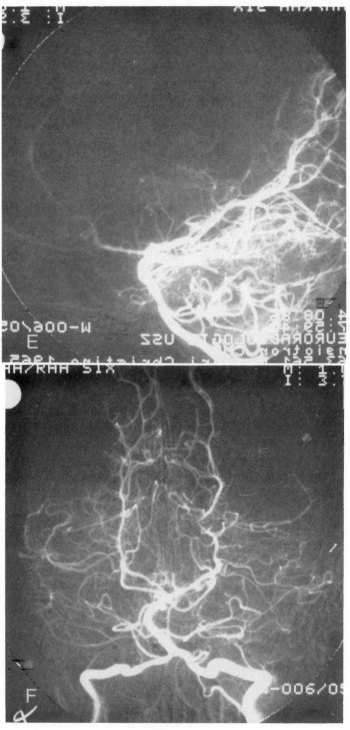

Fig. 3.6*E* and *F*

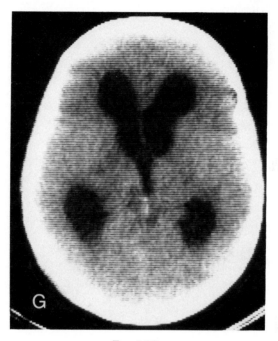

FIG. 3.6G

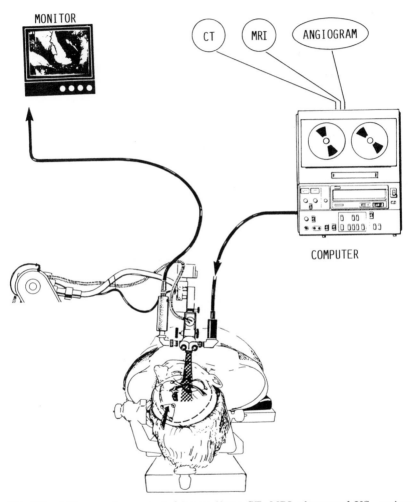

MONITOR

CT   MRI   ANGIOGRAM

COMPUTER

FIG. 3.7.   3-D computer-generated image (from *CT*, *MRI*, ultrasound US, angiogram (A/G) projected into operative field and viewed on monitor).

REFERENCES

1. Apuzzo, M. L. J., and Sabshin, J. K. Computed tomographic guidance stereotaxis in the management of intracranial mass lesions. Neurosurgery., *12:* 277–285, 1983.
2. Ascher, P. W., and Heppner, F. CO_2 laser in neurosurgery. Neurosurg. Rev., *7:* 123–133, 1984.
3. Bergström, M., Böethius, J., Collins, V. P., et al. A combined study of computed tomography and stereotactic biopsy in gliomas. *Excerpta Med Int Congr Ser*, No. 433: 45–50, 1978.
4. Buncke, H. R., Jr., and Schulz, W. P. Experimental digital amputation and reimplantation. Plast. Reconstr. Surg., *36:* 62, 1965.
5. Donaghy, R. M. P. Patch and by-pass in microangeional surgery, edited by R. M. P. Donaghy and M. G. Yasargil, pp 75–86. In: *Micro-Vascular Surgery*, Stuttgart, Thieme, 1967.
6. Jacobson, J. H., and Donaghy, R. M. P. Microsurgery as an aid to middle cerebral endarterectomy. J. Neurosurg., *19:* 108, 1962.
7. Jacobson, J. H., and Suarez, E. I. Microsurgery in the anastomosis of small vessels. Surg. Forum, *11:* 243, 1960.
8. Kelly, P. J., Alker. G. J., Jr., and Goerss, S. Computed-assisted stereotactic laser resection of intra-axial brain-neoplasms. J. Neurosurg., *64:* 427–439, 1986.
9. Kelly, P. J., Alker, G. J., Jr., Kall, B. A., et al. Method of computed tomography-based stereotactic biopsy with arteriographic control. Neurosurgery, *14:* 172–177, 1984.
10. Kelly, P. J., Olsen, M. H., and Wright, A. E. Stereotactic implantation of iridium[192] into CNS neoplasms. Surg. Neurol., *10:* 349–354, 1978.
11. Khodadad, G., and Lougheed, W. M. Repair and replacement of small arteries, microsuture technique. J. Neurosurg., *25:* 61, 1966.
12. Kurze, T. Microtechniques in neurological surgery. Clin. Neurosurg., *2:* 129–137, 1964.
13. Lougheed, W. M., Gunton, R. W., and Barnett, J. J. Embolectomy of internal carotid, middle and anterior cerebral arteries. J. Neurosurg., *22:* 607, 1985.
14. Mazziotta, J. C., and Phelps, M. E. Positron emission tomography studies of the brain. In: *Positron Emission Tomography and Autoradiography: Principles and Applications for the Brain and Heart*, edited by M. Phelps, J. Mazziotta, and H. Schelbert, pp. 493–579. Raven Press, New York, 1986.
15. Saunders, M. L., Young, H. F., Becker, D. P., et al. The use of the laser in neurological surgery. Surg. Neurol., *14:* 1–10, 1980.
16. Takizawa, T., Yamazaki, T., Miura, N., et al. Laser surgery of basal, orbital, and ventricular meningiomas which are difficult to extirpate by conventional methods. Neurol. Med. Chir. (Tokyo), *20:* 719–737, 1980.
17. Tew, J. M., Tobler, W. D. Present status of lasers in neurosurgery. Adv Tech Stand Neurosurg. *13:* 1–36, 1985.
18. Yaşargil, M. G. Experimental small vessel surgery in the dog. In: *Micro-Vascular Surgery*, edited by R. M. P. Donaghy and M. G. Yaşargil, pp. 87–126. Stuttgart, Thieme, 1967.

CHAPTER

4

Surgical Approaches to "Inaccessible" Brain Tumors

M. GAZI YAŞARGIL, M.D., G. F. CRAVENS, M.D., and PETER ROTH

INTRODUCTION

What is an "inaccessible tumor"? The first reaction is that by inaccessible tumors one simply means deeply located tumors within the brainstem. Examples would include tumors within the medulla, pons, midbrain, and diencephalon. However, if by inaccessible tumor one means a tumor which is surgically difficult to approach without damaging vital or eloquent areas of the brain, then one must include regions in the telencephalon as well as brainstem areas. Following Brodman's classification scheme this would include such regions as areas 1–7, areas 40–45, areas 17–19, areas 27–28, and so forth. Soon it becomes apparent that there are no areas of the brain which can be reached safely by surgery without involving some eloquent function of the brain. Following this line of reasoning one is left with the undeniable conclusion that no area in the central nervous system is accessible, an untenable position for the neurosurgeon. Therefore, from a topographical viewpoint the problem is not accessibility but rather approachability with acceptable outcome. Thus to put the title in more precise terms, "Surgical approaches to inaccessible brain tumors with acceptable results" becomes the main theme.

Surgical resection of diagnosed lesions has been performed for over 100 years. Standardization of neurosurgical operating techniques reached a high point in the 20th century with Harvey Cushing and Walter Dandy. Enucleation en block with and/or without lobectomies and piecemeal dissection became the golden standard of neurosurgical technique. These early neurosurgery giants showed the possibilities and limitations of operating on a heretofore inoperable organ. Using the radiographic studies and known neurophysiology and technology of their time, they created operative approaches for essentially all lesions in virtually every location in the brain. When one considers the limitations of medicine at that time, then such operations as Dandy's approach for 3rd ventricular tumors (16), Krause's infratentorial supracerebellar exploration for lesions in the quadrigeminal region (47), and Cushing's transsphenoidal

42

hypophysectomy (14) all seem like heroic advances in neurosurgery. With the vast improvement in neuroanesthesia and operative technology (including both stereotactic and microsurgical fields) coupled with the unprecedented advances in neuroradiology and pharmacology, the neurosurgeon of today is able to further refine the surgical approaches and improve upon the results of our neurosurgical forefathers.

Previously, the diagnosis of brain lesions was possible only with analysis of careful neurological examinations and the aid of air studies and angiography. Computed tomographic (CT) scans and magnetic resonance imaging (MRI), in the past 10 and 5 years, respectively, have revolutionized our ability to diagnose lesions with respect to their specific locations. These studies also give information regarding a lesion's relative tissue characteristics (i.e., infiltrating or well-defined margins or cystic *vs.* solid). Thus from CT scans and MRI we ascertain information such as tumor size, location, and biological behavior which influences the decisions for different methods of treatment.

MRI studies have become essential in the differential diagnosis of some lesions (90). For example, the distinction between a hematoma and a cavernous angioma which has hemorrhaged can often be made prior to surgery. CT scans and MRI have, in many cases, shown tumors to be well demarcated. Therefore with this added information from more sophisticated radiographic studies, surgery has become a viable option. Our attitudes regarding resectability have been changed by these new advancements. Now the burden of answering this challenge is again with the surgeon. If a lesion is localized and well circumscribed but located within a deep-seated position, we as surgeons must have or must develop the surgical skills or techniques to deal with this challenge. The development of new diagnostic modalities and the integration of those modalities with the development of methods of treatment simultaneously advance and perpetuate each other.

Using microsurgical techniques for the past 20 years on more than 5000 cases (which include aneurysms, arteriovenous malformations, and tumors), a method for treatment of a diversity of pathology has been refined (86–88). From the experience with microtechniques has come the knowledge that the construction of the brain allows one to reach deep and hidden areas with acceptable success. Previously many of these locations had been considered "inaccessible." The knowledge and respect of basal cisterns has been rewarding in the surgical treatment of aneurysms, arteriovenous malformations, and tumors at the base of the brain. The cisternal (subarachnoid system) anatomy is not only at the base of the brain but also is in every location around and within the brain. The brain is not an isolated compact structure like an island unto itself; rather it is like a continent with a multifaceted coastline and many water inlets: it floats in a sea of CSF, with rivers of cerebrospinal fluid which allow access to its interior.

In order to master the techniques of microsurgery it is necessary to become familiar with the microanatomy of the cisternal, fissural, sulcal, and neurovascular systems. These systems provide natural pathways for dissection which preserve important adjacent structures. For example, in the management of saccular aneurysms, which in 99% of cases are located within the basal subarachnoid cisterns, the precise anatomic knowledge of cisternal systems in relation to arteries and cranial nerves becomes quintessential.

Microanatomic knowledge is also fundamental for the removal of some tumors at the base of the cranium, brain, and some basal arteriovenous malformations (AVMs). The majority of these AVMs and tumors, however, are localized within the hemispheres and brainstem. For this reason knowledge of the sulcal and fissural microanatomy and the arterial and venous structural arrangements becomes indispensable for proper treatment.

The unique construction of the brain has been recognized and reproduced in literature and art since the early dawn of man's intellectual awakening. Its gross anatomical features have been described by anatomists for centuries and subsequently studied by all students of the nervous system. Although every neurosurgeon is well informed about gyral, sulcal, and fissural anatomy, the classical neurosurgical concepts partition the brain into supratentorial and infratentorial components each composed of hemispheres, lobes, and a connecting brainstem. The gyri and sulci have been excluded from a surgical perspective, as surgeons have not been able to perform manipulations without microtechniques in such small crevices.

The attitude, relative to gyral and sulcal anatomy, has been one of neglect due to the seemingly endless variations. Differences also exist between the two hemispheres. However, neurosurgeons are presently confronted with a similar situation that occurred almost 50 years ago with the advent of cerebral angiography. The recognition of all the arteries and veins and their numerous variations seemed overwhelming at that time. Further study and analysis, however, showed that there were basic rules to the arterial and venous system (20, 34–37, 56, 80, 83). This axiom holds true for gyral and sulcal anatomy. Up until the present time, neurophysiology and gross anatomical studies have shown the diversity and asymmetry of the brain, but the fissural, sulcal, and gyral morphology has not been precisely studied.

Microsurgical experiences necessitated the development of a concept of basal cisterns for aneurysms and also a new neuroanatomical concept to deal with and describe AVMs and tumors. Lesions of the cerebrum and cerebellum have been divided into two groups: convexial and central. This separation may initially seem arbitrary, however, after careful observation and scrutiny, the convexial part of the hemispheres is related more to the anatomy of the gyral and sulcal systems with their unique arrangement of arteries and veins within the sulci. The central areas are more closely aligned with the fissural system, especially the transverse fissure, and its different arterial and venous architecture.

Knowledge of this new concept of neuroanatomy is but one element of microsurgery. Another component is the mastery of the "keyhole" technique. The general belief has always been that microneurosurgery would allow the magnification of structures such that the surgical manipulations would be more precise. The experienced microsurgeon would confirm that magnification is important, but more important is the capability of sharp stereoscopic focus in a deep narrow opening with adequate illumination. The ability to work with depth perception with ideal lighting is indispensable. Due to its optical construction, the microscope creates a telescopic effect which allows the surgeon to work at a depth of 10–12 cm through a small opening 5 mm wide and 16 mm long. In this way, the keyhole technique can be accomplished through sulci and fissures using the microscope.

MICROSURGICAL ANATOMY

Primarily the microanatomy of the cisternal system will be reviewed, followed by the fissural anatomy and, finally, a brief description of sulcal anatomy. Obviously, when applying the above microanatomy in surgical procedures, a combination of any or all of the anatomy for a given region is used. The anatomical descriptions are meant to aid in the understanding of microanatomy and its application to microneurosurgery and are not exclusive of one another.

Cisternal Anatomy

In order to follow standard neurosurgical approaches for various tumors, the subarachnoid cisterns may be divided into two groups. These include supratentorial and infratentorial cisterns. Both groups may be further divided into four subgroups; anterior, lateral, posterior, and superior. Each of these subgroups contain the various individual arachnoid cisterns (see *Microneurosurgery* vol. I, (86)).

The *anterior* or *parasellar group* includes the carotid cistern, chiasmatic cistern, lamina terminalis cistern, olfactory cistern, and Sylvian cistern. The inferior part of the carotid cistern and the superior and lateral parts of the interpeduncular cistern form the lateral part of Liliequist's membrane, the medial part being formed by the common wall of the chiasmatic and interpeduncular cisterns. The carotid cistern contains the carotid artery. The chiasmatic cistern encloses the subarachnoid space around the optic nerves and chiasm, and anteroinferiorly it extends to the infundibulum and pituitary stalk. With an incomplete diaphragma sella, the chiasmatic cistern may extend into the sella. The lamina terminalis cistern is defined by the anterior cerebral arteries. It contains both the anterior cerebral arteries, medial lenticulostriate branches, and the anterior communicating artery complex. The olfactory cistern is formed by the arachnoid over the olfactory tract between the orbital gyrus laterally and the gyrus rectus medially. The cistern may extend in a "slit-like" fashion between the gyri.

The *Sylvian cistern* is unique in that it is a transitional cistern between the basal cisterns and the subarachnoid space along the Sylvian or lateral fissure. The medial and inferior part of the Sylvian cistern contains the proximal portion of the middle cerebral artery. Lateral and more superficial, the frontal and temporal lobes are closely approximated, thus obscuring much of the cistern from direct view. At the level of the middle cerebral artery bifurcation, the cistern is relatively large, corresponding with the underlying limen insulae. In addition to the middle cerebral artery it contains the superficial and deep Sylvian veins.

The *lateral* or *parapeduncular group* includes the crural and anterior ambient cisterns. The crural cistern is located between the parahippocampal gyrus and the cerebral peduncle. It contains the anterior choroidal artery and the medial posterior choroidal arteries and the basal vein of Rosenthal. The ambient cistern covers the lateral aspect of the mesencephalon. It is included in both the supratentorial and infratentorial groups. The cerebral peduncle is medially located; the mesial temporal lobe supratentorially and the lobulus quadrangularis infratentorially are laterally located. The ambient cistern contains segments of the posterior cerebral artery, numerous mesencephalic branches, and the more posterior part of the basal vein of Rosenthal. Parallel to this cistern the superior cerebellar artery and trochlear nerve have their own arachnoid sleeves.

The *posterior* or *tentorial notch cisterns* include the quadrigeminal cistern and the velum interpositum cistern. The quadrigeminal cistern is bordered anteriorly by the dorsal mesencephalon, the quadrigeminal plate, and the pineal gland. The cistern is contiguous with the velum interpositum cistern superiorly and the ambient cistern laterally. The velum interpositum cistern is a small but important cistern which extends from the habenular commissure to the foramen of Monro, anteriorly. It is located beneath the splenium of the corpus callosum posteriorly and beneath the fornical commissure anteriorly. The pulvinar portion of the thalamic area is located laterally to the cistern. The cistern contains the medial posterior choroidal artery, splenothalamic branches of the peri-callosal arteries, and the internal cerebral veins.

The *superior* or *callosal group* is divided again into an anterior and posterior portion. The anterior corpus callosum cistern extends anteriorly to the crista galli. It is bound by the falx cerebri and the pia of the cingulate gyrus. The posterior corpus callosum cistern, which is contig-uous with the anterior portion, extends posteriorly and inferiorly to the quadrigeminal and velum interpositum cisterns at the splenium of the corpus callosum. These two cisterns contain the pericallosal vessels.

The *hemispheric cistern* covers the entire hemisphere. The arachnoid extends across the crest of a gyrus and then splits into two layers in passing across a sulcus. One layer extends across the top of a sulcus, and the other arachnoidal layer follows the pia down the walls and floor of the sulcus (Fig. 4.1).

The *infratentorial cisterns* are grouped into anterior, lateral, posterior, and superior groups. The *anterior group* includes the interpeduncular cistern, the prepontine cistern, and the premedullary cistern. The inter-peduncular cistern is formed between the two cerebral peduncles as they emerge between the two optic tracts. The superior boundary is formed from the mesencephalon and the inferior portion of the lower dienceph-alon. Laterally the cistern joins the ambient, crural, and carotid cisterns. The anterior-inferior portion of the boundary is formed by the clivus. The anterior-posterior extension of the superior wall of the cistern is fused with the chiasmatic cistern medially and the carotid cistern lat-erally to form Liliequist's membrane, as previously mentioned. The inferior portion of the interpeduncular cistern extends to approximately the upper third of the basilar artery. The cistern contains the basilar artery and origins of the posterior cerebral artery and superior cerebellar artery, as well as the origin of the oculomotor nerve and basal veins of

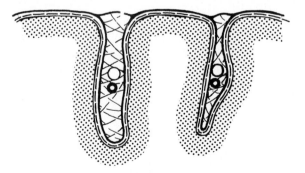

FIG. 4.1   Splitting of arachnoid into two layers with one layer extending deep into the sulcus.

Rosenthal. The prepontine cistern is located between the anterior surface of the pons and the clivus surrounding the lower two-thirds of the basilar artery. The cistern contains the basilar artery, the origin of the anterior inferior cerebellar artery, and the abducent nerve. The premedullary or anterior medullary cistern extends superiorly from the pontomedullary sulcus over the anterior aspect of the medulla inferiorly to the upper cranial spinal cord. It contains the anterior spinal artery and the anterior medullary vein.

The *lateral group* includes the posterior inferior aspect of the ambient cistern, the superior cerebellopontine cistern, and the inferior cerebello-pontine cistern. The ambient cistern was described previously. The superior cerebellopontine cistern attaches to the pons at the ponto-medullary junction. This cistern shares a common arachnoidal wall with the ambient cistern above. Laterally the cistern extends to the origin of the internal auditory canal. Posteriorly it is bounded by the posterior quadrangular and superior semilunar lobules of the cerebellar hemisphere anteriorly. This cistern contains the anterior inferior cerebellar artery, the internal auditory artery, and cranial nerves V, VII, and VIII, as well as the lateral pontomesencephalic vein. Lateral and superior to the cistern is Dandy's vein or superior petrosal vein. The inferior cerebello-pontine cistern or lateral cerebellomedullary cistern lies anterior and lateral to the medulla. It shares an arachnoid wall with the superior cerebellopontine cistern above and extends from the pontomedullary sulcus superiorly to the foramen magnum inferiorly. (It is lateral to the premedullary cistern.) It contains the vertebral artery, posterior inferior cerebellar artery origin, the retro-olivary and lateral medullary veins, and cranial nerves IX, X, XI, and XII.

The *posterior group* includes the cisterna magna and the posterior portion of the superior cerebellar cistern. The cisterna magna is formed as the dorsal spinal subarachnoid space opens into the intracranial cavity dorsal to the medulla. It extends up to the posterior medullary velum. Beneath the vermis and the cerebellar tonsils it communicates with the fourth ventricle via the foramen of Magendie. It contains the vermian branches of the posterior inferior cerebellar artery and the vermian veins. The dorsal arachnoid wall of this cistern can often be vascularized. The superior cerebellar cistern covers the superior vermis and extends be-tween the two hemispheres. Anteriorly it approaches the tentorium to converge with the quadrigeminal and ambient cisterns. It contains distal branches of the superior cerebellar artery and vermian veins.

The *superior group* includes the vermian and hemispheric cisterns. These are located in the midline and above the cerebellar hemispheres. These contain the medial and lateral terminal vessels of the superior cerebellar artery and precentral cerebellar veins as well as draining veins from the tentorial dura and straight sinus.

There are three additional points to be covered related to cisternal anatomy prior to reviewing fissural anatomy and approaches. First, there can be numerous connective tissue strands (or arachnoid fibers) within cisterns which support various arteries, nerves, and veins within the cisterns. Thus, tumors which enlarge into the cisternal space will be invaginated by an arachnoid covering. In addition adjacent vessels and cranial nerves should also have individual arachnoidal sleeves. This fact is important when attempting to dissect lesions within the cisternal areas. Usually an "arachnoid dissection plane" is present, although at times there may be extensive scarring of the arachnoid. Secondly, there are three cisternal junction regions where the walls of the cisterns converge to re-enforce the supporting arachnoid fibers. These include the pineal region, the parasellar region, and the lateral cerebellopontine area at the foramen of Luschka. Finally, in certain areas there is a close approximation of the subarachnoid space and the ventricular system allowing surgical access. These areas include the lamina terminalis, the choroidal fissure, the velum interpositum, and the medial and lateral outlets of the fourth ventricle.

Fissural Anatomy

As noted in the previous section related to cisternal anatomy, the subarachnoid cisterns are located not only at the base of the brain and brainstem but also are found in dorsal, medial, lateral, and superior locations in both the supratentorial and infratentorial compartments. Knowledge of the anatomy of the major fissures allows one to gain access to various subarachnoid compartments and subsequently to various intraventricular regions adjacent to the subarachnoid space. It becomes obvious that one can use this surrounding sea of cerebrospinal fluid to approach various deep anatomical structures within the brain and brainstem.

There are numerous major fissures which can be utilized in microsurgical approaches. In this discussion only the anatomy of the more commonly used major fissures will be discussed. For a better understanding of the anatomical relations of the various fissures, a review of the embryological development of the brain is necessary. As the telencephalon develops at variable rates the process causes the formation of the various fissures. (For a more complete discussion refer to *Microneurosurgery*, vol. IIIA, Chap. 7 (88).

As with the cisternal anatomy, the major fissures can be divided into supratentorial and infratentorial groups. The supratentorial group includes the Sylvian fissure, the interhemispheric fissure (both anterior and posterior), and the transverse fissure. The infratentorial fissures include the cerebellopontine fissure, the mesencephalocerebellar fissure, the pontobulbar or pontomedullary fissure, and the vallecula (at the foramen Magendie) beneath the paired tonsils and nodule and uvula of the vermis.

The *Sylvian or lateral fissure* is a deep transverse furrow from which the middle cerebral vessels arise. It may be 4–6 cm in depth posteriorly and runs anteroposteriorly with an upward inclination to enter the inferior parietal lobule in a T-shaped fashion. The horizontal, anterior and ascending rami of the lateral fissure are well developed and deep. By opening the arachnoid over the Sylvian cistern, at the level of the frontal opercular gyrus, the middle cerebral vessels become apparent. Further opening of the arachnoid and lips of the fissure will allow visualization of the insula within the floor of the fissure. The insular cortex is surrounded by the circular sulcus, except anteroinferiorly, where the insular cortex continues uninterrupted via the limen insulae onto the inferior frontal gyrus. At the base of the brain the vascular anatomy of the Sylvian fissure provides a guideline for proper dissection of the more anterior and inferior aspect of the fissure. Often the orbital frontal gyrus indents the corresponding temporal lobe distorting the more anterior portion of the fissure. By following the proximal middle cerebral artery this portion of the fissure can be opened. This allows the frontal and temporal lobes to fall away from the sphenoid wing and orbital roof to gain better access to basal structures. Through the opened Sylvian fissure the opercular, insular, insulostriate, and insulostriocapsular areas can be explored.

The *interhemispheric fissure,* as its name implies, separates the two hemispheres of the cerebrum. Anteriorly it extends from the base of the frontal fossa at the lamina cribrosa between the gyrus rectus along the corpus callosum and the junction of the falx cerebri and tentorium cerebelli posteriorly. Because of its overall length, this fissure allows access to midline structures along the anterior-posterior axis of the brain. It contains the two leaves of dura of the falx, the associated arachnoid, and pericallosal vessels. It permits exposure of the corpus callosum, including the genu, body, and splenium. Draining veins from the cerebral cortex to the superior sagittal sinus often restrict wide exposures. Beneath the falx the two borders of adjacent cingulate gyri may be juxtaposed to give a false impression of having reached the corpus callosum; however, with separation of the overlying arachnoid one will expose the underlying corpus callosum. Posteriorly the interhemispheric fissure may be used to gain exposure of the more deeply located transverse fissure which is obscured from view by the overhanging splenium and occipital lobes.

The *transverse fissure* has a more complicated anatomical structure. Unlike the other fissures which have primarily a two-dimensional configuration the transverse fissure has extensions in all three planes of a three-dimensional system (Fig. 4.2). Simplistically it is located beneath the splenium of the corpus callosum above the anterior margin of the confluence of the falx cerebri and tentorium cerebelli. Its posteroinferior portion overlies the dorsal mesencephalon. Its lateral margins swing around the mesencephalon to the lateral aspect of the cerebral peduncles, extending anteroinferiorly along the incisura of the tentorium, coming into approximation with the inferior and medial part of the Sylvian fissure. Superiorly and anteriorly it contains the tela choroidea and extends beneath the fornices to the level of the intraventricular foramen. The inferior aspect of this anterior extension gives rise to the choroid plexus of the third ventricle. The lateral margins of this extension, which also contain the tela choroidea, extends into the lateral ventricles as the

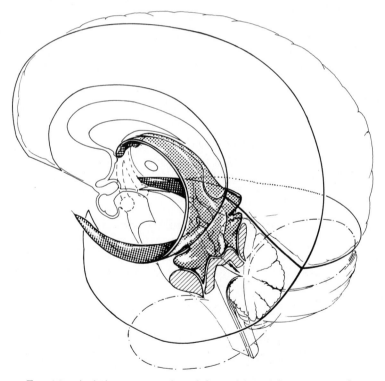

FIG. 4.2.   Artistic representation of the position of the transverse fissure.

choroid plexus. This extension into the lateral ventricles is known as the choroid fissure. The choroid fissure is a potentional slit only, located between the fornix and the lamina affixa on the dorsal side of the thalamus. The choroid fissure also follows the curve of the fimbriae of the fornices as the choroid plexus gains entry into the inferior horns of the lateral ventricles. Thus the choroid plexus of the third ventricle is united with the choroid plexus of the lateral ventricles via the choroid fissure between the thalamus and the fornix. The transverse fissure thus allows access to both dorsal brainstem areas and intraventricular areas.

The infratentorial compartment has numerous anatomical fissures. At the present time only four major fissures will be reviewed. These include the mesencephalocerebellar fissure superiorly, the cerebellopontine fissure laterally, the pontomedullary fissure anteriorly and inferiorly, and the vallecula posteriorly.

The *mesencephalocerebellar fissure* lies above the cerebellar hemispheres (specifically the quadrangular lobule, the ala of the central lobule, and the culmen) beneath the tentorium. Its anterior extent is the inferior portion of the dorsal surface of the mesencephalon and the superior medullary velum below. Branches of the superior cerebellar artery and precentral cerebellar vein are located here and impede the limited exposure by restricting the retraction of superior cerebellum.

The *cerebellopontine fissure*, a remnant of the pontine flexure laterally, lies within the lateral and superior aspect of the posterior fossa in what is known as the cerebellopontine angle. It may be described as being bound medially by the pons; superiorly by the "under aspect" of the brachium pontis medially and the overhanging quadrangular lobe laterally; inferiorly and laterally are the flocculus and biventral lobe of the cerebellum. The anterior margin is the petrous portion of the temporal bone. Cranial nerves V, VII, and VIII, and the anterior inferior cerebellar artery and its branches, are located there.

The *pontomedullary or pontobulbar fissure* is more medial in its location. It is bound by the occipital bone anteriorly and extends medially and inferiorly to give access to inferior pontine structures ventrally. The medial and anterior aspect of the biventral lobule overhangs the approach to this fissure. Cranial nerves IX, X, XI, and XII course laterally to limit the overall exposure. Access to the proximal portion of the posterior inferior cerebellar artery as it arises from the vertebral artery is also possible.

The *posterior fissure* in the infratentorial group is represented by the vallecula. The inferior folia of the vermis project from the vallecula, which separates the two cerebellar hemispheres. Separating the cerebellar tonsils exposes the underlying uvula of the vermis, beneath which lies the opening to the fourth ventricle via the foramen of Magendie. By opening or enlarging the arachnoid opening into the ventricle one gains access to the dorsal medial brainstem and lateral recesses of the fourth ventricle and restiform body.

Sulcal Anatomy

Little has been written relative to the anatomy of the sulci and sulcal vasculature. The following salient points which are relevant to microsurgical approaches will be reviewed. There is considerable individual variation in the patterns of gyri. The two sides of a given brain differ in the arrangement of their convolutions and sulci. However, certain patterns relative to sulcal anatomy can be observed.

There are four types of sulci: axial sulci, limiting sulci, operculated sulci, and complete sulci. Axial sulci are usually located in regions of special growth or special topographical locations and are longitudinal infoldings in homogenous areas. Such an example would be the posterior calcarine sulcus in the visual cortex in the occipital lobes. These sulci are relatively deep. Limiting sulci usually separate the cortex into different areas of function. They are more prominent in their appearance. As they are formed earlier in embryonic development than the axial sulci, they attain even greater depth than the axial sulci. An example would be the central sulcus. An operculated sulcus is one which separates distinct functional areas at its entrance but not at its floor. Often a third area of function is present in the floor or walls of the sulcus. An example would be the lunate sulcus, separating at the surface the striate and peristriate areas and containing the parastriate area within its walls. A sulcus which is so deep that it produces an elevation in the walls of a ventricle is called a complete sulci. Such an example would be the collateral sulcus.

All types of sulci have complex anatomical shapes within their depths. Small finger-like projections can occur at the bottom of a given sulcus. These can often be found to have extensions of several centimeters and can indent proximal and even distal gyri at the bases. With previously used lobectomies and lobulectomies one could thus injure adjacent gyri at the base of a sulcus without appreciating injury to the surface gyral pattern.

The vasculature within the arachnoid cistern of one sulcus may contribute to the perfusion and drainage of several gyri. Thus, when opening the arachnoid of a given sulcus one must pay special attention to avoid injury to the vessels of that sulcus.

The cortical vessels normally transverse the free surface of a gyrus before entering the sulcus to supply that sulcal region. However, an artery within the depth of a given sulcus or finger extension of a given sulcus may enter another communicating sulcus without reappearing on the free surface. Thus adequate exposure of sulcal vessels is important to avoid injury to blood supply to adjacent gyri.

SURGICAL TACTICS

The primary aim of surgery of tumors is twofold. First, one must establish a precise tissue diagnosis for guiding proper treatment. Second, the surgeon must be able to excise the tumor without injuring contiguous vital structures. In formulating a tentative diagnosis one must be able to define the exact location or topography of the lesion. This can be accomplished to a great extent with modern day radiographic techniques. However, it remains only an approximate diagnosis. The exact location of a lesion and its relationship to surrounding tissues can only be ascertained with surgery and the actual visualization of the tumor mass. In addition only surgery can show the type of tumor (or other pathology) which is present and thus establish a prognosis for the patient. This information becomes indispensable when trying to formulate a proper mode of therapy for the patient.

In defining the exact topography of a lesion and its relationship to other structures relative to surgical manipulations, a simplified scheme is used to review the various ways a tumor may present. Tumors involving the hemispheres or convexial lesions may present in one of five ways:

(a) The tumor may be entirely upon the surface.
(b) Only a small portion of the tumor is present on the surface.
(c) The tumor is below the surface but present within a sulcus.
(d) The tumor is completely subcortical (not visible either on the surface or within the sulcus).
(e) The tumor is intraventricular.

Lesions which present completely upon the surface are "attacked" directly and removed from the underlying cortex. When only a small portion of the tumor is present on the surface, with the remaining portion within the sulcus, the tumor is again attacked directly and debulked and subsequently removed, preserving normal cortex.

When a lesion is completely hidden from view, the sulcus which gives the best access and exposure is opened, and the limits of the tumor are identified. The tumor's vascular supply is isolated, and the tumor is subsequently removed. Lesions which are neither visible on the surface nor within a sulcus provide a greater challenge. In order to expose these lesions the microsurgeon must choose the route which will cause the least cortical damage. The tumor is dissected from the surrounding tissue and removed (Fig. 4.3). Intraventricular lesions often arise from a vascular pedicle or from the wall of the ventricle and are often associated with some degree of hydrocephalus. They are reached by using one of the microsurgical approaches discussed below. Following visualization of the tumor the vascular supply is isolated and the lesion is removed. The primary goal in all of the examples above is to localize the lesion and establish the shortest route of exposure and excision which causes the least amount of injury to surrounding structures. Nature usually prepares the brain for microsurgery as lesions invariably are close to a sulcus or fissure and in the case of intraventricular lesions are surrounded by cerebrospinal fluid which provides a route for exposure and resection.

Central lesions may either be intrinsic, extrinsic, or mixed. Using the fissural approaches described in the next section one is able to gain access to these central masses. Intrinsic tumors normally displace normal tissue and invariably are close to the surface at some point. Upon entering the mass, it is imperative that the subsequent dissection and debulking of the tumor be done from within. This allows removal without retraction or stretching of adjacent delicate neural pathways. Extrinsic tumors can usually be attacked directly, but again care is taken to remain within the tumor mass during the debulking procedure. Mixed lesions are approached where they are obvious on the surface, and then by following the lesion as it enters normal neural tissue they are again debulked from within. It is imperative, while removing central lesions, to stay within the tumor mass. The associated bleeding which occurs is controlled by repetitive coagulation and simple suction and occurs only within the tumor and not in adjacent tissue. After the lesion has been completely debulked from within, the margins will begin to collapse inward and then one can remove the tumor. The mass is debulked by successively dissecting away the internal parenchyma of the lesion, like peeling an onion from within (Fig. 4.4).

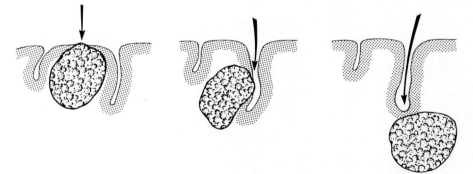

Fig. 4.3.   Different surgical approaches related to various locations of lesions.

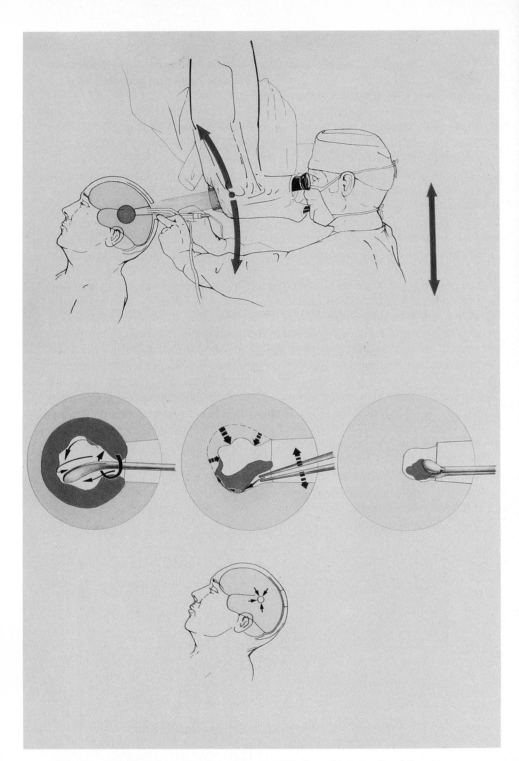

FIG. 4.4. (A) Keyhole approach to deep-seated lesion with help of mobile microscope (mouth switch). (B) Internal decompression, debulking, peripheral dissection, with reexpansion of normal tissue. (C) Complete removal allowing expansion of normal brain.

The second consideration of microsurgery deals with the precise or exact resection of tumor masses. First and foremost every attempt should be made to remove a tumor completely. Implicit in this attempt at complete resection is that little or preferably no damage to surrounding tissue should occur. Additionally, there should be no alteration in central nervous system hemodynamic, cerebrospinal fluid, or metabolic physiology. One must be able to preserve the vasculature to normal structures, maintain normal cerebrospinal fluid pathways, and preserve metabolic functions in surrounding brain. Obviously all tumors cannot be totally excised. However, this ultimate decision can only be made after examining a tumor at the time of surgery. If total removal is not feasible, then the debulking of a tumor mass for subsequent chemotherapy or radiation is essential. Finally, as with all surgical specialties the microsurgeon must be attentive and ensure proper hemostasis and antisepsis to avoid postoperative complications associated with hematomas and infections.

The microtechniques of resection involve the isolation of vessels and tumor debulking and dissection. In the exposure of the vasculature the microsurgeon must be able to isolate and identify normal vessels, transit arteries (which may or may not supply "feeders" to the tumor), and terminal vessels that directly supply the lesion. This entails dissecting and preserving the large normal vessels that are often adjacent to the mass (Fig. 4.5). Contrary to AVMs, which may have large terminal arteries, tumors do not have large terminal arteries. Vessels greater than 1 mm do not act as terminal vessels for a lesion. It is usually supplied by many smaller branches. Thus, preserving large vessels and resecting only "feeder" vessels maintains the normal blood supply to adjacent structures and deprives the tumor of its vascular input (Fig. 4.6). It is also essential that vasospasm of the transit vessels be treated by repeated application of papaverine to avoid ischemia both locally and in distal areas. Resection of the venous drainage of a tumor is also important. This is usually done last. Often the veins are red and dilated relative to the normal venous structures, thus making their identification somewhat easier. When dividing vessels it is judicious to do so close to the tumor mass. This allows for some retraction of the vessel following its being cut.

In debulking a tumor, internal decompression (with preservation of the tumor capsule) allows the shrinkage of the tumor mass with added visibility and allows the microsurgeon a "handle" with which to manipulate the mass. This is especially important with the deeper central lesions. As the tumor becomes smaller, one gains more "working room," and the margins of the tumor can be safely dissected without added retraction of contiguous structures. In addition, vessels which were previously hidden by the tumor can now often be easily dissected free. This tactic of internal decompression requires courage and patience on

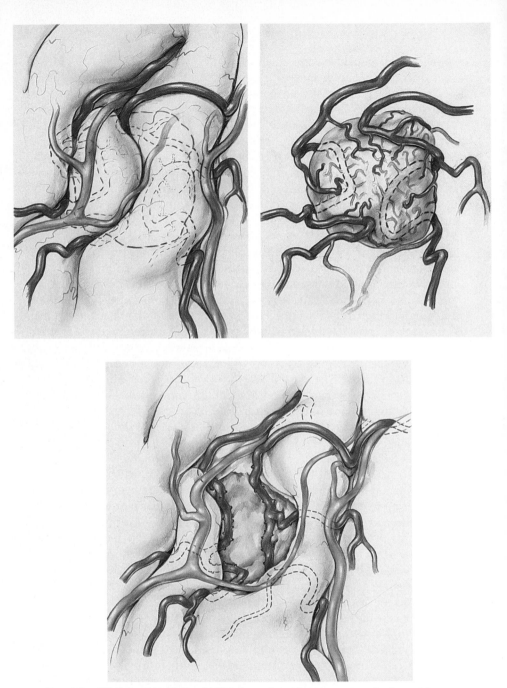

FIG. 4.5.   (A) Subcortical lesion hidden from view prior to opening of sulcus with proper visualization of tumor and hidden normal vessels. (B) Dissection of "feeding" vessels from transit vessels. (C) Preservation of normal vasculature, treatment of vasospasm, and preservation of normal tissue.

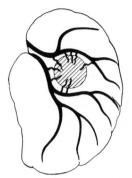
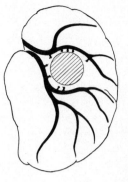
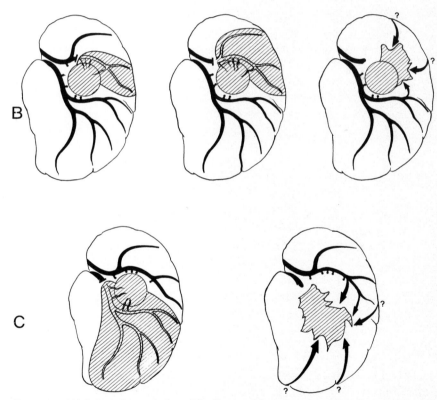

FIG. 4.6.   (A) Selected coagulation of feeding vessels and preservation of normal transit vessels. (B) Coagulation of transit vessel with resultant infarction of normal brain of variable size due to collateral circulation. (C) More proximal coagulation of major vessel with large infarct variable in size. Surgical actions as described in B and C should be absolutely avoided.

the part of the microsurgeon. The aspiration of the tumor contents is invariably associated with bleeding which at times can be rather vigorous. This can be controlled with continuous suction and repetitive bi-polar coagulation. Again this is bleeding within the tumor and not into normal tissue, thus causing no permanent sequelae. The experienced microsurgeon can differentiate between bleeding from tumor vessels and bleeding from adjacent large arteries and should control the former and avoid the latter. As the tumor shrinks, the juxtaposed feeding vessels can be sacrificed preserving normal vessels. Thus by a combination of both internal decompression and circumferential dissection lesions can be effectively isolated and removed while maintaining normal vasculature and structure of adjacent tissue.

Methods in elimination can best be reviewed following the diagrammatic outline below:

    A. Direct Tumor Elimination
        1. Mechanical—excision, suction, rotosuction, ultrasonic aspiration
        2. Physical—laser, cryosurgery
    B. Indirect Tumor Elimination
        1. Vascular supply—direct ligation of feeding vessels, embolization (balloon, plastic beads), polymerization (isobutyl-2-cyanoacrylate)
        2. Irradiation
        3. Chemotherapy
        4. Biological—immunotherapy (interferon, selective antibody, drug to enhance immune system)
    C. Combination of above

From the above outline of various modalities for tumor eradication it becomes obvious that a combination of techniques is used for tumor surgery. However, even more fundamental is the methodology which is used in applying these various techniques. This will be briefly reviewed in the next section.

MICROSURGICAL APPROACHES

Central to microsurgical methods is the "keyhole" approach (Fig. 4.7). This implies using natural anatomical dissection planes such as the arachnoid cisterns, the fissural approaches, or sulcal approaches to gain access to a tumor with minimal or no injury to normal neuroanatomy. There should be minimal retraction of normal tissue. In addition the opening is designed to be only as large as absolutely necessary. Upon initial exposure of the lesion the surgeon then develops a plan of removal.

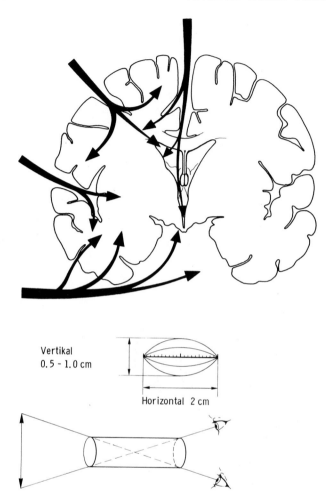

FIG. 4.7. Various fissural, sulcal, and cisternal approaches for inaccessible lesions. Bottom illustration shows necessary opening for the keyhole approach.

Dissection of the peripheral margins of the tumor from adjacent tissue or central decompression followed by dissection of the peripheral margin are two such approaches. Additionally the surgeon must abolish the vascular supply to the lesion. This may be done either prior to surgery or at the time of dissection. Using the above concepts one is able to effectively and safely extirpate the lesion with the least amount of trauma to normal anatomy.

The microsurgical approaches for "inaccessible" tumors entail the utilization and integration of the above microanatomy and microsurgical techniques and tactics (Fig. 4.8). Tumors within various anatomical

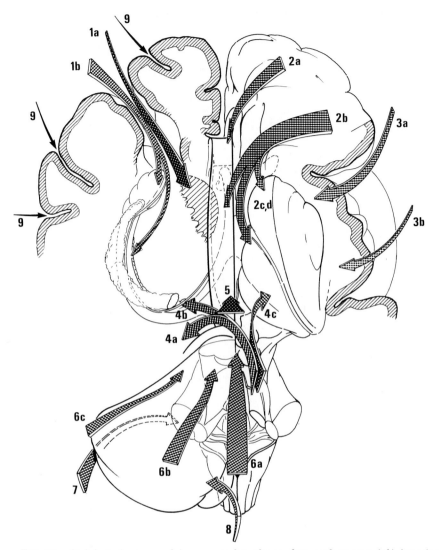

FIG. 4.8. (*1a*) Anterior transsylvian approach to the caudate nucleus area. (*1b*) Anterior transsylvian approach to amygdala and hippocampus. (*2a*) Anterior interhemispheric approach to splenium, corpus callosum. (*2b*) Middle interhemispheric approach to middle portion of corpus callosum, head of caudate nucleus (*2c*), dorsal and anterior thalamus area (*2d*). (*3a* and *b*) Middle and posterior transsylvian approach to the striocapsular-thalamic lesions. (*4a–c*) Posterior interhemispheric approach to parasplenial (*4a*), trigonal (*4b*), and pulvinar thalamic areas (*4c*) along the transverse fissure. (*5*) Posterior interhemispheric approach to medial part of transverse fissure for splenial and pineal lesions. (*6a*) Median supracerebellar approach to dorsal mesencephalon. (*6b* and *c*) Paramedian and lateral supracerebellar approach to superior cerebellar hemisphere lesions. Lateral (*6c*) and paramedian (*6b*) approaches are also shown. (*7*) Lateral approach to lesions in the cerebello-pontine angle. (*8*) Median inferior cerebellar approach to inferior two-thirds of the 4th ventricle. (*9*) Transsulcal approach to various hemispheric lesions.

locations will be discussed relative to the various approaches which can be used to afford exposure with minimal or no compromise of contiguous structures. With each exposure a few representative tumors will be reviewed.

Tumors involving the white matter of the frontal, temporal, parietal, and occipital lobes are resected using the sulcal-cisternal approaches as previously described. Standard craniotomies are placed over the lesions as defined topographically by preoperative radiographic studies. The appropriate sulcus-cistern is then opened over a length which will allow adequate visualization of the lesion. The sulcal vasculature is then exposed and protected, and feeding vessels to the tumor are subsequently eliminated. The lesion is then removed using the microtechniques. If a part of the lesion comes to the surface of a sulcus, then the lesion or tumor is decompressed from within itself. As the tumor wall collapses from the surrounding tissue its vascular supply is visualized and coagulated. The tumor is subsequently extirpated usually in a "piecemeal" fashion. Tumors in these areas include metastatic tumors, gliomas, and oligodendrogliomas and, rarely, tumors of neural cell origin.

The fissural approaches allow the surgeon to take advantage of the cisternal system when exposing deep-seated lesions. Eight basic craniotomies allow proper entry for exposing these lesions via fissural and cisternal approaches. In keeping with the standard neurosurgical procedures these craniotomies are divided into supratentorial and infratentorial procedures. The supratentorial approaches include the pterional or frontotemporosphenoidal craniotomy, the frontal paramedian craniotomy, the subtemporal craniotomy, and the posterior paramedian or parasagittal parietooccipital craniotomy. The infratentorial approaches include the lateral suboccipital craniotomy, the paramedian infracerebellar craniotomy, the median suboccipital craniotomy, and the paramedian supracerebellar craniotomy (refer to *Microneurosurgery*, Vol I, for descriptions (86)).

Utilizing the pterional approach one gains access to the Sylvian fissure. By opening the proximal Sylvian fissure the surgeon can visualize the parachiasmatic and neighboring cisterns to explore the chiasmatic area. Tumors in this region include gliomas of the optic nerve, chiasm, and tract proximally; pituitary adenomas extending out of the sella; craniopharyngiomas; dermoids; epidermoids; lipomas; arachnoid cysts; and hamartomas. Posterior exposure for lesions of the mamillary bodies and peduncular area is easily obtained. Laterally, by opening the cisterns, medial sphenoid wing meningiomas can be isolated and resected. Frontobasilar lesions can be approached by extending the dissection anteriorly. These include gliomas and oligodendrogliomas of the orbital frontal lobes, meningiomas arising from the base of the frontal fossa, and also tumors involving the amygdala and anterior two-thirds of the hippocampus such as gliomas, oligodendrogliomas, gangliogliomas, or gangliocytomas.

Opening the Sylvian fissure more distally (*i.e.*, middle and posterior thirds of Sylvian fissure) allows entry into the capsular and striocapsular regions, and adjacent areas.

The subtemporal approach, which in essence is a posteriorly and inferiorly extended pterional approach, allows exploration of the temporal basal region, the tentorium cerebelli at the incisura, and the parapeduncular areas. Lesions arising in the lateral floor of the middle fossa would include lateral sphenoid wing meningiomas. Additionally, meningiomas arising from the tentorium can be resected. Exophytic gliomas of the cerebral peduncles and medial cavernomas can be adequately exposed and resected as well.

The anterior paramedian frontal craniotomy allows the surgeon to explore the anterior portion of the interhemispheric fissure. Opening the fissure exposes the medial gyri of the frontal lobe and falx cerebri. This exposure also allows access to the anterior portion of the body of the corpus callosum. Extending the exposure transcallosally, the surgeon enters the lateral ventricle at the level of the foramen of Monro. By way of the intraventricular foramen the third ventricle can subsequently be explored. All types and sizes of tumors of the lateral and third ventricles can be reached. This exposure is often aided by the concurrent hydrocephalus with ventricular dilatation that occurs. Additionally lesions within the walls of the ventricles can be resected. These include tumors of the thalamus, caudate, and putamen. Occasionally a combination of the frontal interhemispheric transcallosal approach and the Sylvian fissure approach is used for tumors which have reached enormous proportions, such as a craniopharyngioma.

Through a paramedian parietooccipital craniotomy one can explore the posterior interhemispheric fissure and the more deeply located transverse fissure. By separating the interhemispheric fissure the medial parietal and occipital lobes and posterior part of the cingulate gyrus can be readily visualized. The surgeon also has access to the posterior body and splenium of the corpus callosum, the base of the precuneus and cuneus, and the isthmus of the cingulate gyrus. This allows the surgeon to expose not only the parasplenial area, but also by transcingular or transcallosal entry into the trigonal area, tumors in this region can be resected as well. The transverse fissure allows surgical entry to the dorsal mesencephalon, pulvinar thalami, and lateral and posterior aspects of the cerebral peduncles. The superior extent of the transverse fissure, via the velum interpositum, also allows exposure of dorsal thalamic lesions and posterior third ventricle masses. Lesions would include pineal tumors, thalamic gliomas, and ventricular tumors. The more anterior portions of the lateral extensions of the transverse fissure can be reached using the pterional approach and opening the Sylvian fissure (see previous discussion).

The lateral suboccipital craniotomy allows the visualization of the lateral cerebellopontine fissure and accompanying cisterns. Meningiomas, acoustic schwannomas, cysts, and cholesteatomas make up the majority of tumors in this region.

The paramedian infracerebellar approach utilizes the pontobulbar fissure and the more inferior arachnoid cisterns associated with it. With this exposure the more medial and inferior lesions arising from the pons can be reached. These include intrinsic and exophytic pontine tumors.

The paramedian supracerebellar craniotomy allows access to the cerebellomesencephalic fissure and posterior transverse fissure. Lesions in the inferior part of the dorsal mesencephalon and superior aspect of the cerebellum are explored through this approach. The collicular plate and paracollicular areas as well as the superior cerebellar peduncles and brachium pontis can also be visualized. Lesions in this area include pineal tumors extending beneath the tentorium, meningiomas, and tumors of the superior aspect of the cerebellum, such as metastatic tumors and gliomas.

The median suboccipital approach allows mobilization of both cerebellar tonsils and retraction of the vermis to gain entry into the fourth ventricle. Lesions within the superior and lateral aspects of the fourth ventricle as well as those arising from the floor of the fourth ventricle are visualized with the microscope. Tumors in this area include medulloblastomas, ependymomas, choroid plexus papillomas, and intrinsic tumors arising from the floor of the ventricle, brachium pontis, and restiform body.

CASE REPORTS

The following 22 cases in this report, which are taken more or less randomly from several hundred cases, are presented to help illustrate that lesions from various "inaccessible" areas can be approached using microsurgical techniques and the approaches discussed. A more comprehensive review of the statistical data is scheduled for vol. IV of *Microneurosurgery*. These cases include not only tumors but also other lesions which were originally misdiagnosed prior to definitive surgery and proper treatment. All patients presented are alive and well and actually working. The primary reason for reviewing these cases is to help show that we as surgeons must approach inaccessible lesions with new attitudes.

Case 1

R.H., a 19-year-old female secretary with a long history of right-handed seizures and associated dysphasia. Patient was initially evaluated elsewhere, where a CT scan showed a large cystic lesion in the left posterior insular area. A presumptive diagnosis of tumor was made, and the lesion was felt to be inoperable. The patient subsequently was treated with irradiation. Six months later a repeat CT scan showed progressive enlargement of the cystic tumor (Fig. 4.9A and B). Neurological examination was normal, and the patient had no speech difficulties. Patient underwent a left temporoparietal craniotomy and transsylvian approach (2.0 cm long) with a total gross resection. The cyst was evacuated, and the tumor was dissected from the transit arteries, which were preserved. Postoperatively the patient had no neurological deficits. CT scan was performed (Fig. 4.10) 5 days postoperatively. Histological diagnosis was fibrillary astrocytoma grade I. The patient has no evidence of recurrence after 4 years and is at full working capacity.

Admission: May 8, 1983
Discharge (home): May 16, 1983

Case 2

M.B., a 25-year-old male who suffered from psychomotor seizures of the right arm for 12 years. In 1978 a CT scan showed a left precentral low density lesion. The patient was followed for 7 years with progressive right hemiparesis and dysphasia. A CT scan performed in April 1985 (Fig. 4.11A) showed a cystic change of the lesion. The family then agreed to surgical intervention. A left frontoparietal craniotomy was performed, and the lesion was explored by opening the precentral sulcus and entering (1.0 cm) the cyst from the bottom of the sulcus. Postoperatively the patient improved rapidly with resolution of dysphasia and return of motor strength. A CT scan was done one month postoperatively (Fig. 4.11B). Histological diagnosis was confirmed as an oligodendroglioma. He has returned to full working capacity.

Admission: April 22, 1985
Discharge (home): May 7, 1985

Case 3

A.B., a 49-year-old male patient who suffered with headaches for 4 months and nausea and vomiting for 2 months prior to admission. The patient also complained of recent memory loss and difficulty with sleep. On physical examination he was noted to have ataxia and elements of "organic brain syndrome." CT scan (Fig. 4.12A and B) showed a left

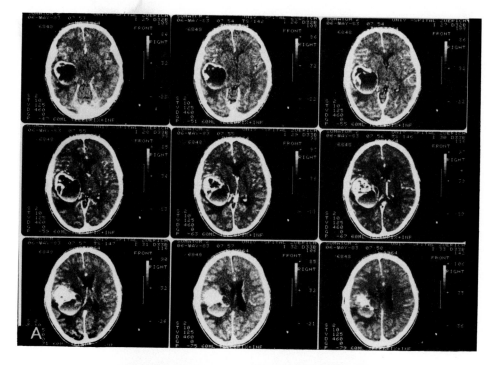

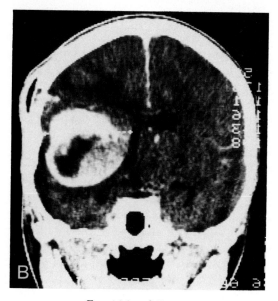

FIG. 4.9*A* and *B*

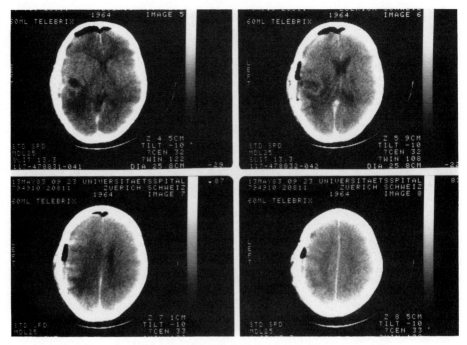

FIG. 4.10

frontobasilar multicystic lesion which extended to and occluded the foramen of Monro with resulting obstructive hydrocephalus. After a shunting procedure was done the patient was explored 3 weeks later via a left pterional craniotomy with total excision of the lesion through a frontobasal lateral incision (2.0 cm). Postoperatively the patient improved remarkably and returned to work 3 months postoperatively. (CT scan 3 months postoperatively, Fig. 4.12C.) The final histological diagnosis was astrocytoma grade II.

Admission: September 11, 1985
Discharge (home): October 7, 1985

Case 4

E.P., an 11-year-old female who 3 years prior to admission experienced mild left arm weakness. A CT scan performed at that time showed a round, hyperdense, right hypothalamic lesion. The patient was followed and developed a progressive left-sided hemiparesis with no sensory deficit. A repeat CT scan (3 dimensional) showed extension of the lesion to the right cerebral peduncle and parahypothalamic area. The thalamus was displaced superiorly and posteriorly (see Fig. 4.13A–C). Surgery was

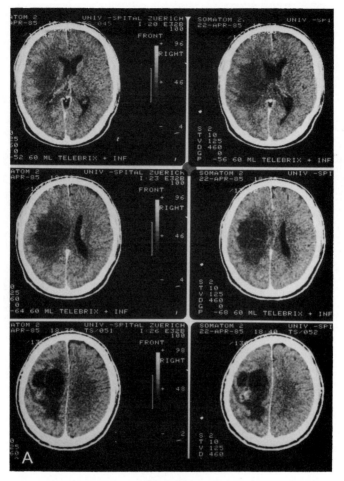

FIG. 4.11*A*

performed via a right pterional craniotomy, transsylvian approach. The tumor was found to be partially bulging into the right subchiasmal space and through the right anterior perforated substance to the subfrontal area. In order to preserve the optic nerve and tract a small incision (1.5 cm long) was made in the anterior perforated substance above the carotid bifurcation. The tumor was highly vascularized and fibrous. Following central decompression the tumor was grossly excised. Postoperatively the patient's hemiparesis gradually improved. Follow-up CT scan one year postoperatively (Fig. 4.13*D* and *E*) shows area of previous lesion with no other radiographic abnormalities. Histological diagnosis was piloid astrocytoma. It is remarkable that the patient had no pre- or

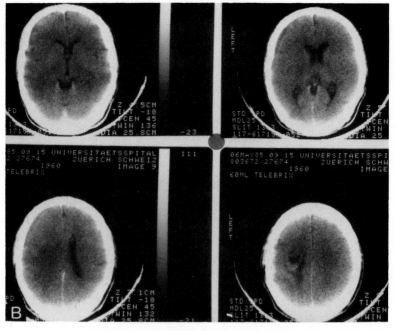

FIG. 4.11*B*

postoperative visual or endocrine problems. The patient has returned to school.

Admission: June 7, 1983
Discharge (home): June 18, 1983

Case 5

R.B., a 10-year-old male who initially presented in 1980 with diplopia. An ophthalmology examination revealed an astigmatism which was corrected with glasses. Six weeks later the patient presented with acute deterioration with disorientation, nausea, vomiting, and ataxia. A CT scan (Fig. 4.14*A* and *B*) showed a hyperdense lesion in the right thalamic area with obstructive hydrocephalus. Following placement of a ventriculoperitoneal (VP) shunt the patient was explored via a right pterional craniotomy and transsylvian approach. The tumor arose from the right optic tract and displaced the right internal carotid artery and the A-1 and M-1 segments. The vascularized tumor was removed in a "piecemeal" fashion for a radical excision. A postoperative CT scan one week later is shown (Fig. 4.14*C*). Postoperative deficit was homonomous hemianopsia which could not be evaluated preoperatively due to the patient's condi-

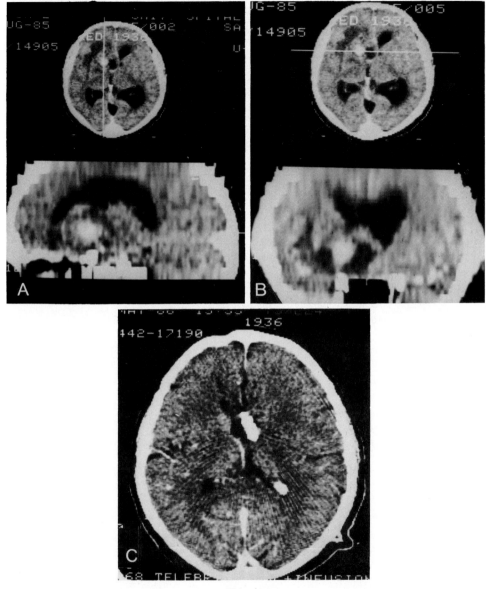

FIG. 4.12

tion. Histological diagnosis was low grade piloid astrocytoma. The patient
is going to regular classes.

Admission: December 14, 1980
Discharge (home): January 8, 1981

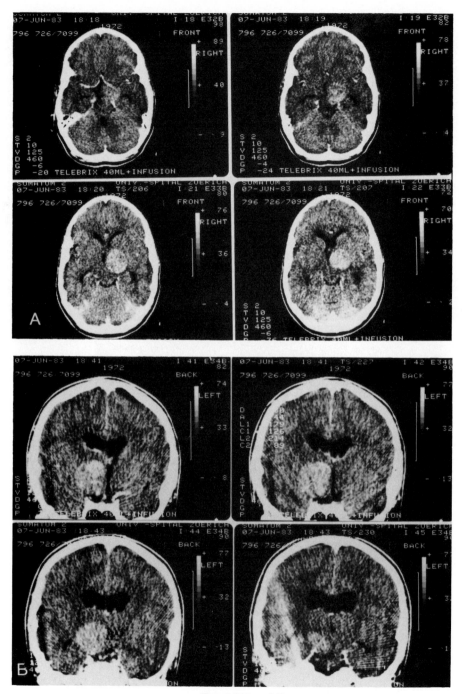

FIG. 4.13*A* and *B*

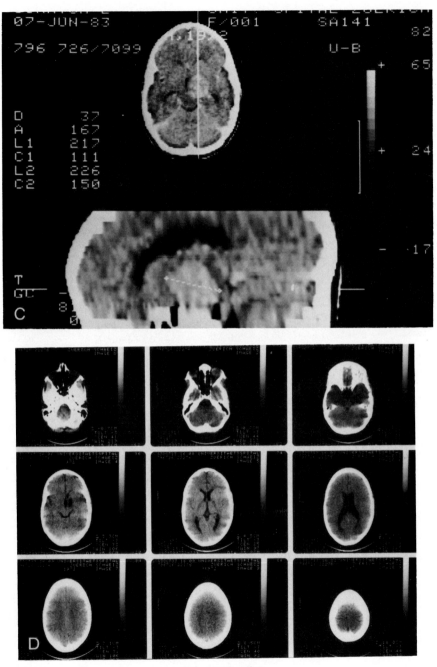

FIG. 4.13*C* and *D*

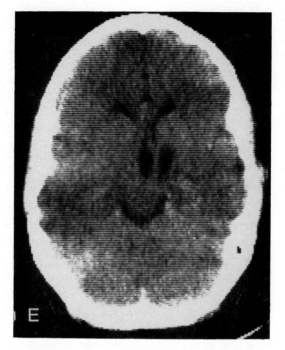

FIG. 4.13*E*

Case 6

A.C., a 7-year-old male child who suffered with left temporal lobe seizures (absence). A CT scan (Fig. 4.15*A* and *B*) showed a left amygdalohippocampal lesion which was well localized with small areas of calcification. Neurological examination revealed no abnormalities. The lesion was explored through a left pterional transsylvian approach (1.6 cm). The lesion was excised totally with no injury to surrounding structures. The postoperative course was uneventful with no neurological deficits and no seizure recurrence. CT scan performed one week postoperatively shows operative site (Fig. 4.15*C*). Histological diagnosis was ganglioglioma. He attends regular school.

Admission: June 20, 1983
Discharge (home): June 30, 1983

Case 7

R.P., a 33-year-old right-handed male teacher who had left temporal lobe epilepsy. The patient suffered from repetitive "somnolent" attacks. A CT scan (Fig. 4.16*A*) showed a hypodense lesion along the amygdala

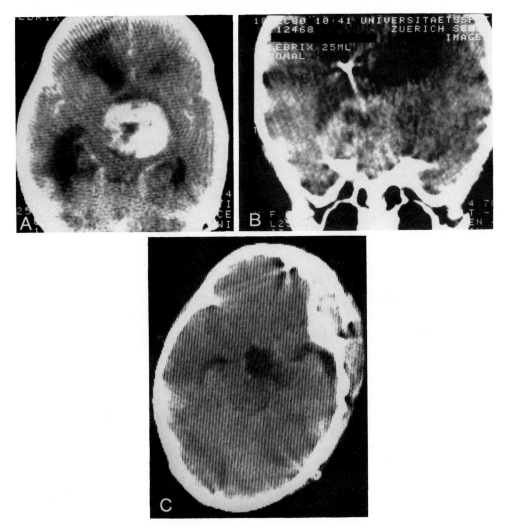

Fig. 4.14

to the parahippocampus and up to the isthmus of the cingulate gyrus
posteriorly. On physical examination the patient had no neurological
deficits. Surgery was performed in two stages. The first operation was
done via a left pterional transsylvian approach (2.0 cm long), and the
anterior third of the lesion within the amygdala and hippocampus was
resected. The second stage of surgery was performed 6 weeks later
through a posterior interhemispheric approach through the transverse
fissure, in the sitting position. The tumor infiltrated the precuneus and

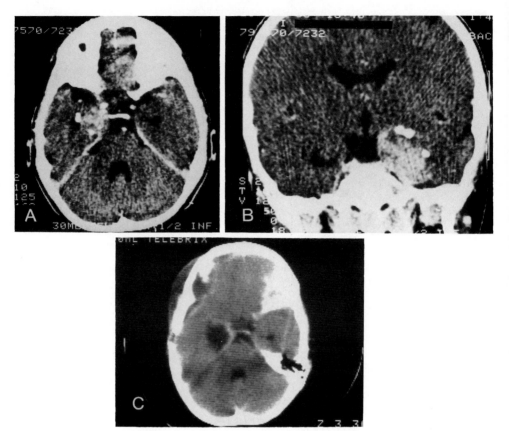

FIG. 4.15

extended under the falx to the right side, and it also extended infratentorially deep to the dorsal mesencephalon. The tumor was transparent and sharply delineated. Dissection along the lateral aspect of the transverse fissure included preservation of the posterior cerebral artery, the basilar vein, and the trochlear nerve. The postoperative course was uneventful with no mental or neurological deficits. Visual fields were preserved. CT scans after 1st stage and 2 weeks after 2nd stage are shown (Fig. 4.16B and C). The histological diagnosis was fibrillary astrocytoma grade II. Patient underwent irradiation and has returned to full-time work.

Admission: October 16, 1985
Discharge (home): November 12, 1985
Re-Admission: November 26, 1985
Discharge (home): December 23, 1985

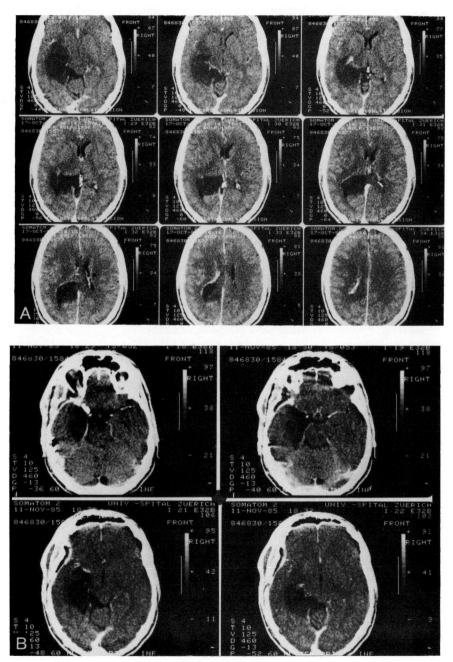

FIG. 4.16*A* and *B*

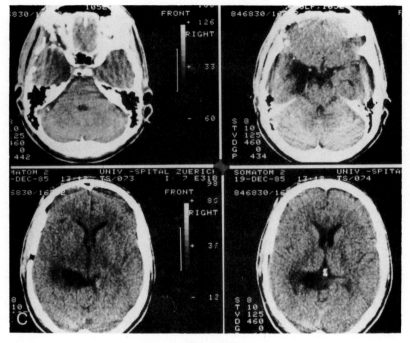

FIG. 4.16C

Case 8

K.J., a 19-year-old female student who developed severe headaches associated with blurred vision. Examination revealed advanced papilledema with choked discs and retinal hemorrhages. The remaining neurological examination was unremarkable. CT scan showed a callosal/subcallosal lesion (Fig. 4.17A). The patient was explored in the sitting position via a right posterior interhemispheric transcallosal approach. The tumor was encountered a few millimeters within the corpus callosum (2.0 cm incision) and was situated over the posterior aspect of the septum pellucidum. The tumor was highly vascularized. A radical resection was performed. The postoperative period was complicated by a hematoma which required reexploration and evacuation. The patient subsequently had no neurological complications and no mental and neurological deficit. Follow-up CT scan 3 months later is shown (Fig. 4.17B). Histological examination revealed an ependymoma. Patient underwent irradiation and has returned to full time studies.

Admission: November 24, 1982
Discharge (home): December 24, 1982

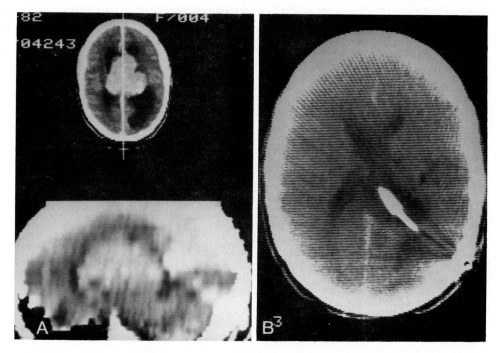

FIG. 4.17

Case 9

G.S., a 58-year-old female who had a 5-month history of progressive depression and "organic brain syndrome." Four weeks prior to admission she developed left arm weakness, and a CT scan was performed which showed right paracallosal lesion (Fig. 4.18A and B). The patient's condition improved with steroids and on subsequent examination she had no neurological deficit. The family was insistent on a surgical attempt for possible cure. The patient was explored in the sitting position through a posterior interhemispheric transcallosal approach. The tumor arose from the corpus callosum and was within the ventricle. A total gross resection was performed. Postoperative course was uneventful, and the patient was discharged after 3 weeks. Histological examination confirmed a glioblastoma. The patient received 6000 rads conventional irradiation. Follow-up CT scan 7 years after surgery is presented (Fig. 4.18C). The patient presently is in the 8th postoperative year, and is working in a bank.

Admission: September 13, 1978
Discharge (home): October 12, 1978

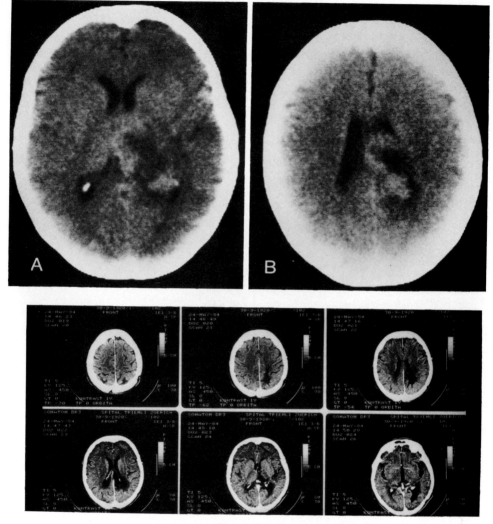

FIG. 4.18A–C

Case 10

M.P., a 31-year-old female who suffered for 3 years with chronic fatigue, apathy, and amenorrhea. Patient also noted mild weakness of left side. A CT scan (Fig. 4.19A) which was performed showed a large, enhancing 3rd ventricular mass. Lesion was felt to be inoperable. Patient subsequently developed progressive left hemiparesis (in the arm greater than in the leg). The patient was then transferred to Zurich and explored through a right anterior transcallosal approach (2.0 cm incision). The lesion was found to be bulging into the right lateral ventricle, which was

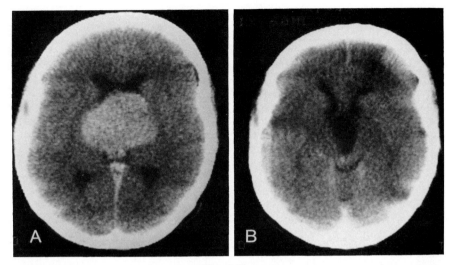

FIG. 4.19

dilated. Tumor was removed in a piecemeal fashion. It arose from the tela choroidea of the 3rd ventricle, displacing the two internal cerebral veins, and was not adherent to the walls of the ventricle. Postoperatively the patient improved rapidly with return of motor function. A follow-up CT scan 2 weeks later is shown (Fig. 4.19B). Histology examination showed a fibrous meningioma. The patient is doing well one year post-operatively and has had a normal pregnancy.

Admission: February 17, 1979
Discharge (home): March 10, 1979

Case 11

C.G., a 24-year-old female with headaches and amenorrhea which began in 1975. CT scan (Fig. 4.20A) at that time showed a lesion in the posterior portion of the 3rd ventricle. The patient had a shunt procedure and was irradiated without biopsy. She was referred to Zurich in 1984 in a cachectic condition. Examination showed severe ataxia, diplopia with Parinaud's syndrome, and a left superior quadrantanopsia. The patient was explored through a posterior interhemispheric parasplenial approach. The lesion was localized in the dorsal thalamic and mesencephalic areas. The tumor was excised radically. She improved rapidly with resolution of ataxic gait and Parinaud's syndrome. CT scan done 2 weeks postoperatively is presented (Fig. 4.20B). Pathology was consistent with ependymoma grade II–III. Two years later, the patient is in good condition without mental and neurological deficit.

Admission: July 19, 1984
Discharge (home): August 7, 1984

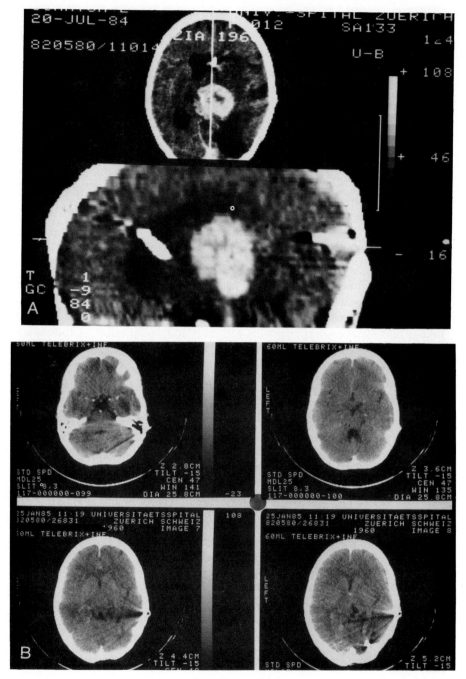

FIG. 4.20*A* and *B*

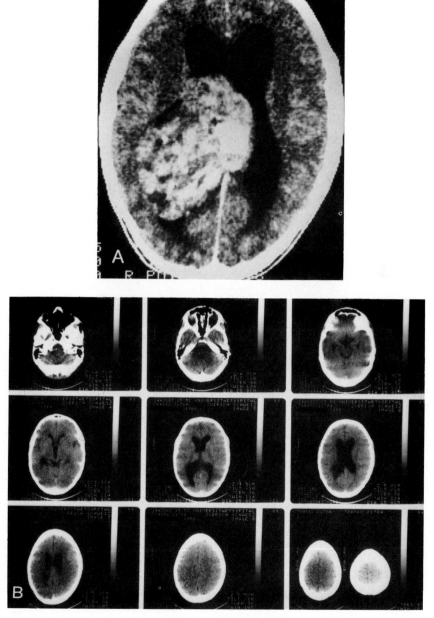

FIG. 4.21*A* and *B*

Case 12

D.F., a 16-year-old male patient with a history of occasional headaches for one year. Four weeks prior to admission he developed dysphasic episodes. A CT scan (Fig. 4.21A) showed a large hyperdense lesion in the posterior aspect of the left lateral ventricle. Examination revealed papilledema, right hand tremor, ataxic gait, and a positive Rhomberg test. The patient was explored via a left posterior interhemispheric parasplenic transcallosal approach (2.0 cm long) which was done in the sitting position. (The posterior corpus callosum had already been partially incised by the falx from pressure from the tumor.) Radical excision was performed. Postoperative course was uneventful with resolution of symptoms. Follow-up CT scan one year later is presented (Fig. 4.21B). Histological diagnosis was fibrillary astrocytoma grade I. Patient is doing well 4 years postoperatively without mental and neurological deficit.

Admission: November 9, 1982
Discharge (home): November 16, 1982

Case 13

E.N., a 38-year-old male who, 10 weeks prior to admission, experienced headaches associated with intercourse. Patient had no other symptomatology. A CT scan (Fig. 4.22A) showed a lesion in the trigone of the right lateral ventricle with an associated hypodense area. The patient's neurological examination was essentially normal. Surgery was performed in the sitting position through a right posterior interhemispheric transcingular approach (2.0 cm long) to the trigone. The tumor was excised in toto. Patient had no neurological deficits after surgery; visual field was preserved. A follow-up CT scan 6 months later showed resolution of the hypodense area (Fig. 4.22B). The final pathology report was meningioma.

Admission: June 20, 1982
Discharge (home): June 30, 1982

Case 14

R. G., a 2½-year-old female who presented with a left-sided tremor and slowed affect. The child was apathetic to all activities. Initially she was seen at Children's Hospital, where a CT scan showed a large intraventricular lesion (Fig. 4.23A). Surgery was performed in the sitting position via a right posterior interhemispheric transcingular approach (2 cm long) to the trigone of the lateral ventricle. A total gross removal was achieved. Postoperatively the child improved dramatically with no obvious neurological sequelae. CT scan one month after surgery showed a

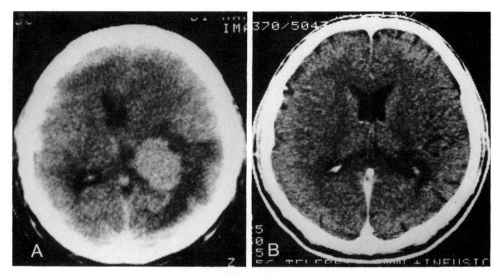

FIG. 4.22

dilated trigone (Fig. 4.23B). Histological diagnosis was fibroblastic meningioma. The child has developed normally during the last 3 years.

Admission: June 27, 1983

Discharge (home): July 5, 1983

Case 15

M.W., a 54-year-old male who had progressive "tiredness" with apathy and an unsteady gait due to right leg weakness which ultimately progressed to complete right-sided hemiparesis. MRI showed a left thalamic lesion with cystic or necrotic changes and peritumoral changes (Fig. 4.24A–C). Differential diagnosis included tumor vs. abscess. The patient was explored in the supine position through a left interhemispheric transcallosal approach (incision 2 cm long in the left medial portion). The thalamus was noted to be bulging, and upon puncture pus was encountered and removed. The cavity was then irrigated with antibiotics. Patient had a full neurological recovery following surgery. The cultures showed *Haemophilus paraphrophilus*, and the patient was treated with appropriate antibiotics. CT scan and MRI scan 4 months postoperatively are shown (Fig. 4.24D–F). MRI scans have been helpful in the preoperative differential diagnosis; however, the CT scan has been more helpful in following the patient's postoperative changes anatomically.

Admission: November 6, 1985

Discharge (home): November 28, 1985

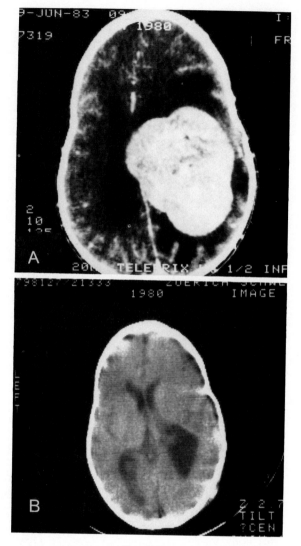

FIG. 4.23

Case 16

L.A., a 35-year-old female teacher with a left progressive 3rd nerve palsy for 10 years. Patient developed a right hemisensory deficit and right hemiparesis 4 years prior to admission. CT scan showed a left peduncular lesion which was sharply delineated on MRI (Fig. 4.25A and B). Patient was explored through a left subtemporal approach and had total gross resection of the lesion. Postoperatively the patient had a

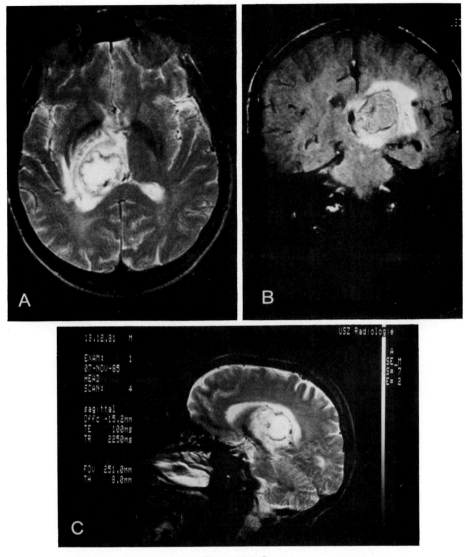

FIG. 4.24A–C

temporary exacerbation of the right hemiparesis which subsequently improved. Postoperative MRI is shown (Fig. 4.25C and D). The histological diagnosis was astrocytoma grade I. Four weeks after surgery the patient was self-sufficient.

Admission: June 23, 1986
Discharge (home): July 24, 1986

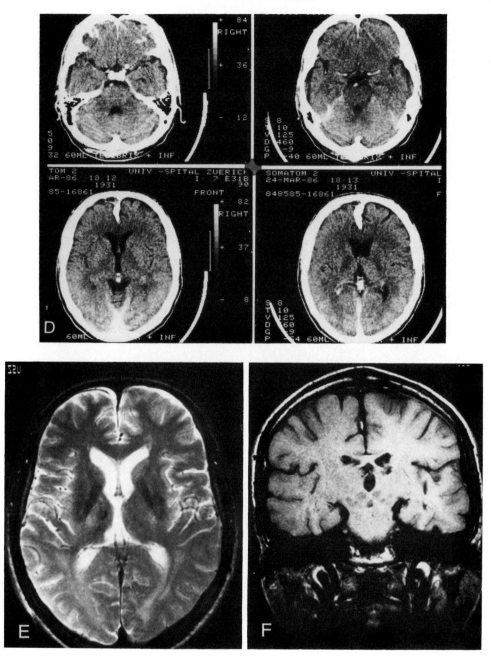

FIG. 4.24D and F

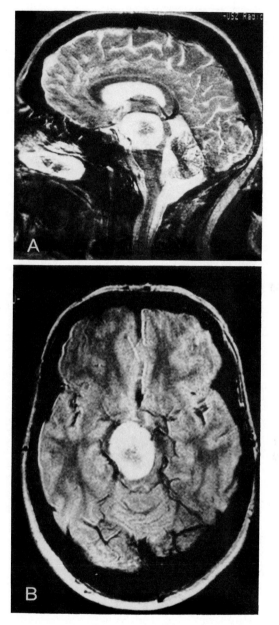

FIG. 4.25A and B

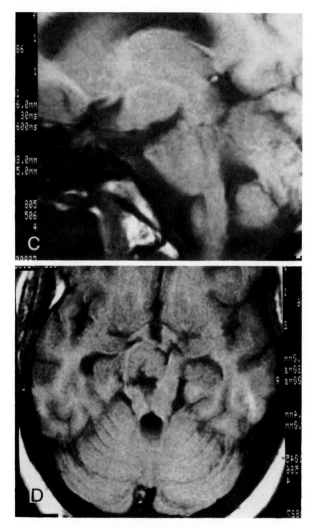

FIG. 4.25C and D

Case 17

S.P., a 4½-year-old male child who developed progressive tetraparesis 9 months prior to admission (right greater than left). On CT scan a mesencephalic lesion was seen (Fig. 4.26A–C). Due to the associated hydrocephalus a shunt was placed with partial improvement of the child's condition. There was progressive deterioration, and the child was transferred to Zurich. On examination there was a right hemiparesis (greater in the arm than in the leg) and severe ataxia with no sensory deficit. Parinaud's syndrome was also present. Surgery was performed via a

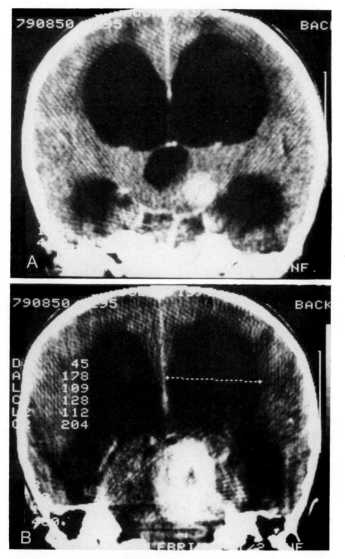

FIG. 4.26*A* and *B*

suboccipital supracerebellar approach in the sitting position. The tumor was resected completely. The patient had an uneventful course following surgery. Histology showed a fibrillary astrocytoma. The follow-up CT scan performed 3 years postoperatively is shown (Fig. 4.26*D*). The patient has no neurological deficits and attends school.

Admission: February 23, 1983

Discharge (home): March 21, 1983

CLINICAL NEUROSURGERY

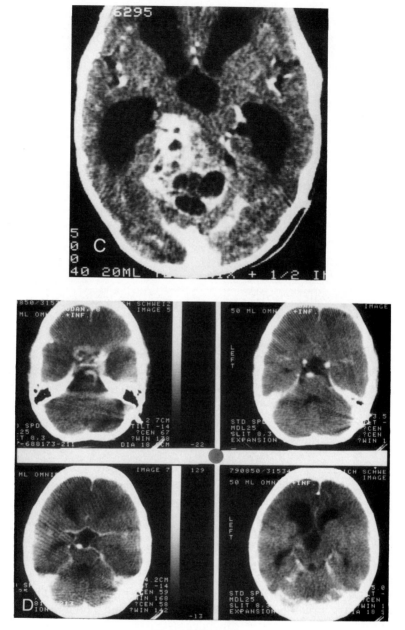

FIG. 4.26C and D

Case 18

J.D., a 24-year-old male who suffered a grand mal seizure in 1982. A CT scan showed a lesion in the dorsal mesencephalon with associated occlusive hydrocephalus. The patient was shunted in 1983. An MRI in 1985 showed progression of the tumor mass (Fig. 4.27A). Examination

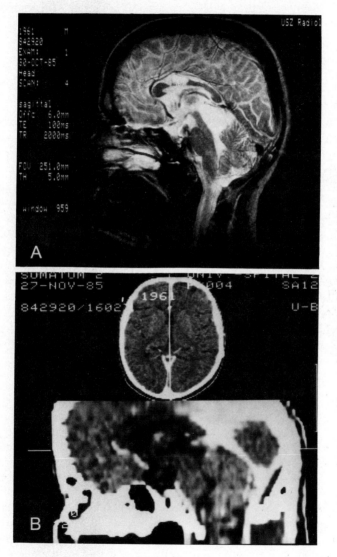

FIG. 4.27

at that time showed the patient to have an intact mental status, horizontal nystagmus, and Parinaud's syndrome with no other neurological deficits. Surgery was performed via a suboccipital paramedian supracerebellar exploration of the dorsal mesencephalon. A firm rubber-like tumor was totally excised. The postoperative course was uneventful. Follow-up CT scan 4 weeks after surgery showed no residual tumor (Fig. 4.27B). Histology was consistent with astrocytoma grade I. At 1-year follow-up the patient still has horizontal nystagmus but has no subjective complaints.

Admission: October 28, 1985
Discharge (home): December 20, 1985

Case 19

R.M., a 4-year-old male who developed left arm weakness 2 weeks prior to admission. On initial presentation he was noted to have a left head tilt. CT scan (Fig. 4.28A and B) showed a hyperdense lesion within the mesencephalon associated with hydrocephalus. The patient had only slight hemiparesis of the left side and was otherwise in remarkably good condition. The lesion was initially felt to be inoperable; however, at the insistence of the parents a tentative exploration was planned. Surgery was performed in the sitting position through a right suboccipital paramedian supracerebellar approach. A 5-mm incision was made beneath the right inferior colliculus above the trochlear nerve where the tumor was in close approximation to the surface. The tumor was resected entirely. (The CUSA could not be used in this small area of exposure.) Postoperatively the patient had regression of his symptoms within several days and was discharged on the 10th postoperative day. Histology confirmed a fibrillary astrocytoma. Follow-up CT scan one year later is shown (Fig. 4.28C). Patient is doing well 3 years after surgery.

Admission: February 7, 1983
Discharge (home): February 23, 1983

Case 20

R.N., a 30-year-old female who had diplopia for 5 years. One year prior to admission she developed dysesthesia of the right hand with hyperacusis and tinnitus of the right ear. A CT scan done at that time (Fig. 4.29A and B) showed a large pontine mass, and the patient was declared inoperable. The patient deteriorated over the next year and was subsequently referred to Zurich. Examination at that time revealed a mild right-sided weakness with decreased sensations on the right, nystagmus, diminished corneal reflexes bilaterally, ataxia, and mild facial nerve palsy on the left. The patient was explored in the sitting position via a median

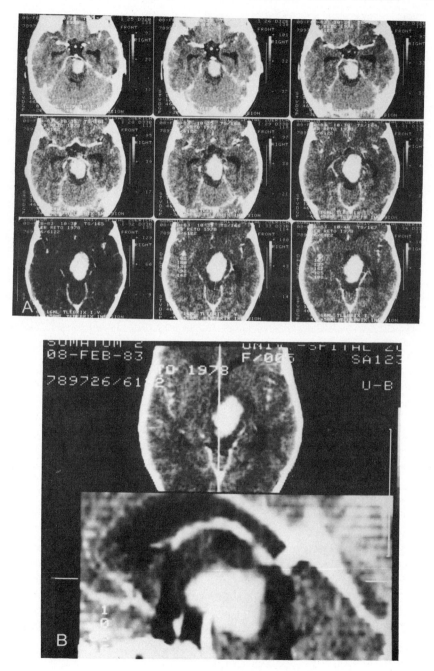

FIG. 4.28*A* and *B*

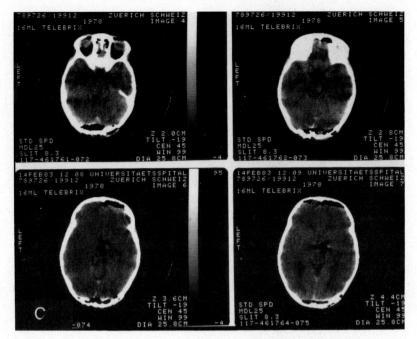

FIG. 4.28C

suboccipital approach. Exposure of the floor of the 4th ventricle revealed a bulging fluctuant mass in the inferior aspect. This was opened (5 mm diameter) with evacuation of fluid and subsequent removal of the capsule wall. The postoperative course was uneventful, and the patient had a complete neurological recovery. Repeat CT scan was performed 10 days postoperatively (Fig. 4.29C). Pathology showed the lesion to be a subependymal cyst. The patient is now at 6 years of follow-up.

Admission: July 20, 1981
Discharge (home): August 13, 1981

Case 21

N.F., a 7-year-old female patient who developed nausea, vomiting, and headaches 2 weeks prior to admission. The patient had a right Horner's syndrome associated with ataxia. On neurological examination the patient was found to have mild right lower cranial nerve palsies (VII, IX, X, XI, XII) and mild sensory deficit in the trigeminal distribution. She had dysphasia and right-sided hypesthesia. CT scan (Fig. 4.30A) showed a hematoma in the right pontine area. She was explored in the sitting position via a midline suboccipital approach. On exposure of the floor of the 4th ventricle a bluish bulging area approximately 3 cm × ½ cm was evident in the right pontomedullary area. An opening was made over the

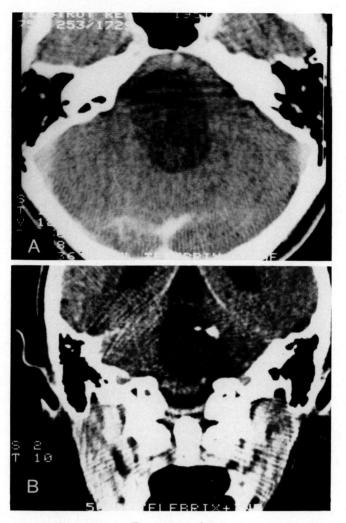

FIG. 4.29*A* and *B*

hematoma, and the clot and angioma were removed. Patient had a rapid recovery postoperatively, and repeat CT scan was performed 3 weeks after surgery (Fig. 4.30*B*). Histological diagnosis was cavernous angioma. Patient is now fully intact neurologically, 2 years later.

Admission: December 12, 1984

Discharge (home): January 1, 1985

Case 22

C.B., a 15-year-old female student who developed headaches, nausea, vomiting, ataxia, and double vision in 1982. A CT scan showed a 4th

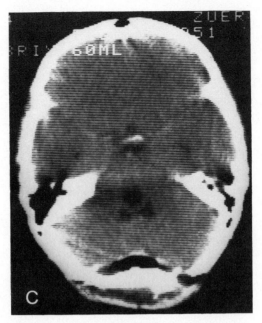

FIG. 4.29C

ventricular mass with obstructive hydrocephalus (Fig. 4.31A). The patient was shunted. One year later the patient had progressive deterioration of the symptoms and became bedridden. Examination at that time
showed nystagmus, dysphagia, dysarthria, and right hypoglossal nerve
palsy. A tracheostomy had been previously performed. A vertebral angiogram showed a vascular lesion consistent with a hemangioblastoma
(Fig. 4.31B and C). Surgery was performed via a suboccipital midline
approach to the 4th ventricle. The resection of the tumor was complicated
by bleeding from an area in the right trigonum hypoglossi which was
controlled with considerable difficulty. The postoperative course was
stormy as the patient had bilateral 12th nerve palsies which gradually
improved over 2 months. The patient was ultimately able to have the
tracheostomy tube removed. The postoperative scan is shown (Fig.
4.31D). Histological diagnosis was hemangioblastoma. Two years later
the patient is neurologically intact except for a mild right 12th nerve
palsy.

Admission: March 13, 1982

Discharge (home): June 2, 1982

DISCUSSION

Every experienced neurosurgeon knows that minimal or no retraction
or compression of the brain is conducive to a better surgical result and

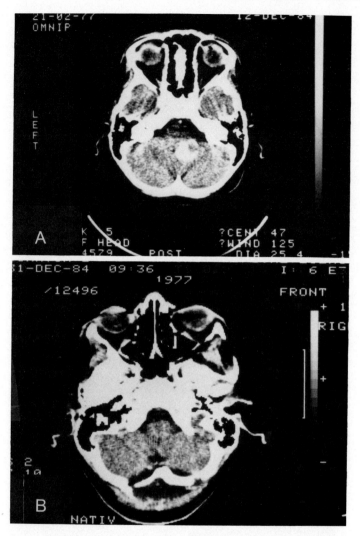

FIG. 4.30

improved postoperative condition of the patient. The opportunity afforded by the microscope to work in small openings with sharp stereoscopic focus has enabled the microsurgeon to be precise in his dissection
and preservation of cerebral vasculature. Accurate dissection of the
arachnoid and the arachnoidal cisterns has also been shown to be
beneficial in the flow dynamics of cerebrospinal fluid. Using the space
provided by a tumor mass and debulking lesions from within has obviated
the need for additional retraction of normal brain parenchyma. Following
these three principles of (*a*) careful vascular dissection, (*b*) using arach-

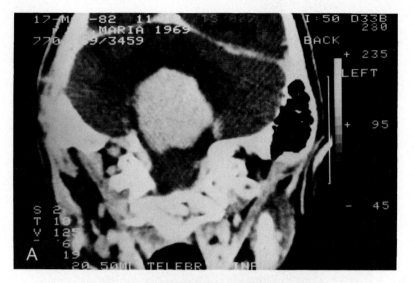

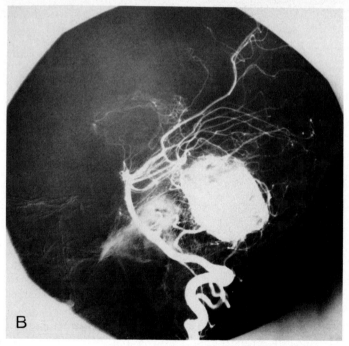

FIG. 4.31*A* and *B*

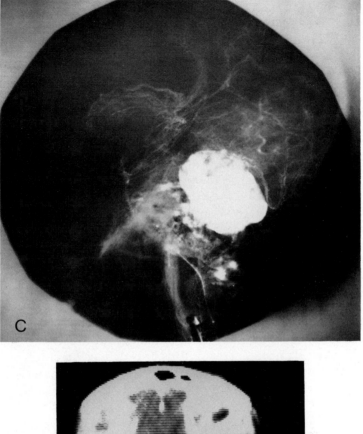

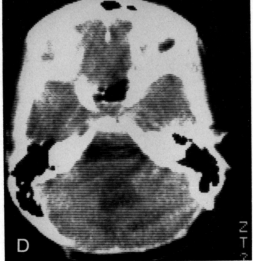

FIG. 4.31*C* and *D*

noidal planes, and (c) avoiding unnecessary retraction and compression of the neural tissue, microsurgical procedures have been applied to increasingly more difficult and inaccessible lesions with encouraging results. The same tactics have also been applied to the so-called simple lesions involving the hemispheres with improved results over the previously performed lobectomies and "generous resections."

After operating on 2500 cases of brain tumors, it has become apparent that our current knowledge concerning the location of various brain functions is inadequate to explain many of the surgical observations. Brain physiology is not static with a fixed anatomical morphology; rather the brain is a dynamic organ with enormous flexibility. It is important to appreciate the established concepts set forth and verified by Penfield and others; however, it is equally important to acknowledge that many times the observed operative results do not coincide with the expected or predicted outcomes (often patients who should have severe or even fatal deficits have none). The work of the many famous neurologists, neurophysiologists, and neurosurgeons which was done to document the localization of function in the brain was for the most part performed on animals or patients with epileptic, ischemic, or traumatic lesions. This was subsequently applied to various other pathological processes in the brain and to normal brain physiology. Normal brain physiology is very different from that which occurs in altered brain tissue and again is a dynamic rather than static process. Precisely defined functions in certain areas of the brain are fully accepted, but there are exceptions to these established principles which cannot be objectively documented. Cerebral changes following resection of a tumor from a given area can be exceptional often with little "objective" alteration.

Many of our present "sophisticated" neuropsychological tests for various brain functions are still grossly inadequate. In addition each disease process involving the central nervous system (Fig. 4.32) has its own pathophysiology and unique metabolism. In evaluating aneurysms we can precisely localize the defect and often document associated vascular changes; however, we have little insight as to the overall mechanisms of pathology. For instance, why do some patients with severe vasospasm have no deficit and others have neurological sequelae at distant sites? With AVMs, we can accurately show the involved vessels and their location, but we cannot predict the degree and quality of adaptation of the surrounding brain or distant structures due to the longevity of the disease process. In trying to understand the physiology of the brain and to localize the specialized areas of function which exist, one is tempted to compare different disease processes which occur within the same location. However, aside from simple mass effect different lesions have different pathophysiological processes. Even tumors in similar locations

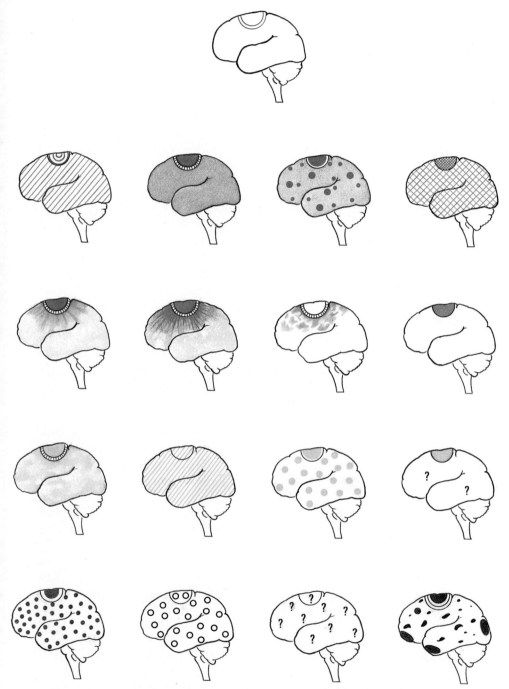

FIG. 4.32.   Various disease processes in the same anatomical location with possible basic metabolical alterations in neurophysiological function.

behave differently. Each lesion, whether vascular, neuronal, or other, has its own unique metabolism and consequently its own unique effect on both surrounding and distant brain tissue. These metabolic processes can also be either active or inactive, thus altering the observed effect in the normal tissue.

Glioblastomas are different from astrocytomas. They are routinely grouped together in pathology however as being of glial cell origin. Experience has shown that glioblastomas behave differently in regards to their overall pathophysiology. Astrocytomas often cause minimal or no change in function when they initially occur in eloquent areas of the brain such as speech or motor control or within brainstem locations (31, 49, 51, 53, 59). Some would rationalize that these observations are a result of the slow growth pattern of astrocytomas relative to glioblastomas. Beyond local symptomatology, however, glioblastomas cause diffuse alterations in brain physiology, especially frontal lobe function, for which there are no accurate tests for evaluating. It is well known that some frontal lesions and some cerebellar lesions may cause vestibular dysfunction, and the corresponding changes in substrates have been well documented. Additionally, lesions in both areas may cause mental changes irrespective of the type or size of lesion involved. Thus, patients with cerebellar lesions may have not only dysdiadochokinesis but bradykinesia of movement and thought as well. Patients with frontal lesions may have not only slowness in mentation but may exhibit vestibular dysfunction.

As clinical researchers, we are accustomed to relating to brain tumors relative to their mechanical effects of compression on brain tissue, brain hemodynamics, and cerebrospinal fluid dynamics. In addition, one must consider that tumors are like organs with their own inherent metabolic, neurochemical, and neuropharmacological processes. These may affect brain function in specific and general ways, in localized and diffuse patterns, and during active and inactive periods. Thus it is imperative to study tumors dynamically rather than in a static manner. This has not previously been possible, but with the aid of new diagnostic technology such as magnetic resonance spectroscopy (MRS) and positron emission tomography (PET) this may become feasible (67, 90).

Previously tumors were often not diagnosed until patients presented with symptoms and were subsequently studied diagnostically. Thus, the tumor growth process and subsequent manifestations were seen and analyzed in the final or end phase of tumor progression. With modern neuroradiographic capabilities (i.e., CT scan and MRI), patients with tumors are being diagnosed much earlier. Tumors in similar locations often present with different symptoms both in quantitative and qualitative degrees. The neuropsychological and neuroradiological studies which are available give information relative to localization but tell little relative to the overall effect on the condition of the brain. The neurologist, neuropsychologist, and neurosurgeon should be more concerned and speculative in that lesions which are discovered incidentally on CT scan or MRI studies do not cause a corresponding neurological or mental status deficit.

It becomes important then to carefully and thoughtfully adapt the neuropathology concepts to the clinical neurophysiology which is observed. As the clinical data base relative to tumors is changed by improved modern diagnostic abilities, the concepts of neuropathological processes will also become more complicated and sophisticated. Our basic parameters for comparison of different disease processes will be different.

Comparison of currently used microsurgical techniques with previously "standard" surgical tactics shows that patients awaken immediately postoperatively. The location of the lesion in the brain is not a factor in the postoperative alertness of the patient. If one can stay within the tumor and not injure or manipulate adjacent areas, it is possible to operate on any area of the brain with no subsequent increase in the neurological deficit.

There are no silent areas in the brain. Every area is eloquent and has its own unique function as well as being integrated with other areas of the brain. It is important, therefore, to respect the microsurgical rules:

(a) Avoid unnecessary compression of neural structures.
(b) Do not injure transit arteries (treat vasospasm).
(c) Use arachnoid dissection planes.
(d) Monitor CSF dynamics and avoid increased pressure due
    to fluid accumulation.

Meticulous attention to details and techniques coupled with proper pulmonary management to avoid obstruction to venous outflow and its associated problems enables the microsurgeon to treat lesions in any location. The brain is not a closed system. It has a highly complex anatomical construction which allows microsurgical approaches to every location. It is both dynamic and flexible, and this allows for accommodation of lesions and their associated structural and functional alterations of normal brain tissue. This same flexibility and dynamism also allows microsurgical resection of these lesions without additional injury to the brain if performed with dexterity, proper technique, and respect for microsurgical principles.

CONCLUSION

If one reviews the former literature, there are reports of small groups of cases of "inaccessible" tumors which have been explored with variable results (7, 9, 13–18, 26, 40, 45, 47, 50, 51, 57–59, 78). Since the introduction of the microscope and microtechniques, there have been increasing numbers of publications dealing with these tumors (1–6, 10, 11, 19, 21, 22, 27, 29–32, 39, 46, 48, 49, 52–54, 56, 59, 62–66, 68–71, 74–76, 79, 82). The development of microsurgery spawned an era which witnessed a rapid growth in our ability to diagnose neurological diseases both earlier and more accurately. This advanced diagnostic capability afforded by MRI and CT scans has presented many new surgical challenges. Microsurgical techniques aligned with CT-guided stereotactic biopsy (12, 24, 25, 33, 44, 61, 73) or implantation of radioisotopes (60, 81), radiosurgery (55, 77), and computerized laser surgery (41, 43) match the advances in neurodiagnostic skills and potentially offer answers to the surgical questions of our time. Only by comparing, improving, and implementing new surgical concepts in relation to anatomical knowledge (8, 20, 23, 28, 35–37, 38, 71, 72, 80, 83–85, 89) can the ultimate solutions for treatment of neurological disease be obtained.

Hopefully the presented cases will help to change the present attitudes not only of neurologists and neuroradiologists but also of neurosurgeons. The previous dictums related to surgical indications should be rethought and changed. Not operating due to "inaccessibility" or following patients who have a lesion but are neurologically intact is no longer reasonable or correct. One cannot aggressively operate in any location in the brain. However, if one is clinically thoughtful and follows the principles of microsurgery, every lesion can be safely approached and removed.

REFERENCES

1. Antunes, J. L., Louis, K. M., and Ganti, S. R. Colloid cysts of the third ventricle. Neurosurgery, 7: 450–454, 1980.
2. Apuzzo, M. L. J. Transcallosal interfornical exposure of lesions of the third ventricle. In: *Operative Neurosurgical Techniques*, H. H. Schmidek, and W. H. Sweet, eds., pp. 585–594. Grune & Stratton, New York, 1982.
3. Apuzzo, M. L., Dobkin, W. R., Zee, C. Surgical considerations in treatment of intraventricular cysticercosis (an analysis of 45 cases). J. Neurosurg., 60: 400–407, 1984.
4. Baghai, P., Vries, J. K., and Bechtel, P. C. Retromastoid approach for biopsy of brain stem tumors. Neurosurgery, 10: 574–579, 1982.
5. Becker, D. H., and Silverberg, G. D. Successful evacuation of an acute pontine hematoma. Surg. Neurol., 10: 263–265, 1978.
6. Bernstein, M., Hoffman, H. J., Halliday, W. C., et al. Thalamic tumors in children. Long-term follow-up and treatment guidelines. J. Neurosurg., 61: 649–656, 1984.
7. Bray, P. F., Carter, S., and Taveras, J. M. Brainstem tumors in children. Neurology, 8: 1–7, 1958.
8. Browder, J., Kaplan, H., and Krieger, A. J. Anatomical features of the straight sinus and its tributaries. Clinical correlations. J. Neurosurg., 44: 55–61, 1976.
9. Cairns, H., and Mosberg, W. H. Colloid cysts of the third ventricle. Surg. Gynecol. Obstet., 92: 545–570, 1951.
10. Camins, M. B., and Schlesinger, E. B. Treatment of tumours of the posterior part of the third ventricle and the pineal region: a long term follow-up. Acta Neurochir.

(Wien), *40:* 131–143, 1978.

11. Castillo, R. G., and Geise, A. W. Meningioma of the third ventricle. Surg. Neurol., *24:* 525–528, 1985.

12. Coffey, R. J., Lunsford, L. D. Stereotactic surgery for mass lesions of the midbrain and pons. Neurosurgery *17:* 12–18, 1985.

13. Cramer, F. The intraventricular meningiomas: a note on the neurologic determinants governing the surgical approach (abstr.). Arch. Neurol., *98:* 1960.

14. Cushing, H. *Pituitary Body, Hypothalamus and Parasympathetic Nervous System.* Springfield, Ill., Charles C Thomas, 1932.

15. Dandy, W. E. Extirpation of the pineal body. J. Exp. Med., *22:* 237–247, 1915.

16. Dandy, W. E. Diagnosis, localization and removal of tumors of the third ventricle. J. Hopkins. Hosp. Bull. Rep.: 33–188, 1922.

17. Dandy, W. E. *Benign Encapsulated Tumors in the Lateral Ventricle of the Brain.* Williams & Wilkins, Baltimore, 1934.

18. Dandy, W. E. Operative experience in cases of pineal tumors. Arch. Surg., *33:* 19–46, 1936.

19. Delandsheer, J. M., Guyot, J. F., Jomin, M., *et al.* Accès au troisième ventricule par voie inter-thalamo-trigonale. Neurochirurgie, *24:* 419–421, 1978.

20. Duvernoy, H. M. *Human Brainstem Vessels.* Springer, Berlin, 1978.

21. Enzian, W. Removal of intrapontine-mesencephalic spongioblastoma. Neurosurg. Rev. *6:* 67–70, 1983.

22. Epstein, F., and McCleary, E. L. Intrinsic brain-stem tumor of childhood: Surgical indication. J. Neurosurg., *64:* 11–15, 1986.

23. Fujii, K., Lenkey, C., Rhoton, A. L., Jr. Microsurgical anatomy of the choroidal arteries: Lateral and third ventricles. J. Neurosurg., *52:* 165–188, 1980.

24. Fukushima, T. Endoscopic biopsy of intra ventricular tumors with the use of a ventriculofibroscope. Neurosurgery, *2:* 110–113, 1978.

25. Galanda, M., Nádvornik, P., Šramka, M., *et al.* Stereotactic biopsy of brainstem tumors. Acta Neurochir Suppl (Wien) *33:* 213–217, 1984.

26. Greenwood, J., Jr. Radical surgery of tumors of the thalamus, hypothalamus, and third ventricle area. Surg. Neurol., *1:* 29–33, 1973.

27. Guidetti, B., Delfini, R., Gagliardi, F. M., *et al.* Meningiomas of the lateral ventricles. Surg. Neurol., *24:* 364–370, 1985.

28. Hardy, D. G., Peace, D. A., and Rhoton, A. L., Jr. Microsurgical anatomy of the superior cerebellar artery. Neurosurgery, *6:* 10–28, 1980.

29. Hirsch, J. F., Zouaoui, A., Renier, D., *et al.* A new surgical approach to the third ventricle with interruption of the striothalamic vein. Acta Neurochir. (Wien), *47:* 135–147, 1979.

30. Hoffman, H., Yoshida, M., Becker, L. E., *et al.* Experience with pineal region tumors in childhood. Neurol. Res., *6:* 107–112, 1984.

31. Hoffman, H. J., Becker, L., and Craven, M. A. A clinically and pathologically distinct group of benign brain stem gliomas. Neurosurgery, *7:* 243–248, 1980.

32. Hoffman, H. J., Bendrick, E. B., and Humphreys, R. P., *et al.* Management of craniopharyngioma in children. J. Neurosurg., *47:* 218–227, 1977.

33. Hood, T. W., Gebarski, S. S., McKeever, P. E., *et al.* Stereotaxic biopsy of intrinsic lesions of the brain stem. J. Neurosurg., *65:* 172–176, 1986.

34. Huang, Y. P., and Wolf, B. S. The veins of the posterior fossa—superior or Galenic draining group. A.J.R., 95 (1965), 808–821.

35. Huang, Y. P., and Wolf, B. S. Precentral cerebellar vein in angiography. Acta Radiol (Diagn.) (Stockh.), *5:* 250–262, 1966.

36. Huang, Y. P., Wolf, B. S. Angiographic features of fourth ventricle tumors with special

reference to the posterior inferior cerebellar artery. A.J.R., *107:* 543–564, 1969.

37. Huang, Y. P., Wolf, B. S., Antin, S. P., *et al.* The veins of the posterior fossa, anterior or petrosal draining group. A.J.R., *104:* 36–56, 1968.

38. Huang, Y. P., Wolf, B. S., and Okudera, T. Angiographic anatomy of the inferior vermian vein of the cerebellum. Acta Radiol. (Diagn.) (Stockh.), *9:* 327–344, 1969.

39. Isamat, F. Tumours of the posterior part of the third ventricle: neurosurgical criteria. Adv. Tech. Stand. Neurosurg., *6:* 171–184, 1979.

40. Kahn, E. A., Crosby, E. L., and DeJonge, B. R. Tumors of the posterior fossa. In: *Correlative Neurosurgery,* edited by E. A. Kahn *et al.* Springfield, Ill., Charles C Thomas, 1969

41. Kelly, P. J., Alker, G. J., Jr., and Goerss, S. Computer-assisted stereotactic laser microsurgery for the treatment of intracranial neoplasms. Neurosurgery, *10:* 324–331, 1982.

42. Kelly, P. J., Alker, G. J., Jr., and Zoll, J. G. A microstereotactic approach to deep-seated arteriovenous malformations. Surg. Neurol., *17:* 260–262, 1982.

43. Kelly, P. J., Kall, B., Goerss, S., *et al.* Precision resection of intra-axial CNS lesions by CT-based stereotactic craniotomy and computer monitored CO_2 laser. Acta Neurochir. (Wien), *68:* 1–9, 1983.

44. Kelly, P. J., Kall, B. A., and Goerss, S. G. Computed assisted stereotactic biopsies utilizing CT and digitized arteriographic data. Acta Neurochir. Suppl. (Wien), *33:* 233–235, 1984.

45. Kempe, L. G., and Blaylock, R. Lateral trigonal intraventricular tumors. A new operative approach. Acta Neurochir. (Wien), *35:* 233–242, 1976.

46. King, T. T. Removal of intraventricular craniopharyngiomas through the lamina terminalis. Acta Neurochir. (Wien), *45:* 277–286, 1979.

47. Krause, F. Operative Freilegung der Vierhugel nebst Beobachtungen uber Hirndruck und Dekompression. Zentrachl. Chr., *53:* 2812–2819, 1926.

48. Kurze, T. Approaches to the incisura. Clin. Neurosurg., *25:* 700–716, 1978.

49. Lassiter, K. R. L., Alexander, E., Jr., Davis, C. H., *et al.* Surgical treatment of brain stem gliomas. J. Neurosurg., *34:* 719–725, 1971.

50. Lassman, L. P. Tumours of the pons and medulla oblongata. In: *Tumours of the Brain and Skull,* Part II, *Handbook of Clinical Neurology,* vol. 17, edited by P. J. Vinken and G. W. Bruyn, pp. 693–706. North-Holland, Amsterdam, 1974.

51. Lassman, L. P., and Arjona, V. E. Pontile gliomas of childhood. Lancet, *i:* 913–915, 1967.

52. Lavyne, M. H., Patterson, R. H., Jr. Subchoroidal trans-velum interpositom approach to mid third ventricular tumors. Neurosurgery, *12:* 86–94, 1983.

53. Laws, E. R., Jr., Taylor, W. F., Marvin, B. C., *et al.* Neurosurgical management of low-grade astrocytoma of the cerebral hemispheres. J. Neurosurg., *61:* 665–673, 1984.

54. Lazorthes, G., Bastide, G., Roulleau, J., *et al.* Les artères du thalamus. Verhandlungen des I Europaishen Anatomische Anzeiger. *Erzanzung Zum, 109:* 828–831, 1960/1961.

55. Leksell, L. Stereotactic radiosurgery. J. Neurol. Neurosurg. Psychiatry, *46:* 797–803, 1983.

56. Long, D. M., and Chou, S. N. Transcallosal removal of craniopharyngiomas within the third ventricle. J. Neurosurg., *39:* 563–567, 1973.

57. McKissock, W. The surgical treatment of colloid cyst of the third ventricle. A report based upon twenty-one personal cases. Brain, *74:* 1–9, 1951.

58. Matson, D. D. *Neurosurgery of Infancy and Childhood,* ed. 2. Charles C Thomas, Springfield, Ill., 1969.

59. Mercuri, S., Russo, A., and Palma, L. Hemispheric supratentorial astrocytomas in children. Long-term results in 29 cases. J. Neurosurg., *55:* 170–173, 1981.

60. Mundinger, F., Birg, W., and Ostertag, C. B. Treatment of small cerebral gliomas with CT-aided stereotaxic Curie-therapy. Neuroradiology, 16: 564–567, 1978.
61. Ostertag, C. B., Mennel, H. D., and Kiessling, M. Stereotactic biopsy of brain tumors. Surg. Neurol., 14: 275–283, 1980.
62. Palma, L., and Guidetti, B. Cystic pilocytic astrocytomas of the cerebral hemispheres. J. Neurosurg., 62: 811–815, 1985.
63. Patterson, Jr., R. H., and Danylevich, A. Surgical removal of craniopharyngiomas by a transcranial approach through the lamina terminalis and sphenoid sinus. Neurosurgery, 7: 111–117, 1980.
64. Pendl, G. Pineal and Midbrain Lesions. Berlin, Springer, 1985.
65. Pendl, G., and Koos, W. Microsurgery of brainstem tumours in childhood and adolescence: A review of past experience. Adv. Neurosurg., 8: 403–408, 1980.
66. Pendl, G., Koos, W., and Witzmann, A. Infratentorial supracerebellar approach to pineal and mesencephalic region in children. Adv. Neurosurg., 11: 263–269, 1983.
67. Phelps, M., Mazziotta, J., and Schelbert, H. Positron Emission Tomography and Autoradiography: Principles and Applications for the Brain and Heart. Raven Press, New York, 1986.
68. Raimondi, A. J., and Gutierrez, F. A. Diagnosis and surgical treatment of choroid plexus papillomas. Child's Brain, 1: 81–115, 1975.
69. Rand, R. W. Transfrontal transsphenoidal craniotomy in pituitary and related tumors. In: Microneurosurgery, edited by R. W. Rand, pp. 93–104. St Louis, Mosby, 1978.
70. Rand, R. W., Lemmen, L. J. Tumors of the posterior portion of the third ventricle. J. Neurosurg., 10: 1–18, 1953.
71. Rhoton, A. L., Yamamoto, I., and Peace, D. A. Microsurgery of the third ventricle. Part 2. Operative approaches. Neurosurgery, 8: 357–373, 1981.
72. Saeki, N., Rhoton, A. L., Jr. Microsurgical anatomy of the upper basilar artery and the posterior circle of Willis. J. Neurosurg. 46: 563–578, 1977.
73. Shelden, C. H., McCann, G., Jacques, S., et al. Development of a computerized microstereotaxic method for localization and removal of minute CNS lesions under direct 3-D vision. Technical report. J. Neurosurg., 52: 21–27, 1980.
74. Shucart, W. A., and Stein, B. M. Transcallosal approach to the anterior ventricular system. Neurosurgery, 3: 339–343, 1978.
75. Stein, B. M. Supracerebellar approach for pineal region neoplasms. In Current Techniques in Operative Neurosurgery, edited H. H. Schmidek and W. H. Sweet, pp. 257–264. Grune & Stratton, New York, 1977.
76. Stein, B. M. Transcallosal approach to third ventricle tumors. In: Current Techniques in Operative Neurosurgery, edited by H. H. Schmidek and W. H. Sweet, pp. 247–255. Grune & Stratton, New York, 1977.
77. Steiner, L., Leksell, L., Greitz, T., Forster, D. M. C., and Backlund, E. O. Acta Chirurg. Scand., 133: 459, 1972.
78. Sweet, W. H., Talland, G. A., Ervin, F. R. Loss of recent memory following section of the fornix. Trans. Am. Neurol. Assoc., 84: 76–82, 1959.
79. Symon, L. The temporal approach for resection of craniopharyngioma. In: Operative Surgery: Neurosurgery, edited by L. Symon. Butterworth, London, 1979.
80. Takahashi, M., Wetson, G., and Hanafee, W. The anterior-inferior cerebellar artery. Its radiographic anatomy and significance in the diagnosis of extraaxial tumors of the posterior fossa. Radiology, 90: 281–287, 1968.
81. Talairach, J., Szikla, G., Tournoux, P., et al. Therapeutic uses of radioisotopes. International Congress Series, II International Congress of Neurological Surgery, Washington, D.C., 1961.
82. Tomita, T. Surgical management of cerebellar peduncle lesions in children. Neurosur-

gery, *18:* 568–575, 1986.
83. Wolf, B. S., Huang, Y. P., and Neuna, C. M. The lateral anastomotic mesencephalic vein and other variations in drainage of the basal cerebral vein. A.J.R., *89:* 411–422, 1963.
84. Yamamoto, I., and Kageyama, N. Microsurgical anatomy of the pineal region. J. Neurosurg., *53:* 205–221, 1980.
85. Yamamoto, I., Rhoton, A. L., and Peace, D. A. Microsurgery of the third ventricle. Part I. Microsurgical anatomy. Neurosurgery, *8:* 334–356, 1981.
86. Yaşargil, M. G. *Microneurosurgery*, vol. I. Stuttgart, Thieme, 1984.
87. Yaşargil, M. G. *Microneurosurgery*, vol. II. Stuttgart, Thieme, 1984.
88. Yaşargil, M. G. *Microneurosurgery*, vol. III. Stuttgart, Thieme, in press, 1987.
89. Zeal, A. A., and Rhoton, A. L. Microsurgical anatomy of the posterior cerebral artery. J. Neurosurg., *48:* 534–559, 1978.
90. Zimmerman, R. A., Bilaniuk, L. T., Johnson, M. H., *et al.* MRI of central nervous system: Early clinical results. *AJNR 7:* 587–594, 1986.

5

Survival of Neurosurgery in Changing Legal and Economic Times

DONALD H. STEWART, Jr., M.D.

INTRODUCTION

A number of years ago, several people decreed that neurosurgery would die. The strange thing is that it hasn't. Neurosurgery is alive and flourishing—it is different now than it was in the past, and we can say with certainty that we will witness great changes in the future. Neurosurgery will definitely survive; the only question is: How will we as Neurosurgeons cope with and manage the changes?

To answer this, it may be of interest to think about the rather phenomenal changes which have taken place in the past 30 years and to look ahead in three areas which you have recently listed in a poll conducted by the Joint Public Information Committee of the American Association of Neurological Surgeons (AANS) and the Congress of Neurological Surgeons (CNS) to be of critical importance in the next 10–15 years. They are medical liability, manpower, and reimbursement.

First, what was our specialty like only 30 years ago—in 1956? There were fewer than 1000 neurosurgeons in the U.S. There were no Taveras chairs for pneumoencephalograms, and three-picture angiograms were the rule. Computed tomographic (CT) scans and magnetic resonance imaging (MRI) scans had not been developed. Dexamethasone was not used. The microscope and its good lighting systems were not commonplace. Neurosurgeons spent most nights looking through small burr holes for surface clots. Residents spent the better part of each day doing myelograms, angiograms, and pneumoencephalograms. Colloid cysts were difficult to diagnose. Operations often took 12 hours in skilled hands. Brains were always swelling out of the box, and morbidity was real and everyday. Neurosurgery was demanding intellectually, physically, and emotionally. Neurosurgeons were tough, so tough that one wag said she would never cease to be amazed at how nice they all were to each other when they came together at meetings. Clinics were run by volunteer staff, and patients had uneven access to care. The Federal and State governments had not entered the picture with respect to payment for services. Research techniques were crude by the standards of today. Deoxyribonucleic acid (DNA) had just been synthesized. We knew of only two neurotransmitters. Neurobiology at the submolecular level was truly embryonic. There was no Joint Council of State Neurosurgical Societies and no Socioeconomic Committee for neurosurgery.

Twenty years later in the mid 1970s, neurosurgeons had begun to demand and create an organizational structure that would meet their rapidly changing needs. Dr. Richard Schneider, in his 1975 presidential address to the AANS, said that the three major concerns of neurosurgery were Education, Manpower, and Professional Medical Liability. He saw the need for neurosurgery to swallow a bitter birth control pill and suggested that it would not be unreasonable for the legal profession, which at that time was producing 30,000 new lawyers a year, to consider similar action. In the next 11 years we created 1300 new neurosurgeons and about 360,000 additional lawyers. He went on to suggest that the battle for Neurosurgery might be lost if in the socioeconomic storms swirling about us we failed to maintain our surgical skills, medical knowledge, and empathy in treating the sick (13).

At about the same time Dr. Robert Ojemann, your past president and current president of the AANS, suggested in his presidential address to this organization that government regulation of medicine was imminent (9). Today, a decade later, we find that it is not only the Federal government but also the private sector—the big corporation—which seek to regulate our daily activities.

MEDICAL LIABILITY

Let us first look at medical liability. There is no question that we are citizens of a highly litigious society. We are trying to make a NO RISK society in which no one assumes any personal risk or, as stated by Frank Trippett in *Time* magazine, we are striving for a utopia "that is free, if not of risks, then of all individual responsibility for those taken and lost" (16). Serious problems have developed with respect to availability and cost of insurance to pay for claims arising from such a system. In addition we are beginning to witness a serious impairment and a disintegration of our treasured social institutions.

In 1985 approximately 50% of 205 Neurosurgeons polled in New York State had been sued at least once in the previous 12 months, and some had been sued 3 times. At that time the cost of medical liability insurance ranged from $30,000 to $62,000. Today the cost of that insurance is about $50,000 per year for Upstate Neurosurgeons and slightly over $100,000 per year near New York City. The costs are higher than a year ago, as they are in most states, because of a failure of the legislative process to adequately address the issues.

Perhaps lessons can be learned from a reform effort which was started by Neurosurgeons and other high risk specialists in New York State. One year ago physicians in New York realized that they were too few in number to warrant any specific attention from the legislature regarding Tort reform. As a result, they developed a strategy which would attract the attention of the public.

It worked! The strategy was directed to influence the only institutions which depended upon physicians—the hospitals. Some physicians indicated that they would no longer take on new patients and thus would admit fewer patients to hospitals. Some chose to move their practice across State lines. Some chose selectively to admit patients only to government-supported hospitals. No attempt was made to curtail emergency services. The hospitals perceived, as a result of these varied activities, that they were in trouble: either their occupancy and income would go down and stress their ability to maintain payrolls, or they would be overwhelmed with work which they could not handle as an institution. Suddenly the Hospital Association, the Boards of Directors of Hospitals, the news media, the people and, finally, the legislators and the Governor perked up their ears. They all perceived that the Institution of the Hospital was threatened. The goal of this agitation was to get the Legislature to enact laws which would significantly change the Tort system.

As a result of this perceived threat to what are considered valued social institutions, the Attorney General of New York actually threatened antitrust suits against several physicians, and there were rumors abounding of telephone surveillance by the Attorney General. This stopped the very effective lobbying effort for reform of the Tort system. As a result no significant changes in the law were made.

However, in the U.S. as a whole there has been a significant beginning to reform of the Tort system, and more reforms will come because the public will demand change. People are slowly but surely coming to the realization that their institutions are beginning to fail. Social service organizations dedicated to providing essential services are threatened by the costs of "protection." Your voluntary dollars are being used to pay premiums rather than support programs. These premiums are used to pay a very small segment of society and their advocates. In New York State in 1985 approximately $720,000,000 was collected by physicians and hospitals from 20,000,000 people and was paid mainly to nonprofit insurance companies for medical liability insurance. This money will be used to indemnify about 2000 alleged victims of malpractice—but the majority of that money will be paid to lawyers. Schools are not able to offer many sports programs and after-school events. A family-owned company no longer rents small boats because in the event of an accident the assumption is that the lessee will attack the lessor, and the protection money is prohibitive for the company.

Millions of people in business, in voluntary organizations, and in government have finally begun to realize that the system put in place by lawyer legislators, despite our objections, is destroying the fabric of our institutions. What we need is a victims committee for the voters. I say it is time to stand up and say: "Enough." It is time to say to these lawyer representing legislators that we will no longer tolerate legislative initiatives which allow a very real form of terrorism in society to flourish. As George Will suggested, the attempt to make social policy by litigation rather than legislation has evaded the democratic due process and further diminished society's already attenuated belief in individual responsibility (16).

California is perhaps ahead of us all in many respects. If the legislature does not express the will of the people, then by a referendum the will of the people can override the legislators' disregard of the will of the voters. This phenomenon was responsible for changing laws dealing with the theory of joint and several liability. Not all states enjoy this democratic tool.

Major educational institutions, particularly those which are privately funded, have begun to realize the terrible impact of liability premiums on their own budgets. Their corporate power is tremendous, and the pressure for reform of the Tort system from this direction is welcome. As budget pressures are felt down the line in the University and as discretionary dollars in University departments dry up, University Neurosurgeons may make their voices heard more loudly in the fight for reform of the Tort system.

Our society is finally beginning to understand that it cannot expect to tolerate a NO RISK SOCIETY and the accompanying social terrorism where just about anyone can hold anyone else hostage with the help of a lawyer—unless it also accepts the concept of unlimited costs, taxation, and the serious impairment of social and cultural institutions which it holds to be of value.

Rabbi Michael Ross, in a letter to the *Wall Street Journal* in July 1986, said: "For millennia my people have correctly understood the concept of an eye for an eye as meaning not more than an eye. The simple meaning is that the punishment for any liability should not exceed the actual damage. In today's legal climate the concepts of deep pocket defendants and obscenely large punitive judgements are finally being shown for the primitive vengeance that they are" (11).

The situation is critical. If changes do not occur in the malpractice mess, Neurosurgeons will become so careful that they will not take on high risk problems. They will flee from the emergency rooms and place cost-benefit concerns above quality service. It will be a sad day, as John Cooper said in another context at a Duke University symposium, if "competition to survive replaces competition to serve."

The worst scenario would be one in which our profession fails to attract the best and the brightest to its ranks. I am concerned that unless we reverse the "NO RISK" syndrome, the adversarial climate, and the obscene cost of insurance, the best and the brightest will choose not to become part of the cadre of Neurosurgeons. It is important that each of you take a stand and work for changes in the Tort system. The profession as we know it will depend on your efforts.

MANPOWER

Many of the questions relating to your second concern, manpower, have been aired quite sufficiently at a symposium sponsored by the Joint Council of State Neurosurgical Societies. There is no question that the number of Neurosurgeons in this country has increased despite the recommendations of our Manpower Commission and the admonitions of Dr. Schneider in the 1970s. No single person or institution has the power to alter the policy of manpower production. Any future changes may ultimately be dependent on economic factors. No one who has a well-established system in place wants to be told that it has to be changed. The graduates of various Neurosurgical Training Programs seem to be getting jobs, presumably of their liking, which is probably a good indicator of the need for their services. Only when there are no jobs will the program directors think that there are too many Neurosurgeons. As competition for neurosurgical cases increases and as department budgets are cut, full-time faculty are moving to assure income for themselves and their departments. This pressure for cash flow and patients could ultimately change the concept of the need for new trainees and the relationship between Neurosurgeons.

Today in 1986 I see several issues at the center of public policy debate on manpower. To many policy makers, the issue is marketplace competition. They see the increase in numbers of Neurosurgeons as positive for the consumer because, theoretically, this should drive prices down. To others the problem is distribution, not numbers. This school of thought urges larger numbers in order to increase access to care. Other policy makers are of the opinion that, as the numbers of Neurosurgeons increase, the cumulative general clinical experience of the individual Neurosurgeon will decrease because he or she will be doing less clinical work. They urge subspecialization as an answer to the decreased availability of a general practice of Neurosurgery.

Perhaps we should seriously pursue the suggestion made by this author to seek an objective third party to study manpower and its relationship to quality Neurosurgery (15). The Washington Committee negotiated with the prestigious Brookings Institute to do just that. For the moment, the Brookings Institute is unable to undertake the study. I do not think we should be deterred. Perhaps we should explore an arrangement with the Robert Wood Johnson Foundation or the Rand Corporation. This effort can build upon our earlier Manpower Commission report and the Graduate Medical Education National Advisory Council (GMENAC) report.

I also think that we should seriously discuss the option of open discussions with the Federal Trade Commission (FTC) about the restraint of trade issue. Merely to assume an adversarial position with the FTC is not in our best interest. Such discussions could lead to an examination of issues of economics and quality of care and could result in an FTC "advisory" which could sort out the fiction and fact.

REIMBURSEMENT

The third concern of Neurosurgeons in the U.S. at the present time is reimbursement. It may not be unreasonable to be concerned about this since in many parts of the country the cost of liability insurance just to open the office door is more than $100,000—a sum which exceeds the annual salary of a United States Senator. However we should remind ourselves of the words of Dr. Arnold Relman: "The essence of being a doctor is not to make money. The essence of being a doctor is to serve the patient ... If doctors don't carry around with them all the time a keen sense of their moral commitment to patients and to society, they can't be good doctors ..." (10).

Whether we like it or not a new, disturbing era has arrived for physicians. It is termed an era of competition and is hailed as a period of awakening of the marketplace to the economics of medical care. It appears that a Health Care System which worked reasonably well has been put into a box and is being shaken fairly hard with the intent to disassemble, reorganize, and modify it severely, but not necessarily for the benefit of the sick. No one has ever proven that the rapidly proliferating new systems which are supposed to be competitive for purchasers and profits in the health care marketplace are the best systems for the patient. They may turn out to be beneficial only for their managers, supermanagers, and stockholders. Dr. Eli Ginzberg, a thoughtful person, has suggested that the current pursuit of the illusion of competition as the savior of a system that in fact doesn't need saving but only modest adjustment is going to prove a disappointing course (6). The final result is difficult to predict, other than to state that there will be a substantially changed system.

Most institutions change slowly, and any institution which consumes $400,000,000,000 ($400 billion!) per year will obviously change very slowly. We are at least fortunate in our country to have maintained a relatively pluralistic approach to the delivery of health care, and it would appear that we have a good mix of private and public sector involvement as discussed by John Lister in his 1986 Shattuck Lecture (8). Both systems seek to reduce the rate of increase of health care expenditures. Both have placed physician reimbursement reform as a top priority.

Regulating compensation for physicians is more difficult for the public sector than the private sector. The government can decrease payments to physicians; however, it runs the risk of alienating physicians and large numbers of voter/purchasers of Medicare insurance if it reduces the payment level so low that the providers refuse to participate.

Government must be careful that it does not deny access to health care for the people it represents. For example, money paid by the State of New York to a Neurosurgeon for rendering the most complex care to a Medicaid recipient is less than the amount of money that the physician must pay for the medical liability insurance for that particular patient. In this circumstance there is no incentive for the physician to participate in the program. Some Neurosurgeons have offered to provide free care to Medicaid recipients in return for the State paying for the liability costs incurred by this group of people. So far, no interest has been shown by the Governor in such a proposal.

Presently there is a crescendo of activity on the part of government to explore and develop new ways to pay physicians. In Canada, the Ontario parliament recently outlawed extra billing. This removed legally, and for political reasons, a contractual freedom that physicians had traditionally enjoyed (4). In Massachusetts the courts have ruled that unless a physician accepts assignment in his dealings with Medicare patients who are partially Federally supported, then he or she may not have a license issued by the State to practice medicine! This apparent coercion and indenturement of physicians by a government that espouses competition in the marketplace is perhaps opening the door in that State for the necessity of a union to represent these quasiemployees. Up to this point unions have not been legal for self-employed physicians. Without certification as a union by the National Labor Relations Board a group of physicians cannot compel any collective negotiations, and its members run the risk of antitrust violations (3).

In our country the customary, prevailing, and reasonable payment method is being dismantled rapidly by both private and public initiatives. Different levels of payment for similar services, depending upon whether or not the physician agrees to accept assignment, is one option being considered. Others are national reimbursement levels for certain procedures and services. A recalculation of the Medicare Economic Index has been proposed. Capitation payments by the government to a physician, or to a Health Maintenance Organization (HMO), or to any other health care care delivery system are being considered. Under such a system the organization receiving the capitation payment may pay the provider in a variety of ways. This could include fee for service, capitation, salary, or profit sharing. The development of a Resource-Based Relative Value Scale is at present a very active project of the Health Care Financing Administration. The payment of assistants at surgery and regional fee variations are also being studied. The difficulties of using a Current Procedural Terminology (CPT) to define payment units for physicians are being addressed. The problems associated with bundling and unbundling of procedures are vexing.

Organized Neurosurgery under the leadership of the AANS and CNS has representatives or liaison persons involved in the discussion of most of these questions. This is being done through a variety of contacts with government, AMA, and other specialty groups. We should strive to obtain the requisite financial support and public policies which will guarantee the continued availability of high quality neurosurgical services.

The background paper on Neurosurgery prepared by the Harvard School of Public Health in June of 1986 for use by the Commission to develop a Resource-Based Relative Value Scale noted that 18% of a Neurosurgeon's income in 1982 came from Medicare and 8% from medicaid sources (11). Seventy-four percent (74%) came from other sources. This suggests that changes made in reimbursement schedules by the private sector, not the public sector, will have the greatest effect on the income of the Neurosurgeon.

It is clear that the for-profit health care enterprises are successful and growing rapidly (7). We are all familiar with the Humana Corporation, a company called National Medical Enterprises, and the entry of various insurance companies into the business of owning HMOs. These businesses face an ethical consideration regarding access to health care, but their special interests do not easily translate into public interests (5). We may well be entering an era in which cost-benefit analysis of health care will override concerns for quality care and access.

The private sector's plan to reduce the cost of health care seems an admirable goal from a public relations perspective. It is in fact striving to redistribute money in order to provide income for health care managers and stockholders or to shore up the failing steel and transportation industries. The three top executives of the National Medical Enterprises, according to a report in the *Los Angeles Times* in September of 1985, received a total of $21 million in compensation for their services (14). The senior executives of other large health care corporations are also not doing badly even by these standards. These individuals and companies state that they are committed to quality health care, but the stockholders do expect a profit, and management skill must be compensated (12).

The marketing of our own services or those of the smaller institutions in which some of us work is manifested by the various letterheads which we use. These quite clearly indicate our specific interests which are directly related to the securing of business and, thus, of income. Even large service institutions have letterheads indicating that they serve as international resources. Some of these institutions are branching out and setting up satellite clinics. They too are concerned with quality care, but they are also concerned with making money. Competition for the opportunity to take care of the sick means increasingly that the operation must take on the trappings of a business. The individual Neurosurgeon can compete with another Neurosurgeon but not so easily with institutional competitors.

Neither the government nor the private sector will be the advocate for the Neurosurgeon's income, as they have other priorities. The Neurosurgeon must become knowledgeable about the specifics of compensation, and he or she must not fail to pay close attention to them. Will Neurosurgeons stand together on these issues, or will they be fragmented and go their own separate ways? Organizations like the CNS and AANS should take very active leadership roles, as they are beginning to do, in order to represent their membership in economic and legal political matters. The critical need for a strong, representative organization of Neurosurgeons has never been more acute.

Thus in these circumstances a fine balancing act by the Neurosurgeon is necessary. On the one hand is a drive to satisfy altruistic and intellectual forces. On the other hand are socioeconomic, legal, and political forces which must be addressed.

CONCLUSION

In the final analysis, the words of Dr. Carola Eisenberg of Harvard Medical School are pertinent:

> The satisfaction of being able to relieve pain and restore function, the intellectual challenge of solving clinical problems, and the variety of human issues we confront in daily clinical practice will remain the essence of doctoring, whatever the changes in the organizational and economic structure of medicine.... If we focus on our primary responsibilities to serve as advocates for our patients, we will both maintain our professional integrity and provide the leadership for a broad public coalition in defense of health care (2).

ACKNOWLEDGMENT

I would like to thank my wife, Anne, for her good judgment, humor, and editorial assistance, which contributed greatly to this paper.

REFERENCES

1. Background Paper on Neurosurgery for Technical Consulting Panel Meetings. Cambridge, Mass., Harvard University School of Public Health, June 11 and 12, 1986.
2. Eisenberg, C. It is still a priviledge to be a doctor. N. Engl. J. Med., *314:* 1113–1114, 1986.
3. Foy, D. J. Should the Medical Society of the State of New York Form a Union? N.Y. State J. Med., *86:* 288–289, 1986.
4. Frum, D. Canada Puts Heat on 'Coldhearted' Doctors, *Wall Street Journal*, p. 17, Aug. 22, 1986.
5. Gamarekian, B. A Lobbyists Quest for Editorial Ink, *New York Times*, A14, July 30, 1986.
6. Ginzberg, E. Is Cost Containment for Real? J.A.M.A., *256:* 254–255, 1986.
7. Gray, B. H., and McNerney, W. J. For-Profit Enterprise in Health Care. The Institute of Medicine Study. N. Engl. J. Med., *314:* 217–222, 1986.
8. Lister, J. Shattuck Lecture—The politics of medicine in Britain and the United States. N. Engl. J. Med., *315:* 168–174, 1986.
9. Ojemann, R. G., Presidential Address: "Moving Ahead." Clin. Neurosurg., *24:* 1–8, 1977.
10. Relman, A. Confessions of a worried doctor. Yankee Magazine, *50:* 84–87, 132–137, 1986.
11. Ross, M. Limits of Justice. *Wall Street Journal*, p. 27, July 1, 1986.
12. Rundle, R. L. American Medical International to Cut Staff, Close Insurer in Reorganization, *Wall Street Journal*, p. 8, August 25, 1986.
13. Schneider, R. C. The 1975 AANS Presidential Address: The "future trends" in neurosurgery are here. J. Neurosurg., *43:* 651–660, 1975.
14. Shiver, J. Job Prognosis Favorable in Health-Care Industry, *Los Angeles Times*, p. 7, September 29, 1985.
15. Stewart, D. H. Presidential Address: "Quality and Neurosurgery." Clin. Neurosurg. pp. 3–12. Williams & Wilkins, Baltimore, 1982.
16. Will, G. F. The "I'm entitled" spirit. In: *The Pursuit of Virtue and Other Tory Notions*, pp. 94–96. Simon & Schuster, New York, 1982.

II

Cerebrovascular Surgery

6

The Future of Carotid Endarterectomy: a Neurologist's Point of View

JOHN P. CONOMY, M.D.

Why should it be that a condition which is rationally demonstrated to be connected with the production of symptoms of disease, that condition being subject to diagnostic illumination and therapeutic correction by safe means, be a subject of perennial controversy? Why should a surgical operation which is capable of postponing or preventing neurological catastrophe be the subject of irresolute debate? Such is the case with carotid endarterectomy. Controversy, at times heated, occasionally instructive, has been the fate of the carotid endarterectomy since its inception. I suspect that its future will, like its past, be marked by debate and seasoned with study and learned discourse. The present, and perhaps the future of carotid endarterectomy, is marked at times with polemics, acrimony, the shedding of more heat than light about the subject, along with allegations of ill-performance and overabundant use (2, 11). Those who are proponents of the procedure will need to continue to contend with those who legitimately, and as a result of more or less scientific inquiry, contend that symptoms of carotid arterial insufficiency are either not connected, or are only connected in some convoluted way, with carotid stenosis or occlusion; that carotid arterial bruits have a negligible importance in the genesis of stroke; that the procedure of carotid endarterectomy is too often needlessly and unsafely performed; that it does not protect its subjects from stroke; and that the entire experience of carotid endarterectomy constitutes a highly undesirable societal dollar cost. The proponents of carotid endarterectomy have no choice it seems but a good defense of their actions in behalf of this procedure.

It seems to me that the future of carotid endarterectomy should be guided by the answers to the following questions: (*a*) Is the procedure rational? (*b*) Is it safe? (*c*) Is it effective? (*d*) Are its benefits greater than its costs and risks? These questions open the portals of the myriad other inquiries, some of which I hope to address in the course of this chapter.

IS CAROTID ENDARTERECTOMY A RATIONAL PROCEDURE?

There are those who would argue, with no little justification, that carotid endarterectomy is a rational procedure if it works, that is, if it prevents stroke and stroke's concomitant death and disability (5). That argument, however, confuses rationality with efficacy, and the two are not the same. Justification based on risk-benefit analysis is another view of efficacy and does not analyze the causal relationship between disease expression and its pathophysiologic basis. Rationale for carotid endarterectomy is demonstrated first of all by demonstration that carotid stenosis and occlusion are related to stroke and that the surgical procedure removes the cause, preempting a morbid effect.

Apoplexy was known to Hippocrates and probably to physicians before him. It seems to me a wonder of recorded human history that nearly 5 millenia elapsed before the condition of apoplexy and its relation to stenosis and occlusion of the carotid arteries was firmly pieced together. The clinicopathological work of C. M. Fisher in Canada and the U.S. (14), Yates and Hutchinson in Great Britain (36), and Lhermitte, Gautier, and Derouesne in France (21) was significant in establishing the causal links. That carotid endarterectomy was performed in 1953 was a logical extension of the established relationship between carotid arterial obstruction and cerebral hemispheric attacks. Given this unclouded point of view, carotid endarterectomy is a rational procedure. There are a number of facts, however, which serve to challenge this rational consideration. First, there is the haunting but unavoidable realization that carotid stenosis and occlusion occur innocuously. Secondly, some operated arteries occlude sooner and more later, with or without the production of neurological deficits (25, 26, 31). Thirdly, stroke occurs even in patients whose carotid endarterectomy is a surgical success.

If rational basis of carotid endarterectomy is to be considered it seems to me that reasoning about the issue needs to be extended to define not only under what abstract circumstances carotid stenosis leads to stroke, but also to which specific patients that set of circumstances pertains. The rational process must not cover the logic of the surgical procedure, but the selection of patients in whom it might be performed.

THE ISSUE OF CAROTID BRUITS

Vascular noises in the neck come from a variety of sources: vascular hyperdynamic states, thyroid disorders, venous hums, and transmitted cardiac noises, to cite the common ones. Once the bruit is demonstrated to be of carotid origin (the pitch increasing with the degree of stenosis, a crescendo-decrescendo quality to the bruit and extension of the rumble into diastole), some degree of carotid stenosis can reasonably be suspected. For some, indeed for many, the presence of carotid noise is an invitation to some imaging procedure, ordinarily an angiogram, and if this is abnormal, a surgical operation. This sequence of events frequently involves an asymptomatic person, or a person also symptomless who is to undergo some high-risk surgical procedure. It is in this category of individual that the risks of the surgical procedure are more clear than the potential benefits (6), at least in my own view of the situation and the view of some others (15, 22, 35). Some have expressed the view that auscultation of the neck should be avoided because it "leads us into temptation but does not deliver us from evil" (20). I believe that that is going too far. The neck of patients should be ausculated as part of the neurological examination, but my own belief is that the cervical bruit should be pursued only in those patients whose bruit is correlated with symptoms or clear compounding risk. To those who would argue vigorously that asymptomatic carotid stenosis should routinely be operated or that prophylactic carotid endarterectomy is effective in stroke prevention, I would answer politely that vigor does not constitute evidence and that evidence is not necessarily proof. A last word regarding carotid bruit. As I labor in an institution where bruits are abundant and vascular illnesses are the order of the day, I have come to regard carotid bruit as an excellent clue to the presence of coronary heart disease. A carotid bruit is a tip-off for a set of cardiac illnesses which are far more lethal to the cerebrovascular disease patient than is stroke itself (18).

IS CAROTID ENDARTERECTOMY SAFE?

If carotid endarterectomy is a rational procedure to be done in the context of rational patient selection, is the procedure a safe one? To answer this question, the same rational process must be applied to the establishment of acceptable risk, to risk minimization, and to the selection of a surgeon and that surgeon's operating team. In the individual case (and that is how candidates for this procedure appear) risk must not only be reflected against figures averaged from the "Poor Outcome" columns of several large, well-known, and widely quoted series, but also against the risks posed by the individual patient (28, 30). These risks include the patient's age, the degree of associated cardiovascular illnesses, the overall state of the cerebral circulation, associated medical conditions, the patient's wishes, and the consideration of the relative risks and benefits of alternative treatments. To these considerations must be added the surgeon's own record as an operator and the performance of the surgical care team. Clearly, the results of many studies disclose wide variation in surgical mortality and morbidity from surgeon to surgeon and from hospital to hospital (12, 25), with some disconsoling figures indicating mortal trouble as a result of operation at date that are some multiple of an order of magnitude greater than the widely used "Poor Outcome" figures of 2 or 3% (17, 31, 32). Given larger morbidity and mortality rates, to which are added the additional individual risks posed to any patient by the condition of his health, some may be better off bearing a stroke rate risk between 2 and 10% per year, and the additional risks posed by one or another form of medical treatment, than they are by the experience of carotid endarterectomy (6, 18, 34).

IS CAROTID ENDARTERECTOMY EFFECTIVE?

It is in this particular area that controversy is most abundant. In general the field has been populated by large numbers of believers and proponents who pit their statistical weapons against an increasingly voluble number of opponents and skeptics. Recently the media, economists, and politicians of some nations have joined the fray. It is becoming increasingly difficult and burdensome to make such sense of arguments regarding effectiveness given the sheer bulk of literature about the topic and the level of noise in the forum. Medical investigations point to the need for randomized, controlled studies to demonstrate both the effectiveness and attendant relative risks of carotid endarterectomy (6, 32). Such persons readily point to the large numbers of patients, the necessarily longer duration of such a study, the difficulty controlling a large number of variables, and the great cost of such an effort. If these things were not reason enough to adopt an alternative strategy for the demonstration of effectiveness and hazard, there are the additional problems of patient and surgeon bias, and ultimate distorted selection. A randomized, controlled study of patients who are somehow not typical of the problem regarding a procedure not done by typical surgeons is misrepresentative of the entire issue and, in the end, will satisfy few. These considerations are, of course, well known to everyone who has been involved in the debate regarding extracranial-intracranial (EC-IC) bypass (13).

What emerges from experience with carotid endarterectomy is the following guide regarding effectiveness, at least from this neurologist's point of view: there seems to be, in very good hands, a 2% mortality rate and 1–6% morbidity rate in patients who are well chosen and operated by experienced surgeons. When successful, carotid endarterectomy prevents transient ischemic attacks (TIA), and prevents stroke, at least for a reasonable period of time, in the distribution of the operated vessel. It does not obviate the stroke problem or cerebrovascular disease risk for the individual having undergone endarterectomy, or obviate the need for ongoing medical treatment with antiplatelet agents or occasionally with other drugs. Carotid endarterectomy does not appear to add years to life, but it clearly may add life to years (23). Patients having undergone carotid endarterectomy need continuing follow-up care not only for subsequent stroke and TIA, but also for coronary heart disease.

There are some factors which, it seems to me, render carotid endarterectomy ineffective and potentially unsafe. They include excessive numbers of operations performed upon the elderly sick; a blanket policy of operations made upon both asymptomatic and insignificant lesions; prophylactic endarterectomy in surgical patients done as a matter of policy; bilateral operations done at a single sitting; endarterectomies done for total occlusion of the vessel; endarterectomies done without angiographic documentation of cerebral circulation; endarterectomies done in patients whose cerebral substance is not known to be free of hemorrhage, tumor, or some other disease; and carotid endarterectomy done at the time of coronary heart surgery. Other conditions for which carotid endarterectomy is needlessly and therefore ineffectively and unsafely done are mentioned only to provide the opportunity to condemn carotid endarterectomy in their treatment. These conditions include, but are not limited to Alzheimer's disease, migraine headaches, multiple sclerosis, carotodynia, and dizziness.

The opportunity to participate in this symposium gave me an opportunity to review what has recently been published in the field of carotid endarterectomy, and I wish to share a small study of this current literature with you. The inquiry was limited to the years 1981 to the present and was accomplished through the Bibliographic Database of the National Library of Medicine. The French and English languages were searched, reflecting my own linguistic limitations. A matrix for database searching was constructed utilizing the following topics: endarterectomy, carotid arteries, carotid artery disease, risk in carotid endarterectomy, prognosis, outcome, late results, follow-up studies, economics, length of stay, and diagnostically related groups related to carotid endarterectomy. A total of 376 articles were identified. Of these, I felt 307 were pertinent to one of the categories below which can be viewed together as looking at where the interest in carotid endarterectomy lies among people who write about the subject. The breakout of topic areas among this literature is shown in Table 6.1.

The allocation of articles into categories was arbitrary but, I believe, fairly done. Some covered more than one topic, leaving me to decide which category was most prominently addressed. Those articles included in the general review category were in general written by vascular surgeons, vascular disease-oriented internists, neurologists, and neurosurgeons. They covered all categories listed above but almost without fail did not address economic issues. Articles dealing with economics were preponderantly authorized by health economists and others in the public

TABLE 6.1

Topic Areas among the French and English Medical Literature Regarding Carotid Endarterectomy (1981–Present)

Economic impact	1.3%
Diagnosis/diagnostic tests	12.4%
Cost-effectiveness/risk benefit	9.1%
Late results	9.8%
Natural history, carotid disease	16.9%
Surgical technique	26.0%
Patient selection	14.7%
Complications of surgery	4.9%
Randomized, controlled medical trials	<1.0%
Randomized surgical studies	<1.0%
General reviews	2.0%

health field, and relied heavily upon grouped epidemiological and financial data. Articles dealing with cost-effectiveness and risk-benefits analysis in carotid endarterectomy were more frequently the work of clinicians, frequently in conjunction with experts in statistics. The embarrassingly few (and given the magnitude of the problem, frighteningly small) randomized therapeutic studies generally had this same constellation of authorship. The publication of late results of carotid endarterectomy, good, bad or indifferent was the work of medical and surgical clinicians. Those articles addressing some aspect of the natural history of carotid arterial disease in the context of carotid endarterectomy were nearly always the work of neurologists and neurosurgeons, and comprised a healthy 16.9% of the publications reviewed. They generally included some suggestions for patient selection, often cautiously stated. The nearly 15% of papers dealing with patient selection, both positive and adverse, were more frequently the work of surgeons than others in the cerebrovascular disease field.

The largest number of articles appearing in this search had to do with surgical technique. Most of them dealt with methods of making the operation safer, at least in the author's opinion. Very frequently the point of these articles was an admonition to accompany the surgical procedure with some neurophysiological monitoring device. The electroencephalographic (EEG) cerebral blood flow (CBF) measurements, evoked response systems, and brain imaging systems figured prominently in this regard. The major contributors to this segment of the current literature were neurologists, neurosurgeons, and anesthesiologists. The literature concerning direct surgical complications comprised 5% of the National Library's bundle. While small in proportion, it attracts wide recognition. Everyone contributes to it. It would be interesting to search a major law library for the contribution of the public and the legal profession in this segment of the literature.

IS THERE A LEARNING CURVE IN THE SELECTION OF PATIENTS FOR CAROTID ENDARTERECTOMY?

In the late spring of 1984 I had the pleasure of serving as a panelist for a study of carotid endarterectomy performed at the Rand Corporation. The study was part of the U.S. government-financed Health Services Utilization Project which was led by Drs. Robert Brook, David Solomon, Mark Chassin, Nancy Merrick, and many other talented people. The project was initiated to study the reasons for significant variation in the performance of medical and surgical procedures, which in addition to carotid endarterectomy, included gastrointestinal endoscopy and coronary angiography (6) and coronary artery bypass graft surgery (8). It would appear that in the sample of Medicare recipients who were the objects of this study, there exists a manyfold difference in the likelihood of experiencing carotid endarterectomy, depending upon one's place of residence. There is, by the way, no manyfold difference in stroke rates based upon domiciliary locus in this country that I am able to ascertain. The impetus for the U. S. government in funding such a study is clear: the interest in the health of the country's citizens is accompanied by the obligation of the nation's Federal government to pay health care bills. I served with a panel of people, most far more expert than I, to see if at least among that group, we were able to reach a consensus regarding the indications for carotid endarterectomy under a variety of hypothetical circumstances, including symptomatic carotid bruit, transient ischemic attack (TIA), completed stroke with or without a completely occluded carotid artery, and in the circumstances of typical and atypical symptoms. We were also asked to consider the plight of persons who were to undergo a major surgical procedure. The panel was drawn from experts representing a variety of medical and surgical specialities. We reached a consensus over the issues involved in patient selection without much difficulty, a very heartening experience.

With the kind permission of the Rand Corporation study group, I obtained permission next to perform the following experiment: testing whether or not the advantages of education and experience played a role in the ability of physicians and surgeons to reach a consensus over the indications for surgery, whether or not that consensus was the same or different than that of a group of "experts" and whether the perceived indications changed as a function of training or experience. The Rand Corporation questionnaire was distributed to each member of the Departments of Neurosurgery and Neurology at the Cleveland Clinic Foundation on July 1, 1984, and the results were summarized in a Grand Rounds presentation of July 27 of that year. In this small and local study, the results were analyzed according to years of training or years of experience. Recall that some of our study sample had been versed in the clinical neurosciences for less than 30 days, and we may never have encountered a patient who presented a problem in decision-making regarding carotid endarterectomy.

The results of this local study demonstrated that our group, as a whole, presented a consensus indistinguishable from that supplied by the experts, which is both heartening and not surprising. We further concluded, based on our small sample, that the indications for carotid endarterectomy were not judged to be any differently by the first year residents than by their more seasoned colleagues. While a number of conclusions based upon this finding may be drawn, it is for me both surprising and disheartening to consider that we may, in the course of professional training, never modify our ideas regarding this procedure, or at least the indications for it, or instruct others to modify our ideas regarding this procedure, or at least the indications for it, or instruct others to modify theirs. I am further led to wonder whether a group of attentive laymen, given a clear and nonpejorative set of facts, may not reach the same conclusions regarding the indications for the performance of this surgical procedure as a more or less sophisticated medical and surgical group. I suspect that the reasons for the lack of demonstration of a "learning shift in our study had to do with the inherently controversial nature of the problem; the lack of help in decision-making reflecting an abundant, but conflictive medical literature; the necessity to appeal to the expressed belief of experts or their statistics who are not present at the bedside as we make decisions; and the negotiated nature of decision-making, including the powerful influence of local habit, as patients are chosen or not chosen for this procedure.

THE FUTURE OF CAROTID ENDARTERECTOMY: A NEUROLOGIST'S POINT OF VIEW

In my view carotid endarterectomy is a rational surgical procedure. In its employment, rational guidelines must extend to the selection of patients used and to the selection of surgeons and surgical teams who perform the procedure and care for patients undergoing it. Carotid endarterectomy is furthermore an effective procedure for the relief of stroke risk in the distribution of the operated vessel (16, 29). Beyond this, effectiveness needs to be proven by the rigorous collection of prospective data, randomized, controlled, or otherwise, as the procedure's future unfolds. The proof of this procedure's effectiveness and the assessment of its benefits and risks, its costs, and its savings cannot be served if among those operated on are patients who are ill-chosen, or if operations are performed under less than optimal circumstances.

The safety of carotid endarterectomy, as well as societal costs of the procedure, are matters which must be forthrightly addressed. The wide variations in geographic performance clearly merit further study. Institutions and individuals with high morbidity and mortality rates related to the procedure require peer review and educational correction. The technical safety of the procedure itself is constantly enhanced by incremental innovations in surgical technique and neurophysiologic monitoring, advances which need to be encouraged, to be tested and, if found efficacious, to be placed into practice.

It seems to me that the interest of current day American society in carotid endarterectomy has been spurred particularly by the issues of effectiveness, safety and cost. Both the public and the medical profession are being asked to inquire whether too many procedures are being done on too many patients by too many operators. Given the cost considerations, it is not difficult to imagine that some form of restraint, perhaps a kind of rationing, will befall the procedure, as is currently the case with efforts on the part of some State, Federal, and similar to other national policies regarding organ transplantation, purchases of large items of medical technology, and the like. Carotid endarterectomy has become a closely scrutinized procedure. Its performance and its hazards, its costs and its benefits merit banner front-page headlines in some of this nation's newspapers (3). Its utility is by no means any longer a matter of academic debate. Along with ocular lens implantation, arthroscopy, gastrointestinal endoscopy, coronary angiography, coronary heart surgery, and other "high volume-high cost procedures," carotid endarterectomy has come under public scrutiny. The national cost for the procedure, estimated to have been done 103,000 times in 1986, has been estimated to be at least $1.2 billion (10) (I believe the figure is too low). It takes the imagination to sense the reaction of the public, many physicians, surgeons, and others in the health care field, third party payers, and regulators who have been told that many of the procedures, perhaps up to 65% of them, are needlessly, uselessly, or badly done. If carotid endarterectomy is to endure, properly organized multiinstitutional studies regarding the rationale, safety, and efficacy of the procedure must be instituted. A strong suggestion that the procedure be done under conditions of proper patient selection by those with specific training, experience, and technical resources needs to be made. These efforts will, I believe, remove a perfectly good operation, properly employed, from the spectre of an imposed interdict.

ADDENDUM

Since the preparation of this manuscript the Rand Corporation publication regarding indications for carotid endarterectomy has appeared. The results may be found in Park, R. E., Fink, A., Brook, R., *et al. Physicians Ratings of Appropriate Indications for Six Medical and Surgical Procedures.* Santa Monica, Calif., The Rand Corporation.

REFERENCES

1. Barnes, R. W., Nix, M. L., Sansonetti, D., et al. Late outcome of untreated asymptomatic carotid disease following cardiovascular operations. J. Vasc. Surg., 2(6): 843–849, 1985.

2. Barnett, H. J. M., Plum, F., and Walton, J. N. Carotid endarterectomy—An expression of concern. Stroke, 15(6): 941–943, 1984.

3. Becker, B. "Study says to avert stroke could result in one," Cleveland Plain Dealer, p. 1, Friday, May 16, 1986.

4. Brott, T., and Thalinger, K. The practice of carotid endarterectomy in a large metropolitan area. Stroke, 15: 950–955, 1984.

5. Bunt, T. J., and Haynes, J. L. Carotid endarterectomy. One solution to the stroke problem. Am. Surg., 51(2): 61–69, 1985.

6. Chambers, B. R., and Norris, J. W. The case against surgery for asymptomatic carotid stenosis. Stroke, 15(6): 964–967, 1984.

7. Chassin, M. R., Kosecoff, Park, E., et al. Indications for Selected Medical and Surgical Procedures—A Literature Review and Ratings of Appropriateness. In: Coronary Angiography. Santa Monica, Calif., The Rand Corporation, 1986.

8. Chassin, M. R., Park, E. R., Fink, A., et al. Indications for Selected Medical and Surgical Procedures—A Literature Review and Ratings of Appropriateness. In: Coronary Artery Bypass Graft Surgery. Santa Monica, Calif., The Rand Corporation, 1986.

9. Donnan, G. A., Bladin, F. F., and Woodward, J. M. The extracranial-intracranial bypass study: How will the outcome affect us? Aust. NZ J Med. 15(3): 386–391.

10. Dyken, M. L. Carotid endarterectomy: A glimmering of science. Stroke, 17: 355–358, 1986.

11. Dyken, M. L., and Pokras, R. The performance of endarterectomy for disease of the extracranial arteries of the head. Stroke, 15(6): 948–950, 1984.

12. Easton, D., and Sherman, D. G. Stroke and mortality rate in carotid endarterectomy: 228 consecutive operations. Stroke, 8: 565–568, 1977.

13. The EC/IC Bypass Study Group. Failure of extracranial-intracranial arterial bypass to reduce the risk of ischemic stroke. Results of an international randomized trial. N. Engl. J. Med., 313(19): 1191–1200, 1985.

14. Fisher, C. M. Occlusion of the internal carotid artery. Arch. Neurol. Psychiatry, 69: 346, 1951.

15. Furlan, A., and Craciun, A. R. Risk of stroke during coronary artery bypass graft surgery in patients with internal carotid artery disease documented by angiography. Stroke, 16: 797–799, 1985.

16. Hertzer, N. R., and Arison, R. Cumulative stroke and survival ten years after carotid endarterectomy. J. Vasc. Surg., 2(5): 661–668, 1985.

17. Hertzer, N. R., Avellone, J. C., et al. The risk of vascular surgery in metropolitan community. With observations of surgeon experience and hospital size. J. Vasc. Surg., 1(1): 23–21, 1984.

18. Hertzer, N. R., and Lees, C. D. Fatal myocardial infarction following carotid endarterectomy: Three hundred thirty-five patients followed 6–11 years after operation. Ann. Surg., 194(2): 212–218, 1981.

19. Ivey, T. D., Strandness, D. E., and Williams, D. B. Management of patients with carotid bruit undergoing cardiopulmonary bypass (Abst.). J. Thorac. Cardiovasc. Surg., 87: 183–189, 1984.

20. Kuller, L. H., and Sutton, K. C. Carotid artery bruit: Is it safe and effective to auscultate the neck? Stroke, 15(6): 944–947, 1984.

21. Lhermitte, F., Gautier, J. C., and Derouesne, C., *et al.* Anatomie et pathophysiologie des stenoses caridiennes. *Rev Neurol* (Paris), *115:* 641, 1966.
22. Loftus, C. M., and Quest, D. O. Current status of carotid endarterectomy for atheromatous disease. Neurosurgery, *13:* 718–723, 1983.
23. Lord, R. S. Survival after carotid endarterectomy for transient ischemic attacks. J. Vasc. Surg., *2*(4): 512–519, 1984.
24. Muuronen, A. Outcome of surgical treatment of 100 patients with transient ischemic attack. Stroke, *15*(6): 959–964, 1984.
25. Piepgras, D. G., Sundt, T. M., Jr., Marsh, W. R., *et al.* Recurrent carotid stenosis. Results and complications of 57 operations. Ann. Surg., *203*(2): 205–213, 1986.
26. Pierce, G. E., Illopoulos, J. I., Holcomb M. A. Incidence of recurrent stenosis after carotid endarterectomy determined by digital subtraction angiography. Am. J. Surg., *148*(6): 848–854, 1984.
27. Roederer, G. O., Langlois Y. E., Jager, K. A. The natural history of carotid arterial disease in asymptomatic patients with cervical bruits. Stroke, *4:* 605–613, 1984.
28. Sundt, T. M., Jr., Ebersold, M. J., *et al.* The risk benefit ratio of intraoperative shunting during carotid endarterectomy. Relevancy to operative and postoperative results. Ann. Surg., *203*(2): 196–204, 1986.
29. Sundt, T. M., Jr., Houser, O. W., Fode, N. C., *et al.* Correlation of postoperative and two-year follow-up angiography with neurological function in 99 carotid endarterectomies in 86 consecutive patients. *Ann. Surg.,* *203*(1): 90–100, 1986.
30. Sundt, T. M., Jr., Sandok, B. A., and Whisnant, J. F. Carotid endarterectomy complications and preoperative assessment of risk. Mayo Clin. Proc., *50:* 301–306, 1975.
31. Thompson, J. R. Carotid endarterectomy, 1982—the state of the art. Br. J. Surg., *70*(6): 371–376, 1983.
32. Trudel, L., Fabia, J., and Bouchard, J. F. Quality of life of 50 carotid endarterectomy survivors: A long-term follow-up study. Arch. Phys. Med. Rehabil., *65*(6): 310–312, 1984.
33. Warlow, C. W. Carotid endarterectomy: Does it work? Stroke, *15*(6): 1068–1076, 1984.
34. Wolf, P. A., Kannel, W. B., Sorlie, P., *et al.* Asymptomatic carotid bruit and risk of stroke. The Framingham Study. JAMA, *245*(14): 1441–1445, 1981.
35. Yatsu, F. M., and Fields, W. S. Asymptomatic carotid bruit. Stenosis of ulceration: A conservative approach. Arch. Neurol., *42*(4): 383–385, 1985.
36. Yates, P. O., and Hutchinson, E. C. Cerebral infarction: The role of stenosis of the extracranial cerebral arteries. London, Medical Research Council Special Report No. 300, Her Majesty's Stationery Office, 1961.

CHAPTER

7

The Past, Present, and Future of Extracranial to Intracranial Bypass Surgery

THORALF M. SUNDT, Jr., M.D., NICOLEE C. FODE, R.N., M.S., and
CLIFFORD R. JACK, Jr., M.D.

INTRODUCTION

The conceptualization and successful demonstration by Yaşargil nearly 2 decades ago of the feasibility of extracranial-intracranial bypass procedures appeared to have opened a new era with considerable promise and hope for the surgical management of stroke victims (33, 34). Since that time a number of reports from various centers have indicated that the procedure could be performed with a high patency rate and low morbidity (1, 11, 15, 21, 23, 24, 28, 31). In the early 1980s the indications for the operation were becoming better defined and, judging from reports in the literature and as is frequently the case with new procedures, a more objective view of the operation's potential had replaced the initial period of enthusiasm. Most surgeons performing the operation felt that it was a low risk, reliable operation, and countless anecdotal experiences seemingly reinforced their opinions. Thus the results of the cooperative trial were shocking to many members of our discipline (9), perhaps not so much because of the negative results of the trial (many of us had assumed that this would be the case because of the complexities of patients with occlusive vascular disease and the major difficulties encountered in categorizing and balancing the many biological variables) but rather because of statements to the effect that no subgroups of patients could be defined in whom the operation was of benefit. The swift reaction of the government and third party agencies to withdraw funding for the operation essentially condemned the operation to one of historical interest, a reaction anticipated by only a very few.

Is the future of bypass surgery as bleak as predicted by some, and will extracranial-intracranial bypass procedures be relegated in the future to a status similar to that of gastric freezing? Some of us believe that the answer to these questions is "no" and that the pendulum will swing back. We believe there will be a resurgence in interest for this procedure in the not too distant future for certain patients. To determine where we are going, let's review briefly where we have been in terms of the rationale for the procedure and some of the reported studies. We will confine our remarks primarily to occlusive disease and only later make some passing references to the management of aneurysms. The operation has fallen under fire primarily for its role in the management of occlusive vascular disease.

RATIONALE FOR BYPASS SURGERY

There is now ample clinical and laboratory work to support the concept that the brain can function on approximately 50% of its normal flow simply by extracting more oxygen and glucose from and delivering more CO_2 and H_2O to the available blood (2, 3, 7, 18, 29, 30). However, when flow drops from 50% to 40 or 30%, changes in the electroencephalogram occur in clinical cases, and abnormalities develop in transport systems monitored in laboratory preparations (30). Thus, the concept that augmentation of cerebral blood flow would be beneficial for patients with marginal ischemia has a sound physiological basis. Theoretically it would restore the capability for normal cerebral autoregulation distal to a point of occlusion and provide the brain with a better reserve of flow for circumstances in which the cardiac output might be diverted to other areas or the perfusion pressure reduced. It has been established that an acute occlusion of the internal carotid artery reduces the perfusion pressure in the ipsilateral cortical circulation by 50% (12).

The controversy regarding the two theories for cerebral ischemic events—*i.e.*, hemodynamic crises distal to major vessel occlusions or stenotic lesions *vs.* microemboli or major emboli from ulcerative lesions— is inextricably entwined with beliefs relative to the usefulness of a bypass procedure in the prevention of stroke. This strikes at the heart of the matter. Proponents of the embolic theory tend to believe that the brain will adapt to its marginal flow status through ample collateral circulation and that if an infarct were to have occurred, it would have already taken place, and thus there is little need for augmenting cerebral blood flow. This is a concept which this reviewer believes is both naive and nihilistic, but it is a belief subscribed to by a great many knowledgeable clinicians. The results of cerebral blood flow measurements during carotid endarterectomy cast considerable doubt on such a position (30). Flow is marginal in a great many cases with a high grade stenosis or occlusion, and there is no doubt about it. An endarterectomy for stenosis and a bypass for occlusion increase flow in zones of marginal perfusion and thus restore a more normal autoregulation and the ability of the brain to accommodate to variations in perfusion pressure (16).

COOPERATIVE TRIAL

In reviewing where we have been, certainly the cooperative trial stands out as the chief study challenging the usefulness of this operation (9, 10).

The extracranial-intracranial bypass study was organized and conducted by Dr. Henry Barnett and colleagues at the University of Western Ontario and McMaster University under a grant from the National Institute of Neurological and Communicative Disorders in Stroke. Data were collected from 71 participating centers in North America, Europe, and Asia during the period from 1977 to 1982. Patients eligible for the study were randomized into medical and surgical arms, and outcomes were measured. There were 714 patients randomized to medical care, and 663 were submitted to bypass surgery.

Results of this study led the investigators to conclude that the extracranial-intracranial bypass procedure was not of benefit in any of the subgroups of patients analyzed and was, in fact, detrimental in two of the subgroups. These studies were published in two parts, the first, dealing mainly with methodology, was published in *Stroke,* and the second containing the results was published in the *New England Journal of Medicine* (9, 10).

AANS Survey

In response to a specific charge from the American Association of Neurological Surgeons (AANS) to respond to this study formally at a meeting of that organization in April of 1986, a telephone survey was conducted of most of the participating centers in the U.S. This telephone survey has been subsequently supplemented with written confirmations from most of the centers and the results published in the *New England Journal of Medicine* (26). The survey also included the major centers contributing from Europe, and it should be noted, parenthetically, that this represented a very large proportion of the cases entered into the study.

Two major concerns prompted this survey:

1. Centers contributing a small number of cases had a bypass patency rate equal to that of those centers with a large number of cases.
2. Clinical material contained: (*a*) a disproportionately large number of patients who were asymptomatic (having one or two transient ischemic events in the 3-month period prior to surgery is not equated to being symptomatic) at the time of surgery (276 cases) and (*b*) a relatively small number of those symptomatic cases that represent the largest group of patients undergoing surgery in the U.S. (287 cases of symptomatic carotid occlusions collected over 5 years from 70 centers equally divided between medicine and surgery equals less than one case per center per year treated surgically).

It has been established that surgical expertise and experience (as emphasized in the report of the cooperative trial itself) have a major bearing on complications in patency of bypass procedures. How could centers randomizing only two to four cases to surgery per year maintain their surgical skills in this area? This led to the above-mentioned survey. Results of the inquiry, summarized in Tables 7.1 and 7.2, have answered the first of the above questions and made it unnecessary to consider further the second as the survey revealed that from 57 of the 71 participating centers randomizing 601 cases to surgery, there were 2572 cases operated on outside of the trial. In the centers from the U.S. alone, contributing 237 patients to surgery within the trial, there were 864 eligible patients operated on outside of the trial. It thus is appropriate to question seriously whether the trial in fact sampled the population at risk or whether it merely analyzed patients who were not considered ideal surgical candidates by most centers.

The impact that this large group of nonrandomized cases would have had on the results of the trial is a matter of conjecture, as no meaningful analysis of this case material is now possible. More important than the absolute numbers of patients operated on outside of the trial are the characteristics and symptoms of these cases. Were patients with frequent ischemic events, vulnerable sources of collateral flow, and good temporal arteries preselected by participating surgeons for a bypass, and other patients with infrequent symptoms, multiple sources of collateral flow, and poor quality temporal arteries randomized? Were these patients significantly different from those randomized? Upon whom rests the burden of proof, investigator or reviewer?

TABLE 7.1

Randomized Cases vs Cases Operated on Outside of Trial: A Survey of 57 of 71 Participating Centers

Location	No. of Centers	Randomized to Medicine	Randomized to Surgery	Operated on Outside of the Trial
U.S. (30 of 33)	30	252	237	1351
Europe (15 of 19)	15	203	190	741
Japan (12 of 14)	12	105	90	480
Canada[a]	5	94	84	?
Total	62	654	601	2572

[a] These centers were not surveyed; randomization was assumed to be complete.

TABLE 7.2

Categorization of Patients Operated on Outside of Trial in U.S. and Japan

Nation	Eligible	Ineligible	Uncertain or Unspecified	Total
Japan	150	207	123	480
U.S.	864	440	47	1351

If the entire population at risk coming under the care of the partici-pants was entered into the randomized trial, the above biological variables would hopefully balance out and be accounted for in the randomization and examination in the clinical material. However, in that the ratio of nonrandomized eligible patients operated on outside of the trial to those operated on inside the trial within the U.S alone was 3:1, it is question-able, indeed doubtful, that these variables did cancel each other out.

Langfitt Committee Report

In order to evaluate the discrepancies between the survey and the report in the randomized trial, Dr. Robert Ojemann, President of the AANS, appointed a prestigious committee to evaluate the results of the study. This committee included Drs. Thomas Langfitt, Nicholas Zervas, and Sidney Goldring, and was chaired by Dr. Langfitt. Their final report was submitted to Dr. Ojemann, who then forwarded it to the *New England Journal of Medicine* in November of 1986.

The results of this investigation are now a matter of record, and it is unnecessary for us to dwell upon the details of that inquiry here (19). It is appropriate, however, to refer to some of its salient features. One of the major discrepancies between the AANS survey and the listing of patients in the randomized trial related to the definition of eligible patients. In the report of the cooperative trial the statement was made: "These lists included 115 eligible patients who refused entry into the trail and 52 patients whose clinicians insisted that they undergo bypass surgery"; for 11 other patients no reason was given. The total of this group is 178 patients, and the conclusion might be inferred that these represented, to the knowledge of the central office, the only eligible patients operated outside of the trail. The committee had difficulty reconciling these categories in the reports for the five column headings on raw data forms submitted by participating centers to the central registry (Fig. 7.1). The report of the cooperative trial made no mention of ineligible patients operated on outside of the trial, but thereafter the central office sent to the committee a list of procedures performed by centers which included a total of 1906 patients operated on outside of the trial.

The committee visited London, Ontario, Canada, in September of 1986. As a result of that visit and subsequent data submitted to the committee, the reasons for the discrepancies were found. The central office developed a category of "Protocol Ineligibility" which referred to patients who were medically eligible for surgery but who refused random-ization. This classification, not specifically discussed in the report of the cooperative trial, or included in the categories on the forms submitted to

EC/IC BYPASS STUDY REPORT OF ALL EC/IC BYPASS PROCEDURES PERFORMED OUTSIDE OF STUDY

Time Period: [6] [1] [0] [2] [8] [2] to [3] [1] [0] [5] [8] [2]

Neurosurgeon: _____

Study Centre: _____

Date of Operation	Patient's Initials	Date of Birth	Sex		Indication for EC/IC Bypass	If Ineligible Indicate Reason	If Eligible By Study Criteria, Check (✓) Reason for Not Being Entered			
			Male	Female			Patient Refused Entry	Referring Doctor Refused Entry	Neuro- logist's Decision	Neuro- surgeon's Decision
3/5/82	JC.	4/26/54	✓		amaurosis fugot intracranial carotid stenosis		✓			

* comments, if desired, can be made on back of page.

When completed, return to: Dr. H.J.M. Barnett, Room 1-18, University Hospital, P.O. Box 5339, Terminal A, LONDON, Ontario, Canada N6A 5A5

FIG. 7.1. This form describes nonrandomized patients and was submitted by all participants to the central office on a quarterly basis. It represents all of the information that was available to the central office from most centers on nonrandomized cases.

London, comprises a group of 475 patients who were medically eligible and protocol ineligible. In addition to this, there were 95 patients who were eligible and not randomized.

Any experienced clinician knows all too well that a patient can be guided into or away from surgery according to the manner in which his or her case is discussed and presented. Thus it is somewhat academic to subcategorize causes for nonrandomization, except for those related to the severity of symptoms and specific disease process. To declare a patient ineligible for inclusion in the randomized trial because he or she refused to be randomized after discussing the case with the surgeon is obviously an administrative decision of questionable validity.

These numbers fall far short of the estimates made by the AANS survey and therefore there is considerable cause for doubt and concern. It is probable that the numbers exceed all estimates, as no records were retained of patients operated on outside of the trial. These revelations may have, for all intents and purposes, essentially invalidated the trial and returned us to square one.

Primary Investigator Response

The primary investigators rendered a persuasive reply to the criticisms raised by the AANS-sponsored survey and audit (5). They favorably compared their study (EC-IC trial) to the Coronary Artery Surgery Study (CASS). However, there are major differences between the two studies. The CASS report included a survey of all patients registered in the study, and the CASS trial itself dealt with only a small subgroup (approximately 12%) of the registered population. Detailed records were available on all cases not entered into the trial. In contrast, we don't have a clue about the characteristics of the patients not randomized into the EC-IC trial.

Editorial—New England Journal of Medicine

Relman's editorial in the *New England Journal of Medicine* places the AANS Survey, the Langfitt Committee Report, and the response from the primary investigator in perspective (22). He indicates that the precise number of eligible patients withheld from the study was less important than the implications of that omission. He concludes that "the conclusions of the EC-IC trial are valid for the population of patients studied, but can these conclusions be extended to all—or even most—patients who might be referred to a neurosurgeon for a bypass operation? In short, how generalizable are the study's results?" Relman states that the only way to resolve the question is to secure follow-up data on patients who underwent surgery outside of the trial.

IMPORTANT STUDIES SUPPORTING THE EFFICACY OF BYPASS SURGERY FOR SUBPOPULATIONS

There are two studies which are of special importance concerning the possible benefit of extracranial-intracranial bypass surgery for patients with advanced occlusive cerebral vascular disease. One of these, by Yanagihara, Piepgras, and Klass from the Mayo Clinic, relates to a subpopulation of patients with ischemic induced movement disorders in which an objective improvement was noted following bypass surgery (32). The other is from a unique group of patients collected by Chater and co-workers from San Francisco (11). These authors collected 39 patients with bilateral internal carotid artery occlusions who also had advanced ischemic symptoms (and this is important to note, as some patients with bilateral internal carotid artery occlusions are asymptomatic) and who underwent unilateral temporal artery to middle cerebral artery bypass procedures. The operative morbidity was significant in this group, and the surgical mortality rate was also high, but this is understandable as these were indeed high risk patients who were neurologically unstable. Parenthetically, a comparison of the surgical morbidity and mortality in the cooperative trial with those of other major series by single institutions suggests that there are differences in the characteristics and severity of symptoms between the population of patients undergoing surgery. The significance of the Chater study is that there were five strokes in follow-up in that group of patients and that all occurred in the unoperated hemisphere. This is a study of special importance, as each case more or less served as its own control.

MAYO CLINIC SERIES—SUPERFICIAL TEMPORAL ARTERY-MIDDLE CEREBRAL ARTERY BYPASS

A brief review of the Mayo Clinic series of temporal artery-middle cerebral artery bypass procedures will illustrate problems encountered in categorizing and analyzing patients with occlusive cerebral vascular disease. It should be emphasized that in order to make such an analysis meaningful, it is necessary to have knowledge of the severity of the patient's preoperative neurological dysfunction and to know something about the underlying vascular pathology and preoperative adequacy of sources for collateral flow.

Case Material

We have detailed previously our operative complications and stroke rate in follow-up among the entire group of 403 patients collected between July 1974 and June 1982 (28, 31). Somewhere toward the middle of our study, we had a patient develop a fixed neurological deficit following postoperative angiography. In this case, the artery was obviously open with a high velocity flow on the Doppler study. This case led to an agonizing reappraisal of our routine policy of performing postoperative angiograms. Thus, we have postoperative angiograms on only 239 of the 403 cases. This does not include angiograms in cases undergoing surgery for giant aneurysms, Moya Moya disease, carotid dissections, and fibromuscular dysplasia.

One hundred sixty-four (164) of these 239 patients had surgery for a symptomatic internal carotid artery occlusion and also had adequate preoperative angiograms available for retrospective review. It is necessary to review this group in order to illustrate the difficulties encountered in correlating the results of surgery with flow through the bypass in patients with occlusive disease and drawing premature conclusions regarding the statistical validity of such an analysis. It was noted in the cooperative trial that there were just as many strokes in follow-up among patients with a high flow through the bypass as among patients with a low flow through the bypass. Parenthetically, although the cooperative trial discusses the method of analyzing postoperative angiograms and addresses this problem in the discussion, there is, curiously, absolutely no information in the "Results" section regarding the results of postoperative angiograms.

There are various causes for high flow and low flow following a bypass procedure. These are dependent upon: (*a*) the pressure gradient between the extracranial and intracranial arterial systems; (*b*) size and distensibility of the donor vessel; (*c*) size of the recipient vessel; (*d*) the construction of the anastomosis; and (*e*) care in which the arterial pedicle was harvested.

When one considers the above variables, it becomes readily apparent that some patients with a very high flow (Fig. 7.2) had this flow because

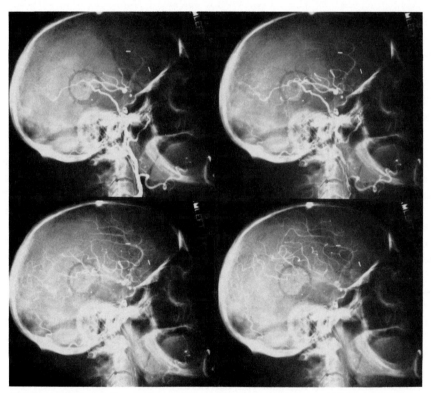

Fig. 7.2. Postoperative angiogram in a patient who had a superficial temporal artery to middle cerebral artery bypass procedure because of a slow stroke syndrome. In this patient, the superficial temporal artery has enlarged to approximately twice its preoperative diameter, and this vessel now serves as a primary source of blood flow to this hemisphere. Forty-five percent of patients having postoperative angiography achieved a high flow (filling of five of the six potential middle cerebral artery vascular territories or more—possible total score of 8 in cases filling the territories supplied by the ophthalmic and anterior cerebral arteries).

there was a major pressure gradient and because collateral flow was so low that the brain readily accepted an alternate source of blood. These were the patients who were particularly vulnerable for a stroke in follow-up without an alternate source of blood flow and thus, although they represent the group of patients most likely to benefit from the surgery, they were also the subgroups most vulnerable for a stroke in follow-up without the operation. Similarly, patients with a low flow may have had this low flow simply because there was no pressure gradient and no real need for the bypass procedure. A third subgroup might have had a low flow because the temporal artery was of very poor quality, and a fourth group could have had a low flow because the arterial pedicle was damaged in its harvesting or because a small cortical vessel was chosen as the recipient artery. These various combinations of groups makes it an exercise of limited usefulness to compare the volume of flow in follow-up with stroke in follow-up unless the other variables are considered (8).

Angiographic Analysis

Details of the pre- and postoperative angiographic analyses in this group of 164 bypasses are being published elsewhere. However, some important findings from this analysis are worthy of notation here: (a) the patency rate of the bypass procedures was 96%; (b) the mean bypass filling score for the patent bypasses was 4.2, meaning that the bypass pedicles supplied 4.2 branches of the middle cerebral artery; (c) eighty percent of the bypasses achieved a medium or high filling score; (d) there was a greater bypass filling in hemispheres in which potential sources for collateral flow were poorly opacified or apparently not present than in hemispheres with readily identifiable sources of collateral flow; and (e) patients who were considered high risks for surgery had a greater risk of stroke in follow-up than those cases not considered a high risk for surgery (however, there are only four hemispheric strokes among the 164 bypass hemispheres).

It is important to distinguish between angiographic opacification and actual cerebral blood flow. However, the fact that 70% of superficial temporal arteries underwent hypertrophy and 80% had a medium or high bypass filling score indicates considerable blood flow augmentation in the majority of the cases and the potential for improved cerebral perfusion.

The EC-IC Cooperative Trial found no difference in the rate of stroke in follow-up between patients with excellent and poor bypass function as assessed at postoperative angiography. No distinction was made in that report between patients who were considered a high risk for stroke prior to surgery and those who were considered a low risk for stroke prior to surgery. It had been the purpose of our study to place this factor into the equation. Only four ipsilateral strokes in follow-up occurred in this group. This small number precluded meaningful generalizations about the relationship between stroke in follow-up and angiographically assessed bypass function. However, it did reconfirm our suspicion that stroke in follow-up did in fact occur among that group of patients who were considered at high risk for stroke and who were neurologically unstable prior to the operation.

ALTERNATIVE OPERATIONS TO SUPERFICIAL TEMPORAL ARTERY-MIDDLE CEREBRAL ARTERY BYPASS PEDICLES

Long Vein Bypass Grafts

If the argument is correct that for normal cerebral function to be maintained, the brain should be supplied with an adequate amount of flow, then vein bypass grafts might very well be the answer in some cases

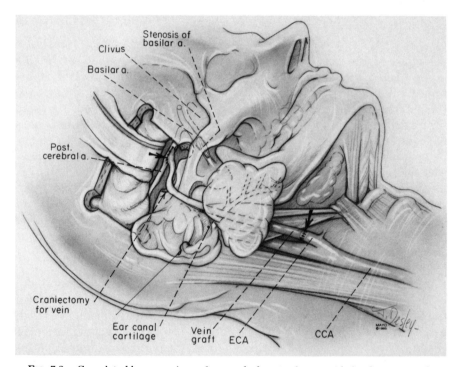

FIG. 7.3. Completed bypass vein graft ascends deep to the parotid gland to enter a deep subcutaneous plane anterior to the tragus of the ear. It then curves over the zygoma and through the temporalis muscle to cross the floor of the middle fossa to the posterior cerebral artery at the margin of the tentorium. *Arrows* point to sites of anastomosis. *CCA*, common carotid artery. *ECA*, external carotid artery.

(25). Space does not permit a detailed evaluation of this subject. It has been published previously (27). It should be underscored, however, that vein bypass grafts have a higher risk and thus far have insufficient long-term follow-up to justify them for cases in which a temporal artery-middle cerebral artery bypass procedure is feasible. The risk of hyper-perfusion breakthrough with intracerebral hemorrhage restricts the technique in patients with progressing ischemic symptoms in the anterior circulation and thus should be used very cautiously in these cases and only when there seems to be no alternative method of management. We have limited the use of this operation in patients with anterior circulation ischemic symptoms to those cases that are not candidates for a temporal

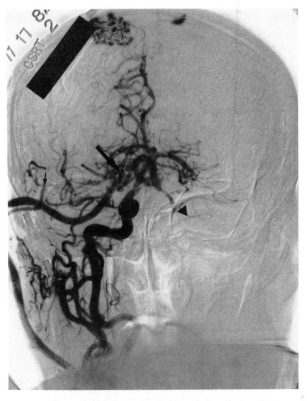

FIG. 7.4.   Postoperative angiogram in a typical case of occlusive disease of the posterior circulation demonstrating a double-barreled saphenous vein bypass graft with one limb (*small arrow*) anastomosed to a branch of the middle cerebral artery. The main trunk of the vein is anastomosed end-to-end to the posterior cerebral artery (*large arrow*). There is retrograde flow in the basilar artery to the point of the anterior inferior cerebellar artery, identified by *arrowhead*.

artery-middle cerebral artery bypass procedure—the primary reasons for not being a candidate for such an operation are a siphon stenosis or an inadequate temporal artery. In our experience and that of others, using a temporal artery-middle cerebral artery bypass procedure for a siphon stenosis, the risk of diversion of flow through the temporal artery pedicle and thereafter precipitating occlusion at the site of the stenosis is not inconsiderable (4, 6, 13, 17). Should the bypass pedicle carry inadequate flow at the time the primary vessel occludes, a major stroke may ensue. Obviously patients with a siphon stenosis must have major symptoms in order to justify a vein bypass graft.

It is not our purpose here to discuss the risks and benefits of saphenous vein bypass grafts for giant aneurysms and intracranial occlusive disease. These have been detailed elsewhere (27). To date, we have treated 79

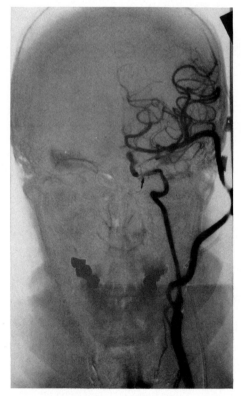

FIG. 7.5. Postoperative angiogram in a patient undergoing a saphenous vein bypass graft for a high grade siphon stenosis (marked by *arrow*). This patient had no cross-flow from the right hemisphere to the left hemisphere, and it was our concern that a superficial temporal artery-middle cerebral artery bypass procedure might precipitate occlusion of the stenotic segment of vessel without adequate flow through the bypass to sustain the hemisphere.

patients for occlusive disease in the posterior circulation, all of whom had failed medical management and showed severe ischemic symptoms prior to surgery; 9 patients with giant aneurysms in the posterior circulation deteriorating from mass effect of the aneurysm; 26 patients with giant aneurysms in the anterior circulation with mass effect or a subarachnoid hemorrhage; and 32 patients with either progressive ischemia in the anterior circulation or continuing ischemic events in the anterior circulation from a siphon stenosis or extracranial aneurysm. Graft patency in the first 65 cases was 74%. However, after significant technical changes of vein graft preparation and construction of the proximal anastomoses, patency in the following 81 cases was improved to 93%.

Excellent or good results (including deficits existing prior to surgery)

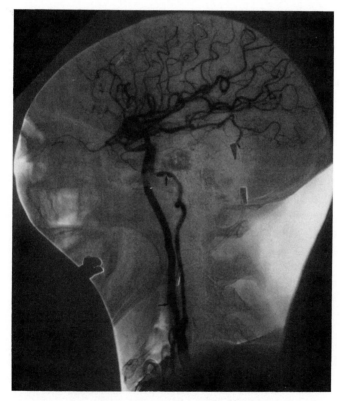

FIG. 7.6.   Lateral angiogram of case in Figure 7.5 demonstrates siphon stenosis (*arrow*) and excellent perfusion of the entire middle cerebral group through the saphenous vein bypass graft along with retrograde flow through the middle cerebral artery to supply the posterior cerebral artery in this patient with a fetal type circulation of internal carotid artery. This individual had sustained multiple ischemic events prior to surgery related to the upright position. He had no complications from the operation and has had no ischemic symptoms in 6 months of follow-up.

were achieved in 78% of patients with advanced occlusive disease in the posterior circulation; 66% of those with ischemic symptoms in the anterior circulation; and 81% of those with giant aneurysms in the anterior circulation. Mean graft flow at surgery in the series was 100 ml/min for posterior circulation grafts and 110 ml/min for anterior circulation grafts. A saphenous vein bypass graft is a major operation and should not be undertaken lightly and obviously has to be restricted for patients in whom there is little doubt about their prognosis without supplementation of cerebral blood flow. The operation is illustrated in Figure 7.3 for a posterior circulation bypass graft and illustrative cases are described in the legends of Figures 7.4–7.6.

Short Vein Bypass Grafts

Little *et al.* have reported their extensive experience with short vein bypass grafts, and we have used this technique in a limited number of cases with good success (20). We have used the operation primarily for

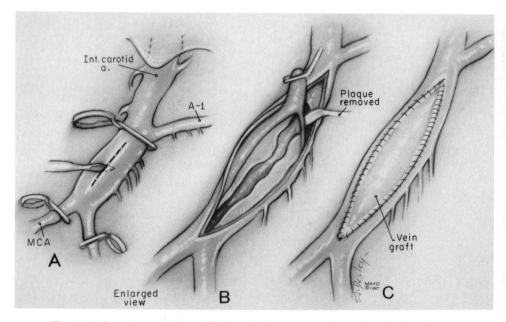

FIG. 7.7. In patients with a middle cerebral artery stenosis, we have had good success with onlay patch grafts with and without endarterectomy. In some instances, it is better to perform a simple onlay patch graft without attempting endarterectomy. This is a surgical decision which must be made at the time of the arterotomy and is dependent upon the characteristics of the atherosclerotic plaque. In those patients with a soft plaque and thrombus in the vessel, endarterectomy is necessary. In cases with pure stenosis related to a fibrous plaque, simple onlay patch grafting without endarterectomy is preferable.

patients with posterior circulation ischemic symptoms in whom an excellent temporal artery was present and in whom an adequate long vein graft was not feasible because of inadequate saphenous veins. This is an option which should be explored more in the future, as it may avoid many problems of cerebral hyperperfusion which we see in the long vein bypass grafts.

Onlay Patch Grafts

This is an operation which we believe will have usefulness for patients with middle cerebral artery stenosis who are symptomatic. The operation is illustrated in Figure 7.7 and the pre- and postoperative angiograms in Figures 7.8 and 7.9. It can be combined with an endarterectomy as was the case in two of our three patients, but in the third patient with a

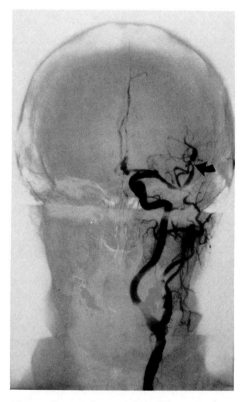

FIG. 7.8. Preoperative angiogram in a patient 76 years of age with a slow stroke syndrome from a high grade stenosis of middle cerebral artery (*arrow*). The patient had a progressive speech disorder of 8-months' duration along with multiple transient ischemic events of right upper extremity weakness and paralysis precipitated by the upright posture. The patient was accumulating both a speech and a motor deficit.

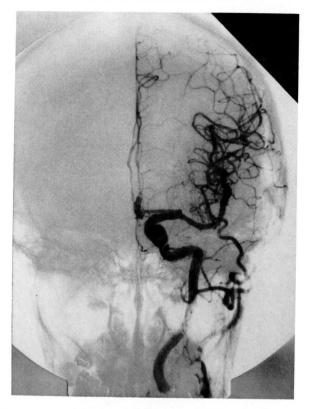

FIG. 7.9.   Postoperative angiogram of the patient in Figure 7.8. In this case the vessel was reconstructed with an onlay patch graft without endarterectomy. Following surgery there was an objective improvement in both motor and speech function.

nonulcerative plaque, the vessel was simply reconstructed with a saphenous vein patch graft.

We have performed endarterectomies and embolectomies without supplementing the operation with an onlay patch graft but, reflecting our preference for patch grafts in carotid artery surgery, we believe patency can be improved by the use of the patch graft.

FUTURE OF TEMPORAL ARTERY TO MIDDLE CEREBRAL ARTERY BYPASS PEDICLES

We believe that there will be an increased use of temporal artery to middle cerebral artery bypass procedures in the future. This is a low risk operation which can achieve very substantial flows in follow-up. It is our experience that the pedicle enlarges with time in patients with a high perfusion gradient and, in these individuals, becomes a substantial source of collateral flow.

Future Indications

In those patients with an adequate temporal artery to serve as a bypass pedicle, we believe that the operation will be indicated in the following groups of patients: (a) patients with continuing transient ischemic events related to an occluded internal carotid artery; (b) patients with a progressing neurological deficit related to an internal carotid artery occlusion; (c) individuals with a slow-stroke syndrome; (d) symptoms of global ischemia related to bilateral internal carotid artery occlusions; and (e) adjunctive procedure for the management of certain intracranial aneurysms (14).

Possible Contraindications

It is hazardous to make arbitrary judgments about proposed methods of management in any group of patients with occlusive vascular disease, as there are so many variables present. However, experience to date suggests that the risk-benefit ratio of the surgery is high for patients with: (a) internal carotid artery siphon stenosis unless the temporal artery is of much greater than average size (4, 6, 13, 17); (b) patients with a large completed infarct; and (c) spontaneous dissections of the internal carotid artery unless the patient is continuing to have transient ischemic events while on anticoagulants.

REFERENCES

1. Andrews, B. T., Chater, N. L., and Weinstein, P. R. Extracranial-intracranial arterial bypass for middle cerebral artery stenosis and occlusion: Operative results in 65 cases. J. Neurosurg, *62:* 831–838, 1985.
2. Astrup, J., Siesjö, B. K., and Symon, L. Thresholds in cerebral ischemia: The ischemic penumbra (editorial). Stroke, *12:* 723–725, 1981.
3. Astrup, J., Symon, L., Branston, N. M., *et al.* Cortical evoked potential and extracellular K^+ and H^+ at critical levels of brain ischemia. Stroke, *8:* 51–57, 1977.
4. Awad, I., Furlan, A. J., and Little, J. R. Changes in intracranial stenotic lesions after extracranial-intracranial bypass surgery. J. Neurosurg., *60:* 771–776, 1984.
5. Barnett, H. J. M., Sackett, D., Taylor, D. W., *et al.* Are the results of the extracranial-intracranial bypass trial generalizable? N. Engl. J. Med., *316:* 820–824, 1987.
6. Chater, N. L., and Weinstein, P. R. Progression of middle cerebral artery stenosis to occlusion without symptoms following superficial temporary artery bypass: Case report. In: *Microvascular Anastomoses for Cerebral Ischemia,* edited by J. M. Fein and O. H. Reichman, pp. 269–271. Springer-Verlag, New York, 1974.
7. Crowell, R. M., Olsson, Y., Klatzo, I., *et al.* Temporary occlusion of the middle cerebral artery in the monkey: Clinical and pathological observations. Stroke, *1:* 439–448, 1970.
8. Diaz, F. G., Chason, J., Shrontz, C., *et al.* Histological structural abnormalities of superficial temporal arteries used for extracranial-intracranial anastomosis. J. Neurosurg., *57:* 328–333, 1982.
9. EC/IC Bypass Study Group. Failure of extracranial-intracranial arterial bypass to reduce the risk of ischemic stroke: Results of an international randomized trial. N. Engl. J. Med., *313:* 1191–1200, 1985.

10. EC/IC Bypass Study Group. The international cooperative study of extracranial/intracranial arterial anastomosis (EC/IC Bypass Study): Methodology and entry characteristics. Stroke, 16: 397–406, 1985.

11. El-Fiki, M., Chater, N. L., and Weinstein, P. R. Results of extracranial-intracranial arterial bypass for bilateral carotid occlusion. J. Neurosurg., 63: 521–525, 1985.

12. Fein, J. M., Lipow, K., and Marmarou, A. Cortical artery pressure in normotensive and hypertensive aneurysm patients. J. Neurosurg., 59: 51–56, 1983.

13. Furlan, A. J., Little, J. R., and Dohn, D. F. Arterial occlusion following anastomosis of the superficial temporal artery to middle cerebral artery. Stroke 11: 91–95, 1980.

14. Gelber, B. R., and Sundt, T. M., Jr. Treatment of intracavernous and giant carotid aneurysms by combined internal carotid ligation and extra- to intracranial bypass. J. Neurosurg., 52: 1–10, 1980.

15. Gratzl, O., Schmiedek, P., Spetzler, R., et al. Clinical experience with extra-intracranial arterial anastomosis in 65 cases. J. Neurosurg., 44: 313–324, 1976.

16. Grubb, R. L., Jr., Ratcheson, R. A., Raichle, M. E., et al. Regional cerebral blood flow and oxygen utilization in superficial temporal-middle cerebral artery anastomosis patients; An exploratory definition of clinical problems. J. Neurosurg., 50: 733–741, 1979.

17. Gumerlock, M. K., Ono, H., and Neuwelt, E. A. Can a patent extracranial-intracranial bypass provoke the conversion of an intracranial arterial stenosis to a symptomatic occlusion? Neurosurgery, 12: 391–400, 1983.

18. Hanson, E. J., Jr., Anderson, R. E., and Sundt, T. M., Jr. Comparison of [85]krypton and [133]xenon cerebral blood flow measurements before, during, and following focal, incomplete ischemia in the squirrel monkey. Circ. Res., 36: 18–26, 1975.

19. Langfitt, T., Goldring, N., and Zervas, N. The extracranial-intracranial bypass study: A report of the committee appointed by the American Association of Neurological Surgeons to examine the study. N. Engl. J. Med., 316: 817–820, 1987.

20. Little, J. R., Furlan, A. J., and Bryerton, B. Short vein grafts for cerebral revascularization. J. Neurosurg., 59: 384–388, 1983.

21. Reichman, O.H. Complications of cerebral revascularization. Clin. Neurosurg., 23: 318–335, 1976.

22. Relman, A. S. The extracranial-intracranial arterial bypass study: What have we learned? N. Engl. J. Med., 316: 809–810, 1987.

23. Rhodes, R. S., Spetzler, R. F., and Roski, R. A. Improved neurologic function after cerebrovascular accident with extracranial-intracranial arterial bypass. Surgery, 90: 433–438, 1981.

24. Samson, D. S., and Boone, S. Extracranial-intracranial (EC-IC) arterial bypass: Past performance and current concepts. Neurosurgery, 3: 79–86, 1978.

25. Spetzler, R. F., Rhodes, R. S., Roski, R. A., et al. Subclavian to middle cerebral artery saphenous vein bypass graft. J. Neurosurg., 53: 465–469, 1980.

26. Sundt, T. M., Jr. Was the international randomized trial of extracranial-intracranial arterial bypass representative of the population at risk? N. Engl. J. Med., 316: 814–816, 1987.

27. Sundt, T. M., Jr., Piepgras, D. G., Marsh, W. R., et al. Saphenous vein bypass grafts for giant aneurysms and intracranial occlusive disease. J. Neurosurg., 65: 439–450, 1986.

28. Sundt, T. M., Jr., Whisnant, J. P., Fode, N. C., et al. Results, complications, and follow-up of 415 bypass operations for occlusive disease of the carotid system. Mayo Clin. Proc., 60: 230–240, 1985.

29. Waltz, A. G., and Sundt, T. M., Jr. The microvasculature and microcirculation of the cerebral cortex after arterial occlusion. Brain, 90: 681–696, 1967.

30. Whisnant, J. P., Sandok, B. A., Sundt, T. M., Jr. Carotid endarterectomy for unilateral carotid system transient cerebral ischemia. Mayo Clin. Proc., *58:* 171–175, 1983.
31. Whisnant, J. P., Sundt, T. M., Jr., and Fode, N. C. Long-term mortality and stroke morbidity after superficial temporal artery-middle cerebral artery bypass operation. Mayo Clin. Proc., *60:* 241–246, 1985.
32. Yanagihara, T., Piepgras, D. G., and Klass, D. W. Repetitive involuntary movement associated with episodic cerebral ischemia. Ann. Neurol., *18:* 244–250, 1985.
33. Yaşargil, M. G. Diagnosis and indications for operations in cerebrovascular occlusive disease. In: *Microsurgery Applied to Neurosurgery*, edited by M. G. Yaşargil, pp. 95–119. Georg Thieme Verlag, Stuttgart, 1969.
34. Yaşargil, M. G., Krayenbuhl, H. A., Jacobson, J. H., II. Microneurosurgical arterial reconstruction. Surgery, *67:* 221–233, 1970.

8

The Management of Intracranial Aneurysms—Prospects for Improvement

BRYCE K. A. WEIR, M.D., F.R.C.S.(C), F.A.C.S.

Our current state of knowledge about intracranial aneurysms has been amply documented (1, 2, 4–18). It would be most suprising if our ability to diagnose and treat such lesions did not go on improving. Patients harboring them are bound to be the recipients of general advances in medical and surgical practice. It remains unclear whether we can extrapolate the rate of progress which has occurred in the past 2 or 3 decades into the coming ones. In the span of almost half a century the technical problems associated with clipping of aneurysms, have largely, if not entirely, been solved through the ingenuity and courage of men such as Dandy, Drake, and Yaşargil. Our knowledge of the natural history of the disease has been built by the labors of those such as Pakarinen, Sahs, and Kassell. Brilliant though their achievements are, the difficulty in placing metal clips across the neck of an aneurysm and rendering an accurate prognosis is an order of magnitude less than the difficulty in reversing the pathologic consequences of rupture or preventing the development of aneurysms in the first instance. It is problematical whether the fundamental challenge of the prevention of vessel wall degeneration can be overcome even by physician-biochemists far in the future. Perhaps it is a more practical exercise to speculate on those areas where our present knowledge base and technology are likely to permit advances (Table 8.1).

Certain facts appear reasonably well founded today which were unknown or in dispute several decades ago. The majority of saccular intracranial aneurysms are not congenital lesions. They develop for the most part at arterial bifurcations subject to repeated hemodynamic stresses, in regions where the tunica media and elastica are absent. The incidence of aneurysms increases steadily with age. Some populations seem to be more afflicted than others, which suggests that there might be linkage to generalized arterial diseases such as arteriosclerosis. Proximally situated intracranial aneurysms are relatively more common among females. Males are relatively more afflicted in the earlier decades.

TABLE 8.1

Prospects for Improvements in Management

Prevention of prehospital sudden death
  Widespread training in cardiopulmonary resuscitation
Prevention of misdiagnosis with the missed opportunity to treat good grade patients after
    "warning leaks"
  Better medical education of students, general practitioners, and other specialists
  Public education regarding the seriousness of the sudden onset, uniquely severe headache
  Widespread employment of CT scanning to investigate such headaches
  Abdandonment of lumbar puncture as the primary diagnostic test
  Early definitive surgery
Prevention of medical and surgical complications
  General improvement in standards of care
Prevention of delayed ischemic deficit
  Avoidance of dehydration, antifibrinolytics, and adverse cardiological, hematological, and
    respiratory events
  Early clot removal and cisternal irrigation, calcium antagonists
  Early treatment with hypertension, hypervolemia, and increased cardiac output at onset
    of signs of ischemia
Prevention of avoidable delayed deterioration
  Early CSF shunting
  Treatment of depression
  Appropriate rehabilitation
Screening for aneurysms in groups at risk
  Digital subtraction angiography or magnetic resonance imaging for cases not definitively
    clipped, such as those treated by carotid ligation
  Familial cases (two or more immediate relatives with known aneurysms)
  Polycystic kidneys, coarctation, fibromuscular dysplasia

Not all patients with cerebral aneurysms die from their rupture. One-half to a third of aneurysms never cause a patient any symptoms. It is likely that there exists a subset of patients with aneurysms, in whom the rate of occurrence within family members exceeds what could be anticipated on the basis of chance alone. In such constellations, aneurysms tend to rupture at an earlier average age and to be more frequently multiple. The average age of patients with bleeding aneurysms is approximately 50. We now know that there are many structural consequences of such a rupture in addition to subarachnoid hemorrhage. Both pathological and computed tomographic (CT) studies have made us more aware of the presence and significance of intracerebral, intraventricular, and subdural hemorrhage as well as hydrocephalus and infarction.

It is now apparent that the lives of patients are at greatest risk following aneurysm rupture immediately thereafter and that the threat diminishes with the passage of time. Approximately one-tenth of patients probably die instantaneously. Others succumb to the direct effect of intracranial hypertension or cerebral destruction by clot or compression. Rebleeding tends to occur more frequently in the first day or so after the initial hemorrhage, and its frequency then tapers off, so that after 6 months the patient has a fairly flat risk curve for the rest of his life.

In those with high volume subarachnoid hemorrhage there is a potential for angiographically demonstrable vasospasm to begin 2 or 3 days after the bleed. It can last for 2 or more weeks. When there is a thick subarachnoid clot this process is often severe and diffuse, and commonly heralds the development of delayed ischemic deficit in those who survive long enough. Neurological sequelae can commence in an interval from 4 or 5 days up to a couple of weeks from the bleed. Whether or not cerebral infarction actually results from angiographically observed vasospasm depends on numerous factors such as the anatomy of the collateral circulation, cardiac output, blood pressure, blood viscosity, the intensity and extent of the constriction, and so on.

The overall outcome for a given patient appears to be related to the volume, rate, and location of the initial hemorrhage; the age of the brain; and other general medical factors. Numerous systems for assigning a neurologic grade to victims of rupture have been devised. In general, the poorer the patient's neurological condition on admission to hospital or immediately prior to surgery, the worse will be the prognosis. In addition it has been shown that the longer the patient has survived after the hemorrhage the better will be the outcome, regardless of the grade of the patient.

It also seems reasonably established that the interval in which the operation is performed is not an overriding determinant of mortality or morbidity. There is, however, strong evidence that there is a "window in time" in the first day or so after the hemorrhage during which surgery can be carried out without much risk of inflicting incremental damage to the already traumatized brain. If successfully accomplished it may reduce the incidence of delayed ischemia by clot removal, and it will certainly reduce the incidence of rebleeding.

We have come to a consensus that definite neck clipping is the best treatment for an intracranial aneurysm which has ruptured. It is no longer in dispute that this approach yields superior results to bed rest and carotid ligation. What is still contentious is the degree to which we should pursue patients who might harbor unruptured and asymptomatic aneurysms. When such lesions should be approached surgically is still a matter of highly subjective judgment. There is a suggestion that they are not prone to rupture if they are relatively small. On the other hand every series of ruptured aneurysms has a size distribution which is bell-shaped and half the lesions are under 8 mm or so in maximum angiographic diameter. We should have an open mind on this question since it is absolutely clear that some morbidity and mortality are inevitable in craniotomy for aneurysm—even for unruptured, technically easy lesions in otherwise healthy patients.

It is not being too optimistic to suggest that means of scanning the entire population for the presence of aneurysms are within our reach. Persons who should perhaps be evaluated first are those who have had previous treatment which is likely to be inadequate, such as carotid ligation or clipping in the premicrosurgical era, patients suffering from diseases such as polycystic kidneys, coarctation of the aorta, fibromuscular dysplasia, and so on. All would be candidates for prophylactic evaluation if the technology were absolutely safe. The calculation of risk-benefit ratios is going to become an increasingly important part of our professional lives. The development of data banks is likely to proceed and should yield increasingly useful guidance in surgical decision-making.

The medical sophistication of the general public will potentially improve matters by bringing patients to neurosurgical attention after relatively small hemorrhages. Despite much being written on the subject of the warning leak, however, the average neurosurgeon still sees many cases in whom the chance of operating on a good grade patient has been irretrievably lost by failure to make the diagnosis. With the availability of computerized tomographic scanning throughout the developed world we will hopefully see the day when all patients with the sudden onset of a severe and unusual headache will have an emergency CT examination. This will relegate the widespread employment of lumbar puncture to the status of an anachronism.

With the advent of magnetic resonance imaging (MRI) and the dramatic improvement in its quality in a very short time we can anticipate that this modality is likely to become an ever more important part of our diagnostic armamentarium, particularly as it is adapted to "angiography" without contrast media (see Fig. 8.1) (3). Magnetic resonance spectroscopy may become a cheaper and simpler way of evaluating certain aspects of brain function than positron emission tomography, although a significant ongoing role for the latter is readily imagined. The technology of digital subtraction angiography will also improve, and we shall see the introduction of relatively inexpensive but accurate systems for the operating room, to assist us in the adequate and safe placement of aneurysm clips.

While we have learned much of the pathophysiology of vasospasm we are far from having solved the problem. The erythrocyte isolated in an alien space becomes metamorphosed from life-giver to life-taker. Whether we can remove it safely, mechanically or pharmacologically, or inactivate its breakdown products, is the subject of intense investigation at the present time. No definite claims can be made. Hundreds of drugs and techniques have been suggested for the prophylaxis or treatment of

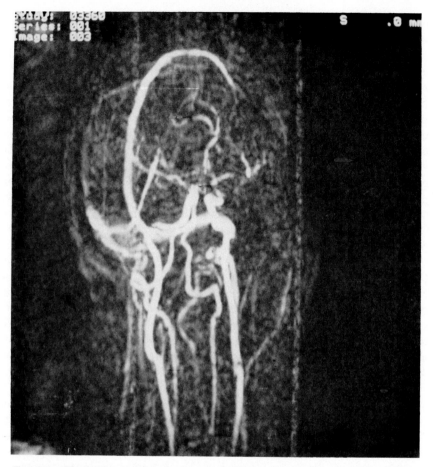

Fig. 8.1.   Magnetic resonance angiograms of a normal volunteer. Projective images of
both arterial and venous structures can be obtained without contrast media. Images are
obtained from velocity information. Pulse sequences have been developed which permit the
selective detection of moving spins. (Courtesy of Charles L. Dumoulin, General Electric
Corporate Research and Development Center.)

vasospasm, but none have proven curative and stood the test of time.
While we have learned not to aggravate the process by using dehydration,
excessive hypotension, or antifibrinolytic agents indiscriminately, it is
becoming evident that hypertension, hypervolemia, increased cardiac
output, optimization of hematologic and metabolic factors, and so on are
still not the complete answer to the problem. All experienced surgeons
have seen patients progressively deteriorate and die despite these measures. Will the future justify the use of some oxygen-carrying compound,
such as the fluorocarbons, given by subarachnoid or ventricular irriga-

tion? Will we call upon radiologists to mechanically distend spastic segments with balloon catheters? It would be infinitely preferable if there were some pharmacological "silver bullet" which could complete the task with less risk and greater ease. The jury is still out regarding the efficacy of calcium antagonists for the prophylaxis and treatment of vasospasm. With the development of animal models we may be able to assess potential therapies more readily.

Our surgical results could probably be largely improved by the wholesale adoption of healthier life styles in the general population. The fat, besotted smoker has already one foot in the grave prior to his subarachnoid hemorrhage.

With the increasing use of the multicenter prospective trials, we may reasonably hope for more reliable data upon which to base our approach to both ruptured and unruptured aneurysm. What criteria should we use to decide that a patient has been irreparably damaged by a hemorrhage, given his age and general state of health? Is heroic surgical intervention justified for all grades and ages of patients at all time intervals after the bleed? We must learn to pay more attention to neurophysiological and psychiatric long-term evaluations of postoperative patients. Neurosurgeons who have dramatically rescued patients from strong currents in the midst of the river Styx can be forgiven for pronouncing an excellent result on the sole basis of the patient's walking into their office sometime later and verbalizing gratitude.

Good grade patients operated on some weeks after hemorrhage can now anticipate an extremely low morbidity and mortality following an operation to obliterate their aneurysms. There is a high likelihood that such procedures will be curative but alas even this does not achieve certainty. For the patients who die within seconds of their bleeding, or for those who arrive at hospital in an agonal state, it seems unlikely that even the technological advances which we may hope for in the next century will have much to offer. It appears to this observer that our glorious calvary charge of progress has come to a halt and that what we must anticipate now is a long siege of trench welfare with small gains, dearly bought.

REFERENCES

1. Auer, L. M. (ed.): *Timing of Aneurysm Surgery*. Walter de Gruyter, Berlin, 1985.
2. Dandy, W. E. *Intracranial Arterial Aneurysms*. Hafner, New York, 1944 (reprinted 1969).
3. Dumoulin, C. L., and Hart, H. R. Magnetic resonance angiography. Radiology, in press, 1986.
4. Fein, J. F., and Flamm, E. S. (eds.). *Cerebrovascular Surgery*, vol. 1–3. Springer-Verlag, New York, 1985.
5. Fox, J. L. *Intracranial Aneurysms*, vol. 1–3. Springer-Verlag, New York, 1983.

6. Hopkins, L. N., and Long, D. M. (eds.). *Clinical Management of Intracranial Aneurysms.* Raven Press, New York, 1982.
7. Ito, Z. *Microsurgery of Cerebral Aneurysms.* Elsevier Science Publishers, B.V., Amsterdam, 1985.
8. Ojemann, R. G., and Crowell, R. M. *Surgical Management of Cerebrovascular Disease.* Williams & Wilkins, Baltimore, 1983.
9. Pia, H. W., Langmaid, C., and Zierski, J. (eds.). *Cerebral Aneurysms: Advances in Diagnosis and Therapy.* Springer-Verlag, Berlin, 1979.
10. Pool, J. L., and Potts, D. G. *Aneurysms and Arteriovenous Anomalies of the Brain.* Hoeber Medical Division, Harper & Row, New York, 1965.
11. Sahs, A. L., Perret, G. E., Locksley, H. B., et al. (eds.). *Intracranial Aneurysms and Subarachnoid Hemorrhage: A Cooperative Study.* Lippincott, Philadelphia, 1969.
12. Sengupta, R. P., and McAllister, V. L. *Subarachnoid Hemorrhage.* Springer-Verlag, Berlin, 1986.
13. Stehbens, W. E. *Pathology of the Cerebral Blood Vessels.* Mosby, St. Louis, 1972.
14. Sugita, K. *Microneurosurgical Atlas.* Springer-Verlag, Berlin, 1985.
15. Suzuki, J. (ed.) *Cerebral Aneurysms: Experiences with 1000 Directly Operated Cases.* Neuron Publishing, Tokyo, 1979.
16. Weir, B. *Aneurysms Affecting the Nervous System.* Williams & Wilkins, Baltimore, 1987.
17. Wilkins, R. H. (ed.). *Cerebral Arterial Spasm.* Williams & Wilkins, Baltimore, 1980.
18. Yaşargil, M. G. *Microneurosurgery*, vols. 1 and 2. Georg Thieme Verlag, Stuttgart, 1984.

9

Spinal Arteriovenous Malformations

EDWARD H. OLDFIELD, M.D., and JOHN L. DOPPMAN, M.D.

In the past several years we, and others, have treated patients with vascular lesions of the spine in whom the clinical findings were identical to those previously considered diagnostic of arteriovenous malformations (AVMs) of the spinal cord. However, in these patients a dural arterio-venous (AV) fistula has been identified which drains into the intradural spinal veins covering the surface of the spinal cord (5, 15, 29, 31, 35, 37, 40, 41, 44, 48). This experience indicates that many lesions previously considered AVMs of the spinal cord are, rather, composed of normal venous channels which have been transfigured by the reception of blood under high pressure and flow and that they are adequately treated by simple interruption of the dural AV fistula (29, 31, 37, 40, 41, 44, 48). Furthermore, the clinical presentation of patients with dural lesions differs from that of patients with intradural AVMs, and this clinical dissimilarity relates to differences in the mechanism of cord injury (40, 41). Moreover, several characteristics of the dural lesions suggest that they have acquired rather than congenital origin (35, 40, 41).

HISTORY

Charles Elsberg performed the first successful operation for a spinal cord AVM in 1914. His patient suffered severe paraparesis and sensory loss to the level of the ninth thoracic dermatome. At surgery Elsberg ligated a dilated posterior spinal vein as it entered the dura adjacent to the eighth thoracic nerve root and removed a 2-cm segment (Fig. 9.1). Over the next 3 months his patient had complete neurological recovery (23).

The early classification of vascular lesions affecting the spine was based on the results of pathological examination and, as in Elsberg's patient, most were considered to be venous in origin. In 1925 Sargent reviewed the previously reported patients with spinal AVMs (42). He considered 19 of the 21 lesions to be venous angiomas. Similarly, Wyburn-Mason in his monograph of 1943 entitled "The vascular abnormalities and tumors of the spinal cord, and its membranes" reviewed 110 patients and described two main types of vascular malformations which affected

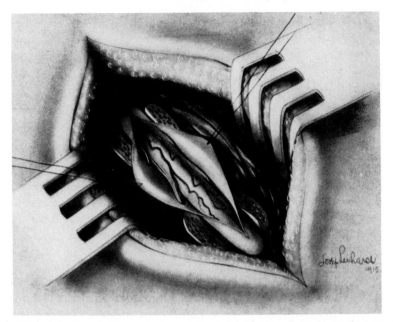

FIG. 9.1. Operative findings at first successful operation for spinal AVM. Elsberg ligated a dilated posterior spinal vein as it entered the dura adjacent to the eighth thoracic nerve root and removed a 2-cm segment. The patient had complete recovery of severe paraparesis and sensory loss below T9. (From Elsberg C. A. *Diagnosis and Treatment of Surgical Diseases of the Spinal Cord and Its Membranes*, pp. 201–204. W. B. Saunders, Philadelphia and London, 1916.)

the spinal cord, AV angiomas and purely venous angiomas. The venous type was described as being formed of an abnormal mass of turgid, blue pial vessels on the cord surface below the midthoracic level. He concluded that 75 of the 110 patients had venous angiomas (46).

With the introduction of selective spinal angiography in the 1960s, the precise anatomy of these lesions could be demonstrated *in vivo*. Spinal AVMs were reclassified on the basis of the vascular anatomy and pattern of blood flow as interpreted from angiography rather than pathology (10, 17, 19). The result was a categorization of spinal AVMs into three types: juvenile, glomus, and the single coiled vessel types (10, 17, 19). In all the nidus of the malformation was considered to be within the spinal cord or pia.

The juvenile type was considered analogous to cerebral AVMs with multiple large feeding vessels supplying a voluminous AVM with rapid blood flow and a spinal bruit. It was noted to occur almost exclusively in children and young adults. The glomus type, quite distinctive in its angiographic appearance, was a localized congerie of smaller blood vessels confined to a short segment of cord with a single feeding vessel. These lesions could occasionally be successfully excised. However, the juvenile and glomus type AVMs comprised only 15–20% of all spinal AVMs. The transition from arterial to venous elements in these lesions was obvious at angiography and the feeding vessel, which had the potential of also supplying the spinal cord, was always an enlarged medullary artery.

The single coiled vessel, the most common type, comprising 80–85% of all spinal AVMs, was characterized angiographically as a single, tightly coiled, continuous vessel on the cord surface. Flow through this lesion was slow, often requiring 16–20 seconds for clearance of the contrast. It was supplied by one, rarely two, feeding vessels which themselves did not supply the cord. In these lesions the arterial to venous transition, unlike the juvenile and glomus types, was not clearly identified; many small communicating vessels between the dorsolateral arterial plexus and the "malformation" were considered likely shunting sites. With the introduction of microneurosurgery the vessels covering the cord surface seemed to be the glomus of the AVM, and surgical stripping of these engorged vessels became the treatment most commonly used (30, 33).

In 1977 Brian Kendall and Valentine Logue described nine patients in whom the site of the AV fistula was identified as the dura covering the proximal nerve root (29). The patients were treated by excision of the dural AV fistula; most enjoyed considerable improvement postoperatively (29, 31). This knowledge has radically changed the approach to and the treatment of these lesions.

It is now recognized that there are two main types of AVM of the spine: dural AV fistulas, in which the nidus of the AV fistula is imbedded in the dural covering of the nerve root, and intradural AVMs, in which the nidus of the AVM is within the cord tissue or the pia. The intradural AVMs are further subclassified into juvenile AVMs, glomus AVMs, and direct AV fistulas (Table 9.1 and Figs. 9.2–9.6) (14).

CLINICAL PRESENTATION, NATURAL HISTORY, AND EVALUATION

Our recent review of 81 patients with spinal AVMs demonstrated that there are distinguishing clinical features between intradural and dural spinal AVMs (40, 41). Those features suggesting an intradural AVM are

TABLE 9.1

Spinal Arteriovenous Malformations

A. Dural arteriovenous fistulas
B. Intradural arteriovenous malformations
   1) Juvenile AVM
   2) Glomus AVM
   3) Arteriovenous fistula

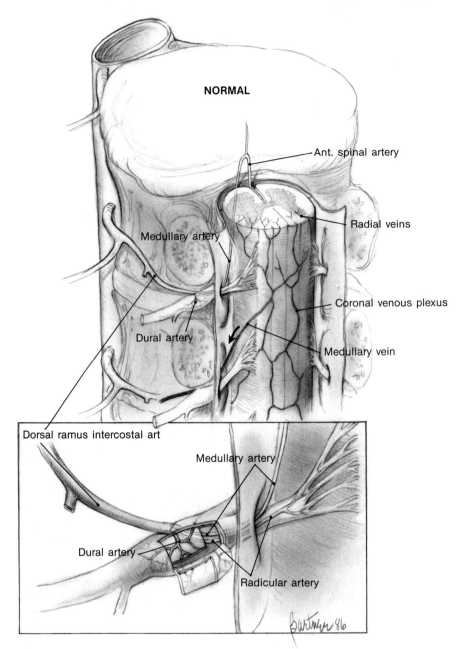

NORMAL

Ant. spinal artery

Medullary artery

Radial veins

Coronal venous plexus

Dural artery

Medullary vein

Dorsal ramus intercostal art

Medullary artery

Dural artery

Radicular artery

FIG. 9.2. At each segmental level the spinal ramus of each intercostal artery divides, after entering the intervertebral foramen and penetrating the outer surface of the dura, into dural arteries, which provide arterial blood to the root sleeve and spinal dura, and radicular arteries, which supply the anterior and posterior nerve roots. In addition, at some levels, and in a sporadic manner, the spinal ramus of an intercostal artery also is the origin of a medullary artery, which enters the dura adjacent to the nerve root ganglion, ascends, and joins an anterior or posterolateral spinal artery to supply the spinal cord. The cord is drained by radial veins, which carry the blood to the cord surface to the coronal venous plexus or longitudinal veins. These veins are drained by medullary veins which pierce the dura adjacent to, but separate from, the dural penetration of the nerve roots.

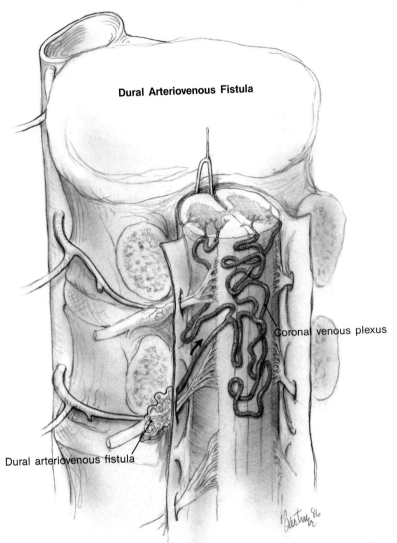

Dural Arteriovenous Fistula

Coronal venous plexus

Dural arteriovenous fistula

FIG. 9.3.   Dural AV fistula is supplied by a dural artery and is drained by a medullary vein, which carries the blood retrograde to the normal direction of venous drainage to the coronal venous plexus, which becomes elongated, tortuous, and dilated by the reception of arterial blood. Increased venous pressure is transmitted to the cord tissue and causes myelopathy.

a patient less than 30 years old, acute onset of symptoms, subarachnoid hemorrhage (SAH), a spinal bruit, and symptoms affecting the arms (Table 9.2). Patients with dural AVMs are usually greater than 40 years of age, have gradual onset and progressive worsening of symptoms,

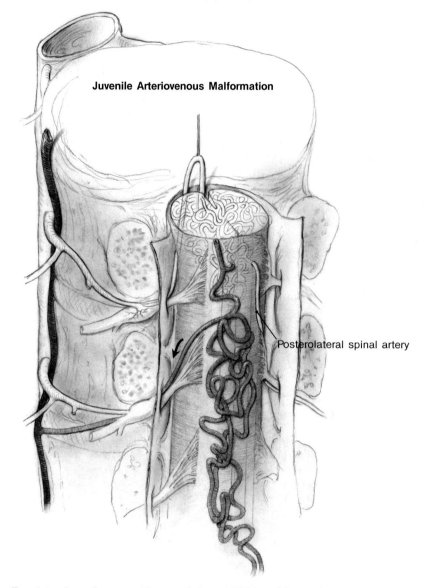

FIG. 9.4. Juvenile type of intramedullary AVM is fed by medullary arteries via the anterior and posterolateral spinal arteries. The nidus of the AVM is large, often fills the spinal canal, and contains cord tissue within the interstices of the vessels of the AVM.

experience exacerbation of symptoms by a change in posture or activity, and the lesions are always in the lower half of the spinal cord and produce symptoms that affect the legs, but not the arms.

Aminoff and Logue in 1974 reported the clinical features and the

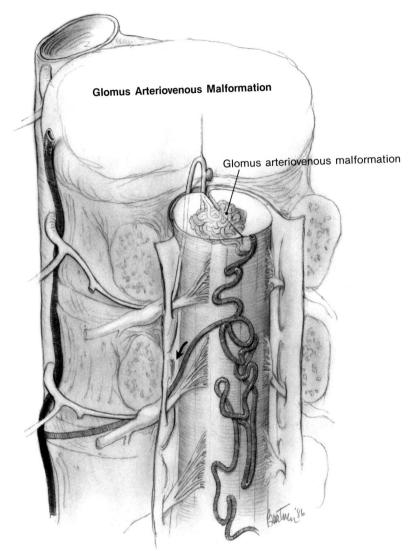

Glomus Arteriovenous Malformation

Glomus arteriovenous malformation

FIG. 9.5. The nidus of the glomus type of intramedullary AVM is a tightly packed congerie of blood vessels confined to a short segment of the spinal cord. These AVMs, which are usually in the anterior half of the cord, are supplied by medullary arteries. Intradural AVMs often have associated arterial or venous aneurysms.

dismal natural history of patients with spinal AVMs (2, 3). Since this study began before the introduction of selective spinal cord angiography, comparison of the natural history of patients with the specific subtypes of AVMs was not possible. However, as most patients now undergo treatment earlier, it may serve as the only good study of the untreated

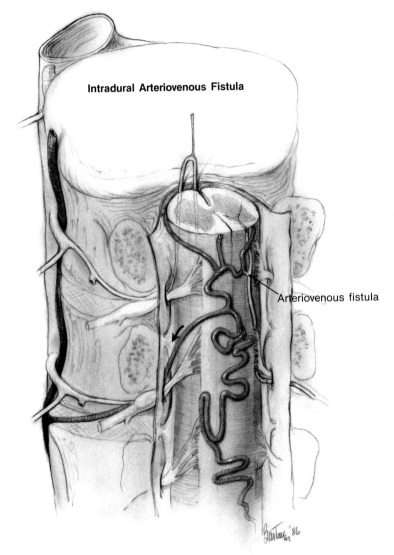

FIG. 9.6.   Intradural direct AV fistula in the pia. Medullary arteries provide the arterial supply.

progression of this disorder. The study was probably strongly prejudiced by the single coiled vessel type, since the great majority of spinal AVMs are of this type. Their patients demonstrated fluctuation of symptoms against a background of steadily increasing disability. By 6 months after the onset of symptoms other than pain, 19% required crutches or were confined to a wheelchair or bed. Ninety-one percent had restricted activity due to a disturbance of gait within 3 years. They concluded that

TABLE 9.2

Clinical Syndrome[a]

	Dural AVM (n = 27)	Intradural AVM (n = 54)
Age	46	24
Onset of symptoms	Gradual (78%)	Acute (37%)
Subarachnoid hemorrhage	0	50%
First symptom	Paresis (44%)	SAH (32%)
Spinal bruit	0	6%
Exacerbation symptoms by activity	70%	15%
Arms affected	0	11%

[a] Reproduced with permission from Rosenblum, B., Oldfield, E. H., and Doppman, J. L. Pathogenesis of spinal arteriovenous malformations. J. Neurosurg., in press, 1987.

"once leg weakness or gait disturbance has developed, it is often progressive with great rapidity until the patient is severely disabled. Within 3 months of functional impairment of the legs, 50% of our patients were severely disabled" (3).

Myelography is the first study performed in patients with clinical evidence of progressive myelopathy and is almost universally abnormal in patients with spinal AVMs. We do not search for a spinal AVM in a patient with a technically acceptable myelogram which does not reveal abnormal vessels. Digital vascular imaging (DVI) after intravenous injection of contrast is occasionally positive, but may miss smaller lesions and often is not of sufficient resolution to identify the origin of the feeding vessels (12, 22). Intraarterial DVI offers increased resolution and if performed before selective spinal angiography limits the area of interest to a short segment of the spinal axis and thus limits the extent of selective spinal angiography required (22). It generally reveals the absence or presence of a spinal AVM and often demonstrates the level of origin of feeding vessels. However, we also have patients with small spinal dural AV fistulas who had a negative DVI study after intraarterial injection of contrast. Moreover, it is important that the arterial supply to the cord in the region of the AVM is identified so that one doesn't inadvertently occlude an anterior medullary artery, such as the artery of Adamkiewicz, when the AVM is occluded. The normal cord vessels are often too small to be identified with DVI after intravenous or intraarterial injection of contrast. Therefore, spinal angiography should be performed in all patients with spinal AVMs, even if the presence of the AVM has been established with other studies.

NORMAL VASCULAR ANATOMY OF THE SPINAL CORD AND DURA

To appreciate the deviant anatomy of spinal AVMs and the different mechanisms of cord injury with the subtypes of AVMs, the normal vascular anatomy of the spinal cord and dura must be understood.

The arteries which supply the spinal cord are divided into two different systems. The anterior spinal artery, which supplies the anterior two-thirds of the cross-sectional area of the cord, including the corticospinal tracts, extends without interruption along the entire anterior surface of the spinal cord. The posterolateral spinal arteries, two plexiform inter-connecting channels running along the posterolateral cord surface, per-fuse the posterior third of the spinal cord (10, 17, 19, 24, 43, 45). In the developing fetus medullary arteries supply the anterior and posterolateral spinal arteries at each segmental level. However, most of these regress well before 6 months of gestational age, and only a limited number of medullary arteries, which provide blood supply only to the spinal cord (24), remain (Fig. 9.2). In adults, spinal rami from the vertebral, subcla-vian and aortic intercostal arteries supply 6–10 anterior medullary arter-ies which inosculate with the anterior spinal artery at intervals. This is especially notable with the artery of Adamkiewicz, which arises from an aortic intercostal artery between T8 and L4.

Two arteries arise as branches of the spinal ramus of the intercostal artery, the same parent vessel as that of the medullary arteries, but persist at each segmental level in the adult. These are the radicular arteries, which supply the anterior and posterior nerve roots but do not provide blood for the cord, and the dural arteries, which provide blood to the root sleeve and spinal dura (Fig. 9.2) (24, 34).

The spinal cord tissue is drained initially by radial veins, which carry the blood from the tissue to the cord surface, where they empty into the coronal venous plexus, a plexiform network of veins in the pia. (Fig. 9.2) (25). The venous blood passes from the coronal venous plexus through the dura to the epidural veins via medullary veins, which penetrate the dura adjacent to, but separate from, the dural penetration of the nerve roots (25). The medullary veins, as the medullary arteries, are not present at every segmental level, but have an inconstant occurrence along the longitudinal axis of the spine. Functional valves at the level of the dura prevent substances injected into the epidural venous system from reach-ing the intradural venous system or the spinal cord (25, 43). However, there are no valves in the intrathecal or intraparenchymal veins; marker substances injected into an intrathecal medullary vein stain the cord tissue (25, 43).

DURAL ARTERIOVENOUS FISTULAS

Dural AVMs arise caudal to the cervical area (Fig. 9.7) (29, 31, 37, 40, 41, 44). Symptoms affect the lower extremities and are frequently exac-erbated by activity. Most patients experience the onset of progressive neurological deficits in the latter half of adult life (Fig. 9.8). Selective spinal angiography demonstrates the nidus of the AV fistula in the

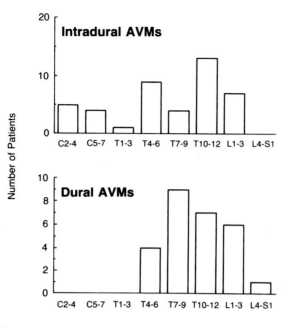

FIG. 9.7.   Site of nidus in patients with dural AV fistulas is below the midthoracic level, whereas intradural AVMs are dispersed along the entire axis of the cord. (From Rosenblum, B., Oldfield, E. H., and Doppman, J. L. Pathogenesis of spinal arteriovenous malformations. J. Neurosurg., in press, 1987.)

intervertebral foramen and the adjacent lateral aspect of the spinal canal and drainage of the fistula into the dilated, coiled pial vessels of the coronal venous plexus on the cord surface (Fig. 9.9).

Figure 9.2 schematically shows the anatomic basis of spinal dural AV fistulas. The dural branch of the intervertebral artery (the spinal ramus of the intercostal artery) supplies the dural AV fistula (37). The medullary vein, the solitary venous outflow of dural AV fistulas, carries blood under high pressure and flow in a retrograde manner to the coronal venous plexus, which becomes dilated, tortuous, and elongated by the reception of excess blood flow under high pressure. Since there are no valves between the coronal venous plexus and the radial veins draining the spinal cord, the high pressure is transmitted directly to the cord tissue, and myelopathy results.

That the blood draining the AV fistula can cause an acquired transfiguration of the normal coronal venous plexus by elongation, dilation, and tortuosity of its component vessels is demonstrated by similar alteration in appearance by lesions that we know are acquired, such as tumors

172

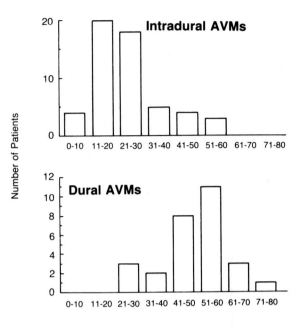

FIG. 9.8. Intradural AVMs predominantly affect children and young adults. Dural AV fistulas usually present in adults over 40 years old. (From Rosenblum, B., Oldfield, E. H., and Doppman, J. L. Pathogenesis of spinal arteriovenous malformations. J. Neurosurg., in press, 1987.)

(hemangioblastomas) with AV shunting (Fig. 9.9), paraspinous gunshot wounds with medullary venous drainage, and intracranial dural fistulas that empty caudally into the venous system of the spinal cord.

It has previously been suggested that vascular steal of blood away from the spinal cord may account for ischemic cord injury in these patients. However, in 23 of our 27 patients with spinal dural AV fistulas, the vessel supplying the dural AV fistula provided no blood supply to the spinal cord (Fig. 9.10) (41). For these fistulas to cause ischemia as a result of arterial steal, they would have to significantly reduce the intraaortic pressure, which is unlikely, since the flow of contrast through these malformations is quite slow, often requiring over 15 seconds to disappear at angiography. Additionally, the pathology of the cord with most spinal AVMs is consistent with venous hypertension and, paradoxically, was described long before it was recognized that most spinal AVMs were dural (1, 4).

The goal of treatment is to eliminate the transmission of venous hypertension to the spinal cord. Stripping the engorged coronal venous

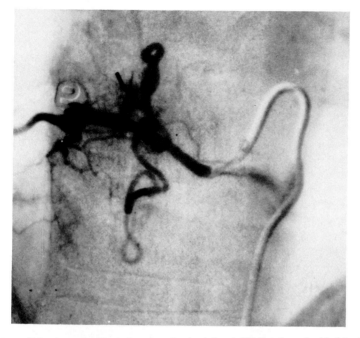

FIG. 9.9.   Selective spinal arteriogram of spinal dural AV fistula embedded in the root sleeve of the ninth thoracic nerve root and the adjacent spinal dura. The nidus of spinal dural AV fistula is typically in the intervertebral foramen (*arrow*) and the lateral aspect of the spinal canal and drains into the dilated, tortuous intradural veins on the cord surface.

plexus from the spinal cord will accomplish this in some patients, but success depends upon inclusion of the vessel between the dural AV fistula and the engorged pial veins in the length of specimen removed. Since these engorged vessels are the normal, but transfigured, veins of the coronal venous plexus, stripping them from the cord surface removes a portion of the normal venous drainage of the cord, and may cause further cord damage. This procedure also often requires an extensive laminectomy and a long, tedious operation, is directed toward an epiphenomenon and not the site of the problem, and is no longer indicated. By obliterating the dural AV fistula, or by interrupting the vessel which carries blood from the dural fistula to the coronal venous plexus, venous hypertension is eliminated, and the cord is allowed to recover and the normal veins of the cord are not sacrificed.

The dural AV fistula can be occluded by embolization during interventional angiography. This has been performed in a large series of patients by Merland *et al.* with success (35). However, this technique cannot be safely employed when the same segmental artery supplies both the dural

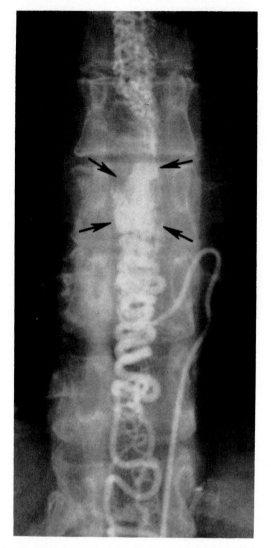

FIG. 9.10.   Selective spinal arteriogram demonstrating hemangioblastoma of the thoracic segment of the spinal cord and the venous drainage of the excess blood flowing
through the vascular tumor. The hemangioblastoma is confined to the area bordered by
arrows. The abnormal appearance with tortuosity, elongation, and dilation of the veins of
the coronal venous plexus is an acquired alteration in these normal vessels which results
from the reception of arterialized blood with high flow and pressure. A similar alteration
in appearance of the normal cord vessels occurs in patients with spinal dural AV fistulas.

AV fistula and the spinal cord, as occurred in 4 of 27 patients with spinal dural AV fistulas (Fig. 9.11). In addition patients occasionally become paraplegic following embolization, possibly due to retrograde thrombosis of the coronal venous plexus (35).

Ideal treatment of spinal dural AV fistulas should obliterate the fistula and interrupt the vein draining intradurally from the dural nidus to the coronal venous plexus to permanently eliminate venous hypertension of the cord. This has been advocated by Logue (31), Oldfield et al. (37), Doppman et al. (15), Symon et al. (44), and Yaşargil et al. (48). Obliteration of the dural fistula may not always be indicated, however, in patients who have a vessel which provides a common origin of a medullary artery supplying the anterior or posterolateral spinal arteries and the dural artery feeding the fistula (Fig. 9.10) (15). The common origin of these vessels from the spinal ramus of the intercostal artery is so close and intertwined that it is not possible to separate the origin of the medullary artery from that of the dural artery feeding the AV fistula without risking occlusion of the medullary artery.

Dural AV fistulas are uniformly amenable to treatment. Of our 27 patients 19 improved after treatment, and in the remaining seven preexisting clinical progression stabilized after surgery (40, 41). No patient was permanently worse as a result of the surgery. Postoperative angiography uniformly suggested complete obliteration of the AV fistulas.

INTRADURAL SPINAL AVMs

In the intradural AVMs of the spinal cord, the juvenile AVMs, glomus AVMs, and the direct intradural AV fistulas, the nidus of the fistula lies within the cord parenchyma or the pia (Table 9.3). One of the feeding vessels of these AVMs is always an enlarged medullary artery that also supplies the spinal cord. These lesions arise as a defect in early vascular embryogenesis.

The clinical and radiographic findings in this group of patients result from rapid blood flow through the AV nidus (40, 41). Compatible with high flow are the presence of widened interpedicular distance on plain x-rays, acute onset of symptoms associated with subarachnoid hemorrhage (SAH), spinal bruit, multiple feeding vessels, and frequent association with spinal aneurysms, all of which are seen only in lesions with rapid flow (40, 41). In our 81 patients with spinal AVMs varices and arterial aneurysms occurred only with the intradural AVMs (40, 41). They are probably caused by the high pressure, high flow rate, and turbulent flow through the intradural nidus and its feeding and draining channels. In contrast to dural AV fistulas, in intradural AVMs myelopathy results from SAH and arterial steal (40, 41). Arterial steal is suggested by the

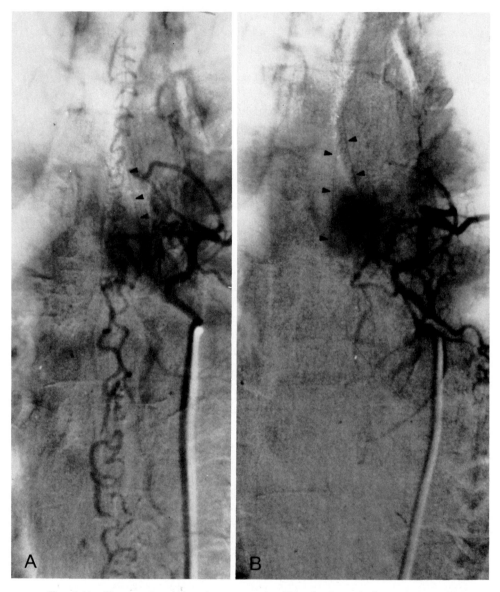

FIG. 9.11. Preoperative (A) and postoperative (B) selective spinal arteriograms in a patient with a spinal dural AV fistula at the seventh thoracic nerve root. (A) The seventh left thoracic intercostal artery provided common origin of the arterial supply to the dural AV fistula (*large arrow*) and to the artery of Adamkiewicz (*arrowheads*). (B) Following surgical interruption of the medullary vein draining the dural AV fistula intradurally, the dural fistula no longer opacifies.

TABLE 9.3

Radiographic Features[a]

	Dural AVM (n = 27)	Intradural AVM (n = 54)
Site of nidus	Lateral canal, 100%	Within cord, 80% Ventral cord surface, 11% Dorsal cord surface, 9%
Level of spine	Lower half	Diffuse
Rapid flow	0%	80%
Associated aneurysm	0%	44%
Shared medullary arterial supply	15%	100%
Route of venous drainage	Rostral, 100% Caudal, 4%	Rostral, 81% Caudal, 72%

[a] Reproduced with permission from Rosenblum, B., Oldfield, E. H., and Doppman, J. L. Pathogenesis of spinal arteriovenous malformations. J. Neurosurg., in press, 1987.

combination of high flow through the AVM and the feeding vessels of the AVM always being medullary arteries that also supply the cord. Sufficient blood flow in the medullary arteries may be diverted from cord parenchyma and into the nonperfusion AV shunt to cause ischemia. As in spinal dura AVMs, the distended draining veins of intramedullary AVMs may also cause ischemia as a result of increased venous pressure. However, the presence and the extent of the bidirectional venous drainage of these lesions suggests that the venous drainage is adequate and that venous hypertension of the cord is unlikely (41).

The ideal therapy for medullary AVMs is complete obliteration of the AV nidus, via microsurgical excision or embolization, while preserving the blood supply of the cord (8, 30, 33, 47). The operating microscope and appropriate microsurgical instrumentation and technique are required for surgery for all spinal AVMs. Operative exposure of intramedullary spinal AVMs is performed in the prone position with a complete laminectomy covering one segment above and below the glomus of the malformation. The dura is opened in the midline using care to preserve the arachnoid intact so that treating of the large, fragile underlying vessels is avoided. This is particularly important in patients with previous SAH when the arachnoid may be quite adherent to underlying vessels of the malformation. In patients with recent hemorrhage into the subarachnoid space, surgery is postponed until enough time has passed for lysis of clots and absorption of blood products from the subarachnoid space. To improve visualization of the component vessels of the AVM, the arachnoid is then removed from the surface of the underlying malformation.

Correlation of the vascular anatomy as seen on the preoperative ιostic studies with that seen intraoperatively is performed so that ₘedullary arteries are preserved during dissection and to aid the early ₑntification and interruption of major feeding arteries as they enter the malformation. Meticulous hemostasis is essential, since blood-stained pia obscures anatomic details. Liberal irrigation during bipolar coagulation prevents coagulated vessel walls from adhering to the tips of the forceps, which can be bothersome at the wrong moment. Larger feeding vessels may require ligatures or clips, but most vessels can be managed with simple bipolar coagulation and interruption. By miscrodissection with the tips of the bipolar forceps in the gliotic plane between the malformation and the adjacent cord tissue and by elevating the malformation as one works from one pole upward or downward, the malformation can be dissected from the surrounding cord. As the margins of the malformation are dissected, gentle bipolar coagulation is used to gradually shrink the AVM and render the periphery of the lesion less friable to manipulation. This also reduces turgidity in the nidus as dissection proceeds. Hypotension occasionally is helpful. Pial traction sutures are used to maintain adequate separation of the cord tissue from the AVM to permit room for dissection. At least one of the major draining veins is preserved patent until dissection around the periphery of the malformation has been completed and all arterial feeding vessels have been occluded. Postoperative spinal anteriography is used routinely to assess the success of complete obliteration of the AVM.

If the juvenile or glomus AVM occupies a considerable portion of the parenchyma of the ventral half of the spinal cord, it may be impossible to remove it without eliciting unacceptable neurological deficit, and surgical excision should not be attempted. Plans to completely excise or obliterate the malformation may also have to be abandoned intraoperatively if it becomes apparent that undue risk to cord function will occur with continued attempts at complete removal. Reduction of flow in these lesions by embolization or ligation of feeding arteries may diminish the incidence of subsequent hemorrhage and may reduce vascular steal and associated ischemia of the cord, but collateral vessels ultimately develop and again supply the AV nidus. Occlusion of the vascular nidus by selective embolization as primary treatment is also frequently beneficial, but the incidence of delayed reestablishment of flow through the nidus of the AVM remains unknown (13, 16, 18, 36, 38).

ETIOLOGY

Our findings in a retrospective review of 81 patients with spinal AVMs (27 dural AV fistulas and 54 intradural AVMs) support an acquired etiology for dural AVMs and a congenital origin of intradural spinal AVMs (Table 9.4) (40, 41). Dural AVMs first became symptomatic in

TABLE 9.4

Etiology[a]

	Dural AVM (Acquired)	Intradural AVM (Congenital)
Onset of symptoms	Latter half of adulthood	Child or young adult
Associated congenital syndromes	No	Yes
Distribution along cord	Lower half	Diffuse
Associated aneurysm	0%	44%
Normal venous pathways	Absent	Prominent

Reproduced with permission from Rosenblum, B., Oldfield, E. H., and Doppman, J. L. Pathogenesis of spinal arteriovenous malformations. J. Neurosurg., in press, 1987.

later adult life, whereas medullary AVMs affected children and young adults (Fig. 9.8). There were associated congenital vascular malformations only with intradural AVMs. If spinal AVMs were congenital malformations of vasculature, one would expect a distribution that is proportional to the distribution of the tissue of the spinal cord. Such a distribution was demonstrated with medullary AVMs, in which there was a uniform distribution along the longitudinal axis of the spinal cord, but not with the dural AVMs, which were all located in the lower half of the spinal canal (Fig. 9.8), a distribution which has been noted by others (29, 31, 35, 42), and which is compatible with an acquired etiology that is dependent on an upright posture (41).

Congenital development of AV fistulas is associated with increased development of draining veins to accommodate the excess blood flow. With intramedullary AVMs, veins drain the excess blood flow rostrally and caudally (41). In contrast, with dural lesions, although they are restricted to the lower half of the spine, inferiorly directed venous drainage seldom occurs (40, 41). All have superiorly directed venous efflux from the AV fistula, frequently filling the distended veins of the transfigured coronal venous plexus all the way to the cranium, drainage against a greater hydrostatic pressure in the upright position than caudal drainage. Thus, venous drainage of the coronal venous plexus via the normal medullary veins appears consistently to be deficient with dural AVMs (35, 40, 41). This suggests that diminished, and not increased, venous drainage of the spinal cord might accompany, or be associated with the etiology of, these lesions, as has previously been suggested by Merland *et al.* (35). We conclude from these observations that spinal dural AV fistulas are probably acquired and that a congenital error in vascular embryogenesis causes medullary AVMs.

The mechanism of the development of an acquired spinal dural AV fistula remains unknown. One possibility is suggested by consideration of structures of the normal dural vasculature. Manelfe described a glomus of blood vessels, a peleton, the function of which is not yet clear, in which a single small arterial branch of the dural artery supplies a tightly packed glomus of dural blood vessels that is drained by a single small dural vein (34). Dural AV fistulas may arise from the development of direct communications between the artery supplying and the vein drainage peletons, possibly a result of thrombosis and recanalization of one of these glomerular-like structures (34), a mechanism similar to that proposed for intracranial dural AV fistulas (6, 7, 28). The etiological significance of the limited medullary venous drainage of the cord in patients with spinal dural AV fistulas remains to be clarified.

CURRENT AND FUTURE DEVELOPMENTS

Although spinal dural AV fistulas are amenable to a simple, safe, and effective surgical therapy and most patients have functionally significant improvement following treatment, most patients do not return to a normal neurological status following obliteration of the AV fistula (29, 31, 37, 40, 41, 44). The final outcome is directly related to the degree of neurological function preoperatively; this is so with dural and intradural AVMs (32, 37, 40, 41, 44). Those patients who are ambulatory preoperatively do well; those with severe, fixed preoperative neurological deficits usually fare less well. Therefore, improvements in the outcome of these patients, particularly those with dural fistulas, in whom the progress of cord injury can be stopped universally by obliteration of the dural AV fistula, should occur with earlier diagnosis and treatment.

Recent technological advances in diagnostic radiology should permit early diagnosis of most patients with spinal AVMs with minimally invasive or noninvasive procedures. Dynamic computed tomographic (CT) scanning, the rapid acquisition of a series of transverse CT images after intravenous injection of contrast, confirms the presence of an AVM and, if the level of the nidus is used for scanning, often demonstrates the intra- or extramedullary location of the AVM (11, 12). The presence of most spinal AVMs can be established by intraarterial DVI (22). A signal void in the spinal cord image in magnetic resonance imaging demonstrates the presence and location of intramedullary AVMs and can also be used to noninvasively sequentially assess the status of flow in these lesions following treatment (9, 20).

A more difficult task is the development of safe and successful treatment for intramedullary AVMs in the caudal two-thirds of the spinal cord. The development and refinement of motor evoked potentials should permit monitoring of the integrity of the corticospinal tracts during occlusion of the nidus at surgery and during therapeutic embolization. The refinement of methods to continuously monitor spinal cord flow intraoperatively to detect sudden alterations in flow with temporary occlusion of vessels, such as laser Doppler velicometry, should make surgical excision of these lesions safer (39). Embolic occlusion may be safer if test infusions of short-acting barbiturates permit prediction of the affect of embolization before the embolic material is introduced (21, 26, 27). Our experience with primates suggests that the duration of paraplegia after infusion of short-acting barbiturates and lidocaine is dose-dependent and fully reversible (21). Continued refinement of currently available techniques and the development of new approaches is certain to permit earlier, safer, and more effect treatment for spinal AVMs in future years.

CONCLUSIONS

With spinal dural AVMs the nidus of the AVM is imbedded in the dura covering the proximal nerve root and in the adjacent spinal dura. Spinal angiography demonstrates an AV nidus of fine vessels in the lateral aspect of the spinal canal and within an intervertebral foramen. Contrast flows through the fistula and intradurally, into a tightly coiled, continuous vessel on the cord surface. It is the dural branch of the spinal ramus of the intercostal artery that supplies the dural AV fistula. Blood flowing through the dural AV fistula is carried through the medullary vein in a retrograde manner to the coronal venous plexus, which becomes dilated, tortuous, and elongated by the reception of excess blood flow under increased pressure. The absence of valves between the coronal venous plexus and the radial veins permits transmission of high venous pressure to the cord tissue, which cause myelopathy.

Medullary and dural AVMs have distinct clinical and demographic differences. The findings suggest a congenital origin for medullary AVMs and an acquired origin for dural AVMs, as has been suggested for cranial dural AV fistulas. The clinical and radiographic features of medullary AVMs suggest that rapid blood flow through the AV fistula is responsible for cord injury, whereas the findings with dural lesions suggest that myelopathy results from venous hypertension. The prognosis for successful treatment in dural and medullary AVMs is a function of the preoperative neurological deficit; most lesions are susceptible to effective therapy.

ACKNOWLEDGMENTS

We thank Howard Bartner for skillfully preparing the illustrations of the spinal cord anatomy.

REFERENCES

1. Aminoff, M. F., Barnard, R. O., and Logue, V. The pathophysiology of spinal vascular malformations. J. Neurol, Sci., 23: 255–263, 1974.

2. Aminoff, M. J., and Logue, V. Clinical features of spinal vascular malformations. Brain, 97: 197–210, 1974.
3. Aminoff, M. J., and Logue, V. The prognosis of patients with spinal vascular malformations. Brain, 97: 211–218, 1974.
4. Antoni, N. Spinal vascular malformations (angiomas) and myelomalicia. Neurology. (Minneap.), 12: 795–804, 1962.
5. Benhaiem, N., Porrier, J., and Hurth, M. Ateriovenous fistula of the meninges draining into the spinal veins: A histological study of 28 cases. Acta Neuropathol. (Berl.), 62: 103–111, 1983.
6. Brainin, M., and Samec, P. Venous hemodynamics of ateriovenous meningeal fistulas in the posterior cranial fossa. Neuroradiology, 25: 161–169, 1983.
7. Chaudhary, M., Sachdev, V. P., Cho, S. H., et al. Dural arteriovenous malformation of the major venous sinuses: An acquired lesion. AJNR, 3: 13–19, 1982.
8. Cogan, P., and Stein, B. M. Spinal cord arteriovenous malformations with significant intramedullary components. J. Neurosurg., 59: 471–478, 1983.
9. Di Chiro, G., Doppman, J. L., Dwyer, A. J., et al. Magnetic resonance imaging of tumors and arteriovenous malformations of the spinal cord. Radiology, 156: 689–697, 1985.
10. Di Chiro, G., Doppman, J. L., and Ommaya, A. K. Selective arteriography of arteriovenous aneurysms of spinal cord. Radiology, 88: 1065–1077, 1967.
11. Di Chiro G., Doppman, J. L., and Werner, L. Computed tomography of spinal cord arteriovenous malformations. Radiology, 123: 351–354, 1977.
12. Di Chiro G., Reith, K. G., Oldfield, E. H., et al. Digital subtraction angiography and dynamic computed tomography in the evaluation of arteriovenous malformations and hemangioblastomas of the spinal cord. J. Comp. Assist. Tomogr., 6: 655–670, 1982.
13. Djindjian, R. Embolization of angiomas of the spinal cord. Surg. Neurol., 4: 411—420, 1975.
14. Djindjian, M., Djindjian, R., Rey, A., et al. Intradural extramedullary spinal arteriovenous malformations fed by the anterior spinal artery. Surg. Neurol., 8: 85–93, 1977.
15. Doppman, J. L., Di Chiro, G., and Oldfield, E. H.: Origin of spinal arteriovenous malformation and normal cord vasculature from a common segmental artery: Angiographic and therapeutic considerations. Radiology, 154: 687–689, 1985.
16. Doppman, J. L., Di Chiro, G., and Ommaya, A. K. Obliteration of spinal cord arteriovenous malformation by percutaneous embolization. Lancet, 1: 477, 1968.
17. Doppman, J. L., Di Chiro, G., and Ommaya, A. K. Selective Arteriography of the Spinal Cord. St. Louis, Warren H. Green, 1969.
18. Doppman, J. L., Di Chiro, G., and Ommaya, A. K. Percutaneous embolization of spinal cord arteriovenous malformations. J. Neurosurg., 34: 48–55, 1971.
19. Doppman, J. L., Di Chiro, G., and Ommaya, A. K. Radiology of spinal ateriovenous malformations. Progr. Neurol. Surg. 4: 329–354, 1971.
20. Doppman, J. L., Dwyer, A. J., Frank, J. L., et al. Magnetic resonance imaging of spinal arteriovenous malformations. J. Neurosurg., in press, 1987.
21. Doppman, J. L., Girton, M., and Oldfield, E. H. A spinal Wada test. Radiology, 161: 319–321, 1986.
22. Doppman, J. L., Krudy, A. G., Miller, D. L., et al. Intraarterial digital subtraction angiography of spinal arteriovenous malformations. AJNR 4: 1081–1085, 1983.
23. Elsberg, C. A. Diagnosis and Treatment of Surgical Diseases of the Spinal Cord and Its Membranes, pp. 201–204. Saunders, Philadelphia and London, 1916.
24. Gillilan, L. A. The arterial blood supply to the human spinal cord. J. Comp. Neurol., 110: 75, 1958.
25. Gillilan, L. A. Veins of the spinal cord. Neurology (Minneap.), 20: 860–868, 1970.
26. Horton, J. A., and Kerber, C. W. Lidocaine injection into external carotid branches:

Provocative test to preserve cranial nerve function in therapeutic embolization. ANJR, 7: 105–108, 1986.

27. Horton, J. A., Latchaw, R. E., Gold, L. H. A., et al. Embolization of intramedullary arteriovenous malformations of the spinal cord. AJNR, 7: 113–118, 1986.

28. Houser, O. W., Campbell, J. K., Campbell, R. J., et al. Ateriovenous malformation affecting the transverse dural sinus: An acquired lesion. Mayo Clin. Proc., 54: 651–661, 1979.

29. Kendall, B. E., and Logue, V. Spinal epidural angiomatous malformations draining into intrathecal veins. Neuroradiology, 3: 181–189, 1977.

30. Krayenbuhl, H., Yaşargil, M. G., and McClintock, H. G. Treatment of spinal cord vascular malformations by surgical excision. J. Neurosurg., 30: 427–435, 1969.

31. Logue, V. Angiomas of the spinal cord: Review of the pathogenesis, clinical features, and results of surgery. J. Neurol. Neurosurg. Psychiatry, 42: 1–11, 1979.

32. Logue, V., Aminoff, M. J., and Kendall, B. E. Results of surgical treatment for patients with a spinal angioma. J. Neurol. Neurosurg. Psychiatry, 37: 1074–1081, 1974.

33. Malis, L. I. Microsurgery for spinal cord arteriovenous malformations. Clin. Neurosurg., 26: 543–555, 1979.

34. Manelfe, C., Lazorthes, G., and Roulleau, J. Arteres de la dure-nere rachidienne chez l'homme. Acta Radiol. Diagn., 13: 829–841, 1970.

35. Merland, J. J., Riche, M. C., and Chiras, J. Intraspinal extramedullary ateriovenous fistulae draining into the medullary veins. J. Neuroradiol., 7: 271–320, 1980.

36. Newton, T. H., and Adams, J. E. Angiographic demonstration and non-surgical embolization of spinal cord angioma. Radiology, 91: 873–876, 1968.

37. Oldfield, E. H., Di Chiro, G., Quindlen, E. A., et al. Successful treatment of a group of spinal cord arteriovenous malformations by interruption of dural fistula. J. Neurosurg., 59: 1019–1030, 1983.

38. Riche, M. C., Melki, J. P., and Merland, J. J. Embolization of spinal cord vascular malformations via the anterior spinal artery. AJNR, 4: 378–381, 1983.

39. Rosenblum, N., Bonner, R., and Oldfield, E. Intraoperative measurements of cortical blood flow adjacent to cerebral arteriovenous malformation using laser doppler velocimetry. J. Neurosurg., 66: 396–399, 1987.

40. Rosenblum, B., Oldfield, E. H., Di Chiro, G., et al. Pathogenesis of spinal arteriovenous malformations. Surg. Forum, 37: 489–491, 1987.

41. Rosenblum, B., Oldfield, E. H., and Doppman, J. L. Pathogenesis of spinal arteriovenous malformations. J. Neurosurg., in press, 1987.

42. Sargent, P. Hemangioma of the pia mater causing compression paraplegia. Brain, 48: 259–267, 1925.

43. Suh, T. H., and Alexander, L. Vascular system of human spinal cord. Arch. Neurol. Psychiatry, 41: 659–677, 1939.

44. Symon, L., Kuyama, H., and Kendall, B. Dural arteriovenous malformations of the spine: Clinical features and surgical results in 55 cases. J. Neurosurg., 60: 238–247, 1984.

45. Turnbull, I. M. Microvasculature of the human spinal cord. J. Neurosurg., 35: 141–147, 1971.

46. Wyburn-Mason, R. The vascular abnormalities and tumors of the spinal cord and its membranes. H. Klimpton, London, 1943.

47. Yaşargil, M. G., DeLong, W. B., and Guarnaschelli, J. J. Complete microsurgical excision of cervical extramedullary and intramedullary vascular malformations. Surg. Neurol., 4: 211–224, 1975.

48. Yaşargil, M. G., Symon, L., and Teddy, P. J. Arteriovenous malformations of the spinal cord. Adv. Techn. Stand. Neurosurg., 11: 61–102, 1984.

III

Spinal Surgery

CHAPTER

10

Somatosensory Evoked Potentials in Neurosurgery

WILLIAM A. FRIEDMAN, M.D.

INTRODUCTION

An evoked potential (EP) is the response of the nervous system to a specific external stimulus. This contrasts with the electroencephalogram (EEG), which may be thought of as the surface summation of all ongoing, "spontaneous" brain activity. Stimuli typically utilized to produce EPs include flash or pattern-shift visual stimuli, click or tone burst auditory stimuli, and electrical, vibratory, or tactile peripheral nerve stimuli. Research applications have included, however, other modalities of stimulation, including olfactory, gustatory, and respiratory (47, 48). Since the nervous system's specific response to these stimuli is much smaller than the summation of all ongoing electrical activity, the EP is of much smaller amplitude than the EEG. In fact the EEG amplitude (approximately 50 μV) is typically an order of magnitude bigger than the largest surface-recorded EPs (5 μV). This means that, without special recording technology, the EP will invariably be obscured by the EEG.

Dawson (49) first reported the existence of human somatosensory evoked potentials (SEPs) in 1947, utilizing the relatively crude technique of superimposing multiple oscilloscope traces. Brainstem auditory evoked potentials (BAEPs) were first reported in 1967 (182). Visual evoked potentials (VEPs) were long known to occur during EEG recording with "photic driving." It was not until the advent, however, of portable, affordable, digital averaging computers, that the application of these techniques in diagnostic clinical neurology became widespread (1970s). Only in recent years has this technology been transported to the operating room and intensive care unit for the express purpose of monitoring, as opposed to diagnosis (78).

Somatosensory evoked potentials have found the most widespread application in the diagnosis and monitoring of neurosurgical diseases. In the following pages, a detailed review of the theory and practice of SEPs will be undertaken.

BASIC NEUROPHYSIOLOGY

All neurons have a resting membrane potential (1). That is, if one inserts a measuring electrode through the cell membrane and inside the cell, the electrical potential will be approximately −70 mV compared to the extracellular environment. This resting potential depends on basic principles of physical chemistry. The predominant intracellular ions are potassium and impermeable anions (negatively charged ions). The predominant extracellular ions are sodium and chloride (see Fig. 10.1). The cell membrane is generally much more permeable to potassium than sodium. In resting conditions, potassium ions tend to diffuse down the concentration gradient, from intracellular to extracellular. This loss of positive ions (cations) renders the interior of the cell relatively more negative than the exterior. The magnitude of the electrical potential required to prevent further diffusion of ions (the equilibrium potential) is related to the concentration gradient via the Nernst equation:

$$\text{Equilibrium potential} = (RT/zF) \; ln \; (K^+ \text{ outside}/K^+ \text{ inside})$$

where R is the gas constant, T the absolute temperature, z the valence of

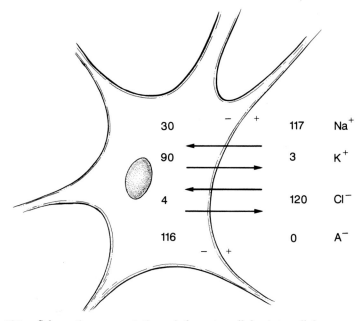

FIG. 10.1. Schematic representation of the extracellular-intracellular concentration gradients for several important ions. In the resting state, the cell membrane is relatively impermeable to all ions but potassium. Flow of potassium down its concentration gradient is primarily responsible for the negative intracellular resting potential. This potential can be closely predicted by the Nernst equation for potassium.

the ion, F the Faraday constant, K^+ outside the concentration of potassium outside the cell, and K^+ inside the concentration of potassium inside the cell. Under standard conditions and base 10 logarithms, the equation can be simplified to:

$$E = 58 \log (K^+ \text{ outside}/K^+ \text{ inside})$$

In the resting state, only potassium approaches its equilibrium potential because the membrane is relatively impermeable to the other important ions. The resting cell potential, therefore, is primarily determined by the potassium concentration gradient.

Neurons transmit information via electrical currents (123). These currents are generated by changes in the permeability of the cell membrane to the various ions. This allows the ions to flow down their concentration gradients to their equilibrium potentials. For example, an excitatory postsynaptic potential (EPSP) is a depolarization of the cell towards less negative interior values thought to result from increased permeability of the membrane to sodium, potassium, and chloride. An inhibitory postsynaptic potential (IPSP) is a hyperpolarization of the cell towards more negative interior values thought to be primarily related to increases in chloride permeability. These permeability changes are generated by the effects of synaptic neurotransmitters on the postsynaptic cell membranes. Because nerves are relatively poor conductors of electricity, EPSPs and IPSPs generally spread very short distances along the nerve (1–2 mm).

If the sum of EPSPs and IPSPs at the synapse reaches a certain critical level of depolarization (threshold), an action potential is generated during which the interior of the cell actually becomes relatively positive because of large increases in sodium conductance. This action potential sets up electrotonic currents. The electrical energy needed to cause the electrotonic currents (which flow from positive to negative) is derived from the inward movement of positive charge at the peak of the action potential. Electrotonic current spread ahead of the action potential causes further depolarization of the membrane, with regeneration of the action potential and undiminished propagation to the next synapse. Behind the action potential, outward potassium current is responsible for repolarization to resting values.

Current flowing across cell membranes gives rise to externally recorded potentials. The shape of such potentials depends upon the conduction of the action potential or synaptic potential through the extracellular fluid. The classic experiments on volume conduction of such potentials were performed by Lorente de No (135). In Figure 10.2A, the neuron is at rest; there is no current flow; and the extracellular electrodes record a potential difference of 0. If an action potential occurs, as the region of intracellular

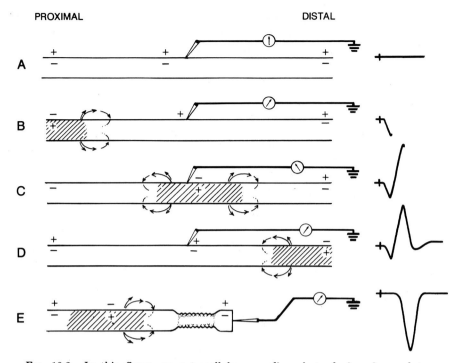

Fig. 10.2. In this figure, an extracellular recording electrode is referenced to an indifferent electrode. In this experiment, a positive potential leads to a downward deflection on the oscilloscope screen. (A) As there is no current flow, the extracellular electrodes record a potential difference of zero. (B) As the electrotonic currents at the leading edge of the action potential approach the recording electrode, a positive extracellular potential is recorded. (C) As the region of depolarization passes directly under the recording electrode, a strong negative potential is recorded. (D) Repolarization again generates a small positive extracellular response. (E) A recording electrode positioned beyond an injured area of nerve ("the killed end effect") records only a biphasic positive potential as the area of depolarization approaches, but never reaches, the electrode. This phenomenon accounts for the shape of many surface recorded evoked potentials.

depolarization approaches the recording electrode, the extracellular electrode records relative positivity, compared to the reference electrode. As the region of maximum intracellular depolarization passes, a relative negativity is recorded. As the area of repolarization passes, a relative positivity is again sensed. Thus the entire waveform is triphasic: positive, reflecting outward, electrotonic current flow toward the approaching region of depolarization; negative, reflecting inward current flow in the region of depolarization; and positive again, reflecting outward potassium current during repolarization.

Volume conductor theory states that the shape of the externally recorded action potential should be porportional to the density of the transmembrane current and fit the negative of the second derivative of the intracellularly recorded action potential (163). This theoretical prediction also yields a triphasic potential. In fact such potentials are routinely recorded from the skin surface overlying peripheral nerves after a somatosensory stimulus. Note well (Fig. 10.2E) that an electrode placed at or beyond the end of the nerve records primarily a positive potential. In this case, the depolarization approaches but does not reach the electrode. The importance of this finding is that a recording electrode placed beyond the termination of a neural pathway will see only a positive potential as that pathway conducts electrical potentials. In fact, many evoked potential recording situations (such as BAEPs) yield primarily biphasic, positive potentials for this reason.

Evoked potentials are frequently referred to as "near-field" or "far-field." A "near-field" evoked potential is one which is generated close to the site of the recording electrodes (*i.e.*, a cortical somatosensory evoked potential). Such potentials are typically relatively large in amplitude and delayed in latency. A "far-field" evoked potential is one which is generated far from the site of the recording electrodes (*i.e.*, brainstem auditory evoked potentials). These potentials are typically small in amplitude, because of the attenuation accrued during volume conduction, and early in latency.

The reader is referred to the references for more information on basic neurophysiology (1, 123).

SEP THEORY

The somatosensory evoked potential is typically generated by applying electrical stimuli to an extremity nerve. A square wave of 0.1–0.2 msec is most commonly used, at an intensity sufficient to produce motor activity. This stimulus has been shown to preferentially activate the largest peripheral nerve sensory fibers (group I). These fibers are also known to primarily mediate vibratory and proprioceptive sensation. The propagated nerve action potentials elicited by this electrical stimulation (*i.e.*, at the wrist or ankle) can be easily recorded more proximally over the peripheral nerve (*e.g.*, Erb's point with medium nerve stimulation). Such a recording will show the triphasic shape predicted by volume conductor theory.

At the point where the nerve roots enter the spinal cord, additional potentials are generated, probably composed of both EPSPs and action potentials (68). Surface spinal cord recordings and skin electrode recordings over the spine yield a consistently reproducible pattern in man and animals. An initial triphasic spike is sometimes seen, which probably corresponds to primary afferent activity. The deflection on the rising phase of the first slow wave is also presynaptic, ascribed to activity in afferent terminals (69). This slow wave (the N wave) has been localized to cellular activity within Rexed's laminae III and IV of the dorsal horn. A subsequent slow positive wave is related to primary afferent depolarization (PAP), a process in which axoaxonic synapses are thought to lead to presynaptic inhibition (156).

Although all of the afferents entering the spinal cord via the dorsal roots project in either the dorsal column or in the dorsolateral fasciculus of the same and adjacent segments, only a small number of the lumbosacral dorsal root fibers in fasciculus gracilis reach the upper cervical cord, and even fewer in the fasciculus cuneatus reach the medulla. Cracco and Evans (38), in an exhaustive study of the effects of asphyxia on various components of the spinal evoked potential, concluded that potentials recorded over the rostral spinal cord arose largely in postsynaptic fibers. Higgins et al. demonstrated conduction failure in the SEP at high rates of stimulation, strongly supporting the contribution of synaptic components to this pathway (99). Thus, the simplified view of a direct transmission line of primary afferents to the sensory relay nuclei is not the case. Interneuronal relay of primary afferent information appears to be the rule rather than the exception.

Whereas most evidence indicates that upper extremity evoked potentials are conducted primarily via dorsal column pathways, much data would suggest that lower extremity EPs are substantially conducted via the lateral funiculus (33). Thus, posterior tibial nerve stimulation at motor threshold intensity primarily activates group I fibers which synapse and travel through the dorsal spinocerebellar tract. After synapsing at the spinomedullary junction (nucleus Z), the pathway projects on to the ventral posterolateral thalamic nucleus (208). Lesion studies in dog, cat, and monkey support the concept that lower extremity SEPs are conducted in all quadrants of the spinal cord but primarily in the dorsal lateral funiculus (54, 67).

Numerous studies have been conducted to identify the sites of origin of the SEP waveforms commonly recorded from the cervical spine, brainstem, and cerebral cortex (7, 8). A number of studies utilize noncephalic, truly inactive reference electrodes. Some, to reduce noise and artifact, utilize cephalic reference electrodes. One must bear in mind that the cephalic electrodes are not truly inactive. They "see" the far-field representation of cervical spinal potentials and various near-field cortical responses. Montages utilizing cephalic references, therefore, generate a complex potential which represents a combination of near-field and far-field recordings. Likewise, though SEP waveforms are frequently referred to as negative or positive (i.e., N13 or P22), the polarity carries no significant physiologic information, as it is totally dependent upon the particular reference electrode selected. It also depends upon the particular convention the investigator follows regarding the display of positive or negative deflection. In our laboratory, all EP recordings are displayed such that a relative positivity (first electrode more positive than the second) results in an upward deflection on the oscilloscope screen. We also arrange our electrode montages such that the more "active" of the two electrodes is the second electrode, and the "reference" electrode is the first electrode. Though most labs follow this convention for BAEPs, many use just the reverse for SEP recordings. The important points to remember are that cephalic "reference" electrodes are often relatively active and that conventions for displaying SEP data currently differ from lab to lab.

SEPs have been extensively studied in normal and abnormal clinical situations, as well as in animal models (51, 56, 97, 121, 122, 144, 149, 152, 172, 178, 180, 188, 199, 207). The following SEP pathway (Fig. 10.3) is presented as a synthesis of currently available information, recognizing that controversy exists as to the precise sites of SEP generation after median nerve stimulation.

Over the lower cervical spine (C7) two potentials are frequently recorded: N12a (meaning negative wave at 12 msec poststimulus), which is thought to correspond to presynaptic afferent impulses, and N13a, which is thought to correspond to postsynaptic dorsal horn interneuronal activity (see spinal potentials above). Similar potentials can be recorded over the upper cervical spine-lower medullary region, at slightly prolonged latencies corresponding to the spinal cord distance travelled. They are called N12b and N13b. Some labs refer to the N12 waves as N11 waves. That these potentials are indeed locally generated within the segmental spinal cord or sensory relay nuclei is supported by the shift of N12 onset latency from lower to upper cervical spinal cord and by a phase reversal of the N13 component when recorded at prevertebral sites (i.e., esophageal leads).

Noncephalic referenced scalp recordings consistently reveal three widely distributed far-field positivities: P9, P11, and P14. The P9 potential corresponds to the afferent impulses recorded over the brachial plexus. The P11 potential corresponds to the cervical spinal cord potential. In lesions of the upper cervical spinal cord and medulla, the P9 and P11 potentials, persist, but the P14 potential is absent. This supports the generally held view that P14 is a nonspinal component generated above the foramen magnum, perhaps in the medial lemniscus. If a cephalic reference electrode is utilized during spinal recordings, the far-field P14 potential becomes inverted ("N14") and interacts in a complex fashion with the near-field N12 and N13 spinal potentials. This may make it very difficult to accurately determine the true central conduction

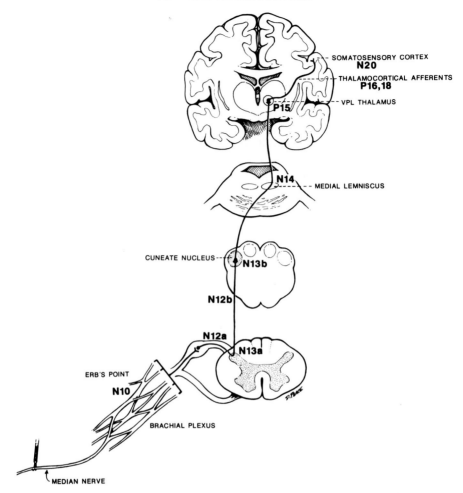

FIG. 10.3.   This figure schematically depicts the putative sites of generation for many of the known components of the median nerve somatosensory evoked potential. These sites include the brachial plexus, middle cervical spinal cord, upper cervical spinal cord, cuneate nucleus, medial lemniscus, sensory thalamus, and somatosensory cortex.

time (CCT, the time from the cervical spinal potential to the cortical potential) (144).

The afferent somatosensory fibers eventually terminate in layer IV of the somatosensory cortex. Multiple potentials can be recorded from the cortical surface (P20, N30, P25, N35) (4, 5). One commonly accepted schema postulates two sources of generation (Fig. 10.4). One source is in area 3b, with activity beginning at about 20 msec. Anterior to 3b a P20–

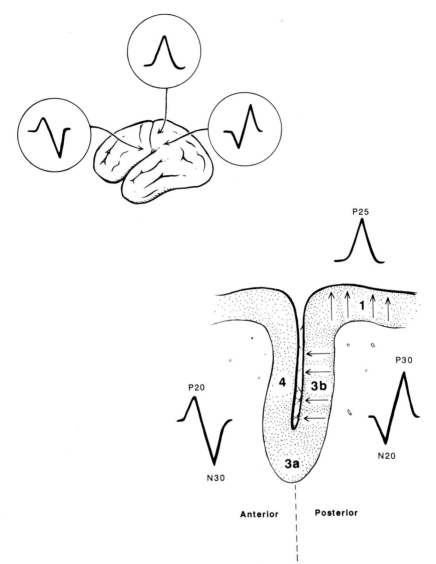

FIG. 10.4   Putative sites of generation of the cortical somatosensory evoked potential. One portion of the potential is generated in area *3b*. The horizontal orientation of the dipole results in a phase reversal of the recorded potential as the central sulcus is crossed. This phenomenon is a very reliable indicator of central sulcus location which can be of great value in certain surgical procedures. Another portion of the potential is generated in area *1* of hand cortex. The vertical orientation of this dipole leads to a potential which is only well recorded very near its site of generation.

N30 wave is recorded; posterior to 3b an N20–P30 wave is recorded (phase reversal as the source is crossed). The other source is in area 1, with activity beginning at approximately 25 msec, generating the P25–N35 component of the cortical SEP. Some workers favor the existence of two separate generator sources for the N30 and P30 potentials recorded anterior and posterior to the central sulcus. Some workers also favor a thalamic or thalamocortical origin for the N20 waveform (30).

It should be noted that scalp recorded cortical SEPs represent a combination of these various potentials. After median nerve stimulation, a cortical potential is typically recorded from the Cz-Cc montage with an upward deflection around 19 msec and a downward deflection around 22 msec (using our polarity conventions, Fig. 10.5) (202). The response to ulnar or radial nerve stimulation is similar, though usually of lower amplitude, presumably secondary to a lesser number of afferent fibers (45). After posterior tibial nerve stimulation, an upward response is usually seen around 39 msec, with a downward response at 41 msec (Fig. 10.6) (13, 176, 200). Sural nerve, saphenous nerve, and peroneal nerve responses can also be obtained (28, 179). Of course, these latency values are highly dependent on the subject's age, limb length, and body height (32, 37, 70, 181, 206). The use of interpeak latencies, such as central conduction time or lumbar to cortical time, can obviate this problem.

DIAGNOSTIC APPLICATIONS IN NEUROSURGICAL DISEASE

SEPs have been used widely in the diagnosis of neurosurgical lesions. They have been of particular interest in two areas, which will be discussed in detail: radiculopathy and brachial plexus injury.

A variety of electrophysiological testing procedures have been used in the diagnosis of cervical and lumbar radiculopathies (6, 55, 59, 92). It was hoped that somatosensory evoked potentials would provide valuable diagnostic data in radicular disease. Unfortunately, the usual nerves stimulated (median or posterior tibial) are comprised of many nerve roots and, therefore, the usual methods of SEP recording cannot be expected to yield sensitive results. Some studies do purport to diagnose lumbar disc disease and/or lumbar stenosis bases on such data (60). Others have failed to demonstrate any diagnostic value, when sound statistical definitions of abnormal SEPs are applied (6).

In an effort to improve the sensitivity of SEPs in diagnosing radiculopathies, two approaches have been used: multiple nerve stimulation and "dermatomal stimulation." In the multiple nerve approach, the tibial, peroneal, sural, and saphenous nerves have been stimulated and the resultant SEPs recorded. The theory is that each nerve has predominant innervation from one nerve root (i.e., peroneal, L5; posterior tibial, S1; saphenous, L4). The dermatomal approach involves directly stimulating the skin overlying each dermatomal area. For example, the web

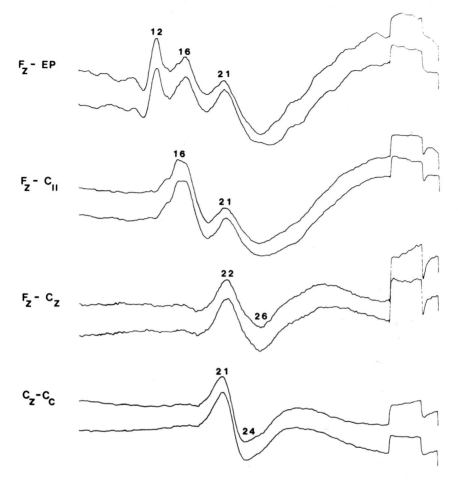

50mS

FIG. 10.5.   A typical median nerve somatosensory evoked potential recorded from four montages. The first montage (frontal scalp-Erb's point) is useful in verifying signal entry into the nervous system. The second montage (frontal scalp-upper cervical spine) yields a spinal potential which is quite resistant to anesthetic effects. The last two montages are commonly employed scalp electrode positions utilized to record the cortical component of the SEP. A 5-msec, 2 μV calibration pulse is seen at the end of each recording.

space between the first and second toes is stimulated for the L5 dermatome. Dermatomal stimulation generally yields smaller and later cortical evoked potentials, since smaller caliber nerve fibers are involved. Spinal potentials, for the same reason, cannot usually be recorded after derma-

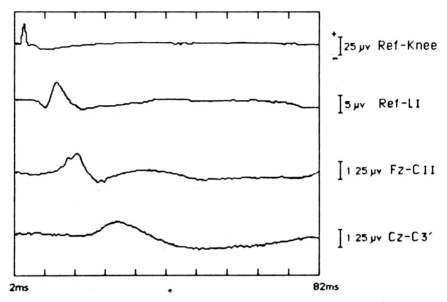

FIG. 10.6. A typical posterior tibial nerve somatosensory evoked potential recorded from four montages. The first montage (reference-knee) verifies signal entry into the nervous system. The second montage (reference-upper lumbar spine) records the potential generated near the conus medullaris. The third montage (frontal scalp-upper cervical spine) shows a cervical spinal potential. This potential is more easily recorded under anesthesia, since electromyographic artifact is absent. The fourth montage is a commonly utilized scalp recording of the cortical SEP. Calibration pulses are seen to the right of each recording. In each case, a positive potential leads to an upward movement on the oscilloscope screen. The most "active" of the two electrodes is the second of each pair.

tomal stimulation. Some studies claim excellent correlation for derma-tomal or multinerve SEPs and myelographic findings (53). Others, using rigorous definitions of abnormality, find them to be less helpful (6). At the present time, the clinical examination is, by far, the most sensitive and accurate tool in diagnosing radiculopathies. The electromyogram appears to be the most useful electrophysiologic test for confirmation of such diagnoses. SEPs, although theoretically promising, currently represent a time-consuming and unproven modality of diagnosis.

SEPs have proven very valuable in the assessment of brachial plexus injuries (31, 125, 141, 215). The primary goal is to identify, either preoperatively or intraoperatively, whether a preganglionic or postganglionic injury exists. If a purely preganglionic injury is present, the dorsal root ganglion will be in continuity with the peripheral nerve (Fig. 10.7). Since the axons remain viable, stimulation of the peripheral nerve will yield a recordable peripheral nerve action potential over the brachial plexus. No potential, however, will be conducted through to the cervical

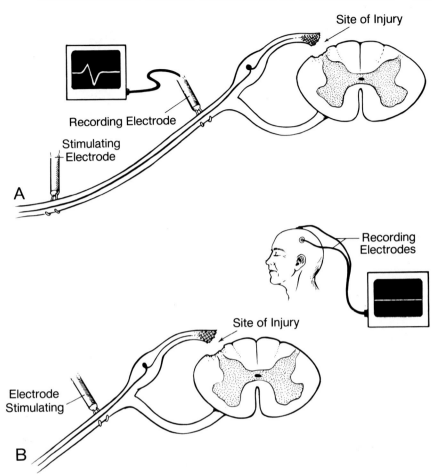

FIG. 10.7.   In a preganglionic injury like this schematic nerve root avulsion, the dorsal root ganglion remains in continuity with the distal nerve. (*A*) Since the axons remain viable, stimulation and recording over the distal nerve will yield a normal sensory nerve action potential. (*B*) Since the nerve root is avulsed, stimulation of the proximal root will not produce a cortical SEP.

spinal leads or cortical leads. If a purely postganglionic injury is present, the axons are not viable, and no peripheral or central potentials can be recorded (Fig. 10.8).

Of course, each peripheral nerve is comprised of multiple nerve roots, so unless a nearly complete brachial plexus injury is present, some conduction of evoked potentials into the central nervous system will occur. Absence of the cortical SEP, with normal peripheral nerve action potentials (NAPs) is diagnostic for preganglionic injury. Absence of the

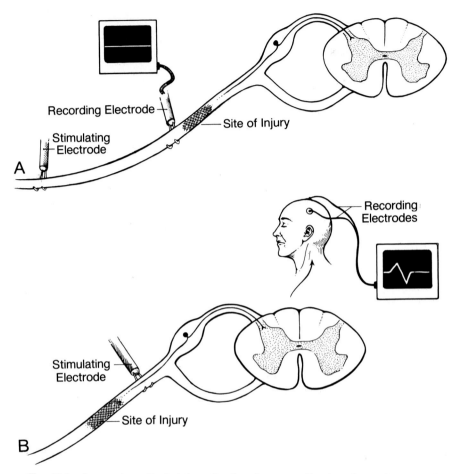

FIG. 10.8.   In a postganglionic injury, the dorsal root ganglion is no longer in continuity with the distal nerve. (A) Since the axons are not viable, stimulation and recording over the distal nerve will yield no NAP. (B) Since the proximal nerve is viable, stimulation of the proximal stump will produce a cortical SEP.

cortical SEP and NAP may be consistent with a purely postganglionic lesion but will also be found with postganglionic injuries combined with preganglionic injuries. Jones *et al.* (107) felt that when the Erb's point potential was attenuated to the same or a greater degree than the cervical potential (median nerve or ulnar nerve stimulation), the lesion was purely postganglionic. When the Erb's point potential was less affected than the cervical potential, an additional preganglionic component was assumed.

During surgical exploration of brachial plexus injuries, the use of SEPs will result in more accurate diagnostic information. Direct stimulation of roots or trunks can be performed. If proximal root stimulation yields no cortical SEP, a preganglionic injury is present. If proximal root stimulation yields a cortical SEP, grafting from this stump area is likely to result in functional reinnervation. Landi *et al.* (125) has suggested that this electrophysiologic assessment is much more accurate than visual inspection.

SOMATOSENSORY EVOKED POTENTIALS IN THE INTENSIVE CARE UNIT

Somatosensory evoked potentials have found increasing application in the evaluation of intensive care unit patients with injuries of the brain or spinal cord. SEPs have been used in an attempt to define the extent of the injury, to monitor patients for evidence of further injury, and to prognosticate regarding chances for neurological recovery (11). In the following paragraphs, information about EP applications in spinal cord trauma and head trauma will be presented.

Spinal Cord Injury

One must use great caution in the interpretation of spinal cord injury experiments or clinical studies involving SEPs (131, 136, 145, 211). Like many studies involving spinal cord injury, the experimental design is not standardized. The techniques used for producing the SEPs vary greatly, and many authors fail to rigorously analyze their results in terms of a statistically valid control data base. The spinal cord injury model or clinical injuries studied often vary considerably. Species used, anesthetic techniques, and postoperative neurological data are highly variable. Nonetheless, certain conclusions may be drawn from a review of the literature.

A great number of experimental studies have investigated the effects of spinal cord injury on the somatosensory evoked potential (2, 40, 46, 83, 126, 175). Experiments utilizing spinal distraction have shown that rapid application of force results in disappearance of SEPs without significant blood flow changes (43, 44). Gradual application of force leads to delayed SEP changes coincident with blood flow evidence of spinal ischemia. Such data indicate that the SEP is a sensitive indicator of spinal cord trauma, often providing evidence of impending injury before it becomes irreversible. The preponderance of experimental data shows that acute changes in SEPs are proportional to the severity of the trauma and are predictive of neurological outcome. For example, Ducker *et al.* demonstrated that 92% of experimentally injured monkeys rendered paraplegic had no SEP within 5 minutes of the trauma (52). Paraparetic animals had initial preservation of the SEP in 40% of cases. In normal animals, the SEP always returned within 3 hours. Similar findings apply to ischemic spinal cord injury models (*i.e.*, aortic occlusion). Such studies have consistently demonstrated a close correlation between SEP changes and neurologic outcome (see below, intraoperative monitoring for spinal cord ischemia). This correlation has been so reliable that the SEP has been used in a number of experiments as a monitor of therapy (61). For instance, Young and Flamm found greatly improved SEPs in cats which received high-dose methylprednisolone 45 minutes after severe contusion injury (212).

Perot greatly stimulated interest in the clinical application of SEPs to spinal cord injury (162). His early studies involved SEP recording in normal subjects and in 47 spinal cord injury patients. No patient with complete injury had lower extremity SEPs. Half of those patients with incomplete injuries had a recordable SEP. At that time it was hoped that SEPs might be useful in distinguishing complete and incomplete injuries, as well as predicting the potential for further recovery.

York *et al.*, however, later studied 71 patients with complete and incomplete spinal injuries (209). They found that while absence of the SEP was indeed associated with a complete injury, presence of the SEP was of little value in predicting the clinical state at the time of examination or in indicating the potential for recovery. In fact, some patients with no clinically detectable sensory function had SEPs. The authors suggest that such SEPs might indicate preservation of sufficient spinal cord continuity for electrical but not for clinical function. Conduction via metal instrumentation was also considered possible.

Dimitrijevic *et al.* studied 66 patients with chronic spinal cord injury and found a correlation between the "quality" of the SEP and clinical sensory function (50). Statistically valid measures of "quality" were not used. In a recent study, Chabot *et al.* evaluated lower extremity SEPs in 27 controls and 34 spinal cord-injured patients (27). They found that patients with normal motor and sensory exams could be reliably distinguished from those with decreased or absent function. The latter two groups could not, however, be distinguished. McGarry *et al.* studied 25 chronically injured patients (45). They found that 4 of 9 patients with normal SEP latencies had "no useful lower extremity function" and 8 of 16 patients with prolonged potentials were able to ambulate.

For reasons enumerated in the opening part of this section, the data presented above does not present a wholly congruent picture. The author's interpretation, based on the data and personal experience, is as follows.

In the acute operative monitoring situation, involving the possibility of global spinal cord trauma (*i.e.*, scoliosis surgery), the SEP is highly predictive of motor and sensory function. That is, an absent SEP after a spinal cord contusion injury will accurately predict a complete injury. A preserved SEP will predict normal spinal cord function. It is important that if the trauma is not global the SEP will only predict sensory outcome. For example, if the corticospinal tract is damaged during microsurgical removal of a tumor, a preserved SEP will probably be seen and will not predict the postoperative motor deficit.

In the subacute or chronic situation, SEP correlation with spinal cord function is less sure. Absent or severely altered SEPs seem to generally indicate complete injury. Preserved SEPs, however, often poorly correlate with motor outcome and, less frequently, are seen with poor sensory function. The disparity of acute and chronic data are thought to be related to the relative resistance of the SEP pathways to permanent injury, such that although they may dysfunction during the acute phase of injury, they survive, recover, and function again (at least electrically), even though more vulnerable cord areas (*i.e.*, central gray) are permanently disrupted.

Head Injury

Evoked potentials have been extensively utilized to study patients after head injury (48). Once again, the reader must utilize caution in interpreting such studies. The methods of EP analysis are often other than statistical. For example, Rappaport *et al.* employ a rating system based on latency and amplitude, but also including "noisiness, interside variability, and replicability (165, 166)." Although such qualitative abnormalities are undoubtably present after central nervous system injury, any rating system which depends upon subjective grading is subject to systematic errors of some magnitude. Likewise, many authors rely upon evoked potentials other than short-latency components. These middle and long latency components are notoriously subject to metabolic variables and, therefore, more likely to be found abnormal for a variety of reasons in the multiply traumatized patient. Despite such problems in analysis, much useful information has been compiled regarding EP changes in head injury.

Greenberg *et al.* (77, 79, 153, 157, 158) conducted a series of studies employing VEPs, SEPs, and auditory evoked potentials (brainstem and longer latency) in the evaluation of comatose patients. Their initial study included data from 51 patients. An impaired BAEP was associated with abnormal oculocephalic responses or pupillary light reflexes. The duration of coma seemed to correlate with measures of hemispheric dysfunction, not measures of brainstem dysfunction (BAEP). In a later study of 100 patients, multimodality evoked potentials were found to predict outcome with 80% accuracy (81). This accuracy improved to 100% if patients dying from causes other than the head injury (*i.e.*, sepsis), were excluded from analysis. In a subsequent study of 109 patients, SEPs were found to have an 88% accuracy rate in predicting outcome if potentials of up to 250 msec latency were included in the analysis (80). The group consistently felt that evoked potentials were the most accurate single prognostic indicant after head trauma—better, for example, than Glasgow coma scale, computed tomographic (CT) findings, intracranial pressure (ICP) data, or clinical information. Importantly, no falsely pessimistic (false-positive EP changes) errors were associated with this indicant.

Hume and Cant studied central conduction time in 94 patients with head trauma and compared the results with a normal data base (103). CCT was determined at multiple times after injury and predicted outcome in 75–84% of patients. Six of seven survivors with hemispheric asymmetry had hemiplegia on the predicted side. Bilaterally absent SEPs predicted death in 8 of 8 patients.

Mackey-Hargadine and Hall (139) have studied EPs in over 500 comatose head trauma patients. Their experience was less encouraging in predicting outcome as opposed to predicting potential for recovery. An abnormal BAEP was found to be an indicator of poor outcome, but a normal BAEP in the acute period had no predictive value—that is, patients with normal BAEPs had an approximately 50% chance of a good outcome. The long-latency auditory response was not observed in the majority of these patients, even those with good neurological outcome. The middle latency response, however, was highly correlated with cognitive outcome. SEPs and BAEPs were found to be helpful in optimizing medical therapy such as hyperventilation. They were of great value in monitoring patients in barbiturate coma, where the neurologic exam was no longer possible. Other animal and clinical studies confirm the resistance of short-latency SEPs and BAEPs to the effects of barbiturates (see section on anesthetics).

EPs have been used increasingly to evaluate pediatric coma from all causes (105, 183). Frank *et al.* found that absence of the cortical SEP, with preservation of the BAEP, correlated with loss of cortical function and chronic vegetative state in five children with anoxic brain injury (64). Lutschg *et al.* examined 43 comatose children with BAEPs and SEPs (138). Absence of the BAEP or SEP indicated an extremely poor prognosis. Latency prolongations were seen in one-third of patients who made an excellent recovery. The BAEP was very resistant in cases of hypoxic brain injury. Goff *et al.* used SEPs to evaluate patients with Reye's syndrome (72). Early components of the SEP were frequently absent or suppressed. Recovery of these components early in the course of the disease was favorable prognostically. These studies present a very consistent picture: absent EPs indicate a poor prognostic outcome; preservation of the SEP or VEP indicates a favorable outcome; and preservation of the BAEP predicts survival but not quality of outcome (especially in hypoxic injuries).

SOMATOSENSORY EVOKED POTENTIAL MONITORING IN THE OPERATING ROOM

In the previous section, the utility of evoked potentials as a diagnostic and prognostic test was discussed. In the following pages, the use of evoked potentials as a monitoring tool will be presented. This application is the newest and most exciting area of EP technology as it relates to neurosurgery. Because short-latency EPs are relatively resistant to anesthetic agents, EPs can be used to monitor neural pathways during surgery. Such monitoring can, theoretically, detect problems hours before the conclusion of anesthesia would allow a neurological examination. This timely information can, in some circumstances, be utilized by the surgical team to alter the course of surgery, resulting in a decreased incidence of neurological complications. Of course, this "monitoring" application of EPs differs markedly from the diagnostic applications previously discussed. One does not depend upon a one-time examination of the evoked potential pathway with comparison to a normal data base. Rather, one monitors the patient's own baseline potential sequentially throughout a time period of many hours, looking for significant changes during the course of surgery. A number of groups have reported on their successful intraoperative monitoring experiences (3, 34, 76, 85–87, 91, 93, 95, 96, 159, 167, 214).

At the time of this writing, the University of Florida Neurosurgical Evoked Potential Laboratory had monitored over 600 cases. The results of this experience, as well as a review of all available literature, will be considered in the following discussion of current SEP applications in the operating room.

Areas Where SEP Monitoring is Currently Indispensible

CORTICAL LOCALIZATION

The precise localization of somatosensory and motor cortex is vital for the successful performance of certain neurosurgical procedures. For example, resection of a suprasylvian epileptic focus near the central sulcus may result in an unwanted motor deficit if the resection includes precentral gyrus. Conversely, fear of causing such a deficit may lead to an inadequate cortical resection. Unfortunately, purely anatomical landmarks are notoriously variable and misleading. The traditional solution had been to perform such procedures under local anesthesia, with electrical stimulation of the cortex and mapping of the elicited reponses. The use of local anesthesia undoubtedly increases the difficulty of the procedure, for the patient and the surgeon, and probably increases the risk.

Kelly *et al.* described, in 1965, the use of cortical evoked potentials to localize somatosensory cortex (114). Subsequently, a number of investigators, including Goldring (73), Goldring and Gregorie (74), Luders (137), and Allison (4) reported their successful experience using the following general technique. The median nerve opposite the operated hemisphere is stimulated. An array of electrodes is applied directly to the brain surface, and montages in front of and behind the presumed hand sensorimotor area are selected for recording. The SEP recorded from somatosensory cortex (postcentral gyrus) consists of N20/P30 potentials. The SEP from motor cortex (precentral gyrus) consists of the mirror image P20/N30 potential. Polarity inversion of this evoked potential is a firmly established, highly reliable criteria for the identification of the central sulcus. An example from the author's laboratory is shown in Figure 10.9.

As discussed in the section on SEP origins, the most likely neurophysiological explanation for this polarity inversion is that the site of generation is area 3b, located on the posterior bank of the central sulcus. One must also recall that a P25 potential is generated in area 1. This potential can be recorded only from the hand area of somatosensory cortex and, thus, may be of aid in determining this locale if the waveform is properly identified. Since it occurs halfway between the N20 and P30 potentials, it may be confused with them, leading to inaccurate estimation of the site of phase reversal.

Goldring and Gregorie reported the use of this technique in 100 epilepsy patients (74). Allison utilized it during surgery on 44 patients (4). The use of evoked potentials to localize sensorimotor cortex is an established aid of indisputable value in neurosurgical procedures involving cortical incisions for resection of certain epileptic foci, vascular malformations, or neoplasms near the central area of the brain.

PERIPHERAL NERVE TRAUMA

The early treatment of closed peripheral nerve trauma is conservative. Should no functional return be detected, clinically or electrophysiologically, within 2–3 months, surgical exploration is often warranted. Such exploration will usually reveal the injured area to be swollen in a fusiform manner. This gross appearance, termed "neuroma-in-continuity," is consistent with widely differing internal pathology. When nerve stimulation failed to elicit muscular contraction, it was formerly very difficult to decide whether to resect such a lesion. With the advent of intraoperative evoked potentials the decision is usually straightforward (110).

The following general technique is used (see Fig. 10.10): A sterile

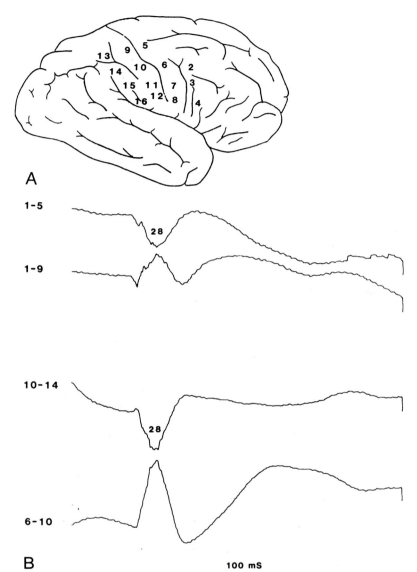

FIG. 10.9.   Epilepsy surgery. (A) Map of intraoperative electrode placement over the central area of the right hemisphere. Electrode 1 (not shown) is on temporalis muscle. (B) Median nerve SEPs recorded from selected montages. As the central sulcus is crossed (between electrodes 5 and 9), a phase reversal is observed. Bipolar recording around electrode 10, verifies this site as near hand somatosensory cortex.

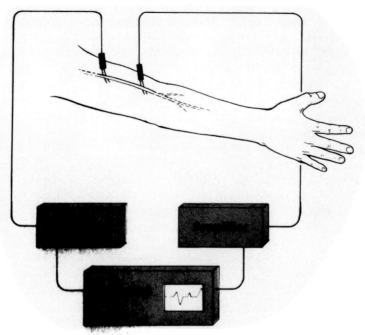

FIG. 10.10. Schematic representation of the stimulating and recording paradigm used to record nerve action potentials. These potentials are often of sufficient size that they can be seen on single oscilloscope sweeps.

stimulating electrode is placed as far proximally on the injured nerve as the surgical exposure will permit. A sterile recording electrode is placed just proximal to the neuroma-in-continuity. Stimulation and recording over this segment of normal nerve should generate "nerve action potentials (NAPs)," which are often large enough to be seen without signal averaging. The production of NAPs over this segment of normal nerve verifies that the EP system is functioning properly. The recording electrode is then moved just distal to the neuroma-in-continuity. If axonal regeneration has occurred across the area of damage, NAPs will still be recorded.

Peripheral nerve injuries are often classified as neuropractic, axonotmetic, or neurotmetic. Neuropraxia is a reversible injury in which there is a variable loss of distal function. The causes are thought to include local electrolyte imbalance, neural ischemia, and compressive-shear forces of an acute or chronic nature. If chronic compression is present, local myelin alterations may be evident ultrastructurally. In this situation neurolysis may be required to restore neural function. Neuropraxia secondary to acute trauma generally improves without surgical intervention within a 6-week period (usually within days). If neuropraxia is present, axonal dysfunction is only found at the site of injury; hence, stimulation of the nerve distal to the injury will produce muscle contraction. Nerve action potentials can be generated above and below the injury site but will not be conducted across that area.

Axonotmesis is a pathological process of increased severity including loss of axons and myelin with preservation of the surrounding connective tissue elements. The continuity of these structures provides a pathway by which axonal regrowth can effectively occur. The time needed for restoration of function after axonal destruction is determined by the rate of regrowth and the distance from the site of injury to the point of muscle innervation. Axonal regeneration is known to progress at approximately 1 mm/day. Thus, at 2 months after injury, sufficient time has passed for growth across a focal area of injury, but not for muscle reinnervation (in most cases). Nerve stimulation will not produce muscle contraction. Nerve action potentials will, however, be conducted across the area of injury. As this natural process of reinnervation is much more efficient than that which occurs in a transected and sutured nerve, a neuroma-in-continuity should not be resected if axonotmesis is identified with NAPs.

The most severe type of peripheral nerve trauma is neurotmesis. Pathologically, the axons and myelin are destroyed with additional disruption of the surrounding connective tissue structures. A nerve transection is a form of neurotmesis, but the same situation may exist within a neuroma-in-continuity. In this case, the potential pathway of neural regeneration has been ablated. Stimulation of the nerve either proximal or distal to the neuroma will not produce muscle contraction. NAPs will not be conducted across the neuroma. As no functional recovery can be expected, the demonstration of a neurotmetic neuroma-in-continuity is an indication for resection with nerve anastamosis or grafting.

Kline and Judice reported a 12-year experience using this technique on 171 patients with brachial plexus injuries (115). Sixty-three of 282 injured nerve elements after gunshot wounds were spared resection because of intact NAPs. Fifty-seven recovered function with neurolysis only. One hundred twenty nerve elements were identified as neurotmetic by the NAP technique—all were confirmed pathologically. A case of popliteal sciatic nerve injury from our laboratory is shown in Figure 10.11. Eighteen months after resection of neuroma, with primary nerve anastamosis, plantar flexion is normal, dorsiflexion is antigravity, and sensation has returned to all but the tips of the toes.

Why not wait for definitive clinical evidence of reinnervation or failure thereof? In most peripheral nerve injuries, the slow rate of axonal regrowth leads to a long period before reinnervation can occur. For example, a sciatic nerve injury at the knee, with axonal destruction, will

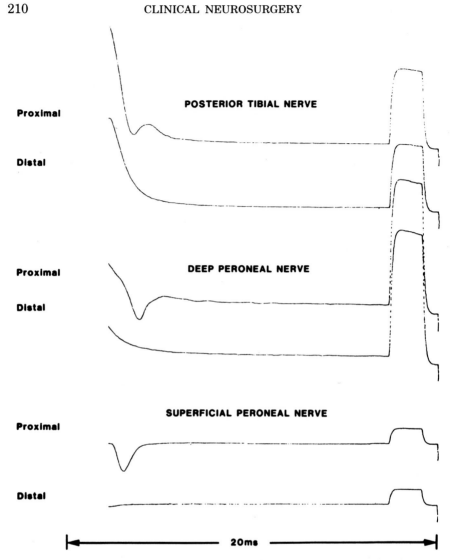

FIG. 10.11.   Evoked potential evaluation of injured sciatic nerve. In this gunshot wound of the popliteal sciatic nerve, neuromas-in-continuity were identified in all three branches three months after injury. Stimulation and recording proximal to the site of injury yielded a nerve action potential in all cases. Stimulation proximal and recording distal to the neuromas yielded no NAPs. This indicated that a neurotmetic injury existed. The neuromas were excised back to normal fascicular anatomy, and nerve anastomoses performed with a good clinical result. Pathologic analysis of the neuroma confirmed the electrophysiologic diagnosis.

require at least a year to grow down the nerve towards the foot, with resultant motor and sensory reinnervation (1 mm/day). If one waits a year, finds no evidence of spontaneous reinnervation, and then explores the injury, resects the neuroma, and reanastamoses the nerve, another year will elapse before reinnervation can occur. By this time, irreversible changes will have occurred within the affected muscles. The timing of these injuries, therefore, dictates that a decision be made between 3 and 6 months after injury regarding surgical repair. It is safe to say that intraoperative EPs are indispensible in making this decision correctly.

Areas Where SEPs Are Often Helpful

CENTRAL NERVOUS SYSTEM ISCHEMIA (INCLUDING ANEURYSM AND AVM SURGERY, CAROTID ENDARTERECTOMY, AND AORTIC SURGERY)

Aneurysm/Arteriovenous Malformation Surgery.   Improvements in diagnostic and surgical techniques have greatly reduced the morbidity and mortality of aneurysm surgery. The most feared complications of such procedures include immediate postoperative deficit secondary to inadvertent inclusion of a major vessel or perforating artery in the aneurysm clip and delayed ischemic neurological deficits from vasospasm. An intraoperative monitoring technique which would reduce the incidence of either of these problems would, undoubtedly, be welcomed by all neurovascular surgeons.

A large body of experimental data exists to support the use of somatosensory evoked potentials as a monitoring tool for intracerebral ischemia (112). In a series of experiments, Symon's laboratory has demonstrated that median nerve EPs are affected at cerebral blood flows of 15 ml/100 g/minute following acute middle cerebral occlusion in the baboon (94, 101, 106, 184, 189, 193). Branston *et al.* have also shown that irreversible changes in cellular metabolism, including failure of the sodium-potassium pump, occur at a lower threshold (approximately 10 ml/100 g/minute) (16–22). The concept of the ischemic penumbra, wherein blood flow is below that required for synaptic activity, like EPs, but is above that needed for basic cellular metabolism, has been popularized by Astrup *et al.* (9, 10) and Symon *et al.* (190, 192, 194). The fact that the SEP disappears at a threshold higher than that for cellular death indicates that it will likely provide a warning of ischemia before irreversible damage occurs (108).

SEP changes also correlate with blood flow changes after experimental head trauma (39) and global ischemia (82). Lesnick *et al.* found that the SEP correlated with cortical and white matter blood flow in 14 cats following bilateral carotid ligation (132). Lopes Da Silva *et al.* found a linear relationship between cerebral blood flow and cortical SEP amplitude between 15 and 60 ml/100 g/minute (134). EP responses varied significantly among animals, dependent upon the extent of ischemia in the hand area of cortex. Similar data confirm the absence of single-unit electrophysiological activity at blood flows less than 18 ml/100 g/minute (98). Others have reported such findings in different animal models (14, 82, 148, 168, 174, 186, 201).

More recently, numerous reports have appeared, documenting the use of SEPs on patients with subarachnoid hemorrhage, either preoperatively or intraoperatively. Symon's group examined SEP latencies, noninvasive xenon cerebral blood flow, and clinical classification (195). A statistically significant difference was found between SEP latencies in grade IV patients and all other grades (170). At a cerebral blood flow of 30 ml/100 g/minute, significant central conduction time (102) changes were found. In addition, a report of 33 patients monitored intraoperatively suggested their applicability in reducing surgical complications (203). Carter demonstrated the feasibility of SEP monitoring and suggested that "when rCBF values fall and the CCT slows, neurological deficit will probably occur" (26). McPherson *et al.* reported a case in which SEPs disappeared during temporary clipping of a middle cerebral aneurysm and returned after this clip was removed (146). A dense hemiparesis resulted but resolved over 24 hours. Owen *et al.* used SEP monitoring to guide the sacrifice of vessels during removal of an intramedullary high cervical arteriovenous malformation (160). Grundy *et al.* lost the lower extremity SEP during resection of a spinal AVM, and this correlated with severe postoperative deficit (89).

Fox recorded central conduction times after aneurysm surgery and found that they "correlated reasonably well with the patient's clinical state at the time of testing" (63). Suzuki *et al.* found a correlation between SEP results and clinical outcome during vasospasm (187). Kostron *et al.* reported a similar correlation in cases of vasospasm after head injury (119).

Symon *et al.* suggested that posterior tibial nerve SEPs might be more appropriate in monitoring anterior communicating and anterior cerebral artery aneurysms, as the leg and foot area of cortex was within the vascular territory at greatest risk (203). Grundy *et al.*, in a case report, described the use of lower extremity SEPs to determine the safety of sacrificing an anterior cerebral artery feeding a larger arteriovenous malformation (90).

At the University of Florida, SEPs or BAEPs have been monitored in over 100 aneurysm cases. The results of those studies performed on 50 patients between July 1983 and May 1985 were recently analyzed (66).

Baseline EPs were obtained shortly after the induction of general anesthesia and were recorded continuously during surgery. Absolute latency, interpeak latency, and cortical EP amplitude were subsequently determined. Statistical analysis confirmed that significant changes in these parameters are routinely seen during aneurysm surgery. Arbitrary definitions of abnormal latency and amplitude changes could, therefore, lead to an excessive false-positive/false-negative rate.

A case involving a 4-cm giant middle cerebral aneurysm is shown in Figure 10.12. The aneurysm was trapped between clips, opened, and emptied of clot. The arterial lumen was reconstructed with a large straight aneurysm clip. A right median nerve somatosensory evoked potential was continuously recorded throughout surgery. The Erb's point potential and cervical potential remained unchanged. The cortical potential began to diminish in amplitude approximately 2 minutes after trapping and, after 11 minutes, had disappeared. The patient awakened with a global aphasia and right hemiplegia. A subsequent CT scan confirmed the presence of a large left middle cerebral artery infarction.

In Figure 10.13, the results of a case involving a giant ophthalmic artery aneurysm are shown. The right median nerve SEP was again monitored continuously throughout surgery. During temporary clipping

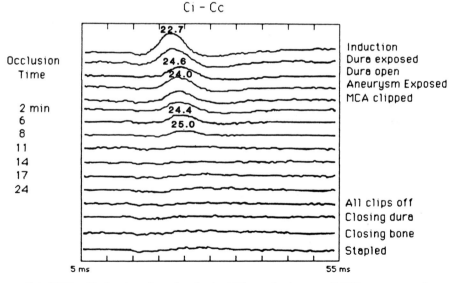

FIG. 10.12.   During trapping of a giant middle cerebral artery (MCA) aneurysm, these median nerve SEPs were sequentially recorded. After an occlusion time of 11 minutes, no SEP could be recorded. Attempts to empty the aneurysm of clot and reconstruct the lumen did not lead to return of the potential. The patient awakened with a severe middle cerebral artery infarction.

Cz - Cc

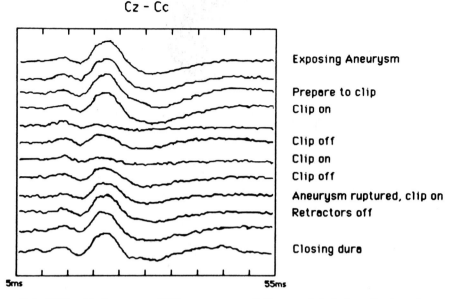

Exposing Aneurysm

Prepare to clip
Clip on

Clip off
Clip on
Clip off

Aneurysm ruptured, clip on
Retractors off

Closing dura

5ms 55ms

FIG. 10.13. Median nerve SEPs were sequentially recorded during clipping of an ophthalmic artery aneurysm. During temporary occlusion of the carotid, the SEP promptly disappeared. After final positioning of the clip, the potential returned. The patient awakened without deficit.

of the carotid, the SEP promptly disappeared. When the clip was readjusted, the SEP promptly returned. The patient awakened without focal deficit.

For the entire series, prolongation of central conduction time, decrease in cortical amplitude, or disappearance of the EP, from the time of dural opening to the time of closure, were predictive of postoperative sensory or motor deficit. Other deficits (*i.e.*, aphasia) could not be predicted, as those areas of brain are not monitored with SEPs. In addition, BAEPs and SEPs failed to reliably predict deficits after basilar aneurysm surgery. Complications of such cases usually involve occlusion of the posterior cerebral arteries or basilar perforating vessels. Such occlusions do not usually embarrass the auditory or somatosensory pathways and, hence, monitoring such pathways is of marginal value.

Carotid Endarterectomy (CEA). Electrophysiological monitoring during carotid endarterectomy is a controversial topic (124, 164). The controversy revolves not so much around the accuracy of monitoring but around its usefulness. Some surgeons shunt every carotid to prevent ischemia during clamp time. Others, citing fears of shunt emboli, never shunt and claim excellent results. Yet another group shunts only those

carotids in which clamping induces electrophysiologic evidence of ischemia. It is this group of surgeons which absolutely depends on accurate
monitoring to direct surgical maneuvers. For those who always or never
shunt, the only remaining therapeutic manipulations, if monitoring suggests ischemia, are elevation of blood pressure or replacement of a
defective shunt.

Sharbrough *et al.* have monitored over 2500 carotid endarterectomies
with continuous electroencephalography and intraarterial xenon cerebral
blood flow (177, 185). They have demonstrated that a decrease in blood
flow during clamping to 18–21 ml/100 g/minute will induce severe EEG
changes. In addition, embolic events will be detected as local changes in
EEG. In their series, no patient has ever awakened with a neurologic
deficit unpredicted by EEG. For those who choose to monitor carotid
endarterectomies, EEG remains the best proven modality. It does require
close cooperation with the anesthesiologist in maintaining an acceptable
level of anesthesia for optimal EEG recording. It also requires the
presence in the operating room of a person skilled in the interpretation
of EEG.

Jacobs *et al.* (104) reported the use of SEPs during CEA in 25 patients.
Two patients lost the cortical SEP during surgery—one of these had a
stroke. Markand *et al.* later monitored 38 CEAs with SEPs. In 10 CEAs
under general anesthesia, three patients developed marked changes, all
of which were reversed with shunting (142). In one of 28 cases performed
under local anesthesia, similar changes developed. They were accompanied by clinical deficit which resolved with shunting. Russ and Fraedrich reported one case in which the cortical SEP disappeared during
carotid clamping (171). The patient awakened with a neurological deficit
which resolved within 24 hours. Others have reported similar experiences
indicating the utility of SEPs in monitoring CEA. Some investigators
also feel that SEP changes of a lesser degree may correlate with postoperative neuropsychological function (23, 42).

Although SEPs are not firmly established as a monitor during carotid
endarterectomy, much experimental evidence and all clinical material to
date indicate their sensitivity and utility in detecting cerebral ischemia
(215). Multichannel EEG is probably more sensitive, in that smaller
areas of altered activity may be detected (*i.e.*, after emboli). EEG changes
are also immediately obvious, whereas EP changes require a period of
averaging lasting up to several minutes. EPs, on the other hand, are less
sensitive to alterations in anesthesia and other metabolic parameters.
They also do not require the presence of an electroencephalographer in
the operating room.

Aortic Surgery.   The arterial supply to the thoracic spinal cord is
typically not well collateralized, thereby making this region prone to
ischemic lesions. A single anterior spinal artery runs the entire length of

the cord in the ventromedial sulcus. This artery originates at high cervicomedullary junction from branches of both vertebral arteries. Throughout its course, numerous radicular branches contribute to its flow, including the thyrocervical trunk and the artery of Adamkiewicz, which arises as a left intercostal aortic branch between the T9-L2 level in most patients.

Two potential mechanisms exist by which the spinal cord may become ischemic during aortic surgery (120). Cross-clamping of the aorta will result in decreased spinal cord blood flow, thereby rendering watershed zones vulnerable to infarction, particularly in the thoracic cord. The second mechanism entails sacrifice of a critical intercostal branch during repair of an aortic lesion. This is most likely to occur during replacement of a low thoracic aortic aneurysm with graft material. Clamping the abdominal aorta almost never causes spinal cord injury, since the vital blood supply is above the clamp.

A number of experimental studies have evaluated the SEP during distal aortic hypotension (100). Coles et al. found that the early component of the SEP was substantially diminished after 4 minutes of aortic exclusion between clamps in the dog (35). If the ischemia was extended to 27 minutes, 66% of the animals awakened paraplegic. Nine of ten animals with preserved sensory function regained a normal SEP within 30 minutes of unclamping. Laschinger, in a series of experiments, has monitored SEPs and microsphere spinal cord blood flow during graded aortic hypotension in the dog (128–130). Maintenance of a distal aortic perfusion pressure of 60 mm Hg or greater resulted in a preservation of spinal cord blood flow and somatosensory evoked potentials in all animals. All but one animal likewise remained stable down to aortic perfusion pressures of 40 mm Hg. Reduction of aortic pressure to below 40 mm Hg resulted in complete loss of SEPs in all animals. Another experiment demonstrated that exclusion of a critical intercostal vessel would lead to disappearance of the SEP, with severe blood flow alterations in an isolated segment of spinal cord. The resultant neurologic deficit in similar experiments has been favorably affected by steroid administration (127), the use of venoarterial shunts (84), and perfusion cooling of the spinal cord (36).

Cheng et al. have systematically investigated the effects of aortic occlusion on the lumbar SEP in a rabbit model (29). Kobrine et al. have studied spinal and cerebral SEPs during graded hypotension (116–118). They found, with hydrogen clearance blood flow techniques, that spinal cord blood flow was essentially zero before the SEP was disrupted. It should be noted that both the microsphere and hydrogen clearance technique have limitations in accurately measuring low flow states.

Kaplan et al. have monitored SEPs during aortic occlusion in 17 dogs

(113). The SEP changes, clinical outcome, and histology were analyzed. Graded occlusion to 40 mm Hg produced no significant changes in SEP. Complete aortic occlusion, producing a distal pressure of 15–25 mm Hg, invariably produced SEP changes. The cortical, cervical, and lumbar potentials were affected. The NAP was relatively resistant to ischemia. Ischemia for greater than 30 minutes beyond SEP change invariably resulted in a neurologic deficit. Ischemia for 15 minutes beyond SEP change produced a variable clinical result (normal, mild deficit, or severe deficit). All animals with intact sensory function experienced prompt return of the SEP after unclamping. The typical histologic lesion, if a clinical deficit was present, involved the central and dorsal gray matter of the spinal cord.

These results correlate well with the available clinical data on SEP monitoring during aortic surgery. Lachinger and colleagues found no SEP changes in patients with distal aortic pressures above 60 mm Hg (41, 129, 130). Two patients were described in which distal pressure was less than 40 mm Hg and the SEP disappeared between 15 and 25 minutes after clamping. In one of these patients the SEP was absent for 60 minutes before unclamping, and the patient awakened paraplegic. In a later series of 25 patients, 5 of 6 in whom SEPs were absent for longer than 30 minutes awakened paraplegic (120). Mizrahi and Crawford monitored 13 patients undergoing aortic aneurysm surgery and found that 10 patients lost the SEP in cortical leads 17–40 minutes after clamping (150). The patient with the longest period of nonrecordable SEPs (59 minutes) awakened paraplegic. At the University of Florida, SEPs were monitored during 22 coarctation procedures (109). Forty-one percent (41%) had changes in the SEP. In one case disappearance of the SEP for 30 minutes was accompanied by paraplegia. Loss of the SEP for 14 minutes in another case resulted in transient lower extremity paresthesiae postoperatively. Loss of the SEP for lesser periods of time was not accompanied by deficit. In another case, test clamping of the aorta resulted in reproducible, rapid loss of the SEP such that an alternative surgical procedure (subclavian-aortic bypass) was selected (see Fig. 10.14). All SEPs returned after unclamping.

Fox et al. found changes in the SEP and the tonic vibration reflex during aortography (62). More recently, Berenstein et al. utilized SEP monitoring during spinal angiography and/or embolization in 41 patients (12). Angiographic opacification rapidly reduced SEP amplitude. SEPs were considered valuable in assessing the potential risk of embolization. SEP improvement paralleled clinical improvement, and permanent SEP loss, in one case, correlated with deficit.

Thus, there are ample experimental and clinical studies which show the SEP to be an effective monitor of spinal ischemia. No animal or

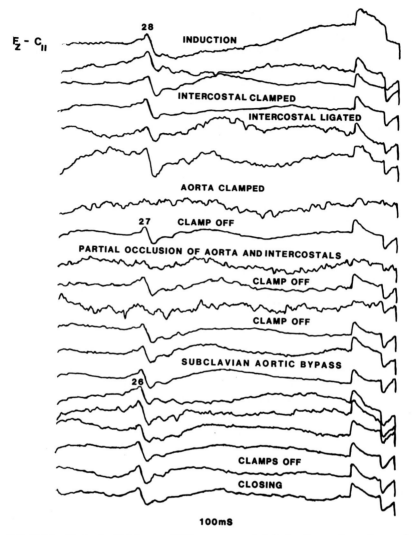

$$\text{F}_{\text{Z}} - \text{C}_{\text{II}}$$

28   INDUCTION

INTERCOSTAL CLAMPED

INTERCOSTAL LIGATED

AORTA CLAMPED

27   CLAMP OFF

PARTIAL OCCLUSION OF AORTA AND INTERCOSTALS

CLAMP OFF

CLAMP OFF

SUBCLAVIAN AORTIC BYPASS

26

CLAMPS OFF

CLOSING

100mS

FIG. 10.14. Posterior tibial nerve SEPs were recorded during thoracotomy for repair of aortic coarctation. The cervical spinal montage is shown. During test clamping of the aorta, the evoked potential disappeared. Removal of the clamp resulted in its prompt return. This phenomenon was observed during two subsequent attempts at aortic clamping. The surgeons elected to perform a subclavian aortic bypass instead of the usual patch graft repair which requires total aortic occlusion. The SEP remained normal, and the patient awakened without deficit.

patient in which SEPs have remained normal during aortic clamping has yet awakened with neurologic deficit. Conversely, all animals and patients with neurologic deficit have had documented changes in the SEP. It appears that irreversible ischemic damage will often occur within a fixed time period (15–45 minutes) after disappearance of the SEP. Although disappearance of the SEP for an indeterminate time period will predict motor outcome, the return of the SEP only signifies preservation of sensory function. Most clinical and experimental evidence indicates that the SEP usually returns after unclamping, regardless of motor outcome.

SPINAL SURGERY (SCOLIOSIS, FRACTURE-DISLOCATIONS, SPINAL TUMORS, DORSAL ROOT ENTRY ZONE LESIONS)

Scoliosis. The surgical treatment of scoliosis involves a small but real risk of spinal cord damage. Although neurologic deficit may occur in <1% of Harrington rod instrumentation cases, the use of sublaminar wiring techniques (*i.e.*, Luque rods) may be associated with a higher risk. The traditional method of preventing such deficits has been the "wake-up test." This test requires that the patient be awakened in the operating room, immediately after insertion of the instrumentation. If the patient can voluntarily move his legs, anesthesia is reinstituted and the wounds closed. If the patient demonstrates some deficit, the distraction is reduced or the instrumentation removed. In several such instances, neurologic deficit has been reversed. Obviously, the "wake-up test" is a stressful experience for the patient, surgeon, and the anesthesiologist.

Orthopaedic surgeons have enthusiastically embraced the concept of SEP monitoring during scoliosis surgery (204). Nash *et al.*, in 1977, reported their early experience with SEPs in 26 orthopaedic and 8 neurosurgical cases (154). The group later investigated the use of deliberate hypotension and continuous opioid anesthesia and found both compatible with SEP monitoring (88, 161). Engler *et al.* also reported early on their successful experience monitoring 55 scoliosis patients (58). Brown, Nash, *et al.* recently reported on SEP monitoring of 300 spinal procedures (24). Three neurologic deficits were detected intraoperatively and confirmed on postoperative neurologic exam. In four cases of altered SEPs, surgical action was taken, with improvement in the SEPs and no postoperative deficits. There were no deficits unpredicted by SEP monitoring.

Bradshaw *et al.* reported on SEP monitoring in 40 patients undergoing scoliosis surgery (15). Temporary neurologic deficit, documented by wake-up test or postoperative neurological exam, correlated with SEP changes in two cases. No other deficits or SEP changes occurred. The authors favored epidural or spinous process recording. Wilbur *et al.* used SEP monitoring in 137 patients undergoing posterior spine fusion for scoliosis (205). Forty-one per cent (41%) of patients undergoing segmental wiring procedures had at least transient changes in the SEP—nine of these had some neurological deficit. Several patients had postoperative paresthesiae which were not predicted by SEP changes, but the three patients with major motor deficit all had significant SEP changes.

Mostegl and Bauer monitored SEPs during 61 scoliosis cases (151). Amplitude changes in the P40 waveform occurred in almost all patients. Several patients had more severe EP changes during surgery which led to immediate wake-up tests, confirmation of deficits, reduction of distraction, and postoperative recovery of function. One patient had normal SEPs during surgery but, when examined 2 hours postoperatively, was paraplegic. SEPs were repeated at that time and were absent. This case seems likely to be a postoperative rather than an intraoperative complication, although the lack of detailed SEP records or neuroexams renders a precise conclusion impossible.

At the University of Florida, all scoliosis cases are monitored with SEPs. If changes are noted in the SEP, an immediate wake-up test is performed. If no changes are detected, no wake-up test is performed. In a series of 34 cases, two have developed significant alterations in the SEP. In Case 1, the SEPs from the lower extremities disappeared during exposure of the spine, well in advance of any instrumentation (Fig. 10.15). Concurrent measurement of upper extremity SEPs disclosed no metabolic or technical problem. An immediate wake-up test was performed, confirming paraplegia. A postoperative emergency myelogram was normal, and the patient subsequently regained antigravity strength in the lower extremities. In Case 2, the lower extremity SEPs disappeared after passage of a sublaminar wire. Again, persistently normal upper extremity SEPs were helpful in excluding technical difficulties. The patient was paraplegic on wake-up test and did not regain lower extremity function. In all other cases, SEPs remained unchanged and patients had no deficits.

Other Spinal Cases.   SEPs have been utilized during surgery for spinal fracture dislocation (155). Definitive series are not available for analysis, although there are many anecdotal reports. At the University of Florida 51 such cases have been monitored. Significant changes have been detected in two. In the first instance, the SEP disappeared for 5 minutes after the passage of a Luque wire. It subsequently returned to normal, and the patient awakened without deficit. In the second case, the SEP disappeared from the right leg during spinal instrumentation (Fig. 10.16). The SEP remained normal from the left leg. Unfortunately, the patient suffered a myocardial infarction near the end of surgery, arrested, and could not be resuscitated. Though neurological exam was not possible, the spinal cord was obtained at autopsy. Pathology revealed acute hemorrhage and mechanical disruption of the right half of the cord, without significant damage to the left.

SEPs have been used during dorsal root entry zone lesions (DREZL) (25, 65). They are helpful in two ways. First, they can be used to

Spinal Instrumentation

Induction, incision

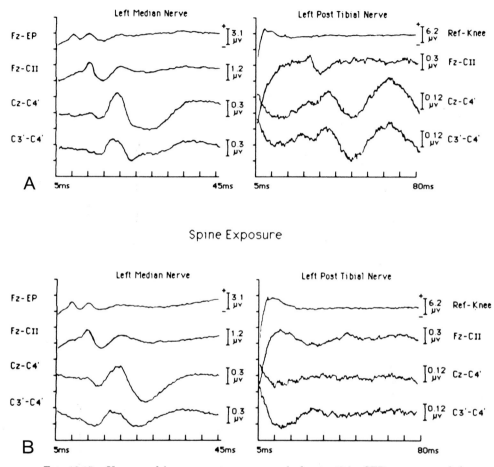

FIG. 10.15. Upper and lower somatosensory evoked potentials. SEPs were recorded sequentially from the left median nerve and left posterior tibial nerve during scoliosis surgery. The left median nerve potentials serve as a "control" for technical and anesthetic problems. At induction (A), good potentials are seen from each extremity in four montages. During spine exposure (B), the cervical and cortical responses from leg stimulation disappeared, although the arm potentials remained unchanged. The surgeons were warned; a wake-up test was performed; and paraplegia was confirmed. Surgery was aborted, and the patient later regained partial lower extremity function.

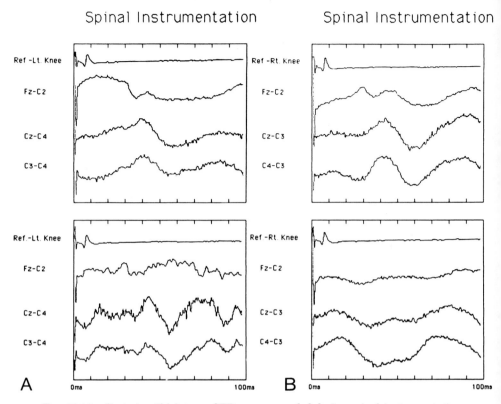

FIG. 10.16.   Posterior tibial nerve SEPs were recorded during spinal instrumentation for a severe osteoporotic fracture. (*A*) Recordings from the left leg, before (*above*) and after (*below*) spinal instrumentation show good potentials in four montages. (*B*) Recordings from the right leg show normal potentials from all four montages before instrumentation (*above*). After placement of the right upper hook, the cervical and cortical responses disappear, although the knee recording verifies signal entry to the nervous system (*below*). (*C*) Spinal cord histology demonstrates multiple hemorrhagic areas throughout the right spinal cord only (H & E, ×10). This case vividly demonstrates the importance of separate recordings from each lower extremity during spinal surgery.

electrophysiologically confirm the precise area of the cord to be lesioned. Stimulating electrodes are positioned on the skin in the painful area or over the appropriate intercostal nerves (if the thoracic area is involved). The recording electrode is placed on the nerve root as it enters the cord. When the electrode is positioned on the correct root, a nerve action potential is recorded (Fig. 10.17). Second, the SEP from the ipsilateral lower extremity can be monitored while the dorsal root entry zone lesions are placed. Preservation of the SEP will allow one to confidently continue lesion-making without fear of significant lower extremity sensory loss.

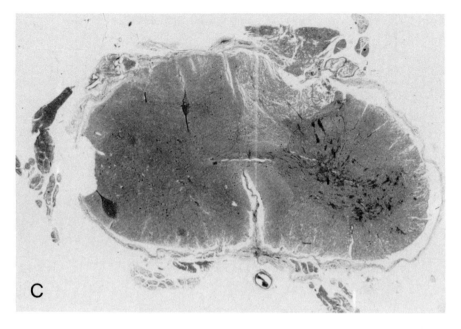

This was formerly the most commonly reported complication of DREZL.

SEPs have also been employed during resection of spinal cord tumors (140). Many spinal cord tumors cannot be monitored with SEPs because the lesion itself severely distorts or abolishes the SEP. One must remember that microsurgical dissection may allow selective removal of motor components of the spinal cord without damage to sensory components. This situation will, on occasion, result in normal or improved SEPs with poor motor outcome (Fig. 10.18). This sharply contrasts with SEPs as used in global spinal cord trauma (such as spinal ischemia or scoliosis surgery) where SEP changes correlate very well with motor outcome. SEPs have been used during diagnosis and surgery for spinal stenosis (57, 75, 143, 147, 197, 198, 213), myelomeningocele (169), arteriovenous malformations (89, 160), and other lesions (111). Though great interest has been generated regarding their predictive power in cases of spondylotic myelopathy, the results of these studies have generally been unimpressive.

REPORTS OF "FALSE-NEGATIVE" SEPS

Four criteria must be satisfied if EP monitoring is to be of value in the operating room (139). First, the neural pathways at risk must be amenable to monitoring. Second, personnel and equipment must be available for

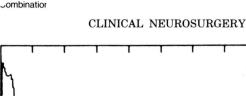

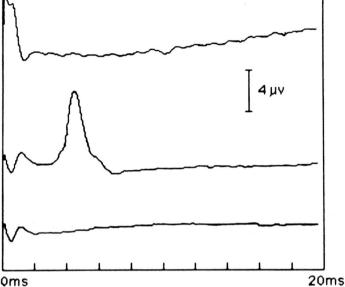

4 µv

Oms   20ms

FIG. 10.17.   During this dorsal root entry zone lesion procedure for thoracic postherpetic neuralgia, the intercostal nerve in the middle of the scarified area was stimulated with needle electrodes. The recording electrode was placed on the exposed thoracic nerve roots after laminectomy and dural opening. When the electrode is placed on the nerve root corresponding to the stimulated intercostal nerve, a large nerve action potential is recorded (*middle trace*).

recording and interpreting the EPs correctly. Third, appropriate sites must be available for stimulation and recording. Fourth, the possibility of corrective intervention, if the EPs change, must exist. Failure to satisfy these basic criteria accounts for all of the so-called "false-negative" EPs thus far reported. Though these reports are extremely few compared to those demonstrating totally satisfactory SEP monitoring experiences, they are of great concern to all physicians working in this area. A detailed discussion of each report, therefore, seems warranted.

Takaki and Okumura reported a case of postoperative paraplegia in a patient with transient obliteration of the lower extremity SEP during repair of a thoracic aortic aneurysm (196). A review of the case confirms that the SEP was absent for two periods of time, totaling at least 40 minutes. After unclamping, the SEP returned to near normal values. The patient subsequently awakened with an "anterior spinal artery syndrome." Apparently unbeknownst to the above mentioned authors,

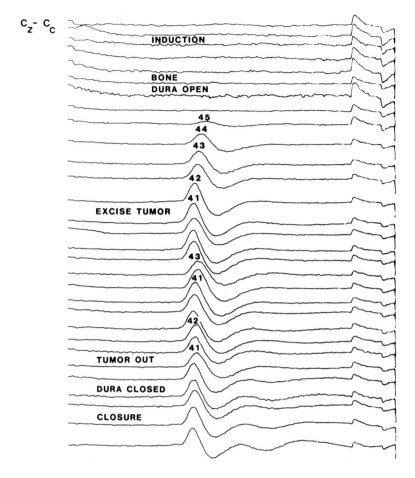

$C_z - C_c$

INDUCTION

BONE

DURA OPEN

45
44
43
42
41

EXCISE TUMOR

43
41

42
41

TUMOR OUT

DURA CLOSED

CLOSURE

100mS

FIG. 10.18.   Spinal cord tumor. Posterior tibial nerve SEPs were recorded during resection of a lower cervical-upper thoracic spinal cord astrocytoma. A cortical montage is shown. During exposure of the tumor, no SEP could be recorded. When the pia was excised, relieving pressure in a grossly distended spinal cord, an evoked potential appeared which was easily recorded throughout the remainder of surgery. The tumor was microsurgically resected. The patient awakened paraplegic with normal sensory function. This case illustrates that focal spinal cord injury (in this case to the motor tracts) will only be monitored effectively by SEPs if the sensory pathways are involved. Global spinal cord injury, however, such as occurs during complicated scoliosis cases, appears to be very effectively monitored by SEPs.

all of the experimental and clinical evidence cited earlier in this text has emphasized that the period of time during which the SEP is absent predicts, with a high degree of accuracy, the motor outcome. No animal or patient monitored in this rather extensive literature has ever awakened with a motor deficit unpredicted by SEP changes. The SEP almost always returns, however, after unclamping, regardless of motor outcome, probably because the white matter pathways are more resistant to ischemia than the central grey matter of the spinal cord. The loss of SEP for the time indicated in this report would lead one, if knowledgeable of this literature, to predict postoperative motor deficit. This case clearly illustrates failure of personnel to correctly interpret the SEPs.

Ginsburg *et al.* recently reported a case of postoperative paraplegia after scoliosis surgery, with preserved intraoperative somatosensory evoked potentials (71). A first stage, anterior release procedure was monitored without incident. Three weeks later, Harrington instrumentation was performed. The initial latencies were prolonged by 5 msec, compared to the first procedure. The SEPs remained abnormally prolonged throughout surgery, and the patient awakened with paraplegia and absence of all sensory modalities in the lower extremities. In subsequent letters to the editor of the *Journal of Neurosurgery*, one reader of the above mentioned article pointed out that the changes in latency shown in the limited illustrations are, by themselves, cause for alarm and that "authors presenting such data should demonstrate that a false-negative result was not obtained because of incomplete or semi-quantitative assessment of SSEP recordings" (173). Another reader was impressed by the poor recording quality and stated that "the traces shown in Fig. 4 representing what the authors call 'well resolved cortical responses' during the second operation when the patient presumably suffered the paralysis, may well be artifacts" (210). These criticisms appear valid.

Lesser *et al.* recently presented six cases of postoperative neurological deficit despite unchanged intraoperative somatosensory evoked potentials (133). An analysis of these cases follows: In Case 1, median nerve SEPs were monitored, and the patient awakened with a deficit implicating the lower cervical and upper thoracic spinal cord. It is obvious, therefore, that the pathway monitored (which includes only the middle and upper portions of the cervical spinal cord) was undamaged, accounting for the normal SEPs. Lower extremity SEPs are needed to predict a deficit in this location. This is a clear example of failure to monitor the pathway at risk.

In Case 2, the patient awakened with right lower extremity weakness and normal posterior tibial SEPs. The authors do not state whether the SEPs were monitored from the left, right, or both lower extremities.

Obviously, only if the correct leg was monitored in isolation can this be termed "false-negative." No case details or evoked potential records are presented. Case 3 is the Ginsburg *et al.* report discussed above.

Cases 4, 5, and 6 all concern patients who awakened totally normal and then, in the postoperative period, developed neurological deficits. A detailed discussion of each case hardly seems necessary, as the intra-operative SEPs clearly accurately predicted the normal neurologic outcome, at the end of the monitoring period, in all cases. Only intraoperative complications can be predicted by an intraoperative monitor. If SEP monitoring had been continued into the postoperative period, changes would have undoubtedly been detected at the time the neurologic complications occurred.

CONCLUSIONS

Somatosensory evoked potential monitoring has a sound and extensive theoretical foundation. SEPs are useful in the diagnostic evaluation of many neurological disorders. Additionally, the relative resistance of short latency SEPs to most metabolic effects renders them a theoretically ideal tool for monitoring neural pathways during neurosurgical procedures. It is very clear that, in the instances of cortical localization and peripheral nerve trauma, SEP monitoring in the operating room is not only helpful but also indispensable. It is equally clear that the preponderance of a burgeoning literature supports their use during many other types of surgery, including cases involving central nervous system ischemia, scoliosis, and other spinal lesions.

The challenges facing SEP monitoring today include continued refinement of the techniques employed for intraoperative monitoring. The use of on-line digital filtering and data trending, for example, will undoubtably lead to improved data interpretation. Much effort will be devoted to the rigorous definition of the latency and amplitude variations in these potentials which will predict a normal or abnormal neurologic outcome. These parameters will need to be determined for each of the many types of surgical diseases, through the accumulation of further human and animal data.

Somatosensory evoked potentials are, for selected indications, a highly reliable monitor of neural function. Though other techniques, such as motor evoked potentials, will provide valuable, complimentary data, SEPs are destined to become part of the standard of care for neurosurgical operative monitoring.

ACKNOWLEDGMENTS

This work was supported by NIH Teacher-Investigator Award 1 KO7 NS00682-01. The author wishes to acknowledge David Peace, M.S., for the medical illustrations and Dietrich

Gravenstein, Scott Hampson, Michael Curran, and Rhonda Richards for dedicated service as evoked potential technicians.

REFERENCES

1. Aidley, D. J. *The Physiology of Excitable Cells*, pp. 7–71. Cambridge University Press, London, 1978.
2. Aki, T., and Toya, S. Experimental study on changes of the spinal-evoked potential and circulatory dynamics following spinal cord compression and decompression. Spine, *9:* 800–809, 1984.
3. Allen, A., Starr, A., and Nudleman, K. Assessment of sensory function in the operating room utilizing cerebral evoked potentials: A study of fifty-six surgically anesthetized patients. Clin. Neurosurg., *28:* 457–481, 1981.
4. Allison, T. Scalp and cortical recordings of initial somatosensory cortex activity to median nerve stimulation in man. Ann. N.Y. Acad. Sci., *388:* 671–678, 1982.
5. Allison, T. Anatomical and physiological foundations of the SEP. In: *Sensory Evoked Potentials*, edited by A. Starr and K. Nudleman, pp. 9–32. Milan, Centro Richerche e Studi Amplifon, 1984.
6. Aminoff, M. J., Goodin, D. S., Parry, G. J., *et al.* Electrophysiologic evaluation of lumbosacral radiculopathies: Electromyography, late responses, and somatosensory evoked potentials. Neurology, *35:* 1514–1518, 1985.
7. Andersson, S. A., Norrsell, K., and Norrsell, U. Spinal pathways projecting to the cerebral first somatosensory area in the monkey. J. Physiol. (Lond.), *225:* 589–597, 1972.
8. Anziska, B., and Cracco, R. Q. Short latency somatosensory evoked potentials: Studies in patients with focal neurological disease. Electroencephalogr. Clin. Neurophysiol., *49:* 227–239, 1980.
9. Astrup, J. Energy-requiring cell functions in the ischemic brain. J. Neurosurg., *56:* 482–497, 1982.
10. Astrup, J., Symon, L., Branston, N. M., *et al.* Thresholds of cerebral ischemia. In: *Microsurgery for Stroke*, edited by P. Schmiedek, *et al.*, pp. 16–21. Springer-Verlag, New York, 1977.
11. Bell, J. H., and Dykstra, D. D. Somatosensory evoked potentials as an adjunct to diagnosis of neonatal spinal cord injury. J. Pediatr., *106:* 298–301, 1985.
12. Berenstein, A., Young, W., Ransohoff, J., *et al.* Somatosensory evoked potentials during spinal angiography and therapeutic transvascular embolization. J. Neurosurg., *60:* 777–785, 1984.
13. Beric, A., and Prevec, T. S.: Distribution of scalp somatosensory potentials evoked by stimulation of the tibial nerve in man. J. Neurol. Sci., *59:* 205–214, 1983.
14. Bourgain, R., and Manil, J. Modifications of the somatosensory evoked cortical potentials in local cortical ischemia. Bibl. Anat., *15:* 359–360, 1976.
15. Bradshaw, K., Webb, J. K., and Fraser, A. M. Clinical evaluation of spinal cord monitoring in scoliosis surgery. Spine, *9:* 636–643,1984.
16. Branston, N. M., Hope, T., and Symon, L. Barbiturates in focal ischemia of primate cortex: Effects on blood flow distribution, evoked potential and extracellular potassium. Stroke, *10:* 647–652, 1979.
17. Branston, N. M., Ladds, A., Symon, L., *et al.* Comparison of the effects of ischaemia on early components of the somatosensory evoked potential in brainstem, thalamus, and cerebral cortex. J. Cereb. Blood Flow Metab., *4:* 68–81, 1984.
18. Branston, N. M., Strong, A. J., and Symon, L.: Extracellular potassium activity, evoked potential and tissue blood flow. J. Neurol. Sci., *32:* 305–321, 1977.

19. Branston, N. M., Strong, A. J., and Symon, L. Impedance related to local blood flow in cerebral cortex. J. Physiol. (Lond.), *275:* 81p–82p, 1978.

20. Branston, N. M., and Symon, L. Depression of the cortical evoked potential with reduction of local blood flow in baboons. J. Physiol. (Lond.), *24:* 98–99P, 1974.

21. Branston, N. M., Symon, L., and Crockard, H. A. Recovery of the cortical evoked response following temporary middle cerebral artery occlusion in baboons: Relation to local blood flow and pO2. Stroke, *7:* 151–157, 1976.

22. Branston, N. M., Symon, L., Crockard, H. A., *et al.* Relationship between the cortical evoked potential and local cortical blood flow following acute middle cerebral artery occlusion in the baboon. Exp. Neurol., *45:* 195–208, 1974.

23. Brinkman, S. D., Braun, P., Ganji, S., *et al.* Neuropsychological performance one week after carotid endarterectomy reflects intraoperative ischemia. Stroke *15:* 497–503, 1984.

24. Brown, R. H., Nash, C. L., Berilla, J. A., *et al.* Cortical evoked potential monitoring. Spine, *9:* 256–261, 1984.

25. Campbell, J. A., and Miles, J.: Evoked potentials as an aid to lesion making in the dorsal root entry zone. Neurosurgery, *15:* 951–952, 1984.

26. Carter, L. P., Raudzens, R. A., Gaines, C., *et al.* Somatosensory evoked potentials and cortical blood flow during craniotomy for vascular disease. Neurosurgery, *15:* 22–28, 1984.

27. Chabot, R., York, D. H., Watts, C., *et al.* Somatosensory evoked potentials evaluated in normal subjects and spinal cord-injured patients. J. Neurosurg., *63:* 544–551, 1985.

28. Chehrazi, B., Parkinson, J., and Bucholz, R. Evoked somatosensory potentials to common peroneal nerve stimulation in man. J. Neurosurg., *55:* 733–741, 1981.

29. Cheng, M. K., Robertson, C., Grossman, R. G., *et al.* Neurological outcome correlated with spinal evoked potentials in a spinal cord ischemia model. J. Neurosurg., *60:* 786–795, 1984.

30. Chiappa, K. H.: Evoked potentials in clinical medicine. Raven Press, New York, 1983.

31. Chodoroff, G., Lee, D. W., and Honet, J. C.: Dynamic approach in the diagnosis of thoracic outlet syndrome using somatosensory evoked responses. Arch. Phys. Med. Rehab., *66:* 3–6, 1985.

32. Chu, N. S., and Hong, C. T. Erb's and cervical somatosensory evoked potentials: Correlations with body size. Electroencephalogr. Clin. Neurophysiol., *62:* 319–322, 1985.

33. Cohen, A. R., Young, W., and Ransohoff, J. Intraspinal localization of the somatosensory evoked potential. Neurosurgery, *9:* 157–162, 1981.

34. Cohen, S. N., Potvin, A., Syndulko, K., *et al.* Multimodality evoked potentials: Clinical applications and assessment of utility. Bull. Los Angeles Neurol. Soc., *47:* 55–61, 1982.

35. Coles, J. G., Wilson, G. J., Sima, A. F., *et al.* Intraoperative detection of spinal cord ischemia using somatosensory cortical evoked potentials during thoracic aortic occlusion. Ann. Thorac. Surg., *34:* 299–306, 1982.

36. Coles, J. G., Wilson, G. J., Sima, A. F., *et al.* Intraoperative management of thoracic aortic aneurysm. J. Thorac. Cardiovasc. Surg., *85:* 292–299, 1983.

37. Cracco, J. B., Cracco, R. Q., and Stolove, R.: Spinal evoked potential in man: a maturational study. Electroencephalogr. Clin. Neurophysiol., *46:* 58–64, 1979.

38. Cracco, R. Q., and Evans, B.: Spinal evoked potential in the cat: effects of asphyxia, strychnine, cord section and compression. Electroencephalogr. Clin. Neurophysiol., *44:* 187–201, 1978.

39. Crockard, H. A., Brown, F. D., Trimble, J., *et al.* Somatosensory evoked potentials, cerebral blood flow and metabolism following cerebral missile trauma in monkeys. Surg. Neurol., *7:* 281–287, 1977.

40. Croft, T. J., Brodkey, J. S., and Nulsen, F. E.: Reversible spinal cord trauma: A model for electrical monitoring of spinal cord function. J. Neurosurg., *36:* 402–406, 1972.

41. Cunningham, J. N., Laschinger, J. C., Merkin, H. A., *et al.* Measurement of spinal cord ischemia during operation upon the thoracic aorta. Ann. Surg., *196:* 285–296, 1982.

42. Cushman, L., Brinkman, S. D., Ganji, S. *et al.* Neuro-psychological impairment after carotid endarterectomy correlates with intraoperative ischemia. Cortex, *20:* 403–412, 1984.

43. Cusick, J. F., Myklebust, J. B., Larson, S. J. *et al.* Spinal cord evaluation by cortical evoked responses. Arch. Neurol., *36:* 140–143, 1979.

44. Cusick, J. F., Myklebust, J., Zyvoloski, *et al.* Effects of vertebral column distraction in the monkey. J. Neurosurg., *57:* 651–659, 1982.

45. D'Alpa, F. Comparison of cervical SEPs on median, radial and ulnar nerve stimulation. Ital. J. Neurol. Sci., *6:* 177–183, 1985.

46. D'Angelo, C. M., Van Glider, J. C., and Taub, A. Evoked cortical potentials in experimental spinal cord trauma. J. Neurosurg., *38:* 332–336, 1973.

47. Davenport, P. W., Friedman, W. A., Thompson, F. J. *et al.* Respiratory related cortical evoked potentials in humans. J. Appl. Physiol., *60:* 1843–1848, 1986.

48. Davis, R. A., and Cunningham, P. S. Prognostic factors in severe head injury. Surg. Gynecol. Obstet., *159:* 597–604, 1984.

49. Dawson, G. D. Cerebral responses to electrical stimulation of peripheral nerve in man. J. Neurol. Neurosurg. Psychiatry, *10:* 137–140, 1947.

50. Dimitrijevic, M. R., Prevec, T. S., and Sherwood, A. M. Somatosensory perception and cortical evoked potentials in established paraplegia. J. Neurol. Sci., *60:* 253–265, 1983.

51. Drechsler, F. Short latency SEP to median nerve stimulation: Recording methods, origin of components and clinical application. Electroencephalogr. Clin. Neurophysiol., *25:* 115–134, 1985.

52. Ducker, T. B., Salcman, M., Lucas, J. T., *et al.* Experimental spinal cord trauma. II. Blood flow, tissue oxygen, evoked potentials in both paretic and plegic monkeys. Surg. Neurol., *10:* 64–70, 1978.

53. Dvonch, V., Scarff, T., Bunch, W. H., *et al.* Dermatomal somatosensory evoked potentials: Their use in lumbar radiculopathy. Spine, *9:* 291–293, 1984.

54. Ealand Snyder, B. G., and Holliday, T. A. Pathways of ascending evoked spinal cord potentials of dogs. Electroencephalogr. Clin. Neurophysiol., *58:* 140–154, 1984.

55. Eisen, A. Electrodiagnosis of radiculopathies. Neurol. Clin., *3:* 495–510, 1985.

56. Eisen, A., and Elleker, G. Sensory nerve stimulation and evoked cerebral potentials. Neurology, *30:* 1097–1105, 1980.

57. El Negamy, E., and Sedgwick, E. M. Delayed cervical somatosensory potentials in cervical spondylosis. J. Neurol. Neurosurg. Psychiatry, *42:* 238–241, 1979.

58. Engler, G. L., Spielholz, N. I., Bernhard, W. N., *et al.* Somatosensory evoked potentials during Harrington instrumentation for scoliosis. J. Bone Joint Surg., *60:* 528–532, 1978.

59. Ertekin, C., Mutlu, R., Sarica, Y., *et al.* Electrophysiological evaluation of the afferent spinal roots and nerves in patients with conus medullaris and cauda equina lesions. J. Neurol. Sci., *48:* 419–433, 1980.

60. Feinsod, M., Blau, D., Findler, G., *et al.* Somatosensory evoked potential to peroneal

nerve stimulation in patients with herniated lumbar discs. Neurosurgery, *11:* 506–511, 1982.

61. Flamm, E. S., Young, W., Collins, W. F., *et al.* A phase I trial of naloxone treatment in acute spinal cord injury. J. Neurosurg., *63:* 390–397, 1985.

62. Fox, A. J., Kricheff, I. I., Goodgold, J., *et al.* The effect of angiography on the electrophysiological state of the spinal cord. Radiology, *118:* 343–350, 1976.

63. Fox, J. E., and Williams, B. Central conduction time following surgery for cerebral aneurysm. J. Neurol. Neurosurg. Psychiatry, *47:* 873–875, 1984.

64. Frank, L. M., Furgiuele, T. L., and Etheridge, J. E. Prediction of chronic vegetative state in children using evoked potentials. Neurology, *35:* 931–934, 1985.

65. Friedman, A. H., Nashold, B. S., and Ovelmen-Levitt, J. Dorsal root entry zone lesions for the treatment of post-herpetic neuralgia. J. Neurosurg., *60:* 1258–1262, 1984.

66. Friedman, W. A., Kaplan, B. J., Day, A. L., *et al.* Evoked potential monitoring during aneurysm surgery—Observations after 50 cases. Neurosurgery, in press, 1987.

67. Gaines, R., York, D. H., and Watts, C.: Identification of spinal cord pathways responsible for the peroneal-evoked response in the dog. Spine, *9:* 810–814, 1984.

68. Gasser, H. S., and Graham, H. T. Potentials produced in the spinal cord by stimulation of dorsal roots. Am. J. Physiol., *103:* 303–320, 1933.

69. Gelfan, S., and Tarlov, I. M. Differential vulnerability of spinal cord structures to anoxia. J. Neurophysiol., *18:* 170–188, 1955.

70. Gilmore, R. L., Bass, N. H., Wright, E. A., *et al.* Developmental assessment of spinal cord and cortical evoked potentials after tibial nerve stimulation: Effects of age and stature on normative data during childhood. Electroencephalogr. Clin. Neurophysiol., *62:* 241–251, 1985.

71. Ginsburg, H. H., Shetter, A. G., and Raudzens, P. A. Postoperative paraplegia with preserved intraoperative somatosensory evoked potentials. J. Neurosurg., *63:* 286–300, 1985.

72. Goff, W. R., Shaywitz, G. D., Goff, M. A., *et al.* Somatic evoked potential evaluation of cerebral status in Reye syndrome. Electroencephalogr. Clin. Neurophysiol., *55:* 388–398, 1983.

73. Goldring, S. A method for surgical management of focal epilepsy especially as it relates to children. J. Neurosurg., *49:* 344–346, 1978.

74. Goldring, S., and Gregorie, E. M. Surgical management of epilepsy using epidural recordings to localize the seizure focus. J. Neurosurg., *60:* 457–466, 1984.

75. Gonzalez, E. G., Hajdu, M., Bruno, *et al.* Lumbar spinal stenosis: Analysis of pre- and postoperative somatosensory evoked potentials. Arch. Phys. Med. Rehab., *66:* 11–15, 1985.

76. Gonzalez, E. G., Hajdu, M., Keim, H., *et al.* Quantification of intraoperative somatosensory evoked potential. Arch. Phys. Med. Rehab., *65:* 721–725, 1984.

77. Greenberg, R. P., Becker, D. P., Miller, J. D., *et al.* Evaluation of brain function in severe human head trauma with multimodality evoked potentials. J. Neurosurg., *47:* 163–177, 1977.

78. Greenberg, R. P., and Ducker, R. B. Evoked potentials in the clinical neurosciences. J. Neurosurg., *56:* 1–18, 1982.

79. Greenberg, R. P., Mayer, D. J., Becker, D. P., *et al.* Evaluation of brain function in severe human head trauma with multimodality evoked potentials. J. Neurosurg., *47:* 150–162, 1977.

80. Greenberg, R. P., Newlon, P. G., and Becker, D. P. The somatosensory evoked potential in patients with severe head injury: Outcome prediction and monitoring of brain function. Ann. N. Y. Acad. Sci., 683–689, 1982.

81. Greenberg, R. P., Newlon, P. G., Hyatt, M., *et al.* Prognostic implications of early multimodality evoked potentials in severely head-injured patients. J. Neurosurg., *55:* 227–236, 1981.

82. Gregory, P. C., McGeorge, P., Fitch, W., *et al.* Effects of hemorrhagic hypotension on the cerebral circulation. Stroke, *10:* 719–723, 1979.

83. Griffiths, I. R., Trench, J. G., and Crawford, R. A. Spinal cord blood flow and conduction during experimental cord compression in normotensive and hypotensive dogs. J. Neurosurg., *50:* 353–360, 1979.

84. Grossi, E. A., Krieger, K. H., Cunningham, J.N., *et al.* Venoarterial bypass: A technique for spinal cord protection. J. Thorac. Cardiovasc. Surg., *89:* 228–234, 1985.

85. Grundy, B. L. Evoked potential monitoring. In: Monitoring in Anesthesia and Critical Care Medicine, edited by Blitt, C. D. New York: Churchill Livingstone, 1985, pp. 345–411.

86. Grundy, B. L. Intraoperative monitoring of sensory-evoked potentials. Anesthesiology, *58:* 72–87, 1983.

87. Grundy, B. L. Evoked potentials in the operating room. Mt. Sinai J. Med., *51:* 585–591, 1984.

88. Grundy, B. L., Nash, C. L., and Brown, R. H.: Deliberate hypotension for spinal fusion: Prospective randomized study with evoked potential monitoring. Can. Anaesth. Soc. J., *29:* 452–462, 1982.

89. Grundy, B. L., Nelson, P. B., Doyle, E., *et al.* Intraoperative loss of somatosensory-evoked potentials predicts loss of spinal cord function. Anesthesiology, *57:* 321–322, 1982.

90. Grundy, B. L., Nelson, P. B., Lina, A., *et al.* Monitoring of cortical somatosensory evoked potentials to determine the safety of sacrificing the anterior cerebral artery. Neurosurgery, *11:* 64–67, 1982.

91. Hahn, J. F., and Latchaw, J. P. Evoked potentials in the operating room. Clin. Neurosurg., *31:* 389–403, 1983.

92. Haldeman, S. The electrodiagnostic evaluation of nerve root function. Spine, *9:* 42–48, 1984.

93. Hargadine, J. R.: Intraoperative monitoring of sensory evoked potentials. In: *Microneurosurgery,* edited by R. Rand, pp. 92–110. Mosby, St. Louis, 1984.

94. Hargadine, J. R., Branston, N. M., and Symon, L. Central conduction time in primate brain ischemia—A study in baboons. Stroke, *11:* 637–642, 1980.

95. Hargadine, J. R., Snyder, E. Brain stem and somatosensory evoked potentials: Application in the operating room and intensive care unit. Bull. Los Angeles Neurol. Soc., *47:* 62–75, 1982.

96. Hashimoto, I., Ishiyama, Y., Totsuka, G., and Mizutani, H. Monitoring brainstem function during posterior fossa surgery with brainstem auditory evoked potentials. In: *Evoked Potentials,* edited by C. Barber, pp. 377–390. Baltimore, University Park Press, 1980.

97. Hashimoto, T., Tayama, M., Hiura, K., *et al.* Short latency somatosensory evoked potential in children. Brain Dev., *5:* 390–396, 1983.

98. Heiss, W. D., Hayakawa, T., and Waltz, A. G. Cortical neuronal function during ischemia. Arch. Neurol., *33:* 813–820, 1976.

99. Higgins, A. C., Pearlstein, R. D., Mullen, J. B., *et al.* Effects of hyperbaric oxygen therapy on long-tract neuronal conduction in the acute phase of spinal cord injury. J. Neurosurg., *55:* 501–510, 1981.

100. Hitchon, P. W., Lobosky, J. M., Wilkinson, T. T., *et al.* Direct spinal cord stimulation and recording in hemorrhagic shock. Neurosurgery, *16:* 796–800, 1985.

101. Hope, D. T., Branston, N. M., and Symon, L. Restoration of neurological function

with induced hypertension in acute experimental cerebral ischaemia. Acta Neurol. Scand. (Suppl.), *56:* 506–507, 1977.

102. Hume, A. L., and Cant, B. R. Conduction time in central somatosensory pathways in man. Electroencephalogr. Clin. Neurophysiol., *45:* 361–375, 1978.

103. Hume, A. L., and Cant, B. R. Central somatosensory conduction after head injury. Ann. Neurol., *10:* 411–419, 1981.

104. Jacobs, L. A., Brinkman, S. D., Morell, R. M., et al. Long-latency somatosensory evoked potentials during carotid endarterectomy. Am. Surg., *49:* 338–344, 1983.

105. Jain, S., and Maheshwari, M. C. Brainstem auditory evoked responses in coma due to meningoencephalitis. Acta Neurol. Scand., *69:* 163–167, 1984.

106. Jakubowski, J., Bell, B. A., Symon, L., et al. A primate model of subarachnoid hemorrhage: Change in regional cerebral blood flow, autoregulation carbon dioxide reactivity, and central conduction time. Stroke, *13:* 601–611, 1982.

107. Jones, S. J., Wynn-Parry, C. B., and Landi, A. Diagnosis of brachial plexus traction lesions by sensory nerve action potentials and somatosensory evoked potentials. Injury, *12:* 376–382.

108. Jones, T. H., Morawetz, R. B., Crowell, R. M., et al. Thresholds of focal cerebral ischemia in awake monkeys. J. Neurosurg., *54:* 773–782, 1981.

109. Kaplan, B. J., Friedman, W. A., Alexander, J. A., et al. Somatosensory evoked potential monitoring of spinal ischemia during aortic surgery. Neurosurgery, *19:* 90–92, 1986.

110. Kaplan, B. J., Friedman, W. A., and Gravenstein, D. Intraoperative electrophysiology in treatment of peripheral nerve injuries. J. Fl. Med. Assoc., *71:* 400–403, 1984.

111. Kaplan, B. J., Friedman, W. A., and Gravenstein, D. Somatosensory evoked potentials in hysterical paraplegia. Surg. Neurol., *23:* 502–506, 1985.

112. Kaplan, B. J., Gravenstein, N., Friedman, W. A., et al. The effects of induced hypotension during experimental vasospasm: A neurologic, electrophysiologic, and pathologic analysis. Neurosurgery, *19:* 41–48, 1986.

113. Kaplan, B. J., Gravenstein, N., Friedman, W. A., et al. Thoracic aortic occlusion: Somatosensory evoked potential monitoring and neurologic outcome in a canine model. Stroke, in press, 1986.

114. Kelly, D. L., Goldring, S., O'Leary, J. L. Averaged evoked somatosensory responses from exposed cortex of man. Arch. Neurol., *13:* 1–9, 1965.

115. Kline, D. G., and Judice, D. J. Operative management of selected brachial plexus lesions. J. Neurosurg., *58:* 631–649, 1983.

116. Kobrine, A. I., Evans, D. E., and Rizzoli, H. Correlation of spinal cord blood flow and function in experimental compression. Surg. Neurol., *10:* 54–59, 1978.

117. Kobrine, A. I., Evans, D. E., and Rizzoli, H. V. Relative vulnerability of the brain and spinal cord to ischemia. J. Neurol. Sci., *45:* 65–72, 1980.

118. Kobrine, A. I., Evans, D. E., and Rizzoli, H. V. The effects of ischemia on long-tract neural conduction in the spinal cord. J. Neurosurg., *50:* 639–644, 1979.

119. Kostron, H., Rumpl, E., Stampfl, G., et al. Treatment of cerebral vasospasm following severe head injury with the calcium influx blocker nimodipine. Neurochirurgia, *28:* 103–109, 1985.

120. Krieger, K. H., and Spencer, F. C. Is paraplegia after repair of coarctation of the aorta due principally to distal hypotension during aortic cross-clamping? Surgery, *97:* 2–7, 1985.

121. Kritchevsky, M., and Wiederholt, W. C. Short-latency somatosensory evoked potentials. Arch. Neurol., *35:* 706–711, 1978.

122. Kudo, Y., and Yamadori, A.: Somatosensory evoked potentials in patients with thalamic lesions. J. Neurol., *232:* 61–66, 1985.

123. Kuffler, S. W., Nicholls, J. G., and Martin, A. R. From Neuron to Brain. Sunderland,

Mass., Sinauer Assoc., 1984.

124. Lam, A. M., and Teturswamy, G. Monitoring of evoked responses during carotid endarterectomy and extracranial-intracranial anastamosis. Br. J. Anaesth., 57: 924–928, 1985.

125. Landi, A., Copeland, S. A., Wynn-Parry, C. B., et al. The role of somatosensory evoked potentials and nerve conduction studies in the surgical management of brachial plexus injuries. J. Bone Joint Surg., 4: 492–496, 1980.

126. Larson, S. J., Walsh, P. R., Sances, A., et al. Evoked potentials in experimental myelopathy. Spine, 5: 299–302, 1980.

127. Laschinger, J. C., Cunningham, J. N., Cooper, M. M., et al. Prevention of ischemic spinal cord injury following aortic cross-clamping: Use of corticosteroids. Ann. Thorac. Surg., 38: 500–507, 1984.

128. Laschinger, J. C., Cunningham, J. N., Isom, O. W., et al. Definition of the safe lower limits of aortic resection during surgical procedures on the thoracoabdominal aorta: Use of somatosensory evoked potentials. J. Am. Coll. Cardiol., 2: 959–965, 1983.

129. Laschinger, J. C., Cunningham, J. N., Nathan, I. M., et al. Experimental and clinical assessment of the adequacy of partial bypass in maintenance of spinal cord blood flow during operations on the thoracic aorta. Ann. Thorac. Surg., 36: 417–426, 1983.

130. Laschinger, J. C., Cunningham, J. N., Nathan, I. M., et al. Intraoperative identification of vessels critical to spinal cord blood supply—Use of somatosensory evoked potentials. Curr. Surg.: 107–109, 1984.

131. Lehmkuhl, D., Dimitrijevic, M. R., and Renouf, F. Electrophysiological characteristics of lumbosacral evoked potentials in patients with established spinal cord injury. Electroencephalogr. Clin. Neurophysiol., 59: 142–155, 1984.

132. Lesnick, J. E., Michele, J. J., Simeone, F. A., et al. Alteration of somatosensory evoked potentials in response to global ischemia. J. Neurosurg., 60: 490–494, 1984.

133. Lesser, R. P., Raudzens, P., Luders, H., et al. Postoperative neurological deficits may occur despite unchanged intraoperative somatosensory evoked potentials. Ann. Neurol., 19: 22–25, 1986.

134. Lopes Da Silva, F. H. F., Van Dieren, A., Jonkman, J., et al. Chronic brain ischemia in the monkey assessed by somatosensory evoked potentials and local blood flow measurements. Behav. Brain Res., 15: 147–157, 1985.

135. Lorente de No, R. Analysis of the distribution of action currents of nerve in volume conductors. Stud. Rockefeller Inst. Med. Res., 132: 384–477, 1947.

136. Louis, A. A., Gupta, P., and Perkash, I. Localization of sensory levels in traumatic quadriplegia by segmental somatosensory evoked potentials. Electroencephalogr. Clin. Neurophysiol., 62: 313–316, 1985.

137. Luders, H., Lesser, R. P., Hahn, J., et al. Cortical somatosensory evoked potentials in response to hand stimulation. J. Neurosurg., 58: 885–894, 1983.

138. Lutschg, J., Pfenninger, J., Ludin, H. P., et al. Brain-stem auditory evoked potentials and early somatosensory evoked potentials in neurointensively treated comatose children. Am. J. Dis. Child., 137: 421–426, 1983.

139. Mackey-Hargadine, J. R., and Hall, J. W. Sensory evoked responses in head injury. CNS Trauma, 2: 187–206, 1985.

140. Macon, J. B., Poletti, C. E., Sweet, W. H., et al. Conducted somatosensory evoked potentials during spinal surgery. J. Neurosurg., 57: 354–359, 1982.

141. Mahla, M. E., Long, D. M., McKennett, J., et al. Detection of brachial plexus dysfunction by somatosensory evoked potential monitoring—A report of two cases. Anesthesiology, 60: 248–252, 1984.

142. Markand, O. N., Dilley, R. S., Moorthy, S. S., et al. Monitoring of somatosensory evoked responses during carotid endarterectomy. Arch. Neurol., 41: 375–378, 1984.

143. Matsuda, H., Kondo, M., Hashimoto, T., *et al.* The prediction of the surgical prognosis of compression myelopathy. Osaka City Med. J., *30:* 91–112, 1984.

144. Mauguiere, E., and Ibanez, V. The dissociation of early SEP components in lesions of the cervicomedullary junction: A cue for routine interpretations of abnormal cervical responses to median nerve stimulation. Electro-Clin. Neurophysiol., *62:* 406–420, 1985.

145. McGarry, J., Friedgood, D. L., Woolsey, R., *et al.* Somatosensory-evoked potentials in spinal cord injuries. Surg. Neurol., *22:* 341–343, 1984.

146. McPherson, R. W., Niedermeyer, E. F., Otenasek, R. D., *et al.* Correlation of transient neurological deficit and somatosensory evoked potentials after intracranial aneurysm surgery. J. Neurosurg., *59:* 146–149, 1983.

147. McPherson, R. W., North, R. B., Udvarhelyi, G. B., and Rosenbaum, A. E. Migrating disc complicating spinal decompression in an achondroplastic dwarf: Intraoperative demonstration of spinal cord compression by somatosensory evoked potentials. Anesthesiology, *61:* 764–767, 1984.

148. Meyer, K. L., Dempsey, R. J., Roy, M. W., *et al.* Somatosensory evoked potentials as a measure of experimental cerebral ischemia. J. Neurosurg., *62:* 269–275, 1985.

149. Meyer-Hardting, E., Wiederholt, W. C., and Budnick, B. Recovery function of short-latency components of the human somatosensory evoked potential. Arch. Neurol., *40:* 290–293, 1983.

150. Mizrahi, E. M., and Crawford, E. S. Somatosensory evoked potentials during reversible spinal cord ischemia in man. Electroencephalogr. Clin. Neurophysiol., *58:* 120–126, 1984.

151. Mostegl, A., and Bauer, R. The application of somatosensory-evoked potentials in orthopedic spine surgery. Arch. Orthop. Trauma Surg., *103:* 179–184, 1984.

152. Nakashima, K., Kanba, M., Fujimoto, K., *et al.* Somatosensory evoked potentials over the non-affected hemisphere in patients with unilateral cerebrovascular lesions. J. Neurol. Sci., *70:* 117–127, 1985.

153. Narayan, R. K., Greenberg, R. P., Miller, J. D., *et al.* Improved confidence of outcome prediction in severe head injury. J. Neurosurg., *54:* 751–762, 1981.

154. Nash, C. L., Lorig, R. A., Schatzinger, L. A., *et al.* Spinal cord monitoring during operative treatment of the spine. Clin. Orthop., *126:* 100–105, 1977.

155. Nash, C. L., Schatzinger, L. H., Brown, R. H., *et al.* The unstable stable thoracic compression fracture. Spine, *2:* 261–265, 1977.

156. Nashold, B. S., Ovelmen-Levitt, J., Sharpe, R., *et al.* Intraoperative evoked potentials recorded in man directly from dorsal roots and spinal cord. J. Neurosurg., *62:* 680–693, 1985.

157. Newlon, P. G. Utility of multimodality evoked potentials in cerebral injury. Neurol. Clin., *3:* 675–686, 1985.

158. Newlon, P. G., and Greenberg, R. P.: Evoked potentials in severe head injury. J. Trauma, *24:* 61–66, 1984.

159. Nuwer, M. R., and Dawson, E.: Intraoperative evoked potential monitoring of the spinal cord: Enhanced stability of cortical responses. Electroencephalogr. Clin. Neurophysiol., *59:* 318–327, 1984.

160. Owen, M. P., Brown, R. H., Spetzler, R. F., *et al.* Excision of intramedullary arteriovenous malformation using intraoperative spinal cord monitoring. Surg. Neurol., *12:* 271–276, 1979.

161. Pathak, K. S., Brown, R. H., Nash, C. L., *et al.* Continuous opioid infusion for scoliosis fusion surgery. Anesth. Analg., *62:* 841–845, 1983.

162. Perot, P. L. The clinical use of somatosensory evoked potentials in spinal cord injury. Clin. Neurosurg., *20:* 367–381, 1972.

163. Phillips, M. I. Unit activity recording in freely moving animals: Some principles and theory. In: *Brain Unit Activity during Behavior*, edited by M. I. Phillips, Charles C Thomas, Springfield, Ill., 1973.

164. Prior, P. E. EEG monitoring and evoked potentials in brain ischaemia. Br. J. Anaesth., *57:* 63–81, 1985.

165. Rappaport, M., Hall, K., Hopkins, H. K., *et al.* Evoked potentials and head injury. 1. Rating of evoked potential abnormality. Clin. Electroencephalogr., *12:* 154–159, 1981.

166. Rappaport, M., Hopkins, H. K., Hall, K., *et al.* Evoked potentials and head injury. 2. Clinical applications. Clin. Electroencephalogr., *12:* 167–176, 1981.

167. Raudzens, P. A. Intraoperative monitoring of evoked potentials. Ann. N.Y. Acad. Sci., 308–326, 1982.

168. Rehncrona, S., Rosen, I., and Smith, M. L. Effect of different degrees of brain ischemia and tissue lactic acidosis on the short-term recovery of neurophysiologic and metabolic variables. Exp. Neurol., *87:* 458–473, 1985.

169. Reigel, D. H., Dallmann, D. E., Scarff, T. B., *et al.* Intra-operative evoked potential studies of newborn infants with myelomeningocele. Dev. Med. Child. Neurol., *18:* 42–49, 1976.

170. Rosenstein, J., Wang, A. D. J., Symon, L., *et al.* Relationship between hemispheric cerebral blood flow, central conduction time, and clinical grade in aneurysmal subarachnoid hemorrhage. J. Neurosurg., *62:* 25–30, 1985.

171. Russ, W., and Fraedrich, G. Intraoperative detection of cerebral ischemia with somatosensory cortical evoked potentials during carotid endarterectomy—Presentation of a new method. Thorac. Cardiovasc. Surg., *32:* 124–126, 1984.

172. Saiki, K. Spinal evoked potential (SEP) obtained by stimulation on the median nerve—Experimental and clinical studies. J. Jpn. Orthop. Assoc., *53:* 1893–1913, 1979.

173. Salzman, S. K., Beckman, A. L., McAtee, S., *et al.* Letter to the editor. J. Neurosurg., *64:* 986–987, 1986.

174. Sato, M., Pawlik, G., Umbach, C., *et al.* Comparative studies of regional CNS blood flow and evoked potentials in the cat. Stroke, *15:* 97–101, 1984.

175. Schramm, J., Shigeno, T., and Brock, M. Clinical signs and evoked response alterations associated with chronic experimental cord compression. J. Neurosurg., *58:* 734–741, 1983.

176. Seyal, M., Emerson, R. G., and Pedley, T. A. Spinal and early scalp-recorded components of the somatosensory evoked potential following stimulation of the posterior tibial nerve. Electroencephalogr. Clin. Neurophysiol., *55:* 320–330, 1983.

177. Sharbrough, F. W., Messick, J. M., and Sundt, T. M. Correlation of continuous electroencephalograms with cerebral blood flow measurements during carotid endarterectomy. Stroke, *4:* 674–683, 1973.

178. Shaw, N. A. A thalamic component of the cervical evoked potential in man. Neurosci. Lett., *57:* 221–225, 1985.

179. Shaw, N. A., and Synek, V. M. Somatosensory evoked potentials following stimulation of the tibial, peroneal, and sural nerves using four different montages. Clin. Electroencephalogr., *16:* 149–156, 1985.

180. Siivola, J. Estimation of the brain and spinal cord conduction time in man by means of the somatosensory evoked potentials and F and H responses. J. Neurol. Neurosurg. Psychiatry, *43:* 1103–1111, 1980.

181. Simpson, D. M., and Erwin, C. W. Evoked potential latency change with age suggests differential aging of primary somatosensory cortex. Neurobiol. Aging, *4:* 59–63, 1983.

182. Sohmer, J., and Feinmesser, M. Cochlear action potentials recorded from the external ear in man. Ann. Otol. Rhinol. Laryngol., *76:* 427–435, 1967.

183. Steinhart, C. M., and Weiss, I. P.: Use of brainstem auditory evoked potentials in pediatric brain death. Crit. Care Med., *13:* 560–562, 1985.

184. Strong, A. J., Goodhardt, M. J., Branston, N. M., *et al.* A comparison of the effects of ischaemia on tissue flow, electrical activity and extracellular potassium ion concentration in cerebral cortex of baboons. Biochem. Soc. Trans., *5:* 158–160, 1977.

185. Sundt, T. M., Sharbrough, F. W., Anderson, R. E., *et al.* Cerebral blood flow measurements and electroencephalograms during carotid endarterectomy. J. Neurosurg., *41:* 310–320, 1974.

186. Sutton, L. N., Bruce, D. A., and Welsh, F. The effects of cold-induced brain edema and white-matter ischemia on the somatosensory evoked response. J. Neurosurg., *53:* 180–184, 1980.

187. Suzuki, A., Yasui, N., and Ito, Z. Brain dysfunction following vasospasm evaluated by somatosensory evoked potentials. Acta Neurochir., *63:* 53–58, 1982.

188. Suzuki, I., and Mayanagi, Y. Intracranial recording of short latency somatosensory evoked potentials in man: Identification of origin of each component. Electroencephalogr. Clin. Neurophysiol., *59:* 286–296, 1984.

189. Symon, L. The relationship between CBF, evoked potentials and the clinical features in cerebral ischaemia. Acta Neurol. Sand. (Suppl.), *78:* 175–190, 1980.

190. Symon, L., Branston, N. M., and Chikovani, O. Ischemic brain edema following middle cerebral artery occlusion in baboons: Relationship between regional cerebral water content and blood flow at 1 to 2 hours. Stroke, *10:* 184–191, 1979.

191. Symon, L., Branston, N. M., and Strong, A. J. Extracellular potassium activity, evoked potential and rCBF during experimental cerebral ischaemia in the baboon. Acta Neurol. Scand. (Suppl.), *56:* 110–111, 1977.

192. Symon, L., Branston, N. M., Strong, A. J., *et al.* The concepts of thresholds of ischaemia in relation to brain structure and function. J. Clin. Pathol. *30* (Suppl. 11): 149–154, 1977.

193. Symon, L., Hargadine, J., Zawirski, M., *et al.* Central conduction time as an index of ischaemia in subarachnoid hemorrhage. J. Neurol. Sci., *44:* 95–103, 1979.

194. Symon, L., Lassen, N. A., Astrup, J., *et al.* Thresholds of ischaemia in brain cortex. Adv. Exp. Med. Biol., *94:* 775–782, 1977.

195. Symon, L., Wang, A. D., Costa e Silva, I., *et al.* Perioperative use of somatosensory evoked responses in aneurysm surgery. J. Neurosurg., *60:* 269–275, 1984.

196. Takaki, O., and Okumura, F. Application and limitation of somatosensory evoked potential monitoring during thoracic aortic aneurysm surgery: A case report. Anesthesiology, *63:* 700–703, 1985.

197. Tamaki, T., Noguchi, T., Takana, H., *et al.* Spinal cord monitoring as a clinical utilization of the spinal evoked potential. Clin. Orthop., *184:* 58–64, 1984.

198. Tamaki, T., Tsuji, H., Inoue, S., *et al.* The prevention of iatrogenic spinal cord injury utilizing the evoked spinal cord potential. Int. Orthop., *4:* 313–317, 1981.

199. Taylor, M. J., Borrett, D. S., and Coles, J.C. The effects of profound hypothermia on the cervical SEP in humans: Evidence of dual generators. Electroencephalogr. Clin. Neurophysiol., *62:* 184–192, 1985.

200. Tsuji, S., Luders, H., Lesser, R. P., *et al.* Subcortical and cortical somatosensory potentials evoked by posterior tibial nerve stimulation: Normative values. Electroencephalogr. Clin. Neurophysiol., *59:* 214–228, 1984.

201. Vajda, J., Branston, N. M., Ladds, A., *et al.* A model of selective experimental ischaemia in the primate thalamus. Stroke, *16:* 493–501, 1985.

202. Walser, H., Mattle, H., Keller, H. M., *et al.* Early cortical median nerve somatosensory

evoked potentials. Arch. Neurol., *42:* 32–38, 1985.

203. Wang, A. D., Cone, J., Symon, L., *et al.* Somatosensory evoked potential monitoring during the management of aneurysmal subarachnoid hemorrhage. J. Neurosurg., *60:* 264–268, 1984.

204. Whittle, J. R., Johnston, I.H., Besser, M., *et al.* Intra-operative spinal cord monitoring during surgery for scoliosis using somatosensory evoked potentials. N.Z. J. Surg., *54:* 553–557, 1984.

205. Wilbur, R. G., Thompson, G. H., Shaffer, J. W., *et al.* Postoperative neurological deficits in segmental spinal instrumentation. J. Bone Joint Surg., *66:* 1178–1187, 1984.

206. Willis, J., Seales, D., and Frazier, E. Short latency somatosensory evoked potentials in infants. Electroencephalogr. Clin. Neurophysiol., *59:* 366–373, 1984.

207. Yamada, T., Muroga, T., and Kumura, J. Tourniquet-induced ischemia and somatosensory evoked potentials. Neurology, *31:* 1524–1529, 1981.

208. York, D. H. Somatosensory evoked potentials in man: Differentiation of spinal pathways responsible for conduction from the forelimb vs hindlimb. Prog. Neurobiol., *25:* 1–25, 1985.

209. York, D. H., Watts, C., Raffensberber, M., *et al.* Utilization of somatosensory evoked cortical potentials in spinal cord injury. Spine, *8:* 832–839, 1983.

210. Young, W. Letter to the editor. J. Neurosurg., *64:* 987–988, 1986.

211. Young, W., Cohen, A., Merkin, H., *et al.* Somatosensory evoked potential changes in spinal injury and during intraoperative spinal manipulation. J. Am. Para. Soc., *4:* 44–48, 1982.

212. Young, W., and Flamm, E. S. Effect of high-dose corticosteroid therapy on blood flow, evoked potentials, and extracellular calcium in experimental spinal injury. J. Neurosurg., *57:* 667–673, 1982.

213. Yu, Y. L., Jones, S. J. Somatosensory evoked potentials in cervical spondylosis. Brain, *108:* 273–300, 1985.

214. Zappulla, R., Greenblatt, E., Kaye, S., *et al.* A quantitative assessment of the brain stem auditory evoked response during intraoperative monitoring. Neurosurgery, *15:* 186–191, 1984.

215. Zverina, E., and Kredba, J. Somatosensory cerebral evoked potentials in diagnosing brachial plexus injuries. Scand. J. Rehab. Med., *9:* 47–54, 1977.

11

The Electrophysiological Monitoring of Motor Pathways

WALTER J. LEVY, Jr., M.D.

INTRODUCTION

Constant attention to whether the surgeon is overly stressing the nervous system in his efforts to help it is a fundamental tenet of surgical method. This has been avoided with carefully accumulated professional experience, and direct visualization by the surgeons. In the last 2 decades the operating microscope has called attention to the value of observation of very small detail. What has remained hidden from direct view was the "magic loom" of electrical signals by which the nervous system controls the body. These are the final determinants of most function. They are at the bottom of the funnel through which forces acting on blood flow, biochemistry, mechanical stress, and disease influence function. It is the desire to directly see and judge those events that has prompted the effort to transform the findings of laboratory neurophysiology into a continuous clinical observation tool in the operating room.

A series of sensory tests (evoked potentials) with high technology instrumentation, making use of computers and very sensitive amplifiers, has evolved into a method for examination of the auditory system (BAER), the somatosensory system (SEP), and the visual system (VEP). The first two of these have found an important place in surgical monitoring. They allow frequent feedback with a degree of reliability many have found of substantial value or even indispensible in difficult cases.

The motor system has, however, largely not been monitored, other than through studies of facial nerve function, and use of focal stimulation of peripheral nerves. This is because there is no effective method for stimulating the brain through the skull. The fact that the axonal impulses cannot cross synapses antidromically prevented stimulation of motor axons in the peripheral nerve from ever effectively traveling in the central nervous system (CNS).

The clinical efficacy of SEPs is a subject of considerable debate. A number of investigators feel that their experience has been one of a small but worrisome rate of failures to predict deficits or false warnings, *i.e.*, when a deficit is not the outcome (16). This also involves important arguments about SEP techniques, which are themselves evolving. But as these debates continue, the need for motor system monitoring is illustrated by the fact that the SEPs travel in the posterior columns and superficial dorsolateral cord, which are supplied by the posterior spinal artery. The motor pathways of critical importance lie in the ventral spinal cord. These include particularly the vestibulospinal and reticulospinal systems, which studies in nonprimate mammals and primates (as well as man) have indicated are essential for ambulation (10). In addition, the corticospinal and perhaps the rubrospinal system in man are essential for fine motor control. All of these motor pathways are supplied by the anterior spinal artery. The existence of well-described clinical syndromes of the anterior cord, anterior spinal artery, and central cord show that differential injury is not uncommon. Furthermore, grey matter functions present in that territory are not well monitored by study of the white matter pathways on the dorsal side of the cord. Finally, there is general agreement that the SEPs in particular have not been a predictor with substantial reliability for long-term prognosis after spinal cord injury.

It is probably unrealistic to expect the SEPs to function alone as a high reliability predictor of motor function, and therefore the need for a motor evoked potential (MEP) is clear. The possibilities for this test were initially suggested but not recognized in 1954, when Gualtierotti and Patterson demonstrated that transcranial stimulation was possible in baboons and one human volunteer, and measured the responses. Transcranial stimulation produced contralateral limb movement, but the patient found it unpleasant (12). Still the currents were similar to those now used by several active groups in Europe. It is likely that this was not followed up on largely because the times were not right for utilization of such a test.

STIMULATION METHODS

Electrical

In 1980, Merton and Morton reported in *Nature*, using a high current (2000 μA) and a short pulse duration (70 μsec) between two electrodes on the scalp, that they had achieved contralateral limb movements and recorded EMG (22). They subsequently found that tensing the peripheral musculature or loading it with a weight would facilitate this response. Unfortunately, this technique was also noxious due to the high currents and close proximity to the brain.

A number of investigators worked on modifications. The principle modification was the introduction of anodal stimulation wherein the anodal electrode is the active electrode producing the effect. The cathodal electrode also stimulates, but at higher current levels. It is postulated that this technique produces predominately indirect excitation of the Betz cells through interneuron pools. Levy *et al.* placed a single anode over the motor cortex on the scalp and a cathode on the palate in anesthetized patients (20). This system has been used in awake patients, but it is usually unpleasant. That method resulted in decreased current requirement to 15–80 mA. Hassan *et al.* placed a belt electrode around the nasion-inion line as a cathode, and Rossini *et al.* used a series of electrodes in a ring-like fashion about the head (13, 24). Amassian *et al.* used a semicircular electrode as an anode together with a separate large cathode for two electrode scalp stimulation (3). The currents of the two scalp electrode systems generally are in the 50–200 mA range.

Each of these methods is unpleasant for the awake patient, with a substantial awareness of superficial scalp muscle contraction and additional tingling and pain. In the case of the cathodal electrode on the palate, current to the teeth is an additional problem. Each of these systems seems to be tolerated by some of the patients (and a number of investigators), sometimes producing only a thump sensation, but by and large they are either cumbersome or too unpleasant to be accepted for general use in awake patients. They are acceptable, however, for use in surgical patients where pain is not an issue. The method predominately activates the Betz cells in the primary motor cortex to give descending responses. A detailed current understanding of the neurophysiology is provided in a review by Amassian (4). Safety standards for brain stimulation have been set by studies using direct cortical stimulation. These have determined that the charge density and current density are key factors determining injury. The electrical stimulation methods are generally well below these limits, in some cases by more than 500 times (1, 2, 17, 20). Stimulation at other sites may produce different evoked potentials. Amassian and Cracco (3) have reported a transcallosal response and Levy *et al.* (21) one from the cerebellum that may be extrapyramidal.

Magnetic

The brain can also be stimulated with magnetic techniques. This was reported by Barker and Jalinous using a magnetic coil placed over the scalp to induce a current in the underlying brain. Stimulation was possible even if the coil was not directly touching the scalp (5). This current loop is significant and can stimulate the brain, resulting in contralateral limb movements. Thus the stimulation is electrical and not magnetic, but is induced by the magnetic field. The loop is approximately the size of the outer diameter of the coil meaning that a substantial area of brain is stimulated since the coil is 13 cm in diameter.

The most prominent feature of the stimulation is that it is not painful. This results primarily from the fact that the magnetic field falls off roughly as the inverse of distance whereas an electrical field falls off as the inverse square, requiring substantially higher fields at the scalp in order to induce neuronal depolarization in the brain. From this fact one can see several advantages and disadvantages of magnetic stimulation. The advantages include the lack of discomfort and the fact that the fields are probably more uniform. They should be less affected by the thickness of the skull or skull defects, whether natural or postsurgical. With electrical stimulation, skull defects may result in unwanted focusing of the current through low resistance pathways. This could result in higher currents than anticipated in small areas. Furthermore, with magnetic stimulation, since the coil does not have to touch the skin, burns should be eliminated as a potential hazard. Heavy metal ion movements from the electrode into the body should also be eliminated.

A major drawback to magnetic stimulation is the fact that a large surface area of the brain is stimulated. This may not be important if monitoring is of general descending pathways in the spinal cord, but could become important if selective testing (e.g., for cortical lesions) is at issue. Additional drawbacks to the device include the fact that it is relatively slow (at present approximately one stimulus every 3 seconds). Testing with magnetic stimulators today has not involved signal averaging, but has used single stimuli of sufficient strength to produce responses.

Another potential limitation concerns the size of the tissue being stimulated. The magnetic stimulator depends upon inducing a current loop in a relatively large area of brain. The smaller the nervous tissue or body tissue being stimulated, the less the induced field current loop. Small-brained animals such as rats are not candidates for magnetic stimulation. Stimulation with cats requires care in the positioning of the coil.

Another consequence of this concerns high impedance barriers (bone) around nervous tissues, which is the case for the spinal cord. Because it is surrounded by bone which blocks induction of a sufficient current loop, the stimulated nervous tissue of the cord is rather small, and at present it is not thought possible to magnetically stimulate the spinal cord. It is possible, however, to use the magnetic stimulator over the spine and activate the roots at their exit from the bony foramina.

A potential drawback of magnetic stimulation which merits careful attention is the fact that the magnetic field can cause any electrically conducting material to move. This would be especially true of materials which form closed loops and are close to the coil. Because the current in the magnetic coil is high (1000 A or more), a piece of metal directly on the coil could move with enough force to injure. This problem should not occur if care is exercised, and loose metal is not left near the coil. The coil should not be placed on metal containers, including the housing of the stimulator, and the patient should not have implanted metal objects. This effect falls off substantially at even a couple of centimeters from the coil. Until the risks are defined it would be wise to exercise caution and avoid testing patients with metal plates, metal prostheses, pacemakers, etc. There is encouragement that the risk for movement of objects (especially small ones) more than a couple of centimeters away from the coil is very small, but this is not yet confirmed.

Finally, regarding magnetic stimulators, the responses obtained are very similar to those of electrical stimulation. The principle difference is that the latencies are a few milliseconds longer. This is thought to be related to the fact that the orientation of the coil is radial rather than tangential to the direction of axons exiting the pyramidal cell layers. Normally, electrical stimulation penetrates down to excite the pyramidal cell outflow of cortex, producing direct excitation of the initial segment or first internode. These are seen as a positive wave called a D-wave. Subsequent waves are the result of indirect excitation from collaterals ending on the neuron and are called I-waves. Therefore in this scenario few D-waves are produced, and predominately I-waves are produced, resulting in slightly longer latencies (see below). This could conceivably result in differential sensitivities of electrical and magnetic stimulation to anesthetics or lesions and merits more investigation. A final note on the magnetic stimulator is that Bickford *et al.* have reported that facilitation can occur between a combination of electrical and magnetic stimulation, so that the net response is greater than the sum of the responses of either stimulus (7). This is another area for interaction and could conceivably get around the problems of the lack of a focal field stimulation.

REVIEW OF CLINICAL TRANSCRANIAL ELECTRICAL STIMULATION

There are several modalities presently in use for transcranial electrical stimulation. It should be noted that those groups in England with access to electric stimulators have set aside this modality in favor of magnetic stimulation, because of the obvious advantage of a lack of discomfort. However, it is likely that electrical stimulation will maintain a place of use in the operating room because it allows stimulation of small areas of the brain. It may also have a place in combination with magnetic stimulation in awake patients. To date, results show that measured responses with electrical stimulation are the same as with magnetic stimulation, with the exception of the slightly increased latencies in magnetic stimulation.

Electrical stimulation produces predominately contralateral responses. An important observation by all groups is that there is rough mapping of the stimulation sites on the scalp with regard to the responding sites in the recording locations. That is to say stimulation over the arm area of motor cortex generally activates the contralateral arm, and medial stimulation over the leg area activates the legs, often bilaterally. There is some uncertainty as to how easy it is to activate the legs, perhaps being more difficult. In transcranial stimulation it is also observed that there are at times bilateral responses. The issue of current spread makes it difficult to know whether this represents an ipsilateral response or spread across the subarachnoid space to the opposite hemisphere. As mentioned later, an ipsilateral response is also observed in direct brain stimulation in animals and man and therefore is likely, at least in part, an ipsilateral pathway (17, 26).

An important observation initially made by Merton and Morton, and studied in more detail by Rothwell *et al.* (26) and Mills *et al.* (23), is that contraction of the muscles (whether voluntary or done by loading) results in a decrease in the latency and an increase in the force of contraction in the recording site musculature (14, 24, 26). However, facilitation can also be observed if contracting other muscles, including those in the opposite hand as reported by Mills. Additionally, it can be observed with prior stimuli given to the hemisphere, whether ipsilateral or contralateral to the stimulation site. Thus a number of modalities of facilitation exist. Furthermore, it has been observed that a prior SEP can also facilitate. These phenomena likely represent lower motor neuron activation via the synaptic pool to prepare neurons for firing, but may have upper motor neuron influence as well.

Rothwell has noted that the direct stimulation of the peripheral nerve provides a force of contraction of the muscle less than that obtained from stimulation transcranially of the cortex (26). He ascribes this to two possible factors. One is that stimulation of the nerve may activate both inhibitory and facilitatory influences on the muscle. The second one, which is likely to play an important role, is that a single stimulus to the cortex results in multiple descending volleys of D- and I-waves. This may well result in the lower motor neuron firing more than once from a single stimulus to the cortex, whereas the muscle receives only one contractural impulse from a single stimulation at the peripheral nerve. A number of groups have reported prolonged latencies, up to 39 msec, with a variety of lesions including multiple sclerosis and disease. Overall there has been encouraging positive correlation of clinical deficits with MEP testing, although the field is obviously young.

Review of Animal Investigations

There has been a small amount of animal investigation in Europe which has not yet been published. In the U.S. and Canada, however, a number of groups have been investigating the MEP. Their findings are that stimulation of the motor cortex produces a descending response which can be picked up in spinal cord, peripheral nerve, and muscle. This has the classically described features of an initial positive deflection followed by a subsequent series of positive waves whose number depends on the stimulus intensity, increasing as the stimulus intensity increases. The initial wave is called a D-wave for the direct response for the pyramidal cell axons at either the initial segment or the first internode, and the subsequent responses are I-waves and depend upon repeated activation of the pyramidal cells by recurrent collaterals or interneurons at roughly 1-msec intervals (2). The resulting spinal cord signal travels at roughly 60–80 meters/second, although some conduction velocities up to and in excess of 100 meters/second have been measured. Substantial caution may well be wise at this point in measuring conduction velocities, even between two points on the spinal cord from cortical stimulation. This is because the components making up the waveform may vary from level to level, which has been suggested from the experimental literature for SEPs. Therefore more investigations are needed that ensure one is measuring the same thing at both electrodes. The spinal cord responses have a lower stimulation threshold than the peripheral nerve responses or muscle responses by a factor of 2–3. Activation of the peripheral nerve occurs at only slightly below the threshold for activation of muscle. Among the muscles, the paraspinal muscles appear to have a lower threshold for activation and substantially longer latencies for as yet unexplained reasons.

The responses from cortical stimulation can be obtained by transcranial stimulation whether done between two scalp sites or alternatively between the scalp and palate using the scalp electrode as the anode located over the motor cortex. Given the same size stimulating electrode in the same position (as nearly as possible) the only difference we have observed in transcranial and direct cortical stimulation is a slightly earlier latency, by 0.5 msec, in transcranial stimulation. This may be due to the greater current spread transcranial stimulation produces, which activates a larger motor neuron pool that therefore fires with a slightly lesser latency. Regarding the pathways activated, classically motor cortex stimulation is described as producing corticospinal responses. Levy et al. (21) and Fehlings et al. (11) at Toronto Western Hospital and Raudzens et al. (16) at Barrow Neurological Institute have found in cats, rats, and baboons, respectively, that pyramidotomy abolishes or nearly abolishes the responses. It has been suggested in the literature, and recently by the

Japanese, that extrapyramidal influences are also present. This may well be the case but has yet to be demonstrated. Spinal cord-lesioning studies using the progressive section of the cord from dorsal to ventral or ventral to dorsal show no effect of dorsal column section on the responses. In addition there is not a loss of the response with sectioning of the superficial 2 mm of the cord representing the spinocerebellar system. There are components traveling in both dorsolateral and ventral cord which may represent both lateral and anterior corticospinal tracts. The signal is present in the spinal cord both contralaterally and ipsilaterally but predominately contralaterally in the dorsolateral cord. In animal studies it is generally observed that at threshold the response is contralateral. Ipsilateral responses have been seen at higher stimulation levels and under some conditions of injury. It has also been noted under conditions of injury that the ipsilateral response may transiently increase. The significance of this fact is unknown at present but may be a useful sign (15, 25).

Regarding Injury

In marginal injury conditions the peripheral responses are the most sensitive, probably because they are mediated by insecure synapses in grey matter sensitive to physical stress, influenced by interneuron pools and changes in vascular supply. In direct comparisons of weight drop with SEPs, the MEPs are consistently more sensitive to injury. In some cases the MEPs disappear with as little as 50 g·cm of force on the cord, more commonly with 100 gm·cm, while the SEPs are usually reported to disappear at approximately 250 gm·cm. The MEP peripheral responses are also sensitive to metabolic events and become unstable or lost with such influences as metabolic acidosis, hypothermia, hypotension, anoxia, and ischemia. Prior to a complete disappearance of the signal, signs of injury include a systematic degradation of the response with repeated stimuli (habituation phenomena). Alternatively the response may simply be unstable and occasionally display some sort of cycling phenomena in which certain blocks of trials will have a response and subsequent blocks will not have a response, followed by return of the response. This raises the question of an interplay between facilitatory and inhibitory factors.

In ischemia MEPs are extremely sensitive, substantially more so than the SEPs when the peripheral responses are measured. In a model of complete ischemia, Konrad *et al.* introduced cardiac fibrillation in dogs and followed the MEPs subsequent to this (15). In a group of 8 dogs the peripheral response disappeared in 30 seconds. A cord response is maintained for 10–13 minutes, which is roughly comparable to that situation seen in the SEP. The cord response may represent white matter resistance in the face of ischemia. It is important to note that the latency of the cord response during this time is only marginally increased, probably too little for use as a good monitoring tool except past a 10-minute interval when the animal is obviously beyond salvage. However, the amplitude of the cord response tripled by 1–2 minutes postfibrillation and then declined. This suggests an increase of amplitude as a warning sign. This can result from increased sensitivity of the axons as a result of ischemia, wherein they are partially depolarized and therefore more susceptible to firing under stimulatory influences. Alternatively, loss of an inhibitory system may occur at lower thresholds of ischemia than the excitatory system being measured.

Oro and Levy examined middle cerebral artery occlusion in the cat as a model of ischemia and found that the peripheral responses change within approximately 1–2 minutes and disappear over a time interval up to several minutes following ischemia (24). The cord responses follow a much slower course for change over several minutes and do not necessarily disappear. Reversible occlusion of the vessel is associated with restoration of the peripheral responses to their original waveform shape and latency, if reopening of the MCA is done shortly after loss of the response. This suggests that MEPs are a possible ischemia monitor. The great sensitivity of the peripheral responses from transcranial stimulation to ischemia and the correlation with blood flow are the principle supports of this concept. The test might well be an effective short-term indicator of compromise of blood flow in the clinical setting.

Several groups, including those of Tator et al. (11) at Toronto Western Hospital and Baskin et al. (6) at Baylor University, have in addition studied chronic spinal cord injury (19). It has been observed that the peripheral responses are quite sensitive to injury. In tracking animals' recovery, when rats and cats of all three groups had peripheral responses, the animals were able to ambulate. When they were absent, the animals did not. While this was true for the animals in our initial experience, we have subsequently observed possible exceptions in the transition of recovery of ambulation, but at this stage neurological grading regarding spinal walking is very difficult, and more work is required. In any event, the peripheral responses were not a long-term predictor of recovery. They appeared only shortly before recovery of the animal or at the time of recovery of ambulation.

A possible clue as to a longer-term predictor may reside with the spinal cord signal. Work in axon counting in the cord in spinal cord injury in cats has shown that with more than 8–10% of axons preserved, cats were able to ambulate. Cats were not able to ambulate with fewer than that preserved. A comparable test of measuring the percentage of amplitude of the spinal cord signal present below the lesion as a function of that above has shown an initial encouraging relationship of higher percentages of the signal transmitted through the lesion with both current ambulation and eventual recovery (19).

METHODS

Our methods have evoked substantially, and our current method with its rationale is described here (17, 20). For clinical studies our methods of stimulation involve either direct cortical or transcranial stimulation. Direct cortical stimulation is used when the brain is already exposed at surgery, obviating the need for transcranial placement. The second circumstance for direct cortical stimulation is when the procedures are done in a sitting or semisitting position with the head elevated above the wound. This results in air rising into the subarachnoid and subdural space, preventing effective transcranial stimulation. In these circumstances, a burr hole is drilled and electrodes placed directly onto the cortex. These electrodes consist of a 0.5–1 cm platinum foil electrode embedded in silicone elastomer. Alternatively 2-cm cotton patties with interwoven stimulating wires acting as cotton wick electrodes can be used. These are placed over the motor cortex in an area appropriate to the sites which need monitoring.

For transcranial stimulation we use a 5 × 8 cm plate consisting of a silastic base and a number of closely spaced blunt gold-tipped contact pins projecting in a brush fashion from the plate. The plate itself is flexible and will conform to the contours of the scalp. The pins penetrate through hair but not scalp to provide uniform stimulating areas. The cathode is placed against the palate. It consists of a semicircular electrode embedded in silastic. A second semicircular electrode is placed on the other half of the hard palate to act as a backup system. This arrangement serves to direct current down through the scalp and skull. Evidence from animal studies and human studies indicates that it is the anode which produces stimulation of a small area of cortex underneath the electrode, supported by the fact that movement of the anode across the scalp can result in selective topographic mapping of the stimulation site into a given limb.

Stimulating currents are set to be just sufficient to produce a stable response with signal averaging in the peripheral musculature. It is not clear at the present time whether it is optimal to use a single stimulus of sufficient magnitude to produce responses or to do many small stimulations and signal average. Both systems are in use. One advantage with averaging is that lower currents are required. There may be more stability of response and easier facilitation between modes, although this requires more investigation. The use of lower amplitude stimuli with averaging reduces potential patient movement during the case, which would be unacceptable to the surgeon.

The currents required for transcranial stimulation of scalp to palate vary from 15 to 80 mA. The stimulators include Cadwell 8400, 7400, and Quantum. A Grass S88 is sometimes used for direct cortical stimulation. The stimulation rates varied from less than 2–28 Hz, but we now prefer 2–7 Hz, which allows the SEPs to be done at the same time. The rate is chosen based on the following tradeoffs. The more rapid the stimulation rate, the less current required, due to facilitation from prior stimuli, and, the faster the feedback to the surgeon. There is a side effect of blood pressure and pulse elevation which results from stimulation which is primarily rate dependent.

The filters are usually 10–2000 Hz, low cut and high cut, respectively. The window is set at approximately 40 msec in width, and the gain is at a low level, 4 μV per division for peripheral responses and generally higher than that for spinal cord, in the range of 10–100 μV per division.

A ground is usually placed in the cervical or shoulder area, and recording electrodes are placed along the cervical spine at C7, T5, and T12 as needle electrodes fed through spinal needles to the level of the ligamentum flavum and lamina. Peripheral electrodes are placed at the ulnar and peroneal nerves, the lateral located by surface stimulation to find the low threshold sites followed by needle electrode insertion. These nerve electrodes may be recording a mix of nerve and muscle responses under some circumstances (even with continuous muscle relaxation), a possibility which needs evaluation. In addition, agonist and antagonistic pairs appropriate to the area of concern are monitored by electromyography (EMG). This generally includes forearm flexor and extensor muscles, abductor pollucis brevis, tibialis anterior, and gastrocnemius. Signals are recorded on a Cadwell 8400 with storage onto hard disc and/or floppy disk as well as being printed out onto paper.

In addition, a variety of information is secured about the patient, including height, weight, interelectrode distance, anesthesia, body temperature, sites of IVs and relevant clinical data which can influence results.

Generally for the MEP stimulation, the electrode is placed over the hand area of the motor cortex unless lower limb responses are required, under which circumstance it is placed over the head in the midline. For cerebellar stimulation the electrode is placed just below the inion, and for SEP stimulation the median and posterior tibial nerves are used. For modulated responses (using one test to condition the response of another), SEP-modulated MEP is done, stimulating the median nerve approximately 20 msec prior to the motor evoked stimulation on the scalp. This produces an artifact at midscreen, but both responses in both tests can be monitored during a procedure using a split screen. For posterior tibial nerve stimulation for lower limbs the SEP is done approximately 40 msec before the MEP. It is likely that modulated interactions occur at the lower motor neuron level to a large extent, and may occur at the upper motor neuron level as well, which needs investigation. Optimal parameters have not been determined.

Anesthetics are either nitrous oxide and narcotic or Forane, which does not seem to have adverse effects on the MEPs in our present experience. Muscle relaxation is an important issue, and this is ensured by continuous infusion. With bolus injections, there is substantial variation in the level of muscle relaxant during the case, and this has two adverse effects. One is instability in the recordings, depending on the level of muscle relaxation given. We have observed that immediately after the bolus, peripheral nerve and cord responses may be depressed, possibly producing a sudden loss of spinal feedback from weak contractions. The second problem with bolus muscle relaxation is that during the periods of lightening the patient may reach a sufficiently low level of receptor block to allow movement from transcranial stimulation. Use of electrical nerve stimulation may not be an adequate guide to complete paralysis, as the MEPs can produce stronger movement than peripheral nerve stimulation (22, 25).

It is important to record impedances. This is especially true if the stimulating impedance is above 2000 ohms. Many commercial stimulators do not produce their rated output at impedances above 1000 or 2000 ohms (even though they may indicate that they do), and therefore may not be capable of doing transcranial stimulation if these impedances are exceeded. Since the impedances above this level are common in biological tissue, it is important to be scrupulous in technique to have a low impedance.

Our percentage of cases in which responses were obtained has increased consistently as our methods have improved over the years. Initially the success rate was 30%, but it increased to about 70% by July 1985. Since then we have obtained responses in every case, but not immediately or from all recording sites. The cord and lower limbs are more often problems, the former because of stimulus artifacts and electrode recording problems, and the latter perhaps due to stimulating electrode position.

CLINICAL EXPERIENCE

Our clinical experience consists of 90 cases. Most studies were carried out in the operating room (OR) but a few were done in the intensive care unit (NICU). We have had limited experience with carotid monitoring but have observed some changes during occlusion in a patient who did not sustain a deficit (Fig.11.1). In the area of the spinal cord, MEP monitoring has been sensitive to injury during manipulation of the cord. Cases include decompression after trauma, cord tumors, laser-induced

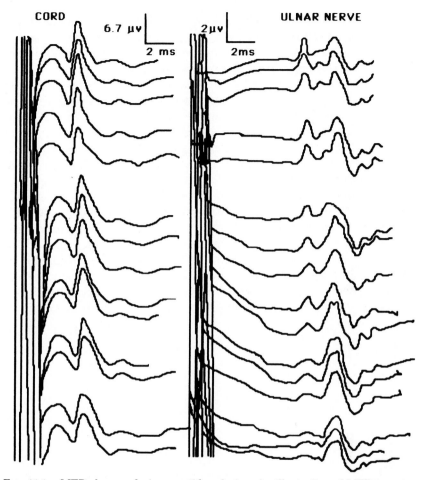

FIG. 11.1.   MEP changes during carotid occlusion. An illustration of MEP responses during monitoring in which a carotid was temporarily occluded. The cord signal is seen on the left, and the ulnar nerve on the right. As the time of occlusion progressed, an early wave disappeared from the ulnar nerve response. The carotid was reopened, and the patient suffered no deficit.

dorsal root entry zone (DREZ) lesions for pain, and anterior cervical disc procedures. We are still in the process of quantitating the analysis of these studies; consequently we cannot make any specific recommendations. Also the methods have evolved too much, and still are evolving, for such questions to be answered. But we have not encountered a case of a permanent deficit where the test has failed to warn us. It displays a great deal of sensitivity to cord manipulation, as it does in the cat. Peripheral responses are more sensitive than spinal, but again a quantitative comparison is not yet available. It is of interest here and in other areas that differential activation of muscle groups may occur (Fig. 11.2). Figure 11.3 shows a patient an anterior cervical disc protrusion with a change in the response during bone plug placement.

Particular questions which remain unanswered include the relationship of the cord and peripheral nerve signals to injury. In the cat, short-term loss of the peripheral nerve response does not result in any deficit. However, cats seldom, if ever, walk without peripheral nerve responses. In man since there is increased control and a lack of autonomous spinal stepping generators, there could plausibly be a closer linkage between motor function and the peripheral nerve responses.

Another question remaining unanswered is the relative role of SEP and MEP. It is clear that the peripheral MEP responses are more sensitive to manipulation in cats than the SEP. The exact consequences of these effects for injury levels, though, are not yet determined. It may well be that a combination of SEPs and MEPs would be optimal for such determinations upon levels of injury. It is certainly a good operating hypothesis that the patient with injury and only marginal function will be impaired by a small change in either sensory or motor modalities.

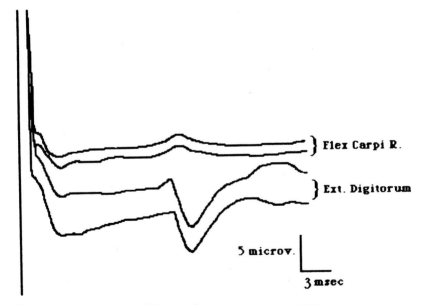

FIG. 11.2.   A comparison of flexor and extensor muscles at MEP threshold. An example of recording from paired flexor and extensor muscles during MEP monitoring. The extensor responses are more pronounced; this is consistent with reported effects of pyramidal activation.

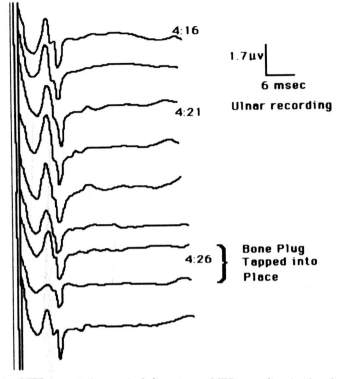

FIG. 11.3.   MEP in anterior cervical discectomy. MEP recording in the ulnar nerve during anterior cervical discectomy. Stable signals are present until the bone plug is tapped into place. The surgeon was notified of the change in the MEP response, and waited for the response to return. The remainder of the procedure used the MEP as a guide to the plug placement. The patient suffered no deficit.

In the posterior fossa we have experience with 15 cases and have used the test on both intraaxial vascular lesions and tumors of the brainstem, cerebellar tumors, and extradural masses. An example is shown in Figure 11.4, where the weakening of an abductor pollicis brevis (APB) response during the removal of a metastatic tumor was associated with increased postoperative weakness on the appropriate side. In these cases the MEP has been sensitive to injury whether the stress involved is that of manipulation or of occlusion of the feeding vessels of arteriovenous malformations (AVMs). In difficult cases such as a hemangioblastoma occupying two-thirds of the brainstem, or an AVM in the floor of the fourth ventricle extending through the pons, the MEP responses were preserved, and the patient did not have an increased deficit below the lesion (15). Manipulations of the AVM or tumor did result in a temporary loss of the response in these cases, however.

For surgery on supratentorial lesions, we have placed the electrode-stimulating patty on an important area of functional cortex near a tumor or other lesion. This is thought to be effective in monitoring that area of cortex. If that area is in a region of the brain which is more likely to be sensitive to injury (*i.e.*, because of its vascular supply, undermining by the tumor, or surgical approach), measuring MEPs from a region of concern may well help protect.

One can also raise the concern that the brain's motor control system is rather diffuse and that monitoring of a single site may not be adequate. For example, both supplementary motor area and primary motor cortex (which itself may need several monitoring sites) are important for motor control. Other areas may also have critical roles. In addition to this problem, if the current is high it may penetrate below grey matter into white matter and therefore not monitor local cortical events. Since the stimulation is thought for tangential current directions to be directly affecting the initial segment or first internode of the pyramidal cell, it is approaching the white matter interface anyway. Another possible source of error is that the current is stimulating a location around a pathological process. Here one could also miss an event.

We have found that the MEP peripheral responses are quite sensitive to manipulation of a tumor adjacent to a stimulating patty, hypotension,

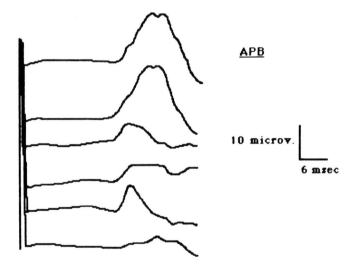

APB

10 microv.

6 msec

FIG. 11.4. MEP responses during removal of metastatic tumor. A patient with a metastatic cerebellar tumor adjacent to the fourth ventricle. During removal the MEP responses in abductor pollicis brevis (*APB*) weakened. The patient had increased weakness on that side and developed a subsequent ventriculitis from which he did not recover.

or other vascular events in the cortex. However, we have not had sufficient experience to be able to confirm its predictability. Figure 11.5 shows the responses during an aneurysm clipping, when induced hypotension lowered the response in the ulnar nerve and increased its latency in the cord. We have had a case of postoperative temporary hemiplegia occurring after removal of a supplementary motor cortex AVM. This was in spite of preservation of signals from stimulating the primary leg area of motor cortex throughout the case (distal to the blood supply of the AVM) (Fig. 11.6). This patient may have developed his deficit postoperatively due to edema or ischemia. It is less likely, but possible, that we stimulated the wrong area. Fortunately the patient made a neurological recovery over 1–2 months. Therefore one does not know if this was a flawed, or useful, test in this case.

In the realm of cerebellar and facilitated modes, we are still evaluating their presence and methodology. Cerebellar stimulation does produce cord, peripheral nerve and muscle responses (Fig. 11.7). We don't have the experience for clinical evaluation of it yet. The modulation of one response by another is also an exciting new area for exploration (Figs. 11.8 and 11.9).

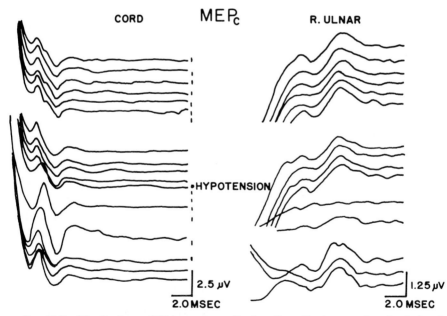

FIG. 11.5.   Monitoring an MCA aneurysm clipping, the patient was undergoing induced hypotension, and the cord responses increased in latency and also in amplitude. The ulnar nerve responses were lost. Both returned with a correction of the hypotension.

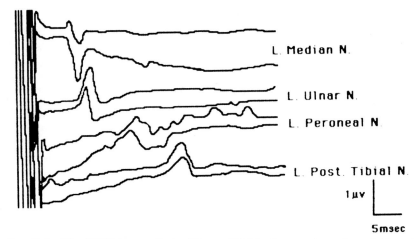

L. Median N.

L. Ulnar N.

L. Peroneal N.

L. Post. Tibial N.

1 μv

5 msec

FIG. 11.6. The MEP in a patient with an AVM in the supplementary right motor cortex. The leg motor cortex area was stimulated. There were responses in several sites. These maintained themselves throughout the procedure. The patient had a temporary hemiparesis from which he completely recovered.

CONCLUSIONS

MEPs appear to be a promising new test. It is in essence a generalization of electrocorticography, but done in such a manner that craniotomy is not a necessary requirement for the testing. Since the stimulation rates are lower than for cortical mapping, and potentially the stimulation current densities are also, the test may well offer advantages over that modality. The patient does not have to be tested awake, and the lower current densities may mean that there is somewhat less of a chance of inadvertent neuronal dysfunction resulting from the stimulation.

Since it appears that these motor tests affect both pyramidal and extrapyramidal functions, and interactions between them, we can expect a difficult and complex development of MEP methodology. Generally, the current techniques appear safe, and the currents are well within the established safety limits for brain stimulation. In the OR the test is probably a variation on the use of cortical stimulation for localization and testing function during lesion removal, with some important potential advantages. Particularly for clinical testing in awake patients (with lower inherent risk-benefit ratios as opposed to the intraoperative, or ICU, situation), work will have to be done to set risk-benefit ratios in both animals and humans. We are optimistic that the MEPs together with the existing clinical tests will enhance the reliability of clinical neurophysiological monitoring, making visible the "enhanced loom" that neurosurgery is endeavoring to preserve.

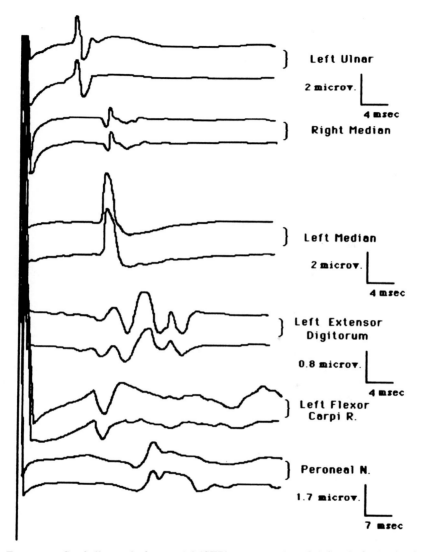

FIG. 11.7.   Cerebellar evoked potential (CEP) responses from left hemisphere stimulation in man. Direct left hemisphere cerebellar stimulation at surgery produces bilateral nerve and EMG recordings, with ipsilateral larger than contralateral in this patient.

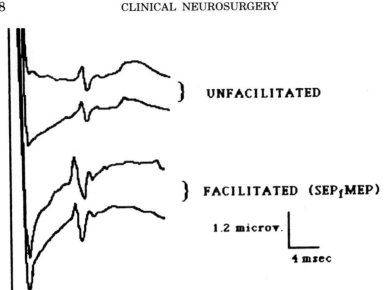

FIG. 11.8.   Facilitation of the MEP by the SEP. Ulnar nerve response of the MEP is enhanced with its latency shortened by the 20-msec prior stimulation of the median nerve to produce an SEP. This interaction may occur at lower or upper motor neurone, probably the former to a large degree. The effect is sometimes inhibitory, and the interactions are not yet specified.

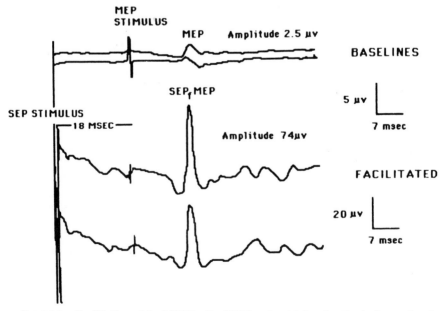

FIG. 11.9.   Facilitation of the MEP by the SEP in a head-injured patient who was barely responsive. The facilitation produced was the most striking we have seen.

REFERENCES

1. Agnew, W. F., Yuen, T. G. H., Pudenz, R. H., *et al.* Electrical stimulation of the brain. IV. Ultrastructural studies. Surg. Neurol., *4:* 438–448, 1975.
2. Agnew, W. F., and McCreery, D. B. Considerations for safety in the use of extracranial stimulation for motor evoked potentials. Neurosurgery, *20:* 143–147, 1987.
3. Amassian, V. E., and Cracco, R. Q. Human cerebral cortical responses to contralateral transcranial stimulation. Neurosurgery, *20:* 148–155, 1987.
4. Amassian, V. E., Stewart, M., and Quirk, G. J., *et al.* The physiological basis of motor effects of a short transient stimulus to cerebral cortex. Neurosurgery, *20:* 74–93, 1987.
5. Barker, A. T., and Jalinous, R. Noninvasive magnetic stimulation of human motor cortex. Lancet, *1:* 1106–1107, 1985.
6. Baskin, D. S., and Simpson, R. K. Corticomotor evoked potentials in acute and chronic blunt spinal cord injury in the rat: correlation with neurological outcome and histological damage. Neurosurgery, *20:* 131–137, 1987.
7. Bickford, R. G., Guidi, M., Fortescue, P., *et al.* Magnetic stimulation of human peripheral nerve and brain (response enhancement by combined magneto-electric technique). Neurosurgery, *20:* 110–116, 1987.
8. Blight, A. R. Cellular morphology of chronic spinal cord injury in the cat: Analysis of myelinated axons by line sampling. Neuroscience, *10* (52):1–543, 1983.
9. Cracco, R. O. Motor pathways: Evaluation of conduction in central motor pathways: Techniques, pathophysiology and clinical interpretation. Neurosurgery, *20:* 199–203, 1987.
10. Eidelberg, E., Story, J. L., and Walden, J. G. Anatomical correlates of return of locomotor function after partial spinal cord lesions in cats. Exp. Brain Res., *42:* 81–88, 1981.
11. Fehlings, M. G., Tator, C. H., and Linden, D. Motor evoked potentials recorded from normal and spinal cord injured rats. Neurosurgery, *20:* 125–130, 1987.
12. Gualtierotti, T., and Paterson, A. S. Electrical stimulation of the unexposed cerebral cortex. J. Physiol. (Lond.), *125:* 278–291, 1954.
13. Hassan, N. F., Rossini, P. M., and Cracco, J. V. Unexposed motor cortex excitation by low voltage stimuli. In *Evoked Potentials, Neurophysiological and Clinical Aspects*, edited by C. Morcutti and P. A. Rizzo, pp. 107–113. Elsevier, Amsterdam, 1985.
14. Hess, C. W., Mills, K. R., and Murray, N. W. F. Magnetic stimulation of the human brain: The effects of voluntary muscle activity. J. Physiol., in press, 1987.
15. Konrad, P., Tacker, W. A., Levy, W. J., *et al.* Motor evoked potential in the dog: Effects of global ischemia on spinal cord and peripheral nerve signals. Neurosurgery, *20:* 117–124, 1987.
16. Lesser, R. P., Raudzens, P., Luders, H., *et al.* Postoperative neurological deficits may occur despite unchanged intraoperative somatosensory evoked potentials. Ann Neurol., *19:* 22–28, 1986.
17. Levy, W. J. Clinical experience with motor and cerebellar evoked potential monitoring. Neurosurgery, *20:* 169–182, 1987.
18. Levy, W. J., McCaffrey, M., York, D., *et al.* Non-pyramidal motor activation produced by cerebellar stimulation in the cat. Neurosurgery, *19:* 163–177, 1986.
19. Levy, W. J., McCaffrey, M., and Hagichi, S. Motor evoked potential as a predictor of recovery in chronic spinal cord injury. Neurosurgery, *20:* 138–142, 1987.
20. Levy, W. J., McCaffrey, M., York, D. H., *et al.* Motor evoked potentials from transcranial stimulation of the motor cortex in humans. Neurosurgery, *15:* 214–227, 1984.
21. Levy, W. J., McCaffrey, M., York, D. H., *et al.* Motor evoked potentials from transcranial stimulation of the motor cortex in cats. Neurosurgery, *15:* 287–302, 1984.
22. Merton, P. A., and Morton, H. B. Stimulation of the cerebral cortex in the intact

human subject. Nature, *285:* 227, 1980.
23. Mills, K. R., Murray, N. W. F., and Hess, C. W. Magnetic and electrical transcranial brain stimulation: Physiological mechanisms and clinical applications. Neurosurgery, *20:* 164–168, 1987.
24. Oro, J., and Levy, W. J. The MEP as a monitor of middle cerebral artery ischemia and stroke. Neurosurgery, in press, 1987.
25. Rossini, P. M., Marciana, M. G., Caramia, M., *et al.* Nervous propagation along "central" motor pathways in intact man: Characteristics of motor responses to bifocal and unifocal spine and scalp non-invasive stimulation. Electroencephalogr. Clin. Neurophysiol., *61:* 272–286, 1985.
26. Rothwell, J. C., Day, B. L., Thompson, P. D., *et al.* Some experiences of techniques for stimulation of human cerebral motor cortex through the scalp. Neurosurgery, *20:* 156–163, 1987.

12

Magnetic Resonance Imaging of Spinal Disorders

PAUL D. DERNBACH, M.D., MEREDITH A. WEINSTEIN, M.D., and JOHN R. LITTLE, M.D.

INTRODUCTION

The increasing sophistication of magnetic resonance imaging (MRI) and its increasing availability have opened new horizons for imaging of the patient with a suspected lesion of the central nervous system. It provides a safe and, in some areas, unsurpassed method of diagnostic accuracy. The interval over which advances in MRI have occurred has been short. It has essentially replaced myelography and computed tomography (CT) in certain areas where these latter techniques were considered "state of the art" only a few years ago. For many of the spinal lesions encountered, there is no "hard" evidence to show the superiority of MRI over conventional means such as CT and myelography. While attempts at quantitating the accuracy of MRI have been made, the number of patients involved has been limited, and the majority of articles are illustrative in nature. The purpose of this article is to provide some guidelines, based on current evidence and experience, for the use of MRI in spinal disorders.

MAGNETIC RESONANCE IMAGING

The process of creating images from the absorption and reemission of radio waves from protons rotating about their axis has been well described in several current reviews (21, 28). Many of the recent advances in MRI are based on variation of the echo-time (TE) and recovery-time (TR) parameters when using the spin-echo (SE) technique. The TE corresponds to the time between transmission of the initial radiofrequency pulse and the reemission of the subsequent echo from the tissue. The TR corresponds to the amount of time between signal sampling. Variation of TR and TE changes the amount of signal from cerebrospinal fluid (CSF) and neural structures. The T2-weighted image obtained with a long TE and TR (*e.g.*, TE, 70 msec; TR, 2000 msec) give CSF an increased signal (appears white) and a T1-weighted image obtained with a short TE and TR (*e.g.*, TE, 32 msec; TR, 500 msec) will show CSF with a decreased signal (appears dark) compared to that of neural tissue. The TE and TR can be varied in order to provide optimal imaging of the area of interest.

The use of surface coils with MRI has provided another major advance in spinal imaging. Prior to the use of surface coils, the signal strength remained relatively constant regardless of the depth of the area of interest. The surface coil, which functions as a receiving coil for signals coming from the object to be imaged, is placed on or near the area of interest. Depending on the coil, the signal intensity may be increased severalfold. The signal-to-noise (S/N) ratio is increased for tissues closer to the surface coil, and tissues farther away will have a low S/N ratio. The improved image quality and detail have become important, especially when evaluating degenerative spine disease.

IMAGING OF SPINAL LESIONS

Degenerative Disc Disease

CERVICAL

Cervical radiculopathy constitutes one of the most common neurologic disorders of the cervical spine. Unfortunately, it is often difficult to obtain adequate visualization of foraminal anatomy in cases of herniated disc or foraminal stenosis. Generally, there is no question when a large disc is seen on CT, CT with intrathecal enhancement (CT/myelography), or myelography. There exists a significant number of cases, however, where the pathology is unclear. The accuracy of CT and/or myelography in these cases has been examined. In a study by Daniels et al., the results of clinical examination, electrophysiologic testing, myelography, and CT in a group of 24 patients was examined in a blinded fashion. They found that CT, with or without intrathecal contrast, was more accurate (specificity 73%) than myelography in identifying symptomatic lesions (11). In an uncontrolled study, Hyman et al. found MRI to be an accurate means of evaluating the degenerative cervical spine but felt myelography was more helpful in fully defining the herniated disc (16). Another small series of patients was evaluated by Modic et al., who found MRI to be less accurate than CT or myelography (24). In a larger series, Bradley et al. demonstrated MRI to be equal or superior to CT for cervical disc disease (7). At the Cleveland Clinic, MRI is often used as the primary form of imaging for the cervical spine after plain radiographs (Fig. 12.1). The process of comparing MRI to CT and myelography is undergoing more extensive evaluation in a cooperative study sponsored by the National Institutes of Health.

In patients with spondylotic myelopathy, MRI is clearly the exam of

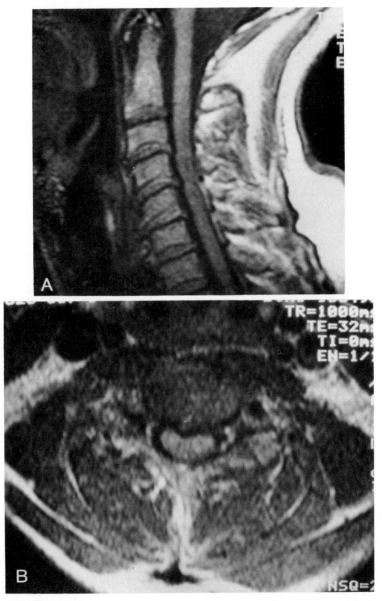

FIG. 12.1.   T1-weighted sagittal image of cervical spine demonstrating deformation of the cord at C4-5 due to disc herniation. (*B*) Transverse image of the C4-5 level demonstrating central disc herniation.

choice. Excellent imaging of the cord and the rostral/caudal extent of the disease is readily apparent (Fig. 12.2). In addition, any intrinsic disease of the cord is seen. The ability of MRI to pick up bony changes is less than that of CT, although bony spurs can be seen with MRI when a medullary cavity is present in the spur.

THORACIC SPINE

Experience with degenerative diseases of the thoracic spine has been limited with MRI. The herniated thoracic disc represents one of the most common degenerative lesions in this area. Prior to MRI, the use of CT with intrathecal contrast enhancement best defined this lesion. With MRI, the level of the disc and any impingement on the cord can be well seen. That one imaging method is superior to the other is unclear at this time, although MRI is the preferred method at our institution.

Another entity involving the thoracic spine is thoracic canal stenosis. This lesion has been described rarely. At the Cleveland Clinic, six cases have been treated in the past 2 years. The most common symptoms are neurogenic claudication and painless myelopathy with the lower thoracic spine appearing to be the most common site for this process. It is characterized by marked hypertrophy of the ligaments and apophyseal joints. Transverse as well as sagittal views are needed to define the pathological changes. Computed tomography appears equally reliable in demonstrating this process, and both MRI and CT have proven superior to myelography (2).

LUMBAR SPINE

The intervertebral disc is composed of the nucleus pulposus, the annulus fibrosis, and the end plate. In a young person, the water content of the nucleus and the annulus is different: approximately 85–90% in the nucleus pulposus and 75–80% in the annulus. As the disc ages and degenerates, the water content of both decreases to approximately 70% (23). By changing the TE and TR length, these changes can be seen with MRI. On a T2-weighted image, the nucleus will show an increased signal relative to the annulus in the young disc due to its relatively higher water content. As the disc degenerates, the difference in signal between the nucleus and the annulus diminishes, and both will show a decreased, but similar, signal on T2 images (Fig. 12.3). The appearance of a herniated disc on MRI is one of decreased signal (T2 image) from the nucleus and annulus with deformation of the thecal sac on axial and transverse images (Fig. 12.4). The herniated disc may show variable decrease in signal intensity, however (23). The finding of disc degeneration alone is insufficient evidence to diagnose disc herniation.

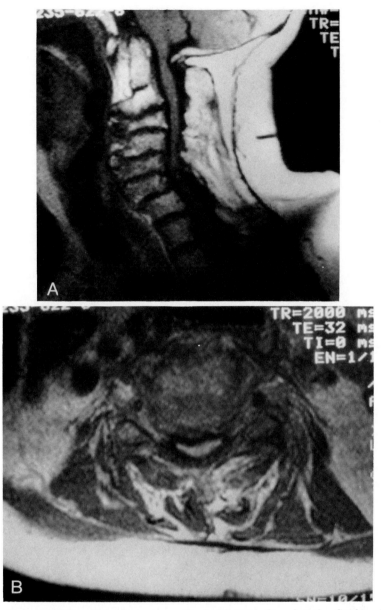

FIG. 12.2.   (A) T1-weighted image in a patient with cervical myelopathy. Cord impingement and deformity is seen at C3-C6, with marked compression at C5-6. Basilar invagination is also evident on this image. (B) Axial image demonstrating canal stenosis with cord
compression in the same patient.

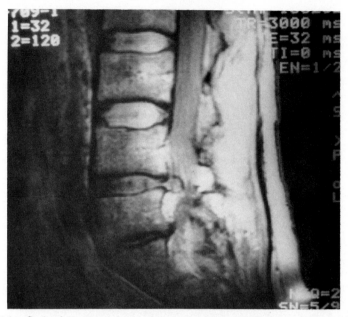

FIG. 12.3.   Sagittal image of the lumbar spine using a balanced technique (short TE, long TR). The discs at L2-3 and L3-4 show increased signals from the nucleus pulposus while the discs at L4-5 and L5-S1 show decreased signal intensity from the nucleus, indicating degeneration of the disc. There is herniation of the nucleus at L4-5. The dark band extending transversely across the midportion of the disc, present here at the higher disc levels, is referred to as the internuclear cleft.

Using CT and myelography, there is considerable debate regarding the optimal means of diagnostic imaging of the lumbar spine (3, 5, 10, 14, 18, 19, 22, 23, 27, 30). Any combination of myelography, CT, or CT/myelography has been shown to provide accuracy of 85–95% in imaging canal stenosis or the herniated lumbar disc. With the early use of MRI, little was added to the investigation of the patient with degenerative lesions. With the use of surface coil imaging and optimal pulse-sequence techniques, MRI provides a noninvasive means of diagnosis, with accuracy equal to that of CT or myelography (14, 22). Excellent images of the lumbar spine are obtained using multiplanar imaging (sagittal and axial), thin slices (7–10 mm), and a combination of T1 and balanced (short TE, long TR) pulse-sequencing. The time needed for a study of this type is about 45 minutes.

A recent article by Modic *et al.* prospectively reviewed MRI, CT, myelographic, and surgical findings in 60 patients with clinical suspicion of lumbar herniated disc or canal stenosis. Of the 48 patients who underwent surgery, there was an 82.3% agreement between MRI and

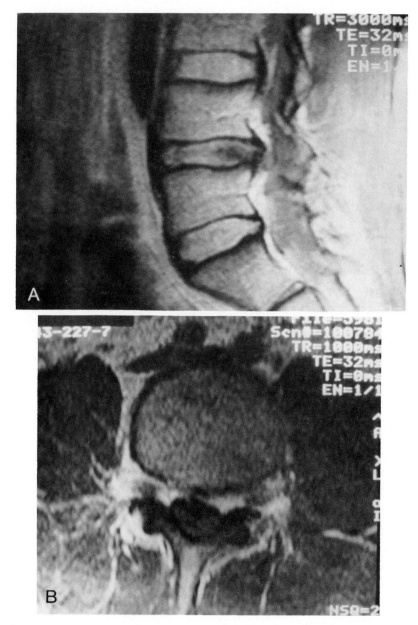

FIG. 12.4.   Lumbar disc herniation. (A) Sagittal image showing herniation of the disc at the L4-5 level. There is deformation of the thecal sac as well as decreased signal intensity from the disc, indicating degeneration at that level. (B) Axial image though L4-5 in the same patient, again showing deformation of the dural on the left. The dark mass anterior to the dura represents the disc fragment.

surgical findings. Between CT and surgery there was an 83% agreement, and between myelography and surgery there was a 71.4% correlation. These figures include both herniated discs and canal stenosis. When comparing radiologic findings, there was an 86.6% agreement between CT and MRI (22). Magnetic resonance imaging is currently used as the primary imaging technique for lumbar spine disease (aside from standard radiographs) at the Cleveland Clinic. The use of myelography and/or CT is reserved for cases in which questions remain unanswered by MRI.

The differentiation between scar tissue and recurrent disc herniation in the postoperative spine remains a difficult problem. Several methods have been evaluated in this area, and despite a range of accuracy from 40 to 70%, CT, with or without intravenous or intrathecal contrast enhancement appears to be the optimal technique (8, 17, 30, 31). Using MRI, it is sometimes possible to image the recurrent disc fragment in continuity with the nucleus pulposus. The disc would appear as an area of decreased signal in association with a mass effect on the nerve root. The scar tissue would show a slightly greater signal than either the nerve root or the recurrent disc (4). This differentiation is best seen with a partially T2-weighted image using a long TR and a short TE.

Other Spinal Lesions

CHIARI MALFORMATION

While myelography or CT alone does not provide the most accurate means of diagnosis, the combination of intrathecal contrast enhancement and CT provides a means of diagnosis only slightly less accurate than MRI (4, 7). In the study by Bradley et al., the accuracy of MRI was equal to that of CT. However, beyond actual diagnosis, the anatomical characterization of the malformation provided by MRI is unsurpassed. The exact location of the caudal extent of the cerebellar tonsils and any associated intramedullary lesion are usually demonstrated clearly. The sagittal and coronal views are best for imaging the position of the tonsils and cord (29). Optimal pulse-sequence techniques should favor a T1-weighted image with a short TE and TR to provide excellent contrast between CSF and neural tissue (Fig. 12.5).

Additional advantages of MRI over other techniques include the multiplanar images obtainable without reconstructive procedures and, more importantly, the lack of bony artifact usually present on CT images in the cervicomedullary junction. Clearly, MRI is the technique of choice for this lesion.

SYRINGOMYELIA

In the past, diagnosis of a syrinx has been difficult relative to imaging. Positive contrast myelography would often show only an enlarged cord

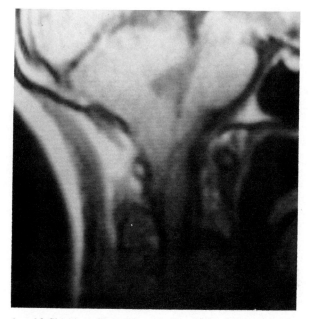

FIG. 12.5.   Arnold-Chiari malformation. A T1-weighted image in the sagittal plane demonstrating herniation of the cerebellar tonsils and caudal migration of the 4th ventricle and brainstem.

without giving further information as to the etiology. Gas myelography would show cord collapse or expansion when placing the position of the patient either head-up or head-down. With the use of delayed (8–12 hours) CT/myelography, the localization and characterization of the cavity improved. With MRI, the cavity is well seen and appears as an area of low signal intensity with smooth borders surrounded by high intensity signals from the cord on T1-weighted images (Fig. 12.6). Although false-positive and false-negative results have been reported with MRI for these lesions (25), it is at least as accurate as CT/myelography. In addition to initial diagnosis, MRI provides the best method for follow-up, although its accuracy in providing information such as position of shunts in the syrinx cavity has yet to be determined. There is little evidence regarding the ability of MRI to delineate septations within a syrinx, although it is possible to visualize these structures.

VASCULAR MALFORMATIONS

As with almost all vascular lesions of the nervous system, an angiogram is best able to provide the definitive diagnosis. The presence of an arteriovenous malformation (AVM), however, can usually be established with a myelogram, provided that a complete study, including supine

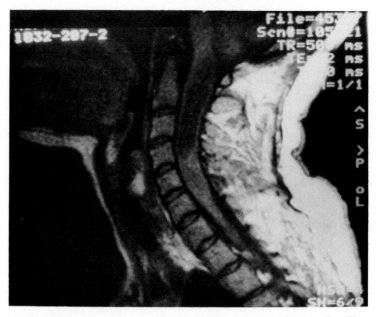

FIG. 12.6. Cervical cord syrinx. The cavity extends from C1-2 to C4. There is also widening of the cord from C4 to C6. The cavity has smooth borders without evidence of edema in the surrounding cord.

views, is obtained (9). In addition to identifying the lesion, it may provide information regarding feeding and draining vessels and generally is safer and less invasive than a spinal angiogram. Several years ago, the use of dynamic CT scanning was felt to be a very useful means of identifying and characterizing these lesions (13). In a recent article, the same authors indicate that MRI may be helpful in the evaluation of these lesions. In three of four cases, they felt that the intramedullary component was better visualized with MRI than CT (12). On T1- and T2-weighted images, areas of high flow would appear as serpiginous areas of decreased signal. The high flow rates quickly remove affected protons from the sampling area, and reemitted signals are not received. With slower flow, the signal becomes more intense. In addition, MRI may be helpful for detecting thrombosis of these lesions which would be seen as an area of high signal intensity on a T1-weighted image. They point out, however, that MRI may not be as accurate in defining dural AVMs, feeding vessels, and small hemangioblastoma nodules.

TUMORS

Intramedullary tumors of the cord are best seen with MRI. They appear as areas of nonhomogeneous signal intensity, with either increased or decreased signal relative to the surrounding cord. Changes in the cord immediately adjacent to the tumor may be present (Fig. 12.7). There may also be evidence for a cystic component to the tumor. Generally, a benign cyst will show smooth, regular margins while a tumor cyst will show

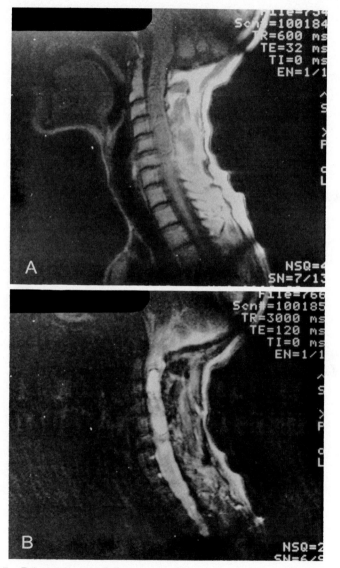

FIG. 12.7.   Primary intramedullary tumor of the cord. (A) T1-weighted image. There is widening of the cord and the tumor appears as an area of irregular signal intensity. (B) T2-weighted image. There is increased signal intensity in the upper cervical cord. A diagnosis of ependymoma was made at surgery.

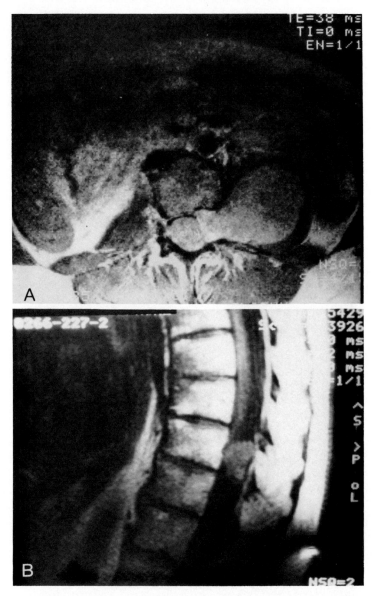

FIG. 12.8. Neurofibroma seen on axial view with balanced pulse-sequencing technique
(*A*). Erosion of the vertebral body is well seen as is the intradural extension. (*B*) Spinal
meningioma, T11. The tumor is well defined on this T1-weighted image. (*C*) The T2-
weighted image of the same lesion shows little change in signal intensity in the tumor.

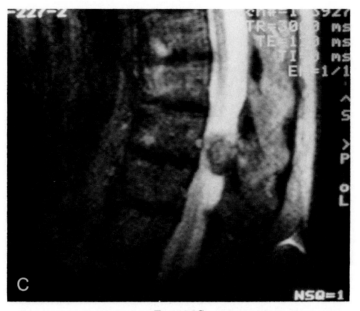

Fig. 12.8C

irregular margins as well as areas of abnormal signal intensity from the cord. While characterization is excellent with MRI, the ability to determine tissue type is poor, as areas of abnormal signal are not specific for a particular disease. Differentiation between benign and tumor cysts can be extremely difficult and at times impossible. For identifying calcifications in tumors, MRI is inferior to CT (12).

The intradural extramedullary lesions, including neurofibromas and meningiomas, are also well seen with MRI. In the case of the neurofibromas, any extraaxial extension is readily seen, and MRI provides outstanding visualization (Fig. 12.8). The area where the use of MRI is much more in question is the search for drop metastases from other tumors rostral to the cord. A common situation would be the postoperative search for spinal metastases in a patient with a medulloblastoma. At present there is little evidence or experience to indicate the superiority of MRI over other methods.

Evaluation of epidural tumor has been augmented with the use of MRI. Subjecting a patient who is usually cachectic and in pain to a myelogram or CT/myelogram is unpleasant for all parties concerned. The MRI provides clear, anatomically correct images of epidural tumor and bony involvement. Affected vertebral bodies appear as areas of decreased signal intensity on the T1-weighted image relative to other vertebral bodies (Fig. 12.9).

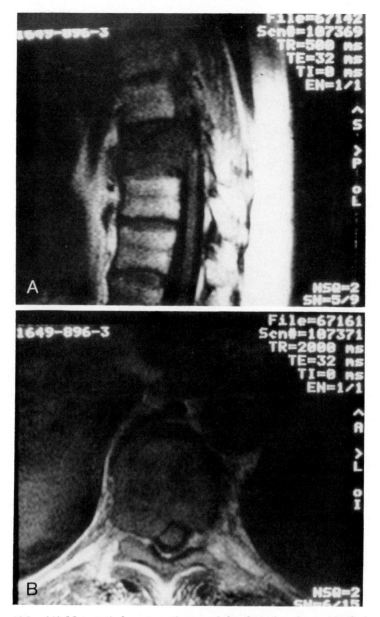

FIG. 12.9. (A) Metastatic breast carcinoma of the thoracic spine, sagittal view. The involved vertebral body appears as an area of decreased signal intensity relative to the other vertebral bodies. (B) Axial view demonstrating cord compression and loss of the subarachnoid space in the area of compression. The vertebral body appears homogeneous, although there is loss of the cortical margin on the posterior and right lateral aspects as well as paravertebral extension on the right.

SPINAL DYSRAPHISM

Imaging of tethered cords, diastematomyelia, lipomas, and meningoceles has also been influenced by MRI. Although accuracy in establishing the diagnosis has remained the same, the amount of additional information gained from MRI remains in question. In several studies comparing MRI with myelography and CT/myelography, MRI gave less information regarding nerve root anatomy and the filum (1, 15). At times, the scoliosis or kyphosis contributed to creating false images of a normal conus and giving the impression of a low-lying structure. Lipomas, however, are easily seen on MRI with T1-weighted images showing the lipoma as an area of increased signal (Fig. 12.10). Despite these drawbacks, MRI appears to provide an excellent means of noninvasive initial evaluation and follow-up. The use of myelography or CT/myelography should be reserved for those cases where the MRI study is inconclusive (1).

Trauma

A high percentage of patients with traumatic spinal injury have multiple system trauma, and use of life support methods such as ventilators, IVs, and special beds for immobilization is common. These particular devices preclude the use of MRI in the acute situation. Once the patient has stabilized, and no longer requires support equipment, there is no doubt that MRI can safely identify the area of trauma and display information regarding the condition of the cord (Fig. 12.11). To correctly diagnose and treat the patient with a spinal cord injury, it is important to evaluate the bony injury as well as the cord. In cases where significant bony impingement on the cord exists, or in cases where it is important to establish the exact extent of bony injury, the use of CT or CT/myelography is superior. An evaluation solely with MRI may be inadequate due to its inability to consistently identify cortical bone.

The evaluation of patients with chronic spinal injuries resulting from trauma is a different situation. The lesions encountered in this group of patients are usually confined to the cord, i.e., spinal cysts, myelomalacia, and syrinx (Fig. 12.12). These lesions are best imaged with MRI (26).

INFECTIONS

Both vertebral osteomyelitis and discitis can be seen on MRI. Initial findings are loss of the internuclear cleft which is normally seen as a dark band extending transversely across the disc space. Next, there is an increase in the signal from the disc and vertebral bodies on the T2-weighted image and a decrease in the signal from the disc and vertebral body on the T1-weighted image (Fig. 12.13). A paraspinal mass may also

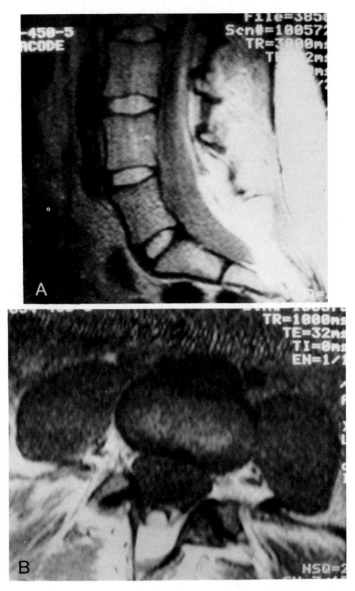

FIG. 12.10.   Tethered cord with lipoma. (*A*) Sagittal and (*B*) axial images demonstrating
the lipoma as an area of high signal intensity in the dorsal aspect of the canal. The filum
is seen as a filament of high signal intensity extending into the mass. For both images: TE,
32 msec. TR, 1000 msec.

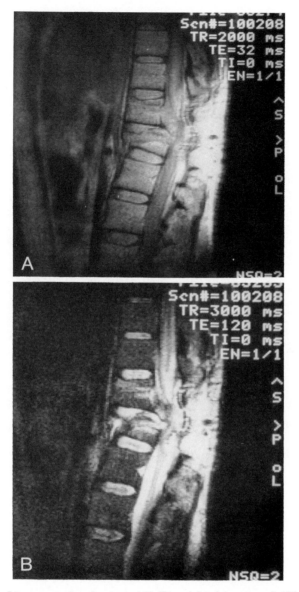

FIG. 12.11.   L1 compression fracture. (A) T1-weighted image and (B) T2-weighted image. The area of injury is readily identified. At the level of injury, there appears to be disc material in the canal as well as bony compression. This is best seen on the T2-weighted image and is represented as a mass with high signal intensity extending into the canal. Disruption of the anterior ligaments is apparent. The discs above and below the injury appear normal on the T2-weighted image.

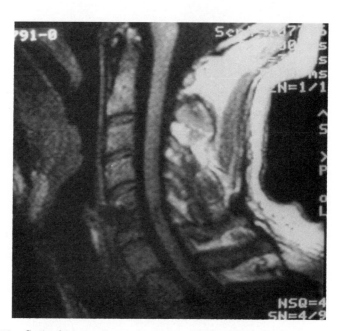

FIG. 12.12. Sagittal image of a posttraumatic syrinx in the cervical region (C5-6). The cavity appears as an area of low signal intensity (similar to that of CSF) with smooth, regular borders. A fusion has been performed at the C5-6 level.

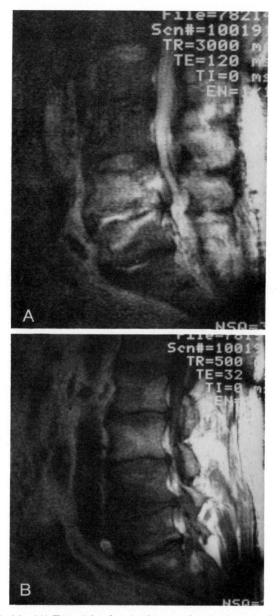

FIG. 12.13.   Discitis. (A) T2-weighted sagittal image showing increased signal intensity in the L4 and L5 vertebral bodies and the L4-5 disc and loss of the internuclear cleft (present in the disc space above). TE, 120 msec; TR, 3000 msec. (B) The T1-weighted image demonstrated decreased signal from the involved vertebral bodies and disc space. TE, 32 msec; TR, 500 msec.

be seen. The accuracy of MRI (greater than 90%) is equal to that of combined bone scanning and gallium scanning and is slightly more accurate than CT in detecting infection (20).

CONCLUSION

The use of MRI has revolutionized our approach to the diagnosis of spinal disease. In almost all areas, MRI has proven to be a beneficial tool in diagnosis. The evaluation of congenital malformations, tumors, cystic lesions, and infections of the spine has been greatly enhanced. The use of MRI in the diagnosis of degenerative disc disease has improved and is beginning to compare favorably with CT and myelography. It is important to point out, however, that MRI is not a panacea for the problems of spinal imaging. Imaging of the patient with scoliosis or with metallic instruments such as pacemakers, aneurysm clips, cardiac valve replacements and spinal instrumentation remains a problem. Also, it is unlikely that MRI will completely replace CT as there are areas where the use of CT provides accuracy equal or superior to that of MRI such as acute trauma and degenerative disc disease. However, with improving quality and consistency of MRI, the rapid development of this tool promises a bright future for imaging of the spine.

REFERENCES

1. Barnes, P. D., Lester, P. D., Yamanashi, W. S., et al. MRI in infants and children with spinal dysraphism. AJNR, 147: 339–346, 1986.
2. Barnett, G. H., Hardy, R. W., Little, J. R., et al. Thoracic canal stenosis: Report of 6 cases and review of the literature. J. Neurosurg., 66: 338–344, 1987.
3. Bell, G. R., Rothman, R. H., Booth, R. E., et al. A study of computer-assisted tomography. II. Comparison of metrizamide myelography and computed tomography in the diagnosis of herniated lumbar disc and spinal stenosis. Spine, 9: 552–556, 1984.
4. Berger, P. E., Atkinson, D., Wilson, W. J., et al. High resolution surface coil magnetic resonance imaging of the spine: Normal and pathologic anatomy. Radiographics, 6: 573–602, 1986.
5. Bosacco, S. J., Berman, A. T., Garbarina, J. L., et al. A Comparison of CT scanning and myelography in the diagnosis of lumbar disc herniation. Clin. Orthop. Related Res., 190: 124–128, 1984.
6. Bosley, T. M., Cohen, D. A., Schatz, N. J., et al. Comparison of metrizamide computed tomography and magnetic resonance imaging in the the evaluation of lesions at the cervicomedullary junction. Neurology, 35: 485–492, 1985.
7. Bradley, W. G., Waluch, V., Yadley, R. A., et al. Comparison of CT and MR in 400 patients with suspected disease of the brain and cervical spinal cord. Radiology, 152: 695–702, 1984.
8. Braun, I. F., Hoffman, J. C., Davis, P. C., et al. Contrast enhancement in CT differentiation between recurrent disk herniation and postoperative scar: Prospective study. AJNR, 145: 785–790, 1985.
9. Buchan, A. M., and Barnett, H. J. M. Vascular Malformations and Hemorrhage of the Spinal Cord. In: Stroke: Pathophysiology, Diagnosis, and Management, edited by H.

J. M. Barnett, pp. 721–729. Churchill Livingstone, Edinburgh, 1986.

10. Chafetz, N. I., Genant, H. K., Moon, K. L., et al. Recognition of lumbar disk herniation with NMR. AJNR, 5: 23–26, 1986.

11. Daniels, D. L., Grogan, J. P., Johansen, J. G., et al. Cervical radiculopathy: Tomography and myelography compared. Radiology, 151: 109–113, 1984.

12. Di Chiro, G., Doppman, J. L., Dwyer, A. J., et al. Tumors and arteriovenous malformations of the spinal cord: Assessment using MR. Radiology, 156: 689–697, 1985.

13. Di Chiro, G., Rieth, K. G., Oldfield, E. H., et al. Digital subtraction angiography and dynamic computed tomography in the evaluation of arteriovenous malformations and hemangioblastomas of the spinal cord. J. Comp. Assist. Comput. Tom., 4: 655–670, 1982.

14. Edelman, R. R., Shouckimas, G. M., Stark, D. D., et al. High-resolution surface-coil imaging of lumbar disk disease. AJNR, 6: 479–485, 1985.

15. Jan, J. S., Benson, J. E., Kaufman, B., et al. Demonstration of diastematomyelia and associated abnormalities with MR imaging. AJNR, 6: 215–219, 1985.

16. Hyman, R. A., Edwards, J. H., Vacirca, S. J., et al. 0.6T MR imaging of the cervical spine: Multislice and multiecho techniques. AJNR, 6: 229–236, 1985.

17. Irstam, L. Differential diagnosis of recurrent lumbar disc herniation and postoperative deformation by myelography: An impossible task. Spine, 9: 759–763, 1984.

18. Ketonen, L., and Gyldensted, C. Lumbar disc disease evaluated by myelography and postmyelography spinal computed tomography. Neuroradiology, 28: 144–149, 1986.

19. Maravilla, K. R., Lesh, P., Weinreb, J. C., et al. Magnetic resonance imaging of the lumbar spine with CT correlation. AJNR, 6: 237–245, 1985.

20. Modic, M. T., Feiglin, D. H., Piraino, D. W., et al. Vertebral osteomyelitis: Assessment using MR. Radiology, 157: 157–166, 1985.

21. Modic, M. T., Hardy, R. W., Weinstein, M. A., et al. Nuclear magnetic resonance of the spine: Clinical potential and limitation. Neurosurgery, 4: 582–592, 1984.

22. Modic, M. T., Masaryk, T., Boumphrey, F., et al. Lumbar herniated disk disease and canal stenosis: Prospective evaluation by surface coil MR, CT, and myelography. AJNR, 7: 709–717, 1986.

23. Modic, M. T., Pavlicek, W., Weinstein, M. A., et al. Magnetic resonance imaging of intervertebral disk disease: Clinical and pulse sequence considerations. Radiology, 152: 103–111, 1984.

24. Modic, M. T., Weinstein, M. A., Pavlicek, W., et al. Magnetic resonance imaging of the cervical spine: Technical and clinical observations. AJR, 141: 1129–1136, 1983.

25. Pojunas, K., Williams, A. L., Daniels, D. L., et al. Syringomyelia and hydromyelia: Magnetic resonance evaluation. Radiology, 153: 679–683, 1984.

26. Quencer, R. M., Sheldon, J. J., Post, M. J. D., et al. Magnetic resonance imaging of the chronically injured cervical spinal cord. AJNR 7: 457–464, 1986.

27. Raskin, S. P., and Keating, J. W. Recognition of lumbar disk disease: Comparison of myelography and computed tomography. AJR, 139: 349–355, 1982.

28. Spetzler, R. F., Zabramski, J. M., and Kaufman, B. Clinical role of magnetic resonance imaging in the neurosurgical patient. Neurosurgery, 16: 511–524, 1985.

29. Spinos, E., Laster, D. W., Moody, D. M., et al. MR Evaluation of Chiari 1 malformations at 0.15T. AJR, 144: 1143–1148, 1985.

30. Teplick, J. G., and Haskin, M. E. Computed tomography of the postoperative lumbar spine. AJR, 141: 865–884, 1983.

31. Weisz, G. M. The value of CT in diagnosing postoperative lumbar conditions. Spine, 11: 164–166, 1986.

13

Intraoperative Spinal Ultrasonography

JONATHAN M. RUBIN, M.D., PH.D., GEORGE J. DOHRMANN, M.D., and WILLIAM F. CHANDLER, M.D.

The precise preoperative and intraoperative localization of lesions of the spine and spinal cord is vital for neurosurgeons. Because the spinal cord is an extremely delicate organ, the surgeon must be acutely aware of the site of his operative field, and the direction in which he is headed at all times.

Preoperative localization of spinal cord abnormalities has reached a high technological level with examinations such as myelography, computed tomography (CT), and magnetic resonance imaging (MRI). MRI has become the diagnostic modality for imaging the spinal cord and spinal subarachnoid space (9, 16, 29). It directly images the spinal cord with high contrast and resolution, and yet MRI does not require the injection of contrast material to achieve this visualization as is necessary in CT and myelography. Further, unlike MRI, CT and myelographic examinations have often been disappointing in the quality of their detail of the spinal cord even with contrast material in the subarachnoid space (6–8, 13, 27).

Unfortunately, despite its exquisite detail of the spinal cord, MRI is of no use as an intraoperative tool. Once in the operating room, the neurosurgeon must use his best judgment when determining the position and extent of lesions based on the MRI-displayed abnormalities. Further, it is clear that any maneuvers performed during an operation will not be depicted on preoperative diagnostic scans. It is at this point that real-time ultrasonography has its greatest utility.

Real-time ultrasonography has turned out to be a sensitive and reliable intraoperative device. Once the bone has been removed, ultrasonography is an excellent localizing instrument, since by merely pointing the scanhead at an abnormality, all of the 3-dimensional coordinates characterizing the location of a lesion relative to the scanhead are determined (4, 22). Because the method proceeds in real time and is safe, ultrasonography can be used frequently to monitor the progress of an operation. Neurosurgeons can not only localize spinal abnormalities, but also they can confirm immediately during an operation that a manipulation has actually produced the intended result (4, 24).

TECHNIQUE

All of the operations to be described were performed on patients in the prone position. In a prone patient, the laminectomy can be filled with sterile saline, providing a fluid path several centimeters deep through which scanning can be performed (Fig. 13.1). The saline path has several functions: it prevents the near-field cap artifact of the scanhead from intersecting the image of the spinal cord; it increases the amount of spinal cord that can be visualized within a sector; and it permits scanning of the intraspinal contents without having to touch the intrathecal contents themselves (4, 24). Lastly, the scanhead can be positioned so that its zone of best focus falls within the spinal cord.

The technique can be performed as well from an anterior approach through a corpectomy (19). The method for scanning the spinal cord is similar to that described above. The space formerly occupied by the resected vertebral body is filled with saline, producing a fluid path—the only difference being that now the more anterior anatomic structures are nearest to the scanhead.

Since the spinal cord is a thin object, high frequency transducers should be used for imaging. We have generally used a 7.5-MHz short focus mechanical sector scanner (Advanced Technology Laboratories, Bothel, WA), but we have also employed a 10-MHz linear array scanner

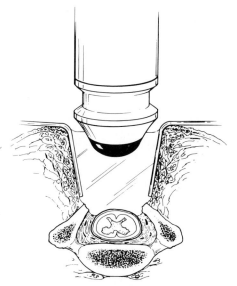

FIG. 13.1. Diagram showing a laminectomy with a scanhead inserted. The saline produces a fluid path so that the spinal cord can be scanned without touching it. (From Dohrmann, G. J., and Rubin, J. M. Intraoperative ultrasound imaging of the spinal cord: Syringomyelia, cysts and tumors—a preliminary report. Surg. Neurol., *18:* 395–399, 1982.)

successfully. In general, any high frequency transducer small enough to fit into the laminectomy should function.

NORMAL ANATOMY

On transverse scans (Fig. 13.2), the posterior dura mater is first to be visualized as a curve convex toward the scanhead. The dura mater extends to both margins of the laminectomy. Under the dura mater, the posterior subarachnoid space is seen as an anechoic space. The spinal cord, imaged immediately under the posterior subarachnoid space, appears as an oval mass in cross-section. The exact shape of the spinal cord differs depending on the part of the cord being scanned. Yet, the central canal is seen as a dot within the ventral half of the spinal cord (4, 23, 26) and is a

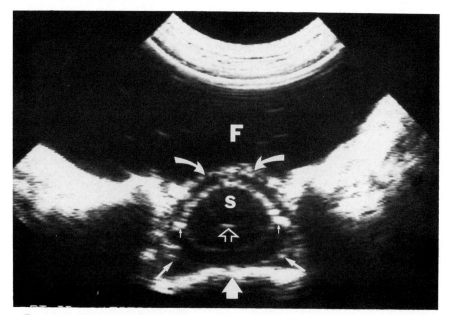

FIG. 13.2.   Normal transverse scan of a spinal cord. A fluid path (*F*) is present in the near field separating the scanhead from the posterior dura mater (*curved arrows*). (Posterior will always be positioned at the top of the images.) The posterior subarachnoid space is the clear space between the posterior dura mater (*curved arrows*) and the spinal cord (*S*). The dentate ligaments (*small arrows*) are the small lines on each side of the spinal cord. The central canal (*hollow arrow*) is represented by a localized reflection in the ventral half of the spinal cord. In this scan, the anterior dura mater (*medium arrows*) is resolved at about 5 o'clock and 8 o'clock, respectively. However, the dura mater cannot be resolved along the posterior surface of the vertebral body (*large arrow*). The anterior subarachnoid space appears as an anechoic area between the spinal cord and vertebral body. (From Rubin, J. M., and Dohrmann, G. J. Intraoperative sonography of the spine and spinal cord. Semin. Ultrasound CT MR, *6:* 48–67, 1985.)

useful landmark. When there are masses present displacing the spinal cord, the cord can frequently be recognized by the presence of the central canal. The canal can be traced down to the conus medullaris, where the spinal cord disappears into groups of nerve roots (Fig. 13.3). Lateral to the spinal cord are the dentate ligaments (Fig. 13.2). They are visualized as lines extending from the lateral edges of the cord. The anterior spinal artery and other marginal arteries are seen pulsating along the periphery of the spinal cord on the real-time images, although they are rarely visible on static images.

In front of the spinal cord, the anterior subarachnoid space and the posterior surface of vertebral bodies and discs are imaged. Even though the sound does not go through bone and poorly penetrates disc material, the effects of an anterior compression made by bony or disc fragments are clearly visible.

The anatomy is also simple to evaluate on longitudinal scans (Fig. 13.4). The posterior dura mater appears as a straight line coursing through the laminectomy. The posterior subarachnoid space is an anechoic zone between the dura mater and the spinal cord. The spinal cord is seen extending within the subarachnoid space between the posterior dura mater and the vertebral bodies—disc spaces. Again the central canal

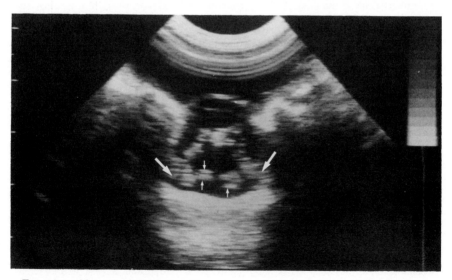

FIG. 13.3. Normal cauda equina. Transverse scan through the cauda equina demonstrating individual nerve roots (*small arrows*) in cross-section. Two large groups of nerve roots (*large arrows*) are visible near the neural foramina. (From Rubin, J. M., and Dohrmann, G. J. Intraoperative spinal ultrasonography J. Belge Radiol. Belg. Tijdschrift Voor Radiol., *69:* 9–27, 1986.)

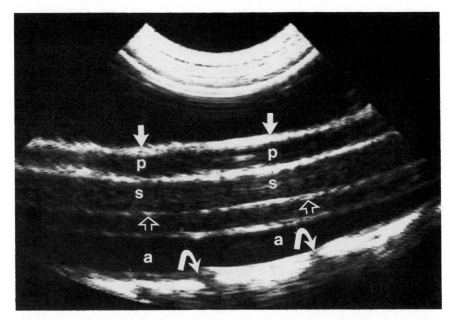

FIG. 13.4. Normal longitudinal scan of spinal cord. The posterior dura mater (*arrows*) is the first reflection beneath the scanhead. (On longitudinal scans, cephalad will always be on the left side of the image.) The spinal cord (*s*) appears as a long ribbon beneath the anechoic posterior subarachnoid space (*p*). The central canal (*hollow arrows*) is a line running through the ventral half of the spinal cord. The posterior surfaces of the vertebral bodies are discontinuous reflections separated by disc spaces (*curved arrows*). The anterior subarachnoid space (*a*) lies between this line of discontinuous reflections and the spinal cord. (From Rubin, J. M., and Dohrmann, G. J. Intraoperative sonography of the spine and spinal cord. Semin. Ultrasound CT MR, *6:* 48–67, 1985.)

is visible, this time as a line, running through the ventral half of the cord. The diameter of the spinal cord depends on the portion of the spinal cord being scanned. It starts out wide in the cervical region, narrowing to a line, the filum terminale, in the lumbar area (Fig. 13.5).

The anterior subarachnoid space is again seen as an anechoic area in front of the spinal cord. Sometimes adhesions or pia arachnoid webs are visible within the subarachnoid spaces. The posterior surfaces of the vertebral bodies are bright echoes interspersed with discontinuities representing the disc spaces (Fig. 13.4). Almost no sound enters the bony vertebrae, but some sound may penetrate the discs. Clearly again, although basically only the posterior surfaces of discs and vertebrae are visible ultrasonically, the effects of compression of the spinal cord by these structures is easy to evaluate (see below).

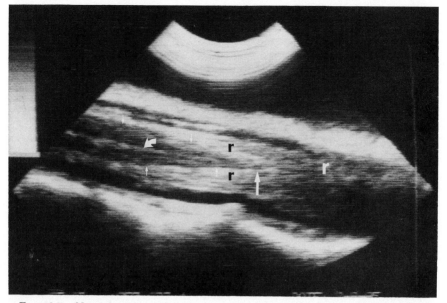

FIG. 13.5. Normal conus medullaris. Longitudinal scan showing the conus medullaris narrowing into the filum terminale. The boundary of the spinal cord (*small arrows*) and the site of origin of the filum (*large arrow*) are visible. Multiple nerve roots (*r*) can be seen surrounding the conus and extending into the cauda equina. The central canal is again demonstrated on this scan (*curved arrow*).

INTRAMEDULLARY TUMORS

Tumors

Intraoperative ultrasonography has been shown to be very useful in the localization and resection of intramedullary spinal cord tumors (1, 4, 10, 15). With the great advances in diagnostic imaging techniques for spinal cord tumors (*i.e.*, MRI) the neurosurgeon usually knows the position and extent of an abnormality before the operation begins. However, once the laminectomy has been performed and the dura mater or spinal cord has been exposed, the ability of ultrasonography to accurately characterize these lesions is of great utility. These masses have been universally more echogenic than the normal spinal cord (1, 4, 10, 15) (Fig. 13.6). They generally expand the cord while disrupting the normal intramedullary anatomy, in particular the central canal echo (26).

Further, intraoperative ultrasonography can, in many ways, display the intramedullary anatomy with greater clarity than even MRI. In particular, intramedullary cysts are imaged much better by ultrasonography than by any other method (Figs. 13.6 and 13.7) (4, 15, 19, 21). It

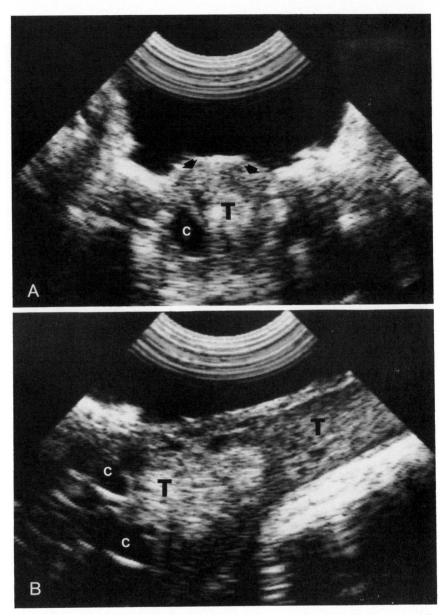

FIG. 13.6. (A) Malignant astrocytoma. Transverse sonogram through a markedly enlarged upper cervical spinal cord. The subarachnoid space has largely been obliterated by the tumor-filled spinal cord; however, there are points where there is contact between the cord and posterior dura mater (*arrows*). An echogenic nodule of tumor (*T*) located centrally in the spinal cord and a cyst (*c*) are also demonstrated. (B) Several areas of echogenic tumor (*T*) and cysts (*c*) are visible in the expanded, upper cervical spinal cord in this longitudinal scan. No cysts were seen on the preoperative CT scan. (From Rubin, J. M., and Dohrmann, G. J. Intraoperative sonography of the spine and spinal cord. Semin. Ultrasound CT MR, *6:* 48–67, 1985.)

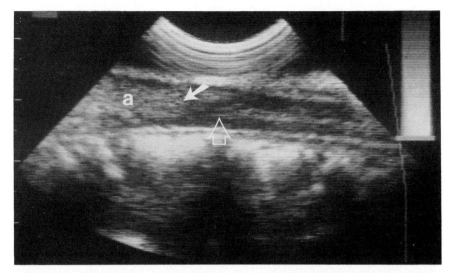

FIG. 13.7.   Intramedullary astrocytoma. Longitudinal scan showing the inferior portion of a diffuse echogenic astrocytoma (*a*) of the spinal cord. Notice that the inferior margin of the tumor (*arrow*) can be defined relative to the comparatively anechoic normal neural tissue and the appearance of the central canal (*hollow arrow*). This is probably a gross boundary, however, since microscopic tumor infiltration cannot be imaged ultrasonically.

is a generally accepted fact that ultrasonography is the technique of choice for evaluating cysts in the body (20), and this has also been the case in the spinal cord (4, 15, 19). Sonography exquisitely images the internal structure of cysts, showing multiple septae and solid nodules along the walls. The surgeon can choose the most direct and safest approach for drainage, thus decreasing the trauma to the spinal cord.

Cysts associated with intramedullary tumors can occur cephalad to the mass, producing symptoms and signs suggesting syringomyelia (17). Besides draining the apparent syrinx (see below), the identification of the tumor is vital. Ultrasonography can accomplish this (Fig. 13.8).

As all neurosurgeons know, the recognition of cystic spaces within a lesion may be of great importance to the progress of an operation. The drainage of cysts in tumors can significantly decrease the mass effect of a lesion, and even if the entire mass cannot be removed, a patient's symptoms may be alleviated exclusively due to a cyst drainage. Further, by opening directly into a cyst, a neurosurgeon gains immediate access to the heart of a tumor, thus diminishing the difficulty of the dissection. Hence, the identification of cysts is definitely of more than academic interest. Yet, all of the present day diagnostic tests are flawed in their ability to demonstrate cysts. There have been many documented examples of false-positive intramedullary cysts on delayed metrizamide CT scans (Fig. 13.9) (19). In these cases, generally of myelomalacia of the

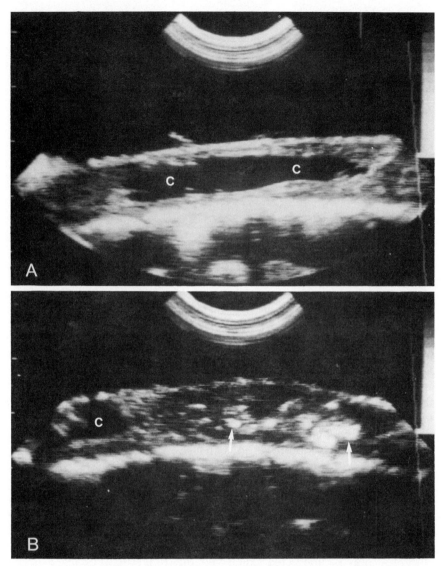

FIG. 13.8. Astrocytoma with central cyst, syrinx. (A) Longitudinal scan of thoracic spinal cord with centrally located cyst (c). (B) Inferior scan showing an echogenic intramedullary astrocytoma. Multiple calcifications are present; some of which have been labeled with *arrows*. Surprisingly, none of the calcifications shadowed. There is a portion of the cyst (c) seen cephalad to the tumor. (From Rubin, J. M, and Dohrmann, G. J. Intraoperative spinal ultrasonography. J. Belge Radiol.-Belg. Tijdschrift Voor Radiol., *69:* 9–27, 1986.)

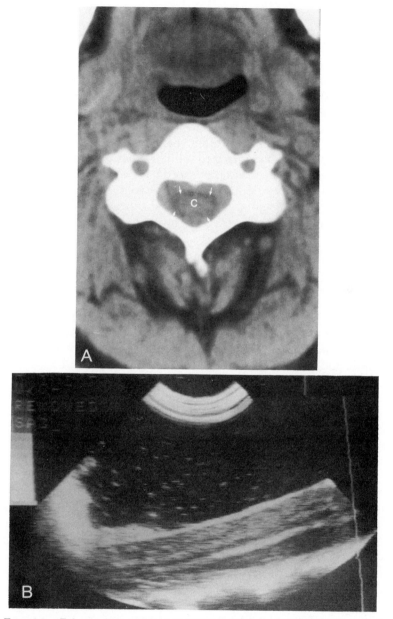

FIG. 13.9.   False-positive syrinx. (*A*) Uptake of metrizamide within the spinal cord (*c*) on a delayed CT scan. Based on this scan, it was presumed that there was an intramedullary cyst. The rim of lower density neural tissue (*arrows*) is present around the "fluid." (*B*) Intraoperative ultrasonogram demonstrating only uniformly echogenic spinal cord with no evidence of a cyst.

spinal cord, metrizamide was believed to have been taken up by small channels in the neural tissue itself. When scanned ultrasonically, no cysts were found. Hence, ultrasonography prevented precarious myelotomies and explorations for cysts. As for MRI, ultrasonography is again showing an increased sensitivity and specificity for cysts. Recent articles have demonstrated that the standard long T1 and long T2 times used to diagnose cysts on MRI only hold when there is a significant water component present (11, 21). Up to one-third of cysts, particularly those containing large quantities of protein, may not have these properties (11). Hence, *a priori* it is very hard to tell if a mass is really a cyst. Such examples of cystic tumors of the spinal cord have recently been described (Fig. 13.10) (21). Both cystic areas that appeared solid and solid areas that looked cystic were demonstrated. Finally, ultrasonography can show multiple cysts in a tumor whereas CT, myelography, or MRI may not show any (4, 15, 19, 21).

Syringomyelia

Ultrasonography has significantly altered the therapy and understanding of syringomyelia. It was generally thought that the cystic spaces within a syrinx were interconnected. Yet, ultrasonography has shown this not to be true (4). At the very least, there are often large numbers of septae dividing the main cavity (Fig. 13.11). In extreme cases, there may be multiple, discrete spaces that do not communicate. These spaces have to be drained individually in order to decompress the syrinx (Fig. 13.12). Besides characterizing the complex structure of these cavities before insertion of shunts, ultrasonography can be employed to confirm the effectiveness of the operative decompression once a drain has been implanted (Fig. 13.13).

Extramedullary Masses

Extramedullary tumors are usually easily visualized by ultrasound. As with intramedullary tumors, they are more echogenic than the spinal cord (Figs. 13.14 and 13.15). In particular, schwannomas, meningiomas, and metastases have all met this criterion. The classic observation with cervical and thoracic extramedullary tumors is an echogenic mass pushing the spinal cord to the side on transverse scans and either anteriorly or posteriorly on sagittal scans (Fig. 13.14). Besides its easily identifiable shape, the spinal cord can also be identified by the presence of the central canal echo in it. Although destroyed by intramedullary tumors, extramedullary masses usually spare this reflection (12, 26). Unfortunately, in cases of extramedullary masses causing severe spinal cord trauma or contusion, the central canal echo can be obliterated (12, 18, 26).

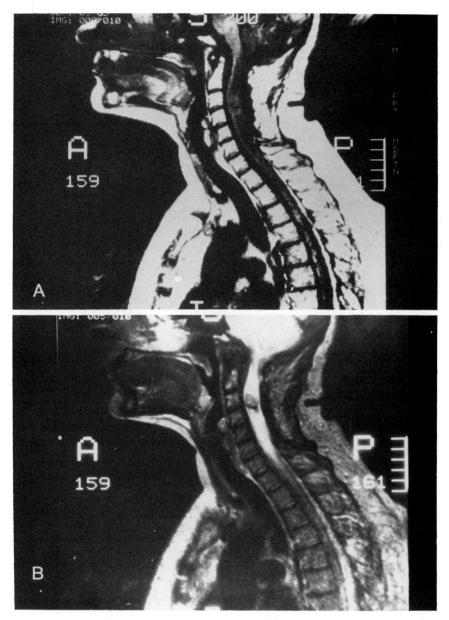

FIG. 13.10.   Erroneous cyst on MRI. 1.5-Tesla MRI scans and intraoperative ultrasound
scans demonstrating an expansile lesion of the cervical spinal cord which was prospectively
diagnosed as a large cystic collection with a solid, central nodule. (A) T1-weighted (TR,
400 msec; TE, 25 msec). (B) T2-weighted (TR, 2000 msec; TE, 25 msec). (C) TR, 2000.

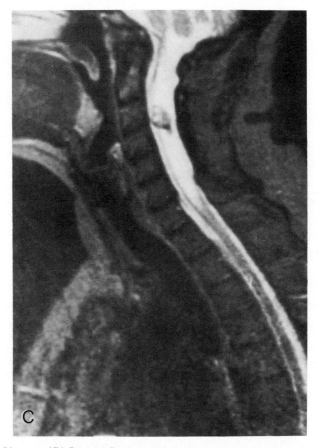

msec; TE, 50 msec. (*D*) Longitudinal intraoperative ultrasound scan showing a diffusely infiltrating, mainly solid lesion of the cervical spinal cord with a localized, septated cystic area (*arrows*) corresponding to the presumed "solid" nodule on MRI. (*E*) Transverse scan again demonstrating localized cystic area (*arrows*) on the left-hand side of the spinal cord. (From Rubin, J. M., Aisen, A. M., and DiPietro, M. A. Ambiguities in MR imaging of tumoral cysts in the spinal cord. J. Comput. Assist. Tomogr., *10:* 395–398, 1986.)

From the point of view of the neurosurgeon, ultrasonography can greatly facilitate operations on extramedullary tumors. Lesions located posteriorly are generally easy to find, although sonography will still determine the point on the dura mater closest to the lesion, thus facilitating the opening of the dura mater. However, the resection of anterior masses is much more difficult (3, 12). Often the neurosurgeon must retract the spinal cord in order to see these lesions. Spinal cord retraction is a dangerous technique, one which most neurosurgeons would rather not perform. With ultrasonography, anterior masses can easily be local-

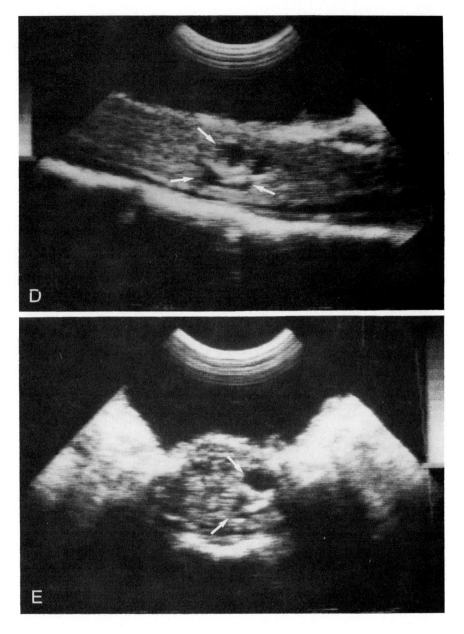

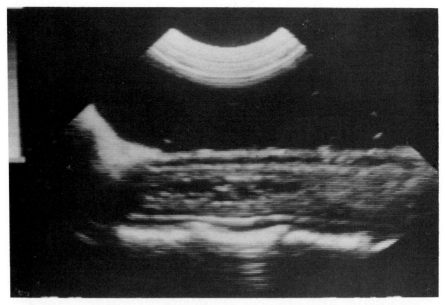

FIG. 13.11.   Syringomyelia. Multiple septations within a syrinx on sagittal scan.

ized and mapped without moving the spinal cord. Lastly, the surgeon can use sonography to image the operative field after resecting the mass to verify the completeness of the operation.

Other medullary masses are also easily identified with ultrasonography. Arachnoid cysts are just as readily visible as intramedullary cysts (Fig. 13.16) (19). These cysts appear as large anechoic spaces displacing the spinal cord. At times tumors can be found within these cysts (Fig. 13.16). Hematomas act as any other extramedullary mass by displacing the spinal cord (Fig. 13.17). They can look either echogenic or anechoic, depending on their age. The older the hematoma, the fewer echoes it contains (2, 5, 14). Abscesses can also be localized. At times, a fluid-filled center is visible as an anechoic area on the ultrasound scan, thus localizing the most likely site for drainage (Fig. 13.18). Along with the fluid-containing portions, more echogenic necrotic debris around the margins can also be seen. Finally, although ultrasound cannot image through bone, the posterior margins of the spine are visible. In a case of a vertebra destroyed by osteomyelitis with an abscess, the irregular destroyed bone caused an abrupt change in the curvature of the spine that was readily visible ultrasonographically (Fig. 13.19).

In a like fashion, it is easy to identify bulging discs or bony bars (Figs. 13.20 and 13.21). The point of compression of the disc or bar is readily visible by ultrasound even though the disc or bar cannot be seen in its

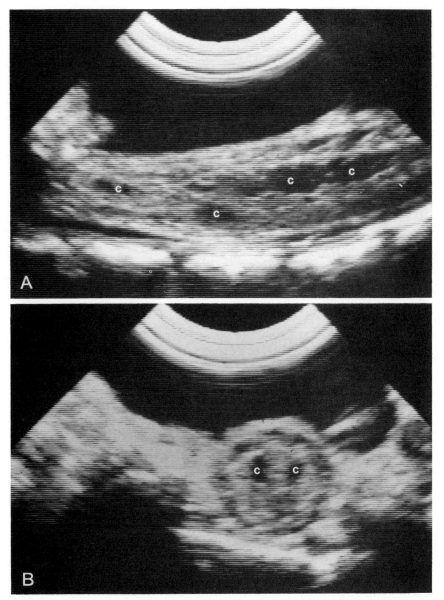

FIG. 13.12. Syringomyelia. (A) Longitudinal ultrasonogram demonstrating multiple
cystic spaces (c) in the spinal cord. (B) Two dorsal cystic areas (c) are shown in this
transverse slice. (C) An oblique scan demonstrating a small catheter (arrows) in a collapsed
dorsal cyst. Notice, however, that a ventral cyst (c) on the other side of the spinal cord has
not collapsed. This patient showed improvement on the right but not the left. (From
Dohrmann, G. J., and Rubin, J. M. Intraoperative ultrasound imaging of the spinal cord:
Syringomyelia, cysts, and tumors—a preliminary report. Surg. Neurol., 18: 395–399, 1982.)

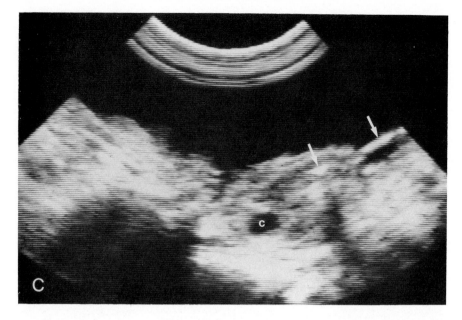

entirety. In many cases, it is possible to differentiate between the two by using their sound-transmitting properties. Sound is totally reflected by bone while only partially reflected by discs. Therefore, if there is through transmission, the mass is likely a disc (Fig. 13.20). Unfortunately, this maxim does not always hold true. Some discs are so attenuating that almost no sound penetrates them, making it difficult to distinguish these discs from bars. Despite these shortcomings, the neurosurgeon can still use sonography to evaluate the operative results. Whatever means is used to decompress the spinal cord or nerve roots, ultrasonography can be used to evaluate the effects of the decompressive procedure. Ultrasonography can often document the need for further decompression of nerve roots or the spinal cord even though they are grossly decompressed on visual inspection (18).

In trauma cases, bone fragments are detectable since they alter the path of either the spinal cord or nerve roots crossing over them (Fig. 13.22). Like bony bars, the highly reflective fragment causes posterior acoustic shadowing, a very characteristic appearance. Shadowing makes identification of individual fragments quite easy. A recent report by Quencer et al. (18) has confirmed the usefulness of ultrasonography in these cases. In 45% of the cases in which ultrasonography was used to document the straightening of gibbuses in thoracic or lumbar fractures

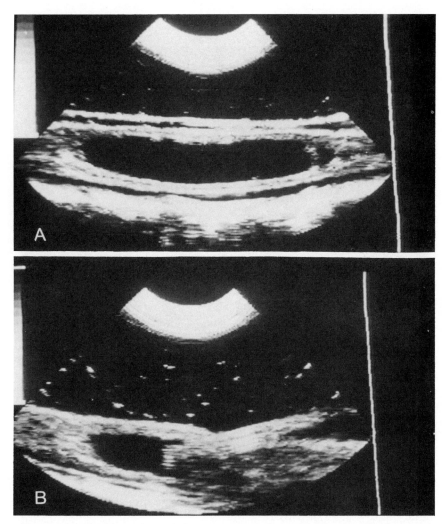

FIG. 13.13.   Syringomyelia. (*a*) Large syrinx on longitudinal scan. (*b*) Shunt tube entering the syrinx posteriorly. (*c*) Slightly later scan showing the shunt tube extending through the entire length of the cavity. (From Rubin, J. M, and Dohrmann, G. J. Intraoperative spinal ultrasonography J. Belge Radiol.-Belg. Tijdschrift Voor Radiol., *69:* 9–27, 1986.)

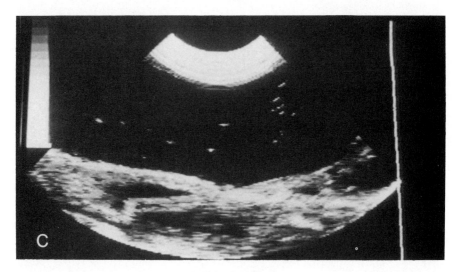

FIG. 13.13C

with Harrington rods or impaction of fragments, the initial procedure was inadequate, *i.e.*, there was residual compression of the spinal cord or nerve roots. Another corrective procedure was necessary to correct the neural impingement. Without ultrasonography, such information could not have been obtained in the operating room. It would have, therefore, required another postoperative diagnostic procedure and possibly reoperation.

Bullet fragments produce shadows as well, but the appearance of the shadow is very different and quite characteristic (28). Rather than completely scattering or absorbing the ultrasound energy that hits it, the sound causes the metal to ring like a bell. This ringing sends multiple echoes back to the transducer. The ultrasound scanner places each echo behind the reflecting object generating a series of bright lines like a "comet tail" (28). This appearance is virtually diagnostic of metal and can be very helpful in locating metallic fragments (Fig. 13.23).

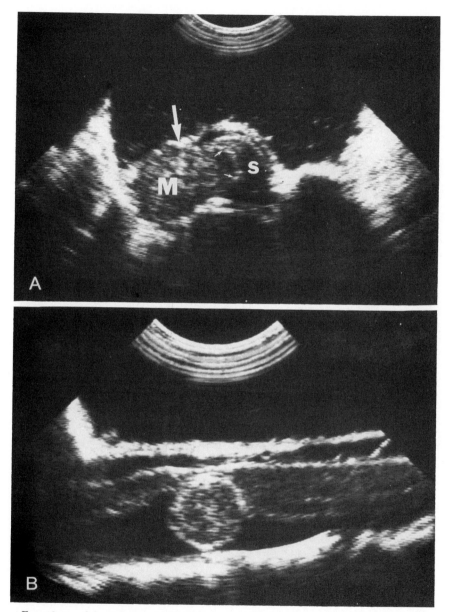

FIG. 13.14.   Schwannoma. (a) Transverse scan showing an intradural, extramedullary mass (M) displacing the spinal cord (s) laterally. The boundary between the cord and mass is well depicted (*small arrows*). Also, the dural reflection of the mass is identified (*large arrow*). (b) Longitudinal sonogram showing the tumor displacing the spinal cord. (From Rubin, J. M., and Dohrmann, G. J. Intraoperative ultrasonography of the spine. Radiology, *146:* 173–175, 1985.)

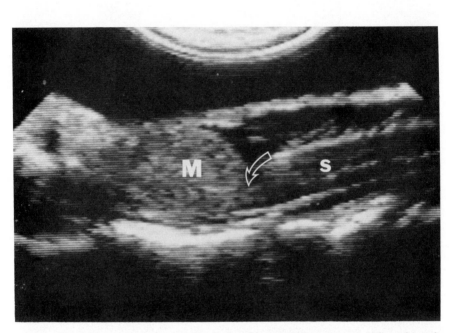

FIG. 13.15. Meningioma. Longitudinal scan showing the tumor mass (*M*) pushing the spinal cord (*s*) anteriorly. The point of compression is easily identified (*arrow*). (From Rubin, J. M., and Dohrmann, G. J., Intraoperative ultrasonography of the spine. Radiology, *146*: 173–175, 1983.)

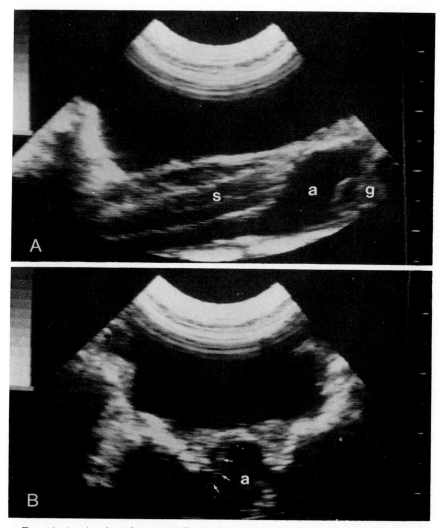

FIG. 13.16.   Arachnoid cyst. (A) Sagittal scan showing the spinal cord (s) with a large
cyst (a) caudal to it. Most of the spinal cord has been pushed out of the slice by the cyst.
A ganglioneuroma (g) was discovered within the cyst. (B) Transverse sonogram showing
the arachnoid cyst (a) displacing the spinal cord laterally. The cyst-spinal cord boundary
is seen (arrows). (From Rubin, J. M., and Dohrmann, G. J. Intraoperative sonography of
the spine and spinal cord. Semin. Ultrasound CT MR, 6: 48–67, 1985.)

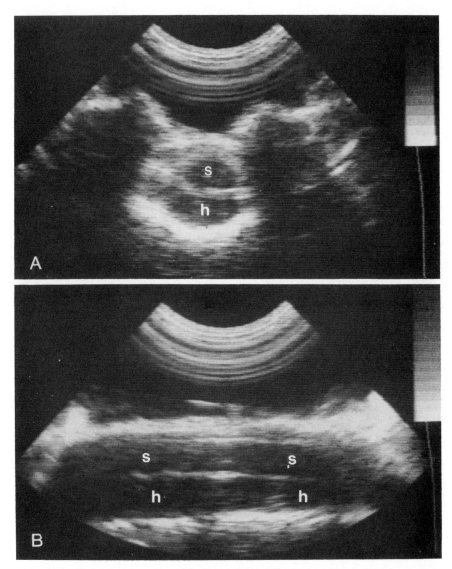

FIG. 13.17. Chronic hematoma. (A) Relatively anechoic mass (h) ventral to the spinal cord (s) on this transverse scan. (B) Longitudinal scan demonstrating that the hematoma (h) extends the entire length of the laminectomy. The spinal cord (s) is pushed posteriorly. (From Rubin, J. M., and Dohrmann, G. J. Intraoperative sonography of the spine and spinal cord. Semin. Ultrasound CT MR, 6: 48–67, 1985.)

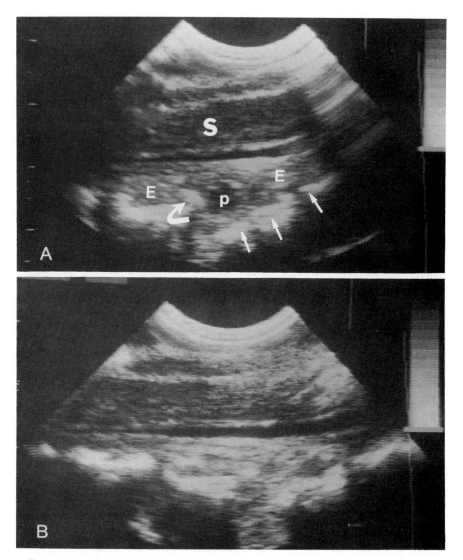

FIG. 13.18.   Epidural abscess. (A) Longitudinal scan showing an epidural mass (E) anterior to the spinal cord (s). A localized anechoic area (p) which was a collection of pus is seen within the mass. Several bone fragments (arrows) due to a vertebral body fracture with devitalized bone are seen. A fragment is seen within the mass itself (curved arrow). The patient had osteomyelitis. (B) Postdrainage scan demonstrating that the pus collection is gone. Staphylococcus aureus was cultured out in this intravenous drug abuser.

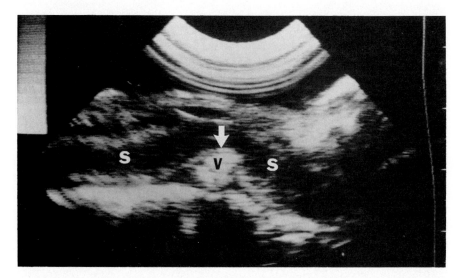

FIG. 13.19. Collapsed vertebral body. Longitudinal scan in a young female with tuberculosis. A collapsed vertebral body (*v*) has protruded posteriorly and is compressing the spinal cord (*s*) at a well-defined point (*arrow*). Some sound has penetrated this collapsed bone for unknown reasons, possibly due to its devitalized nature and lack of calcified matrix. After the placement of Harrington rods, repeat ultrasonography demonstrated that the compression had not been relieved. (From Rubin, J. M., and Dohrmann, G. J. Intraoperative sonography of the spine and spinal cord. Semin. Ultrasound CT MR, *6:* 48–67, 1985.)

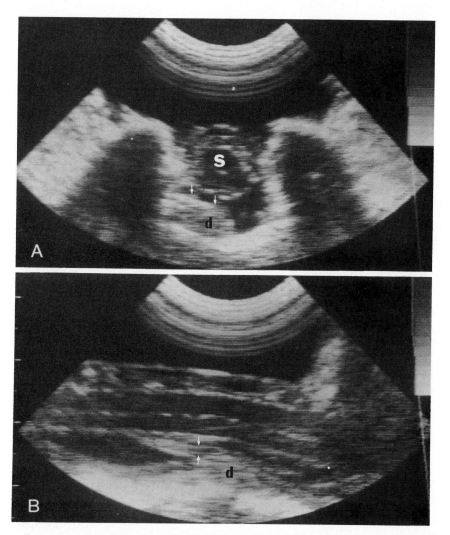

FIG. 13.20.   Protruding disc. (A) Thoracic disc fragment (d) displacing the spinal cord
(s) from anteriorly and laterally. Nerve roots (arrows) are draped over the disc as well.
Notice that sound is able to penetrate the disc. (B) Longitudinal scan of the disc (d)
trapping a nerve root (arrows). (C) Postresection transverse scan showing removal of the
compressing disc fragment. The nerve roots (arrows) are now no longer compressed, and
the spinal cord has rotated back to its normal position. (From Rubin, J. M., and Dohrmann,
G. J. Intraoperative sonography of the spine and spinal cord. Semin. Ultrasound CT MR,
6: 48–67, 1985.)

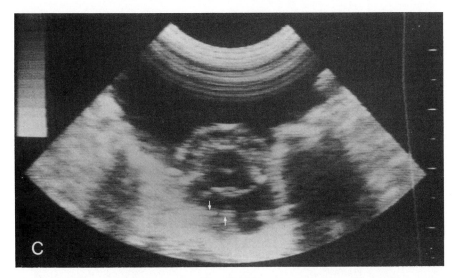

Fig. 13.20C

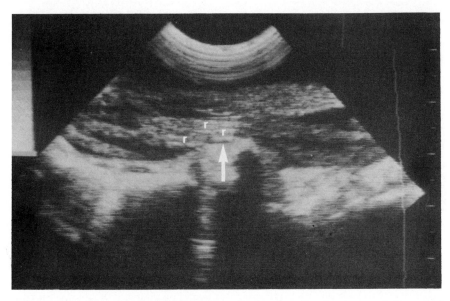

Fig. 13.21. Bony bar. Longitudinal scan showing the site of entrapment (*arrow*) of several nerve roots (*r*) of the cauda equina by a bony bar. As compared to disc fragments (see above), no sound passes through the bone.

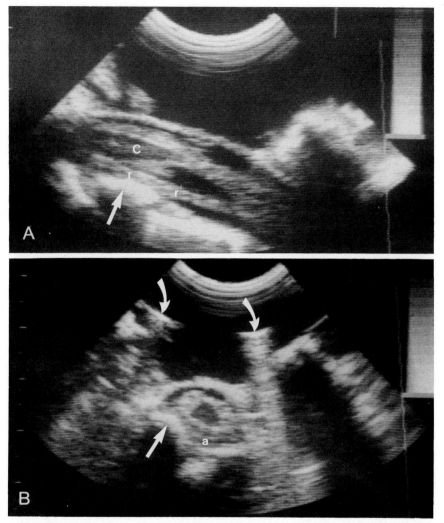

FIG. 13.22.   Bony compression due to trauma. (A) Longitudinal scan showing posterior displacement of the conus medullaris (c) and a directly compressed nerve root (r) by a collapsed vertebral body (arrow). Note the abrupt change in the smooth curvature produced by the posteriorly displaced bone. Even though the bone is not seen in its entirety, the effect on the neural elements is obvious. (B) Transverse scan performed after instillation of Harrington rods (curved arrows) shows that some of the compression has been relieved on the left side with the appearance of subarachnoid space (a) between the spinal cord and vertebral body. However, there was continued compression on the right from a bone fragment (arrow). (C) Longitudinal scan along the right side of the neural canal after rods had been placed showing a site of continued compression of nerve roots (arrow) anterior to the conus medullaris (c). This area corresponded to the site of compression shown in the transverse scan above.

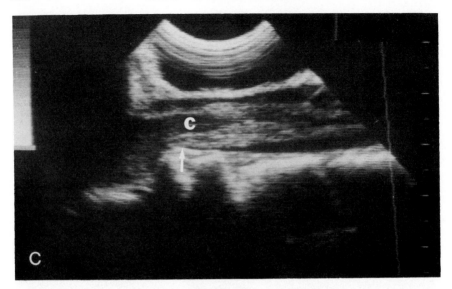

FIG. 13.22C

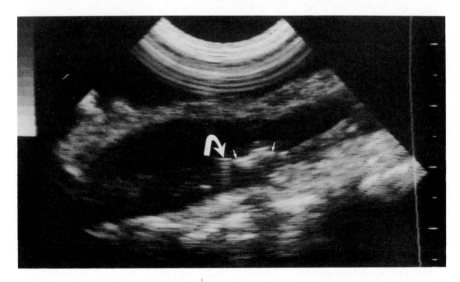

FIG. 13.23. Bone and bullet fragments. Scan through the cauda equina in a young male after a gunshot wound to the back. An echogenic bone fragment (*small arrows*) was localized among the roots of the cauda. Cephalad to the bone fragment, a small bullet fragment (*curved arrow*) with a characteristic "comet-tail" artifact is seen. (From Rubin, J. M., and Dohrmann, G. J. The spine and spinal cord during neurosurgical operations: real-time ultrasonography. Radiology, *155:* 197–200, 1985.)

REFERENCES

1. Braun, I. F., Raghavendra, B. W., and Kricheff, I. I. Spinal cord imaging using real-time high resolution ultrasound. Radiology, *147:* 459–465, 1983.
2. Coelho, J. C. W., Sigel, B., Ryva, J. C., *et al.* B-mode sonography of blood clots. J. Clin. Ultrasound, *10:* 323–327, 1982.
3. Connolly, E. S. Spinal cord tumors in adults. In: *Neurological Surgery,* edited by J. R. Youmans, pp. 3211–3212. Philadelphia, Saunders, 1982.
4. Dohrmann, G. J., and Rubin, J. M. Intraoperative ultrasound imaging of the spinal cord: Syringomyelia, cysts, and tumors—a preliminary report. Surg. Neurol., *18:* 395–399, 1982.
5. Enzmann, D. R., Britt, R. H., Lyons, B. E., *et al.* Natural history of experimental intracerebral hemorrhage: Sonography, computed tomography and neuropathology. A.J.N.R., *2:* 517–526, 1981.
6. Gonsalves, C. G., Hudson, A. R., Horsey, W. J., *et al.* Computed tomography of the cervical spine and spinal cord. Comput. Tomogr., *2:* 279–283, 1978.
7. Hammerschlag, S. B., Wolpert, S. M., and Carter, B. L. Computed tomography of the spinal cord. Radiology, *121:* 361–367, 1976.
8. Haughton, V. M., Syvertsen, A., and Williams, A. L. Soft tissue anatomy within the spinal canal as seen on computed tomography. Radiology, *134:* 649–655, 1980.
9. Huk, W., Heindel, W., Deimling, M., *et al.* Nuclear magnetic resonance (NMR) tomography of the central nervous system: Comparison of two imaging sequences. J. Comput. Assist. Tomogr., *7:* 468–475, 1983.
10. Hutchins, W. W., Vogelzang, R. L., Neiman, H. L., *et al.* Differentiation of tumor from syringohydromyelia: Intraoperative neurosonography of the spinal cord. Radiology, *151:* 171–174, 1984.
11. Kjos, B. O., Brant-Zawadzki, M., and Kucharczyk, W. Cystic intracranial lesions: Magnetic resonance imaging. Radiology, *155:* 363–369, 1985.
12. Knake, J. E., Gabrielsen, T. O., Chandler, W. F., *et al.* Real time sonography during spinal surgery. Radiology, *151:* 461–465, 1984.
13. Lee, B. C. P., Kazam, E., and Newman, A. D. Computed tomography of the spine and spinal cord. Radiology, *128:* 95–102, 1978.
14. Lillehei, K. O., Chandler, W. F., and Knake, J. E. Real-time ultrasound characteristics of the acute intracerebral hemorrhage as studied in the canine model. Neurosurgery, *14:* 48–51, 1984.
15. Machi, J., Sigel, B., Jafar, J. J., *et al.* Criteria for using imaging ultrasound during brain and spinal cord surgery. J. Ultrasound. Med., *3:* 155–161, 1984.
16. Modic, M. T., Weinstein, M. A., Pavlicek, W., *et al.* Nuclear magnetic resonance imaging of the spine. Radiology, *148:* 757–762, 1983.
17. Poser, C. M. The relationship between syringomyelia and neoplasm. In: *American Lecture Series No. 262, American Lectures in Neurology.* Springfield, Ill., Charles C Thomas, 1956.
18. Quencer, R. M., Montalvo, B. M., Eismont, F. J., and Green, B. A. Intraoperative spinal sonography in thoracic and lumbar fractures: Evaluation of Harrington rod instrumentation. A.J.R., *145:* 343–349, 1985.
19. Quencer, R. M., Morse, B. M. M., Green, B. A., *et al.* Intraoperative spinal sonography: Adjunct to metrizamide CT in the assessment and surgical decompression of post-traumatic spinal cord cysts. A.J.R., *142:* 593–601, 1984.
20. Rosenfield, A. T., Taylor, K. J. W., and Jaffe, C. C. Clinical applications of ultrasound tissue characterization. Radiol. Clin. North Am., *18:* 31–58, 1980.
21. Rubin, J. M., Aisen, A. M., and DiPietro, M. A. Ambiguities in MR imaging of tumoral

cysts in the spinal cord. J. Comput. Assist. Tomogr., *10:* 395–398, 1986.

22. Rubin, J. M., and Dohrmann, G. J. Intraoperative ultrasonography of the spine. Radiology, *146:* 173–175, 1983.

23. Rubin, J. M., and Dohrmann, G. J. Intraoperative sonography of the spine and spinal cord. Semin. Ultrasound CT MR, *6:* 48–67, 1985.

24. Rubin, J. M., and Dohrmann, G. J. The spine and spinal cord during neurosurgical operations: Real-time ultrasonography. Radiology, *155:* 197–200, 1985.

25. Rubin, J. M., and Dohrmann, G. J. Intraoperative spinal ultrasonography. J. Belge Radiol. Belg. Tijdschrift Voor Radiol., *69:* 9–27, 1986.

26. St. Amour, T. E., Rubin, J. M., and Dohrmann, G. J. Ultrasonic identification of the central canal of the spinal cord. Radiology, *152:* 767–769, 1984.

27. Taylor, A. J., Haughton, V. M., and Doust, B. D. CT imaging of the thoracic spinal cord without intrathecal contrast medium. J. Comput. Assist. Tomogr., *4:* 223–224, 1980.

28. Wendell, B. A., and Athey, P. A. Ultrasonic appearance of metallic foreign bodies in parenchymal organs. J. Clin. Ultrasound, *9:* 133–135, 1981.

29. Young, I. R., Bailes, D. R., Burle, M., *et al.* Initial clinical evaluation of a whole body nuclear magnetic resonance (NMR) tomograph. J. Comput. Assist. Tomogr., *6:* 1–18, 1982.

CHAPTER

14

What Constitutes Spinal Instability?

MANOHAR M. PANJABI, PH.D., D. TECH.,
LEE L. THIBODEAU, M.D., JOSEPH J. CRISCO, III, M.S., and
AUGUSTUS A. WHITE, III, M.D., D. MED. SCI.

The biomechanical and clinical aspects of spinal instability have been recently reviewed (32, 33, 44, 47, 48), but clinical spinal instability remains a relative term that can be ambiguous, imprecise, and confusing. An accepted working definition of clinical instability is "the loss of the ability of the spine under physiological loads to maintain relationships between vertebrae in such a way that there is neither damage nor subsequent irritation to the spinal cord or nerve roots, and, in addition, there is no development of incapacitating deformity or pain due to structural changes" (45). In this definition, physiological loads refer to stresses incurred by the spine during normal activity for a given patient; an incapacitating deformity is one that the patient finds intolerable; and incapacitating pain is defined as pain intractable to nonnarcotic medication. The neurosurgeon is frequently confronted with the question of spinal instability arising from trauma, surgical procedures, tumors, or some other pathological condition of the spine. In some cases the diagnosis is obvious. However, a precise clinically proven diagnostic method is not available to identify definitively the less apparent cases.

The goals of this report are threefold: (*a*) to present a brief review of basic spinal biomechanics; (*b*) to describe the evolution of a proposed systematic approach for the diagnosis of clinical instability in the lower cervical, thoracic, and thoracolumbar spines; and (*c*) to discuss how a systematic application of clinical and biomechanical information can help the physician evaluate clinical instability in the cervical, thoracic, and thoracolumbar regions.

BIOMECHANICAL CONCEPTS

Kinematics is the study of motion irrespective of the forces involved and, more specifically, spinal kinematics is the study of spine motion without directly considering the associated muscular and ligamentous forces. Several terms inherent to spinal kinematics will be briefly discussed.

Translation. An object undergoes pure translation when the paths of all points located on the object are parallel to one another.

Rotation. A motion contains a rotation when points located on the object do not move in parallel paths.

Displacement. Displacements quantify the motion of an object from one position to another. Displacements may be in the form of a translation, a rotation, or any combination of the two.

Degrees of Freedom. Degrees of freedom are the number of independent displacements of an object. An object constrained to motion in one plane has three degrees of freedom: two translations and one rotation. Objects in 3-dimensional space have six degrees of freedom: three translations and three rotations. To completely define the motion of the cervical spine in space requires the determination of 42 independent displacements (*i.e.*, seven vertebrae, each with 6° of freedom).

Functional Spinal Unit (FSU). The functional spinal unit is the smallest unit of the spine that still exhibits the biomechanical characteristics of the spine. It is composed of two adjacent vertebral bodies and the intervening ligamentous structures. The upper vertebral body of the FSU has six degrees of freedom with respect to the lower vertebral body (*i.e.*, translations in the anterior-posterior, inferior-superior, and lateral directions; and rotations in the flexion-extension, lateral bending, and axial directions). An orthogonal coordinate system can be used to visualize displacements. A coordinate system is shown in Figure 14.1; the origin is at the geometric center of the vertebral body, and the axes are oriented in the anatomical planes.

Coupled Motion. Coupled motion refers to the behavior of the spine to move in translations or rotations independent of the induced motions. The movements of a screw provide an example of coupled motion. A screw is tightened or loosened by rotation, which results in the translation of the screw in or out of the threaded hole. The translation of the screw is said to be coupled to its rotation through the geometry of the threads.

BASIC BIOMECHANICS OF THE SPINE AND SPINAL COMPONENTS

An in-depth discussion of the basic biomechanical characteristics of the spine and its components has recently been published (46). Under physiological loads, the motions of the FSU are governed by the anatomy and mechanical properties of the osseous and ligamentous structures. The difference between two extreme physiological positions is referred to as the range of motion. The ranges of motion for the three primary rotations have been determined for all regions of the spine and are shown in Figure 14.2 (45). In the cervical spine flexion-extension is evenly distributed; however, axial rotation and lateral bending are not. A signif-

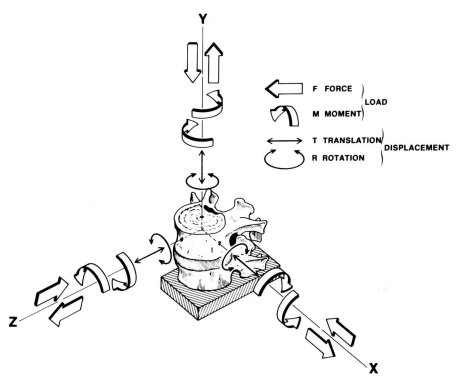

FIG. 14.1. A 3-dimensional coordinate system is used to document the complete mechanical behavior of the functional spinal unit. Six forces along the axes and six moments about the axes of the coordinate system are shown with the three translations and three rotations. (From White, A. A., and Panjabi, M. M. *Clinical Biomechanics of the Spine.* Lippincott, New York, 1978.)

icant amount of axial rotation occurs between C1 and C2, while virtually none occurs between the occiput and C1. Essentially no lateral bending takes place at C1-C2. In the thoracic spine, lateral bending is evenly distributed, while there is more axial rotation in the upper thoracic and more flexion-extension in the lower thoracic regions. This is consistent with the thoracic spine acting as a transition zone between the cervical and the lumbar regions. The limits of physiological translations will be discussed below.

Many of the motions of the spine are coupled through the anatomy of the facet joints, discs, and ligaments. In the upper cervical spine there is a coupling between axial rotation and axial translation. In the lower cervical spine lateral bending to the right will result in an axial rotation of the vertebrae to the left (Fig. 14.3). The lumbar spine also exhibits a

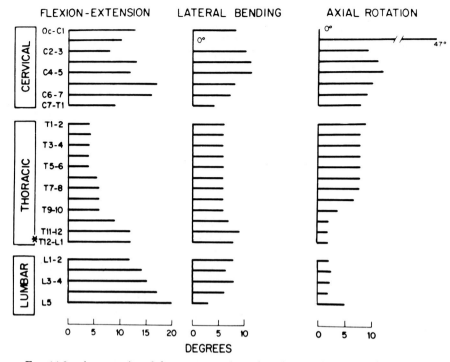

FIG. 14.2.   A composite of the representative values for rotation at the different levels
of the spine in the traditional planes of motion. It is designed to allow a ready comparison
of the motions in the various regions of the spine, as well as of the different types of
movements in each region. (From White, A. A., III, and Panjabi, M. M. The basic kinematics
of the human spine: A review of past and current knowledge. Spine, *3:* 12–20, 1978.)

coupling between lateral bending and axial rotation. However, the pattern
is opposite to that of the cervical spine such that bending to the right
results in axial rotation of the vertebrae to the right (Fig. 14.3). The
upper thoracic region is similar to the cervical region in its coupling
behavior, and the lower thoracic region is similar to the lumbar region.
The midthoracic spine has an inconsistent coupling behavior.

The intervertebral disc is relatively resistant to failure in axial
compression. Although the mode of failure may vary, failure under a
compressive load usually occurs first in the osseous structures for both
the normal and degenerative discs (9). In the spine with a normal disc,
failure occurs in the central portion of the end plate. However, in the
spine with a degenerative disc, failure usually initiates in the cortical
walls of the vertebral body or in the peripheral region of the end plate

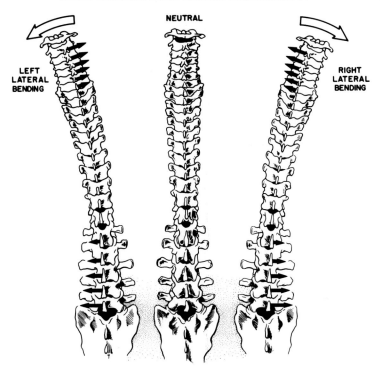

FIG. 14.3. The coupling patterns of the spine change from the cervical to the lumbar regions. In the cervical spine, axial rotation to the left is coupled to lateral bending to the right. In the lumbar spine axial rotation to the right is coupled to lateral bending to the right. The patterns in the thoracic regions are inconsistent. (From Panjabi, M. M., Pelker, R. R., and White, A. A. Biomechanics of the spine. In: *Neurosurgery*, edited by R. Wilkins and S. Rengachary, Chap. 284, pp. 2219–2228. McGraw-Hill, New York, 1985).

(25). Tests have shown that the annular portions of the disc, and not the osseous structures, fail first in axial torsion (14).

The ligamentous structures of the spine must permit physiological motion and prevent neurologically damaging motion by maintaining the spatial integrity of the vertebrae. An example of how these functions are performed is provided by the ligamentum flavum. It has been shown that there is a 10% decrease in the length of the ligamentum flavum in extension (29). However, it does not buckle into the canal when the spine is placed in extension because it is under 15% of pretension in its neutral position. In full flexion the ligament elongates by 35%. The representative stress-strain curve (Fig. 14.4) shows that the ligament is relatively flexible within the physiological range. Beyond this range (50% strain in

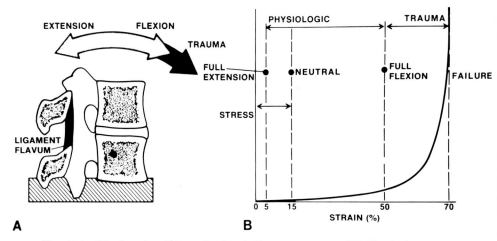

FIG. 14.4.   The functional biomechanics of a ligament are exemplified by the ligamentum flavum undergoing spine motion. (*A*) In flexion it is stretched, and in extension it contracts. In hyperflexion it may be stretched beyond its elastic limit to failure. (*B*) A stress-strain curve of deformation of the ligamentum flavum. (Based upon data from Nachemson, A. L., and Evans, J. H. Some mechanical properties of the third lumbar interlaminar ligament (ligamentum flavum). *J. Biomech., 1:* 211–220, 1968.)

the case of the ligamentum flavum) the ligament becomes very stiff and restricts further motion of the spine.

The anatomy of each vertebra reflects an optimum balance between the load it must withstand and the motion it must perform. This bio-mechanical adaptation accounts for the increasing size of the vertebral bodies and the changing orientation and shape of the facet articulations from the cervical to the lumbar region. The cervical vertebrae can carry a static load of 1500 newtons (350 lbs of force), and lumbar vertebrae can withstand a load of 8000 newtons (1800 lbs of force) before failure. Much higher loads are supported in dynamic loading situations, such as the sudden impact of trauma, due to the viscoelastic properties of bone.

The load that each vertebral body must bear is carried partly by the cancellous core and partly by the cortical shell. In a person under the age of 40, the cancellous bone carries 55% of the load and the cortical bone 45% (29). In someone over the age of 40, the proportions are reversed, and the cancellous bone carries only 35%, while the cortical bone carries 65% of the load. This decrease in strength of the cancellous bone with age may be attributed to a relative loss of osseous tissue. A relatively small loss of osseous tissue (*i.e.*, 25%) can produce a large decrease in bony strength (approximately 50%) (6).

The cancellous bone has other interesting properties. In tests on blocks of cancellous bone subjected to compressive loads, three patterns of failure were found (26). After the initial mechanical failure, the vertebral strength either diminished (type I), stayed the same (type II), or increased (type III). It was found that 87% of the experimental fractures were of types II or III and that there was a higher percentage of males than females in these two groups.

While most of the load on the spine is borne by the vertebral body, 18% of a compressive load (28) and 45% of a torsional load are carried by the facet joints (14). The amount of stability provided by the facet articulations depends on their shape, orientation, and level within the spine.

DEVELOPMENT OF A SYSTEMATIC APPROACH TO DIAGNOSIS OF SPINAL INSTABILITY

While spinal deformities and their potential for causing neurological and musculoskeletal dysfunction have been recognized since antiquity, modern concepts of spinal instability have evolved since the advent of clinical roentgenography. The greatest contribution to our understanding of clinical instability has come from clinical studies which have identified various patterns of spinal injury in terms of their radiographic appearance, mechanism of injury, association with acute neurological deficits, and proclivity for subsequent deformity and/or neurological damage. Additional insight has been provided by *in vitro* biomechanical studies which have defined the functional characteristics of the spine. In this section we describe the evolution of our understanding of spinal instability and how this has led to the development of a systematic approach to the diagnosis of clinical instability.

In 1949, Nicoll published a series of 166 fractures and fracture-dislocations of the thoracic and lumbar spine and suggested that the injuries be divided into stable and unstable groups (30). Stable injuries were those with no danger of increasing deformity or spinal cord damage. The unstable group consisted of those likely to have progressive deformity and cord damage.

Holdsworth elaborated upon Nicoll's classification and proposed a classification of stable and unstable injuries applicable to the entire spine (20). He emphasized the importance of the posterior ligamentous complex in determining stability and stressed the diagnostic value of physical examination and radiography. "Diagnosis is easy if it is appreciated firstly that stability of the injury depends upon whether or not the posterior ligament complex remains intact, and secondly that each type of fracture and fracture-dislocation has a characteristic radiographic appearance ... To recapitulate: fractures, dislocations, and fracture-dislocation of the whole spine can be divided into stable and unstable types. The diagnosis of each type of fracture by clinical examination and by radiography is simple (20)."

Holdsworth (19), Whitesides (50), Bradford (7), and others based their classifications and concepts of spine stability on a 2-column structure (the anterior weight-bearing column resisting compression and the posterior column resisting tension). Based on information from computed tomographic (CT) scans and biomechanical studies, Dennis (12) expanded the two-column concept into the three-column concept of spinal instability. The posterior column was essentially the same as that described by Holdsworth and consisted of the posterior bony arch and the posterior ligamentous complex (supraspinous and interspinous ligaments, facet capsules, and ligamentum flavum). The middle column was defined as the posterior longitudinal ligament, the posterior portion of the annulus fibrosus, and the posterior vertebral body wall. The anterior column was considered to be the anterior longitudinal ligament, the anterior portion of the annulus fibrosus, and the anterior aspect of the vertebral body. The middle column was added because "subluxation, dislocation, and simple instability appear only when the posterior longitudinal ligament and part of the disc are torn in conjunction with the posterior or the anterior ligamentous complex" (12).

Initial biomechanical research focused on either the intact FSU or individual spinal components. Over the past decade, more clinically relevant biomechanical studies have been done on the lower cervical (C2-C7), thoracic, lumbar, and lumbosacral spines (31, 34, 37, 44). Although the experimental paradigm was similar for each region, the methods used to interpret the data from the lumbar and lumbosacral studies differed significantly from those used for the cervical and thoracic spines. Because of this inconsistency, the results of the lumbar and lumbosacral studies will not be discussed.

An understanding of the basic experimental design is crucial to the interpretation of the results and their application to the clinical situation. FSUs were obtained from fresh autopsy material, and the experiments were carried out in high humidity chambers. The lower vertebra was fixed while the upper vertebra was subjected to the experimental loads. The mid-disc plane was orientated in the horizontal plane to negate spinal variations and achieve reproducibility. After applying loads simulating flexion and extension, the motions of the upper vertebral body were measured.

The protocol for each study consisted of two parts. The first involved applying maximum physiological flexion and extension loads to intact

FSUs to determine the upper limits of physiological motion. The maximum physiological loads used were 25 and 43% of body weight in the cervical and thoracic regions, respectively. A physiological load is well within the elastic limits of the anatomical structures. After the application of a load, a minimum of 3 minutes was allowed prior to recording the motion of the FSU in order to allow for creep (additional displacement over time). The maximum displacements for the intact FSUs were considered to represent the upper limits of physiological motion and are given in Table 14.1.

The second part of the experiment consisted of loading the FSUs in flexion and extension with the maximum physiological load and sequentially transecting the anatomical elements until failure occurred. The sequence of transections is given in Figure 14.5. For extension the components were cut from anterior to posterior (*i.e.*, from the top of Fig. 14.5 down). In flexion the order of transection was from posterior to anterior (*i.e.*, from the bottom of Fig. 14.5 up). The anterior elements are defined as the posterior longitudinal ligament and all elements in front of it. The posterior elements consist of all structures behind the posterior longitudinal ligament. The failure of the FSUs was defined as either complete separation, 45° of rotation, or 10 mm of horizontal displacement of the upper vertebra with respect to the lower vertebra. The last element transected prior to failure is defined as the failure element. The *bars* in Figure 14.5 originate at the intact state, show the path of each transection, and terminate at the respective failure element. It is interesting to note that the posterior longitudinal ligament is a failure element in both the cervical and thoracic regions. The motion prior to failure is defined as the motion recorded prior to transection of the failure element.

The values for the upper limits of physiological motion in the intact FSUs and the motion prior to failure of the transected FSUs for the cervical and thoracic regions are shown in Figure 14.6*A–C*. In Figure 14.6*A*, the horizontal displacements (in mm) have been adjusted for the 30% magnification factor of a standard radiograph. The displacements

TABLE 14.1

Upper Limits of Physiological Displacements Including 30% X-ray Magnification for Translations (in mm)

Relative Sagittal Plane Motions	Cervical	Thoracic
Translation		
in mm	>3.5	>2.5
in percent of vertebral body diameter	>20	>10
Rotation		
in degrees	>11	>5

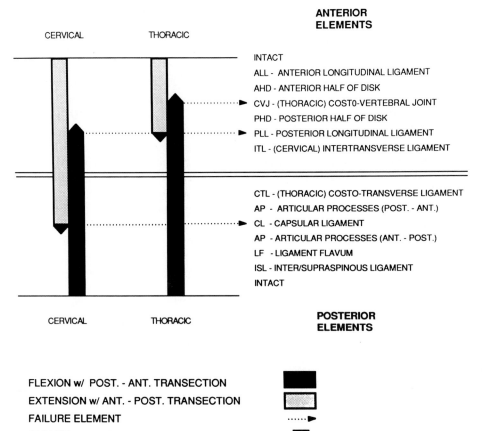

FIG. 14.5. Results of the biomechanical experiments. The elements which produced failure and the transection sequences for the functional spinal units are shown for flexion loading with posterior to anterior cutting and for extension loading with anterior to posterior cutting.

are presented in Figure 14.6*B* as percentages of the anterior-posterior vertebral body diameter. The results of rotation are given in Figure 14.6*C*. Displacements, measured in percentage of vertebral body diameter and degrees, are unaffected by radiographic magnification. It is extremely important to note the overlap between the intact and the prior to failure data shown in Figures 14.6*A–C*. In the cervical spine, for example, 65% of intact and 34% of prior to failure FSUs have horizontal displacements between 10 and 22% of the vertebral body diameter. Due to this overlap, it is not possible to select a displacement value that separates the intact spines from the prior to failure spines. Therefore, in the clinical situation,

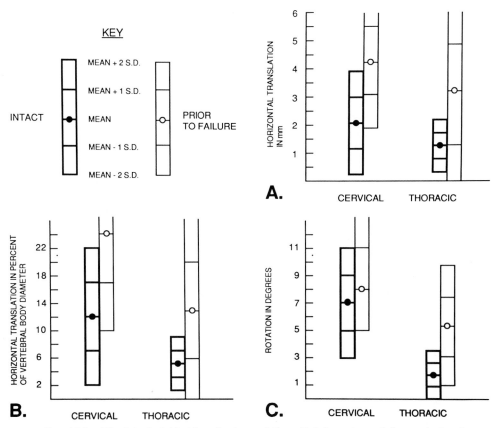

FIG. 14.6.   Physiological (dark) and prior to failure (light) motions of the cervical and thoracic spines are depicted. Shown are the means and SDs (±1 and ±2). (A) Horizontal translations in mm. (B) Horizontal translations in percentage of lateral vertebral diameters. (C) Rotation in degrees.

values of relative displacement cannot definitively differentiate between stable and unstable spines.

Although these biomechanical studies provide important information about the mechanical characteristics of the spine, it is difficult to apply them directly to the clinical situation. The most obvious limitation is that they are *in vitro* studies. It is also important to note that the experiments were performed on FSUs, not complete spines, and only in flexion and extension. An experimental approach to evaluate the contributions of muscle on spinal stability has not yet been developed; thus the effects of musculature were neglected in these studies. Given these limitations and the overlap of the data, additional factors must be considered in the evaluation of clinical spinal instability.

THE CHECKLISTS

Based on what has been learned from clinical and *in vitro* studies, a comprehensive systematic approach has been developed to aid in the diagnosis of clinical instability in the cervical and thoracic spines. Clinical experience has shown that the most important factors to consider when evaluating spinal stability are the radiographic appearance of the lesion, the forces responsible for the injury, the anatomical structures involved, and the presence or absence of neurological deficits. *In vitro* studies have improved our ability to judge which displacements are abnormal and have helped determine which structural components are important for FSU stability. Given the multifactorial nature of the problem and the necessity to consider all relevant factors, clinically applicable checklists for the lower cervical, thoracic, and thoracolumbar regions have been developed (45). Because no single factor should be preeminent in the diagnosis, the checklist has been designed to include internal checks and balances, and the various factors have been weighted based on their relative clinical importance and reliability. The clinician also has the option of partially weighting any single factor (*i.e.*, giving a 1 instead of a 2 or 3 for a borderline finding or interpretation) and in so doing tailors the checklist to the individual patient and increases the clinical applicability.

The checklists for evaluating clinical instability are shown in Table 14.2. The patient is evaluated for each factor in the list as described in the next section. If the findings have an assigned point value totaling 5 or more, the spine is considered to be clinically unstable. A value of 5 was chosen in an attempt to set the sensitivity of the system to the

TABLE 14.2

Checklist for the Determination of Clinical Instability[a] for the Cervical, Thoracic, and Thoracolumbar Regions

Factors	Cervical	Thoracic
Anterior elements destroyed or nonfunctional	2	2
Posterior elements destroyed or nonfunctional	2	2
Relative sagittal plane translation	2	2
Relative sagittal plane rotation	2	2
Positive stretch test	2	
Spinal cord damage	2	2
Nerve root damage	1	
Abnormal disc narrowing	1	
Dangerous loading anticipated	1	2
Disruption of costovertebral articulation		1

[a] A total of 5 or more points equals an unstable spine.

proper level (45). The original authors of the checklists felt that a set-point above 5 would result in undertreatment of a number of unstable spines and a set-point below 5 would result in overtreatment of a number of clinically stable spines. The checklists represent suggested clinical guidelines which will be refined and revised as future clinical and bio-mechanical studies increase our knowledge of spinal instability.

REGIONAL ANATOMY, BIOMECHANICS AND INSTABILITY CRITERIA

Anatomically, biomechanically, and clinically the upper cervical spine (occiput to C2) is distinctly different from the lower cervical spine (C3–C7) and will be discussed separately. The biomechanical and clinical information required to formulate a checklist for the diagnosis of upper cervical spine clinical instability is not yet available. To describe the criteria for upper cervical spine instability, a discussion of the common types of injury in this complex region is necessary.

OCCIPITOATLANTAL COMPLEX

The occipitoatlantal complex has received much less attention than other spinal articulations. The majority of the structural stability at this level is provided by the "cup and saucer"-shaped occipitoatlantal joints, their capsules, and the anterior and posterior atlanto-occipital membranes. Additional support may come from ligaments running between the axis and the occiput (tectorial membrane, alar, and apical ligaments) (17).

Flexion is normally limited by contact between the anterior lip of the foramen magnum and the odontoid tip. Extension is limited by the tectorial membrane (18, 43). The horizontal distance between the occipital basion and the odontoid tip is normally 4–5 mm (48). A study of lateral flexion-extension radiographs found the normal range of sagittal translation to be no more than 1 mm (measured from the occipital basion to the odontoid tip) (51).

The majority of patients with occipitoatlantal hypermobility or sub-luxation present following trauma, but abnormal motion at this level can occur in individuals with congenital fusions of the upper cervical spine, rheumatoid arthritis, or ankylosing spondylosis (13, 27). In a study of fatal craniospinal injuries, occipitoatlantal injuries were not uncommon (11); however, clinical experience with injury at this level is limited, as the patients rarely survive.

The literature contains very little to provide a detailed definition of clinical occipitoatlantal instability. However, based on the anatomy and biomechanics of this joint and the unacceptable risks associated with its displacement one should consider any abnormal positioning (*i.e.*, a horizontal distance of more than 5 mm between the occipital basion and the odontoid tip and/or more than 1 mm of translation in flexion-extension) to be clinically unstable. Neurological signs or symptoms referable to this level also indicate clinical instability (48).

ATLANTOAXIAL COMPLEX

The atlantoaxial complex is the most complicated articulation in the spine, which explains why the literature dealing with this subject is so often controversial. The facet joint has a biconvex configuration and a loose capsule designed to permit a large range of motion and contributes relatively little to clinical stability. The stability of this complex is primarily provided by the odontoid and its osseoligamentous ring composed of the atlas anteriorly and laterally, and the transverse ligament posteriorly. All other structures play a secondary role in atlantoaxial stability (45).

The amount of sagittal plane translation is of clinical significance. The distance between the posterior margin of the anterior ring of C1 and the anterior surface of the odontoid in normal adults is 2–3 mm and remains constant with flexion-extension (15). In children, up to 4.5 mm with some forward movement in flexion is considered normal (21). Studies have shown that the transverse ligament prevents more than 3 mm of anterior sagittal translation. If only the transverse ligament is disrupted, up to 5 mm of anterior translation can occur. Anterior displacements greater than 5 mm indicate that the alar ligaments are also disrupted (15).

The comminuted fracture of the atlas, as described by Jefferson, consists of four parts: the posterior arch; the anterior arch; and the two sides of the ring (22). The mechanism of injury is a direct axial loading of the skull which forces the occipital condyles in a wedge-like fashion into the lateral masses of C1, bursting it into four fragments. Most occur without neurological injury and are clinically stable. However, if the sum overhang of the lateral masses of C1 relative to the lateral borders of C2 is 7 mm or greater the transverse ligament has probably been disrupted, and the injury is considered clinically unstable (42). The rare combination of a Jefferson fracture and an odontoid fracture produces extreme instability (45).

ODONTOID FRACTURES

The classification of odontoid fractures into three types based on the location of the fracture line has been found by most authors to be a useful guide for predicting stability and their potential for union (2). Type I fractures occur through the superior aspect of the odontoid and most likely represent an alar ligament avulsion fracture. Type II fractures occur at the junction of the odontoid and the axis body. Type III fractures extend from the odontoid base into the body of the axis and often involve the superior facets.

The type I odontoid fracture is considered clinically stable because the fracture line is above the transverse ligament. Although both type II and type III fractures are considered acutely unstable, controversy exists over their definitive treatment due to their potential for nonunion with chronic instability. In this discussion of spinal instability it is not our intention to include clinical management and treatment; however, an understanding of chronic instability can be gained by mentioning the frequency of nonunion with conservative therapy. In series of odontoid fractures treated without surgical fusion, type II fractures were much more prone to nonunion than type III fractures with representative values of 30–40% and 10%, respectively (1, 2, 4, 36).

TRAUMATIC SPONDYLOLISTHESIS OF THE AXIS

A traumatic spondylolisthesis of the axis, usually referred to as a hangman's fracture, is a bilateral pedicle fracture of C2. This was the ideal lesion for judicial hanging and was produced by placing the knot in a submental position (10). Today the fracture is most commonly the result of automobile or diving-type accidents which cause axial loading and hyperextension of the head and C1 upon C2. This forces the posterior arch of C2 inferiorly and produces bilateral fractures through the pars interarticularis. Stability is maintained at this stage because little displacement has occurred, and the major ligamentous support remains intact. If the deforming load continues to hyperextend the area further, then disruption of the anterior elements of C2-C3 may occur, and the spine becomes unstable. Because the typical hangman's fracture effectively opens the neural arch of C2 and the spinal cord normally has ample canal space at this level, the patient usually escapes significant neurological injury. Even though the posterior ligamentous structures usually remain intact they cannot provide support due to the pars fracture. With adequate immobilization, the fracture usually heals well, and stability is re-established. If radiographs show significant displacement of the fracture or of the C2-3 vertebral bodies, then a ligamentous disruption is likely, and the injury should be considered unstable (45).

ATLANTOAXIAL SUBLUXATIONS AND DISLOCATIONS

In addition to the three classic injuries of the C1-2 area discussed above, there are a number of other less common patterns of atlantoaxial displacement. These can be divided into five types: anterior translation, posterior translation, unilateral anterior rotation, unilateral posterior rotation, and unilateral rotation combined with anterior or posterior translation (Table 14.3).

TABLE 14.3

Summary of C1-C2 Subluxations and Dislocations

Type	Causes	Physical Findings	Radiologic Studies	Clinical Stability	Treatment
I Bilateral anterior	Dysplastic dens, trauma, infection +z translation (*forward*)	Neutral or cock robin position of head	Lateral of C1, CT scan → anterior displacement of C1 on C2	Anterior displacement of 3 mm, neurologic deficit—clinically unstable	Fusion or trial of conservative therapy
II Bilateral posterior (very rare)	Fractured, absent, or destroyed dens −z translation (*backward*)	Patient may hold head in hands	Lateral of C1, CT scan → posterior displacement of C1 on C2	Clinically unstable	Fuse C1-C2
III Unilateral anterior (most common)	Arthritic conditions and infections ±y axis rotation; instantaneous axes of rotation at opposite joint (*axial rotation*)	Cock robin position of head; difficulty in rotating head away from direction in which it faces; not difficult to move farther in that direction; anterior tubercle of C1 may be shown to be displaced laterally by palpation of posterior pharynx	Lateral of C1, CT scan → anterior displacement of C1 on C2 AP open-mouth laminagrams, C1-C2 → lateral masses in different planes Ciné or several roentgenograms of axial rotation → no motion of C1 or C2	With no neurologic deficit, these are probably stable situations	Trial of reduction and conservative treatment; if symptoms require it, fuse C1-C2

IV Unilateral posterior (rare)	Usually associated with a deformed or fractured dens ±y axis rotation; instantaneous axes of rotation at opposite sides (*axial rotation*)	Cock robin position of head	Lateral of C1, CT scan → *no* anterior displacement of C1 on C1; AP open-mouth laminagrams, C1-C2 → lateral masses in different positions; Ciné or serial roentgenograms of axial rotation → no motion of C1 or C2	With no neurologic deficit, these are probably stable situations	Attempt reduction and, if symptoms require it, fuse C1-C2
V Unilateral combined (anterior and posterior)	Trauma ±y axis rotation; instantaneous axes of rotation at dens (*axial rotation*)	Cock robin position of head	Lateral of C1, CT scan → *no* anterior displacement of C1 on C2; AP open-mouth laminagrams, C1-C2 → lateral masses in different positions; Ciné or several roentgenograms of axial rotation → no motion of C1 or C2	If no neurologic deficit, it may be clinically stable	Trial of reduction and conservative treatment; if not satisfactory, fuse C1-C2

There is limited information available to accurately analyze the various C1-C2 subluxations and dislocations. The definitive diagnosis of their clinical instability remains speculative and controversial. It is known that for abnormal rotatory displacement to occur, the transverse ligament and at least one facet capsule must be disrupted. The C1-C2 complex should be considered unstable if the sagittal plane translation on standard lateral radiographs exceeds 3 mm in adults or 4 mm in children and/or if there is evidence of spinal cord impingement. Table 14.3 lists important information about the five types of atlantoaxial subluxations and dislocations. Table 14.4 lists the instability criteria for the C1-C2 complex (48).

LOWER CERVICAL SPINE (C3-C7)

The annulus fibrosus, the posterior longitudinal ligament, and the facet joints are the most important elements to stability in the lower cervical spine. The ligamentum flavum is well developed in this region of the spine and contributes to stability in flexion. Although the role of the paraspinous musculature in clinical stability has not been determined, it provides a significant degree of support to the lower cervical spine, especially in the acute phases of injury when the muscles are in spasm. The supraspinous, interspinous, and nuchal ligaments are relatively insignificant factors in clinical stability (45, 48).

Biomechanical studies on lower cervical FSUs using the paradigm of sequential transection of supportive elements (as described earlier) provide useful information about the anatomical correlates of instability in this region (see Fig. 14.6). Under maximum physiological loads, failure did not occur if all the anterior elements plus one posterior element or if all the posterior elements plus one anterior element remained intact.

In a second series of cervical spine experiments, a single level laminectomy caused only an 18% reduction in flexion strength. After single level laminectomy and bilateral facetectomy the flexion strength was reduced by 60%, demonstrating the importance of the facet joints in providing stability in flexion (24).

TABLE 14.4

C1-C2 Instability Criteria

Spence's more than 7 mm total
Ring[a] (C1) ↔ Odontoid space more than 3 mm
Avulsed transverse ligament
Neurologic deficit

[a] At 3–5 mm displacement, transverse ligament is out, and alar ligaments are intact. At more than 5 mm displacement, transverse and alar ligaments are out. (Modified from Fielding, J. W., Cochran, G. W. B., Lancing, J. F., *et al.* Tears of the transverse ligament of the atlas: A clinical biomechanical study, J. Bone Joint Surg. (Am.), *56A:* 1683, 1974.)

The biomechanical and clinical factors suggested for use in diagnosing clinical instability in the lower cervical spine are listed in Table 14.2. The first two factors in the checklist deal with the status of the anterior and posterior elements and are based on clinical history and radiographs. The *in vitro* studies suggest that instability may occur if either all of the anterior elements or all of the posterior elements are disrupted or unable to function. Although the decision the clinician makes regarding the status of the anterior and posterior elements will be qualitative, a thorough evaluation of the underlying process greatly improves the accuracy of this decision. For traumatic injuries this includes consideration of the mechanism of injury. For example, one must suspect damage to the posterior elements in cases of flexion injury. When dealing with other processes such as tumors and infections, consideration must be given to the status of the bony and ligamentous structures that have been or are likely to become compromised.

Situations that destroy or render the anterior elements nonfunctional include: (a) hyperextension injuries that rupture the anterior longitudinal ligament, disrupt the annulus fibrosus, or separate the end plate from the vertebral body; (b) flexion injuries that cause comminuted or transverse vertebral body fractures; and (c) bilateral facet dislocations which usually disrupt the posterior longitudinal ligament and the annulus fibrosus. A history of cervical intervertebral discectomy does not necessarily indicate incompetence of the anterior elements; however, one must consider the possibility as the posterior longitudinal ligament may be weakened or destroyed by the degenerative process or by the surgery.

The supportive function of the posterior elements is severely compromised by unhealed bilateral fractures of the neural arch (*i.e.*, bilateral pedicle or facet fractures). The weakness and frequent absence of the supraspinous and interspinous ligaments compound the problem (23). Unilateral facet dislocations often occur without causing significant ligamentous damage and are usually stable. However, when unilateral facet dislocations are associated with facet fracture and/or neurological deficits, extensive posterior ligamentous damage is usually present, and clinical instability is likely. The amount of force required to reduce these injuries is helpful in estimating the degree of structural damage.

When the spatial relationship between two vertebral bodies exceeds the values for the upper limits of physiological motions, clinical instability should be suspected (see Table 14.1). In the clinical situation, measurements of sagittal plane translation and rotation are done on neutral or flexion-extension lateral radiographs. Sagittal translation is determined by measuring the anterior or posterior horizontal distance between the posterior-inferior aspect of the vertebral body above and the posterior-superior aspect of the vertebral body below the interspace in question

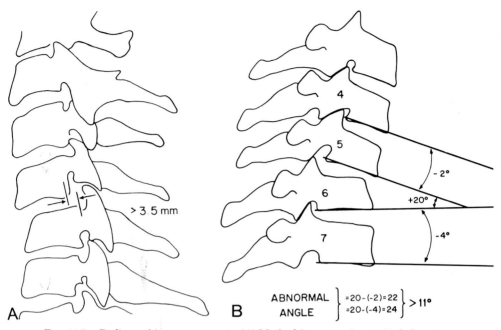

FIG. 14.7. Radiographic measurements. (A) Method for measuring sagittal plane translation. A point at the posteroinferior aspect of the vertebral body above the interspace in question is marked. A point at the posterosuperior aspect of the vertebral body below the interspace in question is also marked. The horizontal distance between the two points is measured (*arrows*). In the lower cervical spine, a distance of greater than 3.5 mm is suggestive of clinical instability. (B) Method for measuring sagittal plane rotation. First, measure the angle formed by the lines drawn from the inferior end plates of the vertebral bodies that form the interspace in question. Then measure the angles of the adjacent interspaces in the same manner. The relative sagittal plane rotation is obtained by comparing the angle of the interspace in question to the angle of either adjacent interspace. In the lower cervical spine a difference of greater than 11° suggestive of clinical instability.

(see Fig. 14.7A). A value greater than 3.5 mm is considered abnormal. To avoid radiographic magnification artifacts, one can relate the horizontal translation to the anterior-posterior width of the vertebral body; a ratio of greater than 20% is abnormal. The sagittal plane rotation is determined by measuring the angle formed by lines drawn from the inferior end plates of the vertebral bodies adjacent to the interspace in question (see Fig. 14.7B). The relative sagittal plane rotation is obtained by comparing the angle of the interspace in question to the angle of either adjacent interspace; differences of greater than 11° are considered abnormal. Comparing the angles of rotation for adjacent segments compensates for spinal curvature. Measurements of rotation are devoid of radiographic magnification artifacts.

In situations wherein the diagnosis of instability cannot be made based on other factors, functional radiographs are helpful to evaluate ligamentous integrity. Flexion-extension studies are commonly employed for this purpose but carry the risk of potential neurological damage. In some cases, the stretch test may be used to evaluate ligamentous integrity and is felt by some to be safer than flexion-extension studies (44, 45, 48). *In vitro* studies have shown that the spinal cord can tolerate considerable amounts of axial displacement without permanent deformation (8). It seems reasonable to expect the spinal cord to tolerate a given axial deformation better than the same deformation applied transversely; however, this has never been studied. The stretch test involves application of increasing amounts of axial traction under carefully controlled conditions (frequent neurological examinations) while looking for displacement on serial lateral radiographs. *In vitro* biomechanical studies on cadaveric cervical spines subjected to axial distraction loads equal to one-third of the body weight have shown that abnormal motion occurs after transection of all of the anterior or all of the posterior elements (35, 49). Based on normal subjects, the stretch test is considered abnormal if there is a change in the intervertebral height of greater than 1.7 mm or a change in the angle between two adjacent vertebral bodies of greater than 5.7° with axial traction of up to one-third of the patient's body weight (40). The test is contraindicated when clinical instability is present by other criteria, and when performed the recommended protocol must be strictly followed (45).

Cervical spinal cord injury strongly indicates a clinically unstable spine, whereas nerve root injury is a much less important factor. In general, if the magnitude of the initial injury is sufficient to produce damage to the neural elements, the spinal structure has probably been disrupted enough to allow further neurological injury, and the situation should be considered clinically unstable. However, there are notable exceptions to this premise. The most common example is the central cord syndrome in patients with cervical spondylosis who sustain a hyperextension injury with compression of the cord between the hypertrophied ligamentum flavum and the anterior osteophytes (41). An example of nerve root injury without spinal instability is the unilateral facet dislocation that injures the foramenal portion of the root while causing minimal ligamentous disruption. Studies of cervical spine trauma in monkeys have shown that the spinal cord injury can occur without concomitant damage to the spine (16). The mechanism proposed is shear strain transmitted to areas of relative cord fixation. It is also conceivable that the spine could deform enough to cause neurological injury while remaining within its elastic range and recoil back to its normal state. These exceptions not withstanding, in most circumstances one must strongly suspect clinical instability when neurological injury is present. The weighting given to cord and root injury in the checklist reflect the fact that neurological deficits are not an absolute indication of instability and should be used in conjunction with other clinical information to arrive at a definitive diagnosis of clinical instability.

An abnormal interspace narrowing seen in the posttraumatic cervical spine may indicate disruption of the annulus fibrosus and possible instability (5). This finding is especially important in younger patients whose other disc spaces are normal.

The final item in the list of criteria for diagnosis of lower cervical spine instability relates to the magnitude of physiological loads expected for a given patient after the injury has healed. Anticipated physiological loading for a professional football player or a manual laborer will be distinctly greater than that for an elderly, sedentary person. Instability is a relative term, and its diagnosis and treatment must be individualized. The physician's judgment as to anticipated spinal loading can be extremely helpful when other criteria for instability are inconclusive and is an important consideration in management decisions.

THORACIC (T1-T10) AND THORACOLUMBAR (T11-L1) SPINE

The thoracic (T1-T10) and thoracolumbar (T11-L1) spines have several unique characteristics that must be considered in the evaluation of their clinical instability. The vertebral articulations and thoracic cage are the major stabilizing structures and make the region mechanically stronger and more rigid than the cervical or lumbar spine. Although the thoracolumbar area is included in the discussion of the thoracic spine, in reality it represents a transition zone between two regions of the spine with significantly different anatomic and biomechanical properties. The concentration of forces in this transition zone accounts for the high incidence of thoracolumbar fracture and/or dislocation and explains their tendency for instability.

The anterior and posterior longitudinal ligaments and the annulus fibrosus are well developed and stronger in the thoracic region than in the cervical region. The thoracic facet capsules are thin and loose and provide much less support than the stronger, tighter cervical facet capsules. The spatial orientation of the facets in the upper and middle thoracic spine are nearly coronal and provide stability mostly against anterior-posterior displacement while allowing axial rotation (the predominant motion in this region). This orientation changes in the lower thoracic area (usually at T11 or T12) to the more sagittally oriented facet characteristic of the lumbar spine. This configuration provides stability against axial rotation while allowing flexion-extension and lateral bending.

The biomechanics of the thoracic and thoracolumbar spine are primarily determined by the shape of the vertebral bodies, their articulations, and the thoracic cage. The normal thoracic kyphosis (20–40°) is related to the slightly wedged configuration of the vertebral bodies. This kyphosis and the fact that the center of gravity is situated well anterior to the spine in this region explains the propensity for the thoracic spine to be unstable in flexion. The support and stability provided by the thoracic cage can be separated into two components: (a) the strong ligamentous attachments between the ribs and the thoracic vertebra (the radiate, costotransverse, and costovertebral ligaments), and (b) the large diameter of the thoracic cage that expands the effective transverse dimensions of the spinal structure and substantially increases the resistance to motion in all planes. The coexistence of a major thoracic cage disruption with a thoracic spine injury has obvious clinical implications in terms of spinal instability (45).

The transection sequence used in the biomechanical studies of the thoracic spine are shown in Figure 14.6 (31). The ribs were cut about 3 cm from the vertebral bodies to allow evaluation of the costovertebral attachments. When loaded to simulate maximum physiological flexion and the elements were transected in the posterior to anterior direction, failure occurred when the posterior half of the disc and costovertebral joints were cut. When loaded to simulate maximum physiological extension and the elements transected in the anterior to posterior direction, failure occurred when the posterior longitudinal ligament was cut (see Fig. 14.6). When applying these *in vitro* values to the clinical situation, it is important to remember that the experiments were done without an intact thoracic cage. A study comparing thoracic range of motion before and after removal of the thoracic cage found that the thoracic cage increased spinal stiffness by 27% in flexion and 132% in extension (3).

The list of factors for diagnosis of clinical instability in the thoracic and thoracolumbar spines is shown in Table 14.2. To make optimal use of these factors the physician must have an understanding of the structures involved by the lesion. The anatomic information provided by standard radiographs of this region of the spine (especially the upper thoracic area) is usually inadequate, and additional radiographic studies such as laminagraphy, myelography, and CT are necessary.

When evaluating the status of the anterior elements, it is helpful to consider their importance to thoracic stability as demonstrated by the *in vitro* studies. Although one can not directly apply this to the clinical situation, the information is conceptually important and indicates the relative contribution that the anterior elements make to *in vivo* thoracic stability. Vertebral body compression and burst fractures are the most common injuries in thoracic and thoracolumbar region (38). These fractures usually occur without significantly disrupting the anterior ligamentous complex. However, if the loss in anterior vertebral height is greater than 50% of the estimated original vertebral body height, progressive kyphotic deformity may develop, and the anterior structures should be considered dysfunctional (50). Another example of anterior element damage is the rotatory fracture dislocation which is well known for its extreme instability. The stabilizing role of the thoracic cage and its attachment to the spine make consideration of these structures important when evaluating the anterior elements.

Evaluation of the status of the posterior elements includes physical examination of the injury as well as radiographic interpretation. Holdsworth suggested "that stability after injury depends upon whether or not the posterior ligament complex remains intact" and stressed the importance of palpating the spine (20). Extensive injury of the posterior elements is usually associated with local tenderness and swelling. A palpable separation between the spinous processes indicates ligamentous disruption, and a lateral malalignment indicates a rotatory component. Holdsworth wrote: "A palpable gap almost always means an unstable spine even if roentgenograms prove equivocal" (19). Radiographic evidence of posterior element subluxations, dislocations, and/or fracture usually indicates posterior element dysfunction.

Measurement of relative sagittal plane translation and relative sagittal plane rotation is made from standard lateral radiographs in the same manner as that described for the lower cervical spine (Figs. 14.7A and B). A relative translation of greater than 2.5 mm and/or a relative rotation of more than 5° are suggestive of instability.

Thoracic or thoracolumbar cord injury is a strong indicator of clinical instability and has been assigned a high weighting value in the checklist. Because the ratio of cord diameter to canal diameter in this region is greater than in the cervical region, the tolerance for abnormal displacement in the thoracic area is less than that in the cervical area. For the same reasons mentioned in the discussion of lower cervical spinal cord injury, additional evidence for instability should be present to make the diagnosis of clinical instability in the thoracic and thoracolumbar regions.

The rationale for including the magnitude of anticipated loading in determining clinical instability has been discussed. In the thoracic and thoracolumbar regions it is given a higher priority than in the lower cervical region due to the inherently greater loads and stresses found in this region.

CONCLUSIONS

We have attempted to integrate salient biomechanical and clinical information and to show how this information can be logically and systematically applied to the evaluation of spinal stability in the clinical situation. However, our understanding of "what constitutes spinal instability" and our ability to definitively differentiate the stable from the unstable spine in the clinical setting is much less precise than is implied by much of the literature on the subject. Further research will hopefully improve our ability to define acute instability and allow a more accurate prediction of chronic instability. A checklist similar to that described for the cervical and thoracic regions is being formulated for the lumbar and lumbosacral regions. We are currently investigating the effects of healing on spinal stability. Finally, prospective controlled clinical trials with long-term follow-up are needed to validate and/or modify the proposed checklists.

ACKNOWLEDGMENT

This research was supported in part by NIH Grants AM 30361 and AM 34699.

REFERENCES

1. Anderson, L. D. Fractures of the odontoid process of the axis. In: *The Cervical Spine*, edited by Robert, W. Chap. 6. Cervical Spine Research Society.
2. Anderson, L. D., and D'Alonzo, R. T. Fractures of the odontoid process of the axis. J. Bone Joint Surg. [Am.], *56A:* 1663, 1974.
3. Andriacchi, T. P., Schultz, A. B., and Belytscko, T. B. *et al.* A model for studies of mechanical interactions between the human spine and rib cage. J. Biomech., *7:* 497–507, 1974.
4. Apuzzo, M. L. T., Heiden, J. S., Weiss, M. H., *et al.* Acute fractures of the odontoid process. J. Neurosurg., *48:* 85, 1978.
5. Bailey, R. W. Observations of cervical intervertebral disc lesions in fractures and dislocations. J. Bone Joint Surg. [Am.], *45A:* 461, 1963.
6. Bell, G. H., Dunbar, O., Beck, J. S., *et al.* Variations in strength of vertebrae with age and their relation to osteoporosis. Calcif. Tissue Res., *1:* 75–86, 1967.
7. Bradford, D. S. Spinal instability: Orthopedic perspective and prevention. Clin. Neurosurg., *27:* 591–610, 1980.
8. Breig, A. Biomechanics of the central nervous system: Some basic normal and pathological phenomena. Stockholm, Almquist & Wiksell, 1960.
9. Brown, T., Hansen, R. J., and Yorra, A. J. Some mechanical test on the lumbrosacral spine with particular reference to the intervertebral discs: A preliminary report. J. Bone Joint Surg. [Am.], *39A:* 1135, 1957.
10. Cornish, B. L. Traumatic spondylolisthesis of the axis. J. Bone Joint Surg. [Br.], *50B:* 31, 1968.
11. Davis, D., Bohlman, H. H., Walker, A. E., *et al.* The pathological findings in fatal craniospinal injuries. J. Neurosurg., *34:* 603–613, 1971.
12. Dennis, F. The three column spine and its significance in the classification of acute thoracolumbar spinal injuries. Spine, *8:* 817–831, 1983.
13. Englander, O. Non-traumatic occipito-atlanto-axial dislocation. Contribution to the radiology of the atlas. Br. J. Radiol., *15:* 341, 1942.
14. Farfan, H. F. *Mechanical Disorders of the Low Back.* Philadelphia, Lea & Febiger, 1973.
15. Fielding, J. W., Cochran, G. W. B., Lancing, J. F., *et al.* Tears of the transverse ligament of the atlas: A clinical biomechanical study. J. Bone Joint Surg. [Am.], *56A:* 1683, 1974.

16. Gosch, H. H., Gooding, E., and Schneider, R. C. An experimental study of cervical spine and cord injuries. J. Trauma, *12:* 570, 1972.

17. Hecker, P. Appareil ligamenteux occipito-atloido-axiodiem: Etude d'anatomic comparee. Arch. Anat. Hist. Embryol., *2:* 57–95, 1923.

18. Hohl, M. Normal motion in the upper portion of the cervical spine. J. Bone Joint Surg. [Am.], *46A:* 1777, 1964.

19. Holdsworth, F. Fractures, dislocations, and fracture-dislocations of the spine. J. Bone Joint Surg. [Am.], *52A:* 1534–1551, 1970.

20. Holdsworth, F. Fractures, dislocations, and fracture-dislocations of the spine. J. Bone Joint Surg. [Br.], *45B:* 6–20, 1962.

21. Jackson, H. The diagnosis of minimal atlanto-axial subluxation. Br. J. Radiol., *23:* 672, 1950.

22. Jefferson, G. Fracture of the atlas vertebra. Br. J. Surg., *7:* 407, 1920.

23. Johnson, R. M., Crelin, E. S., White, A. A., *et al.* Some new observations on the functional anatomy of the lower cervical spine. Clin. Orthop., *111:* 192, 1975.

24. Johnson, R. M., Owen, J. R., Panjabi, M. M., *et al.* Biomechanical stability of the cervical spine using a human cadaver model. Orthop. Trans., *4:* 46, 1980.

25. Kurowski, P., and Kubo, A. The relationship of degeneration of the intervertebral disc to mechanical loading conditions on lumbar vertebrae. Spine, *11:* 726, 1986.

26. Lindahl, O. Mechanical properties of dried defatted spongy bone. Acta. Orthop. Scand., *47:* 11–19, 1976.

27. Marfel, W. Occipito-atlanto-axial joints in rheumatoid arthritis and ankylosing spondylistis. Am. J. Roentgenol. Radium Ther. Nucl. Med., *86:* 223, 1961.

28. Nachemson, A. L. The lumbar spine: An orthopaedic challenge. Spine, *1:* 50–71, 1976.

29. Nachemson, A. L., and Evans, J. H. Some mechanical properties of the third lumbar interlaminar ligament (ligamentum flavum). J. Biomech., *1:* 211–220, 1968.

30. Nicoll, E. A. Fractures of the dorso-lumbar spine. J. Bone Joint Surg. [Br.], *31B:* 376–394, 1949.

31. Panjabi, M. M., Hausfeld, J. N., and White, A. A. A biomechanical study of the ligamentous stability of the thoracic spine in man. Acta Orthop. Scand., *52:* 315–326, 1981.

32. Panjabi, M. M., Pelker, R. R., and White, A. A. Biomechanics of the spine. In: *Neurosurgery,* edited by R. Wilkens and S. Rengachary, Chap. 284, pp. 2219–2228. McGraw-Hill, New York, 1985.

33. Panjabi, M. M., and White, A. A. Basic biomechanics of the spine. Neurosurgery, *7(1):* 76–93, 1980.

34. Panjabi, M. M., White, A. A., and Johnson, R. M. Cervical spine mechanics as a function of transection of components. J. Biomech., *8:* 327–336, 1975.

35. Panjabi, M. M., White, A. A., Keller, D., *et al.* Clinical biomechanics of the cervical spine. Am. Soc. Mech. Eng. Paper:75-WA/BIO-7, 1975.

36. Paradis, G. R., and James, J. M. Postraumatic atlanto axial instability: The fate of the odontoid process fracture in 46 cases. J. Trauma, *13:* 354, 1973.

37. Posner, I., White, A. A., Edwards, W. T., *et al.* A biomechanical analysis of the clinical stability of the lumbar and lumbosacral spine. Spine, *7(4):* 374–388, 1982.

38. Riggins, R. S., and Kraus, J. F. The risk of neurologic damage with fractures of the vertebrae. J. Trauma, *17(2):* 126–133, 1977.

39. Rockoff, S. D., Sweet, E., and Bluestein, J. The relative contribution of trabecular bone to the strength of the human lumbar vertabrae. Calcif. Tissue, *3:* 163–175, 1969.

40. Schlicke, L. H., White, A. A., Pratt, A., *et al.* A quantitative study of vertebral displacement and angulation in the normal cervical spin under axial load. Clin. Orthop., *140:* 47–49, 1979.

41. Schneider, R. C., Cherry, G., and Pantek, H. The syndrome of acute central cervical spinal cord injury. J. Neurosurg., *11:* 564, 1954.
42. Spence, K. F., Decker, S., and Sell, K. W. Bursting atlantal fracture associated with rupture of the transverse ligament. J. Bone Joint Surg. [Am.], *52A:* 543, 1970.
43. Werne, S. Studies in spontaneous atlas dislocation. Acta Orthop. Scand. (Suppl.) 23, 1957.
44. White, A. A., Johnson, R. M., Panjabi, M. M., *et al.* Biomechanical analysis of clinical stability in the cervical spine. Clin. Orthop., *109:* 85–96, 1975.
45. White, A. A., and Panjabi, M. M. *Clinical Biomechanics of the Spine.* Philadelphia, J. B. Lippincott, 1978.
46. White, A. A., III, and Panjabi, M. M. The basic kinematics of the human spine. A review of past and current knowledge. Spine, *3:* 12–20, 1978.
47. White, A. A., and Panjabi, M. M. The role of stabilization in the treatment of cervical spine injuries. Spine, *9:* 512–522, 1984.
48. White, A. A., Panjabi, M. M., Posner, I., *et al.* Spinal stability: Evaluation and treatment, AAOS Instructional Course Lectures, Vol. 30. C. V. Mosby, St. Louis, 1982.
49. White, A. A., Panjabi, M. M., Saha, S., *et al.* Biomechanics of the axially loaded cervical spine: Development of a safe clinical test for ruptured cervical ligaments. J. Bone Joint Surg. [Am.], *57A:* 582, 1975.
50. Whitesides, T. E. Traumatic kyphosis of the thoracolumbar spine. Clin. Orthop. Related Res., *128:* 78–92, 1977.
51. Wiesel, S. W., Rothman, R. H. Occipitoatlantal hypermobility. Spine, *4:* 187, 1979.

15

Stabilization Procedures for Thoracic and Lumbar Fractures

GEORGE W. SYPERT, M.D.

INTRODUCTION

The management of acute unstable fractures of the thoracic (T1-T10), thoracolumbar (T11-L1), and lumbar (L2-S1) spine remain controversial subjects. Management techniques of thoracic and lumbar spine injuries vary widely from a totally nonoperative approach (12, 29) to an approach in which spinal surgery is nearly always employed. During the 1950s and 1960s, surgical therapy largely consisted of posterior decompressive laminectomy. The latter procedure was demonstrated to be ineffective in achieving preservation or return of neurological function. In fact, patients having undergone decompressive laminectomy were found to suffer a greater incidence of delayed complications including spinal deformity and intractable pain (29). These results of laminectomy alone are not surprising since the offending neural compressive lesion is usually a bone fragment located anteriorly from a vertebral body fracture. Moreover, as a result of flexion angulation, the spinal cord and nerve roots are stretched over the anterior deformity. Excision of the posterior elements during laminectomy further contributes to the inherent instability of the original spinal column injury.

The role of surgical management in acute injuries of the thoracic and lumbar spine, however, has continued to evolve such that its goals of maximizing neurological function, stabilizing the spine, and preventing chronic pain states are now generally accepted. One of the most important advances has been the development of stabilizing spinal implant systems. The first truly successful spinal implant adopted and modified for the surgical treatment of thoracolumbar spine injuries was the Harrington rod system (11, 13, 18, 19, 26, 28, 30, 35, 67, 74). Subsequently, a variety of new posterior and anterior stabilizing spinal implants have been successfully applied in the surgical management of thoracic and lumbar fractures. Concurrently, improved anterolateral and posterolateral surgical approaches to the injured thoracic and lumbar spine have been developed which permit decompression of the neural elements with reconstruction of the compromised spinal canal (8, 9, 41, 49, 58, 60, 66).

The other important advance was the development of radiographic imaging, such as polytomography and, more recently, computed tomograph (CT) scans. With the development of precise imaging techniques, particularly CT myelography (11, 39, 59), in conjunction with advances in the biomechanical understanding of the normal and injured spine (4, 15–17, 33, 34, 74), appropriate application of the available neural decompressive technique and spinal stabilizing instrumentation is now possible. Knowledge of the benefits, biomechanical limitations, and complications of presently available spinal instrumentation is requisite for successful surgical management.

GENERAL CONSIDERATIONS

The goals of surgical management of injuries of the thoracic, thoracolumbar, and lumbar spine that produce neural injuries or spinal instability are decompression of the neural elements by returning the configuration of the spinal canal to its normal configuration and restoration of the normal biomechanical characteristics of the spinal musculoosseous-ligamentous structures. Accomplishment of these goals is dependent on knowledge of the mechanisms of the injury, the level of the injury (thoracic/T1-T10, thoracolumbar/T11-L1, or lumbar/L2-S1), the location of any neural compression, and the biomechanical nature of the inherent instability of the spinal column injury. Conventional anteroposterior and lateral spinal radiography, high-resolution CT scanning with sagittal reconstruction (10), and CT myelography in combination with a detailed history, general physical, and neurological examination are generally sufficient to gain this knowledge. Occasionally, magnetic resonance imaging (MRI) may also be helpful in special circumstances. The spinal surgeon can then select an appropriate surgical procedure to decompress the neural elements and reconstruct the spinal column. The type of spinal instrumentation selected will depend upon the methods used to achieve neural decompression and the nature of the spinal injury. Generally, the spinal implant used should produce optimal correction of any spinal deformity and give rigid internal fixation as this offers the greatest probability of a successful outcome. Each of the presently available spinal implants has advantages and disadvantages. It must further be kept in mind that when used improperly all of the spinal instrumentation systems can result in significant complications. Finally, the spinal implant should be considered as a temporary device. Given time and stress, all of the implants will fail if solid osseous union across the instrumented area is not ultimately achieved. Therefore, strict attention to bony fusion must be made simultaneously with the application of the spinal instrumentation.

Prior to a discussion of the specific types of thoracic and lumbar spinal stabilizing systems, a word of caution and plea for judgment in the management of thoracic and lumbar spinal injuries needs to be made. Despite our substantial increase in the knowledge of spinal anatomy, physiology, biomechanics, and instability, the improvements in spinal imaging techniques, and the advances in surgical decompression and reconstruction of the spinal canal and spinal stabilizing devices, scientifically sound data is often insufficient for clinical decision making regarding the advisability of surgical management in many patients suffering injuries of the thoracic and lumbar spinal column. Long-term studies of the physical and occupational limitations incurred by patients who have undergone spinal instrumentation for the correction of thoracic and lumbar spinal injuries do not exist. It is reasonable to consider the possibility that delayed complications such as early spondylotic degeneration and spinal pain syndromes may be a consequence of these instruments (28, 42), particularly if long spinal segments are fused. The rod-long, fuse-short technique (19, 35) and instrumentation without fusion (3) have been proposed to minimize the number of permanently arthrodesed segments and provide increased mobility of the thoracic and lumbar spine. The results of these approaches, however, have not been proven with long-term follow-up studies. Furthermore, spinal segments that have been temporarily instrumented for 9–12 months have not been shown to become mobile. In fact, evidence from experimental animal studies and studies of instrumented human spines demonstrates degenerative facet changes that occurred within a few months of the instrumentation (42).

Of specific relevance is the issue of a compromised spinal canal found on CT scan in a patient with a spinal injury who is neurologically intact, an area of great controversy (9, 13, 26, 40, 44, 73, 74). The natural history of such patients has not been adequately studied. Prior to contemplating prophylactic surgical therapy to prevent a potential problem such as delayed spinal deformity or delayed neurological deterioration, one must keep in mind the fact that numerous U.S. military service men sustained such injuries during their course of duty in the armed services, yet the Veterans Administration Medical Centers have not reported any large numbers of such patients seeking management for these potential complications. Furthermore, these major spinal surgical procedures carry with them the potential for significant acute and chronic complications. It is very difficult to improve on the neurologically normal spine-injured patient. Therefore, given the preceding considerations, it would appear most rational to manage thoracic and lumbar spine fractures in patients with no neurological deficit nonoperatively and wait to see if the canal compromise causes problems. Delayed spinal canal decompression via an anterolateral (7, 8) or posterolateral (54) approach can be performed with a very low risk and excellent preservation of neurological function. In the later situation, the decompression can often be accomplished with a one or two segment arthrodesis, preserving the normal biomechanical function of the remainder of the spinal column.

POSTERIOR SPINAL INSTRUMENTATION

To date, posterior spinal instrumentation has received the greatest application in the correction and stabilization of the injured thoracic and lumbar spine (6, 11, 19, 26, 31–33, 35, 36, 38, 45, 48, 54, 56, 67, 68, 71, 75). In many cases, proper use of such instrumentation reduces the fracture/dislocation, which is of benefit in achieving spinal stability and may occasionally improve neurological function by restoring vertebral alignment and reconstructing the spinal canal (4, 26, 35, 45, 47, 68, 74). Although improvement in neurological function following incomplete spinal cord injury remains to be proved (14, 19, 27, 51, 65, 67, 70), available evidence indicates that realignment and internal fixation decrease spinal deformity and subsequent pain while neural decompression prevents later deterioration in neurological function (7, 8, 26, 35, 51, 56, 70, 75). Surgical stabilization may also permit earlier mobilization of the patient, encouraging rapid progress in rehabilitation and decreasing the incidence of complications related to prolonged bedrest and immobilization (26, 67, 70, 75).

A wide variety of devices have been developed for posterior spinal element stabilization. Some of these implants, including various plates and screws, have not withstood the test of time. In contrast, Harrington distraction and compression rods, Luque intersegmental rods, and modified Weiss springs have been utilized with excellent results. A recently developed system, the Universal instrumentation of Cotrel and Dubousset, is undergoing clinical trials and may play a substantial role in the surgical management of certain thoracic and lumbar spine injuries.

Each of the available posterior spinal implants has both advantages and disadvantages that must be considered carefully in determining the appropriate instrumentation for a particular patient. In general, compression systems are used for isolated posterior ligamentous injuries where the anterior bony column is largely intact. Distraction systems are generally used for isolated anterior vertebral column injuries such as burst fractures. Combined injuries in which the posterior ligamentous complex as well as the anterior vertebral column are both significantly injured cannot be satisfactorily stabilized with distraction instrumentation alone. Luque segmental instrumentation fails to support the vertical compressive load and may be associated with collapse of the vertebral body fracture due to sliding of the wires down the rod. Hence, a variety of surgical strategies have been proposed to address these complex spinal injuries. In addition to an understanding of the biomechanics of the vertebral injury and its requirements for reduction and stabilization, consideration must be given to the experience of the surgical team, the ease of application of the spinal implant, patient factors, and the potential of the surgical procedure selected for complications (6, 11, 27, 31, 32, 36, 48, 55, 56, 58). Complications related to the stabilizing spinal instrumentation include injury to the spinal cord, nerve roots, and vertebral column; pain and disability related to the rigidity of the implant; and late implant failure leading to delayed instability and/or neurological deterioration (6, 19, 26, 28, 32, 35, 36, 47, 55, 56, 58, 75).

With respect to the application of posterior stabilizing spinal instrumentation to thoracic and lumbar spine injuries, one major decision that needs to be considered is the issue of neurological decompression, specifically regarding the patient suffering an incomplete neurological injury. The spinal surgeon can elect to decompress the spinal canal before internal reduction and fixation implants are applied, thus potentially preventing the neural elements from being stretched over the protruded bone fragments or lacerated by bony spicules (8, 48, 49, 54, 58, 67, 70). Another approach is to use the spinal instrumentation at the first step to achieve reduction and realignment of a seriously distorted spinal canal prior to attempting a direct surgical decompression of the neural elements (24a, 26, 35, 60, 74a). The latter may be accomplished via a single stage operation (posterior instrumentation-posterolateral decompression) or two-stage procedures (posterior instrumentation-delayed anterolateral decompression). Presently available data is insufficient to determine which of these approaches is the most appropriate for the patient suffering an incomplete neurological injury associated with a thoracic, thoracolumbar, or lumbar spine injury.

Harrington Spinal Instrumentation

The Harrington spinal instrumentation system consists of either distraction rods or compression rods. The distraction rod system has received the greatest use in the treatment of thoracolumbar fractures. The distraction rods apply axial forces through two sublaminar hooks attached to the rods by means of a hub on one end and a ratchet locking mechanism on the other. Two different mechanisms are provided by the distraction rod-hook complex to correct a spinal deformity: (a) a pure distraction force and (b) 3-point bending (Fig. 15.1). It is through both the longitudinal spinal distraction and the application of sagittal bending movements that the spinal malalignment and deformity are corrected (26). The compression system consists of thinner threaded rods, hooks, and small nuts. Compression and 3-point bending forces are generated by tightening the nuts threaded onto the rod above each hook. As this

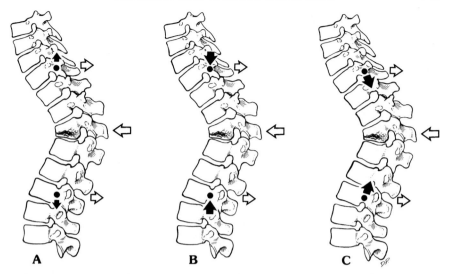

FIG. 15.1. (A) The forces applied by a Harrington or Universal distraction rod system. (B) The forces applied by a Harrington or Universal compression rod system. (C) The forces applied by modified Weiss springs compression system. The *black arrows* represent axial forces. The *open arrows* represent the forces caused by 3-point bending of the spine as the rod is inserted between the two hooks (or springs) attached to the laminae.

system acts in a sagittal plane (Fig. 15.1), the 3-point bending tends to correct a kyphotic deformity whereas the action of compression is to increase the angulation of the deformity (74). The bending moments created by the distraction system are more efficient in the correction of a traumatic kyphotic spinal deformity whereas the compression system has the ability to provide more stability by means of impaction, particularly in the situation of the severely disrupted spine (68, 74). Hence, in situations where substantial instability exists, especially with disruption of the anterior longitudinal ligament, and strong correctional forces are needed, combined compression and distractions rods have been recommended (62, 74).

Harrington Distraction System.   The ligaments of either the anterior or posterior column, particularly the anterior column (anterior longitudinal ligament), are extremely important with regard to maintaining the structural integrity of the spine when using distraction systems (2, 62, 74). A combined injury of the anterior, middle, and posterior columns (15, 16) presents a major problem for the application of a distraction system. While resisting bending of the spine and restoring vertebral body height, Harrington distraction instrumentation requires some intact structure to provide the necessary counterforce in order to hold the laminar hooks and prevent overdistraction. Therefore, Harrington dis-

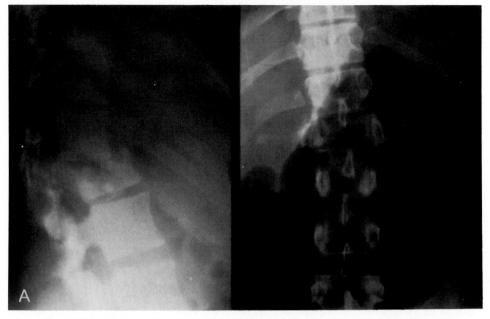

FIG. 15.2. Catastrophic complication related to inappropriate use of Harrington distraction rod system. The patient was a young adult male who sustained a severe fracture-dislocation with disruption of all three spinal columns at T12-L1 (A) and a mild incomplete spinal cord injury. The patient was treated with Harrington distraction rods. An intraoperative radiograph was not obtained. The patient awoke with a complete transverse T12 myelopathy. Note the postoperative radiographs that demonstrate marked overdistraction of the T12-L1 segment (B). Although the surgeon returned the patient to the operating room and corrected the overdistraction with a compression system (C), the patient has remained permanently paraplegic.

traction instrumentation should be used with great caution whenever disruption of the anterior longitudinal ligament is present (Fig. 15.2). It should always be kept in mind that disastrous overdistraction and neural injury can be produced by this device. In most clinical situations, the Harrington distraction rods should be used primarily to produce bending movements to correct the deformity and then serve as internal splints. The distraction force is primarily employed to lock the rods in place via the sublaminar hooks.

Generally, Harrington distraction instrumentation is applied via a posterior midline longitudinal incision. This requires that the patient be carefully turned on a four-poster frame, permitting the spine to go into some extension without compression of the abdominal cavity. Awake positioning of the patient may be helpful to insure that the positioning does not result in compromise of the neural elements. An intraoperative

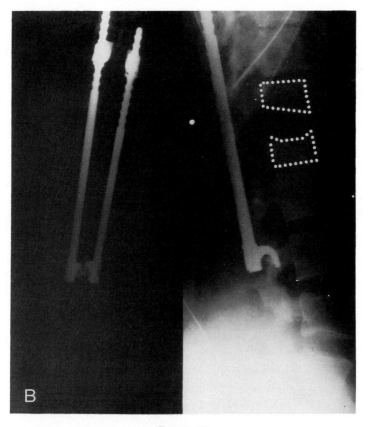

FIG. 15.2B

lateral radiograph should be obtained to be absolutely sure that the correct levels are being exposed and that spinal alignment has not been adversely affected by the patient's position. Once the correct levels are identified, a careful subperiosteal exposure of the spine is performed, which allows the erector spinae muscles to be retracted laterally. Further dissection is carried out to the tips of the transverse processes of the fractured vertebra and its rostral and caudal vertebrae if the "rod long-fuse short" technique is to be used (35).

In general, the spinal exposure should extend in the rostral direction sufficient to allow placement of the superior ratcheted hook (no. 1262) under the lamina of the second or third vertebra above the fractured level. Similarly, the exposure in the caudal direction should permit placement of the inferior square-slotted hook (no. 1254) under the superior margin of the lamina of the second or third vertebra below the fractured vertebra. A small laminotomy is often necessary to achieve

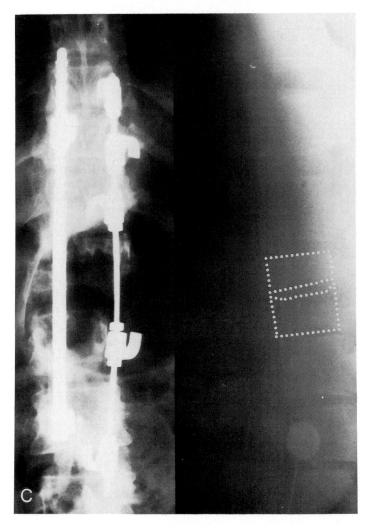

optimal placement and orientation of the hooks. Since the Harrington distraction system is principally used as an antibending device, the rods must be carefully contoured to achieve a normal spinal curvature that maintains appropriate thoracic kyphosis and lumbar lordosis. Moreover, the rod should be *contoured* in a manner that the maximal bending force be applied to intact lamina either rostral or caudal to the involved segment to preclude posterior laminar intrusion into the spinal canal with a resultant neurological catastrophe. Maintaining the plane of the rod curvature in the sagittal plane of the spine necessitates some form of fixation of the rods to the hooks that will mitigate rotation of the rods. This may be accomplished by using the Moe modification of the Harrington distraction rods having square-ended rods and square-holes in the caudal hooks. The latter system does require very precise determination of the final position of the hooks prior to contouring the rods. If these relationships are not maintained, then the plane of the rod curvature may not be in the plane of the spinal curvature such that the normal spinal shape cannot be restored or maintained. Another modification of the Harrington distraction rod system that appears to overcome many of the limitations of the original system is the locking hook spinal rod system pioneered by Jacobs and colleagues (36, 37). The Jacobs rod system features special hooks that permit rotational adjustment and lock around the rostral lamina to reduce dislodgement. Jacobs *et al.* (35) has also provided reasonably strong data in support of the rod long-fuse short technique. The advantages of the rod long-fuse short technique include: (*a*) improved precision of reduction, (*b*) stronger fixation (less force of the hook on the lamina is required), and (*c*) a shorter fusion resulting in improved biomechanics of the lumbar spine. The minor disadvantage is that this technique requires removal of the instrumentation when the fracture and fusion are solid, approximately 9 months later.

An approach that the author has found to be very successful in the operative management of axial loading injuries of the thoracolumbar spine, particularly burst fractures with retropulsed bone compressing the spinal cord and cauda equina, is to perform a partial or complete single level laminectomy at the level of fracture with removal of the pedicle and facet complex on the side of maximal neural compression. A well-machined drill with a cutting burr is very useful in safely accomplishing this decompression. This allows direct visual inspection and intraoperative real-time ultrasound evaluation of the spinal canal during the internal reduction and, if needed, decompression of the spinal canal via a posterolateral transpedicular approach. Using the rod long-fuse short technique, an appropriate contoured Harrington or Universal distraction rod is applied to the contralateral side to achieve an optimal reduction of the traumatic spinal deformity (Fig. 15.3). Optimal reduction and fixation are confirmed with an intraoperative radiograph. In most cases where significant compromise of the spinal canal existed preoperatively, the distraction system failed to reconstruct the spinal canal verified by inspection and intraoperative ultrasound (Fig. 15.3). Using a specially designed set of spinal tamps, beginning with the smallest and shortest tamp and proceeding stepwise to the next larger size tamp, the anteriorly located retropulsed bone fragment(s) is carefully pushed forward back into the vertebral body (Fig. 15.4). The largest or longest tamp will reach completely across the spinal canal. Upon achieving decompression of the

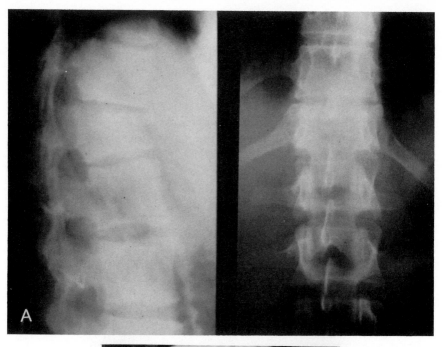

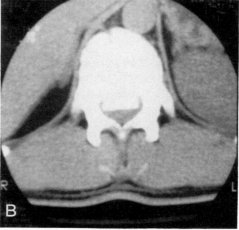

FIG. 15.3. Combined posterolateral decompression with Harrington distraction rod reconstruction of spinal canal and spinal deformity. The patient was an 18-year-old male who was involved in a motor vehicle accident sustaining an incomplete spinal cord-cauda equina injury secondary to a flexion-burst fracture of L1 (*A*) with a retropulsed bone fragment completely blocking the flow of subarachnoid contrast on CT myelography (*B*). (*C*) At surgery, a hemilaminectomy and pediculectomy was performed with a microtron burr, and intraoperative ultrasound was used to visualize the retropulsed bone fragment, prior to distraction (*C1*), after optimal reconstruction of the spine deformity with a contralateral Harrington distraction rod (*C2*) (Note that the correction did not decompress the neural elements), and after posterolateral reconstruction of the spinal canal using spinal tamps (*C3*). Postoperatively, the patient completely recovered all neurological functions (*D*). Nine months later, the Harrington rods were removed as the rod long-fuse short technique was used (*E*). A follow-up CT scan (*F*) revealed excellent reconstruction of the spinal canal in this neurologically intact young man.

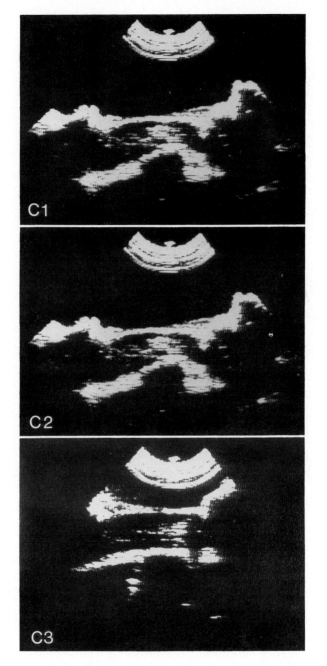

FIG. 15.3C

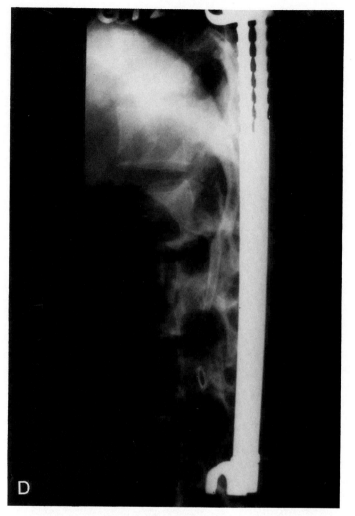

FIG. 15.3D

neural elements and reconstruction of the spinal canal, verified both by palpation and intraoperative ultrasound, the second ipsilateral distraction rod is applied, and a radiograph is obtained to verify the reduction. If the reduction is satisfactory, then the C washers are applied. A short fusion is performed using iliac autograft matchstick grafts obtained with an AO gouge, and the wound is closed in layers over a Hemovac drain. The patient is then mobilized in a polyform clam-shell orthosis on or about the third postoperative day. Follow-up CT scans performed after delayed removal of the rods at about 9 months following surgical recon-

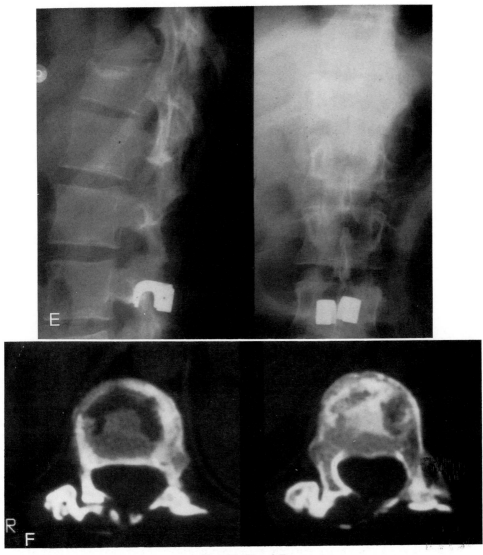

FIG. 15.3*E* and *F*

struction have documented excellent reconstruction of the spinal canal
and decompression of the neural elements (Fig. 15.3). This surgical
approach has been used in 26 patients to date. There have been no
complications related to the posterolateral decompression and reconstruction of the spinal canal. All of the patients with incomplete neural
injuries (18) demonstrated some return of neurological function at follow-

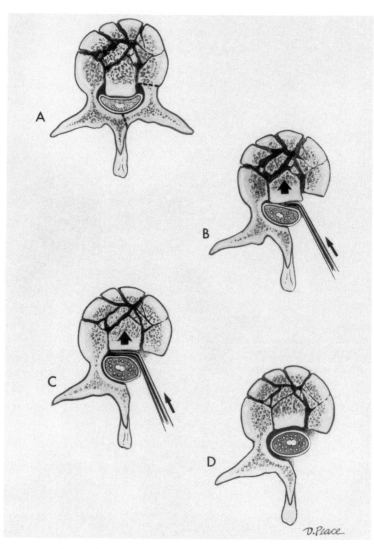

FIG. 15.4. Technique for gradually reconstructing the spinal canal using graduated spinal tamps via a posterolateral approach.

up. Moreover, those patients with normal neurological function preoperative were normal at follow-up. It is our impression this approach has been very rewarding; however, these data are insufficient to scientifically prove the hypothesis that operative decompression of the neural elements and reconstruction of the spinal canal improves neurological function in patients suffering incomplete injuries of the thoracic spinal cord or cauda equina.

Harrington Compression System. Injuries of posterior ligamentous complex secondary to flexion and distraction forces where the anterior columns of the thoracic and lumbar vertebrae are sufficiently intact for supporting anterior compression loads are ideal for the application of posterior compression systems, such as the Harrington compression system. Clinical experience indicates that the application of hooks to the intact lamina immediately above and below the segment of injury to bilateral threaded Harrington compression rods or Knodt rods used in a compression mode (Fig. 15.5), with a fusion across the level of instrumentation, are generally effective in reducing the dislocation and providing a good rigid, stable internal fixation (35, 69). The results of biomechanical studies are consistent with the clinical experience (37). Direct inspection of the spinal canal either via careful ventral palpation or intraoperative ultrasound is essential to be sure that fragments of the intervertebral disc are not displaced into the spinal canal, either by the injury or by the internal reduction. In addition, when the rostral hooks are applied to the superior margins of the lamina, particularly in the thoracic region with its small spinal canal, great care needs to be taken to ensure that the hooks do not compromise the spinal canal and produce an injury of the neural elements.

When compression rods are used to span multiple vertebral levels of the thoracic and lumbar spine, the rostral compression rod hooks are generally attached to the thoracic vertebral transverse processes. These rostral hooks should seat easily under the transverse processes at the junction of the process and the lamina. Often two or three hooks above and below the level of maximal kyphotic deformity are applied to each compression rod. Below T11, the transverse processes are not suitable for application of the compression rod hooks and the hooks must be placed under the lamina as close as possible to the facet joints. Harrington compression rods are supplied in two sizes (1/8th inch and 5/16th inch). The smaller rod is more flexible and easier to use for posterior internal reduction and fixation. After the hook sites have been prepared, the treaded compression rod with the hooks and locking nuts attached is inserted. The compression rod assembly is tightened using rod and hook holders and spreaders similar in principle to the distraction system. The hooks are tightened and fixed in position with locking nuts. After final tightening of the nuts, it is recommended that the threads adjacent to the nuts be crushed to prevent the nuts from loosening with a loss of reduction and fixation.

Harrington Distraction System with Sublaminar Wiring. Improved

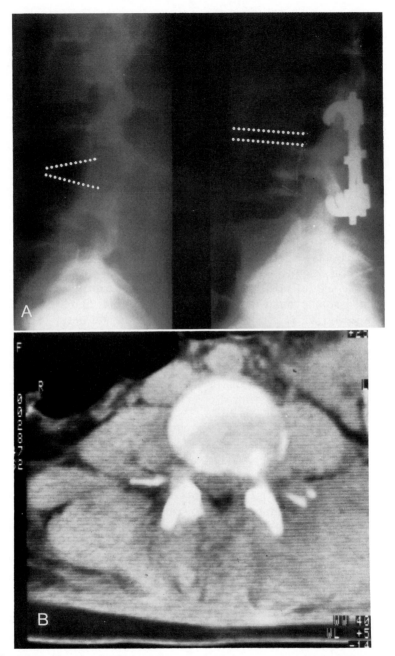

FIG. 15.5.   Use of a simple posterior compression system in a young adult female who sustained a flexion-distraction injury (A) with a large herniated intervertebral disc (B). This patient suffered a partial (incomplete) cauda equina syndrome which completely recovered after neural decompression and compression rod reconstruction.

torsional and translational stability can be obtained with a combination of multiple sublaminar wiring affixed to the Harrington distraction rods (modified Luque). Biomechanical testing has documented the improvement in spinal stability provided by Harrington distraction rods supplemented with sublaminar wires in severely unstable experimental spine fracture models (61). This construct was found to resist axial and forward flexion loading, lateral bending, and rotation when compared to Harrington rods without sublaminar wires. The Harrington distraction rod sublaminar wiring system appears to have its greatest application for severely unstable fractures with gross comminution or certain fracture-dislocations with major translocations. Preliminary clinical results using this construct appear excellent with respect to implant failure (hook displacement, rod breakage, broken wires) or pseudoarthrosis. However, sublaminar wires carry substantial risk for either acute or delayed neurological injury if the implant fails (55). Moreover, Luque has demonstrated that rod failure with segmental sublaminar wires occurs at the apex of the deformity often within 20 to 30 months (53). Neurological injury may also occur with rotation of the rostral hooks into the spinal canal. Another disadvantage of this technique is that the fusion must encompass the entire length of the implant. On the other hand, satisfactory reduction and fixation with this implant may be accomplished using fewer segments when compared with the rod long-fuse short technique and may not necessitate planned delayed removal of the implant.

Harrington Rod-Sleeve System. Since many injuries of the thoracolumbar spine are the result of a combination of forces (flexion, axial compression, and rotation) that leave the spine unstable in multiple planes of motion, Edwards modified the Harrington rod system in order to apply corrective forces in all directions (23–25). This rod-sleeve technique generally uses three elements to apply corrective forces: rods, sleeves, and special anatomic laminar hooks. The design of the rod-sleeve system is such that the distraction rods apply axial corrective forces and provide posts from which various-sized polyethylene sleeves exert the other corrective forces. The rod-sleeve system is supposed to provide comparable stability to contoured Harrington rods with sublaminar wires with greater ease of application and margin of safety (25). Edwards and Levine (24) have reported the results of a prospective protocol using this system in 135 consecutive cases of unstable T5-L3 spine injuries treated within 1 month of injury. All reported cases were at least one year from surgery. Comparing their data to that of studies using alternative techniques published in the literature, the authors claim that this technique resulted in superior postoperative reductions and less loss of correction. Furthermore, they suggest that the rod-sleeve method yields comparable neurological results to primary direct anterior decompression and represents a substantial improvement over the recovery rates reported for posteral reduction or the original Harrington rod technique.

Segmental Spinal Instrumentation

Segmental spinal instrumentation (SSI) was developed by Edwardo Luque in the early 1970s and refers to a spinal implant system that fixates the spine at each vertebral level instrumented (52). The original procedure involved attaching sublaminar wires to a Harrington distraction rod system. Unfortunately, this system frequently failed related to the Harrington rods fracturing at the ratchet-rod junction as a result of stress created at the stepoff. This approach was replaced with a smooth rod which eventually led to the familiar double smooth rod system in which the ends of the rods were bent into an "L" shape such that a rectangle is formed preventing rotation and migration of the rods (Fig. 15.6). Experience with the L rod system when applied to trauma demonstrated a high rate of wire breakage with loss of fixation in some patients, high reoperation rate, and poor vertical stabilization of the spine (25). Subsequently, a C-shaped rod and, more recently, a rectangular rod system have largely replaced the earlier designs for use in trauma and in spine tumor surgery. These latter implants have greater torsional resistance than the earlier implants. The SSI rectangular rod system is presently the implant used when SSI (excluding the Harrington distraction rod with sublaminar wires) is deemed appropriate for spinal reconstruction and stabilization in adult patients at the University of Florida.

A variety of surgical techniques have been used to apply SSI (1, 25). Generally, the spine is approached by a midline incision with subperiosteal dissection of all soft tissue from the posterior elements (the spinous processes may be removed and used as bone grafts. The bases of the spinous processes should be preserved to help prevent possible migration of the rod across the midline. The interspinous ligaments and the ligamentum flavum are removed. It is essential that all of the ligamentum flavum be carefully removed with angled currettes and small-angled Kerrison rongeurs so that the wires will not catch on residual ligament and be diverted into the spinal cord. A double loop of 16- or 18-gauge stainless steel wire is passed beneath the lamina (caudal to rostral) with only fingertip pressure. Care must be taken to ensure that the wire is kept snugly against the undersurface of the lamina and that the wire passes easily without any resistance. If any resistance is met, the wire should be removed and the undersurface of the lamina cleaned of any residual ligamentum flavum. Once the ball tip of the wire has been passed and appears rostral to the superior margin of the lamina, the ball is

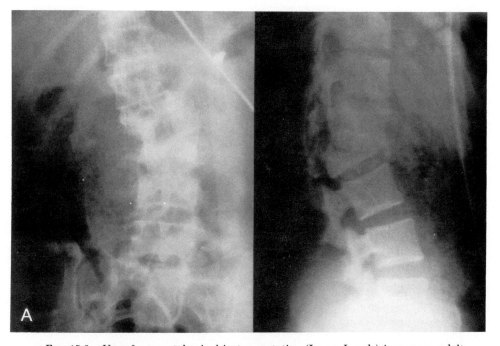

FIG. 15.6.   Use of segmental spinal instrumentation (Luque L rods) in a young adult female who sustained a severe 3-column injury of L2 with lateral translocation of rostral L2 relative to caudal L2 (A) and severe cauda equina syndrome. The patient was so unstable that the slightest attempt to reposition her during nursing care resulted in transient loss of all neurological function below L2. Therefore, an emergency reconstruction of the spinal deformity was performed using SSI (B). During the reconstruction, posterolateral decompression of the spinal canal could not be satisfactorily accomplished. Postoperatively, the patient failed to demonstrate any recovery of neurological function. A CT scan revealed a large retropulsed intradural bone fragment (C). An anterolateral approach was used to perform an L2 corpectomy with removal of the bone fragment, which was intradural. Postoperatively, the patient made a dramatic recovery of neurological function. When last seen 2 years later (D), the patient was pregnant with full return of all neurological functions, except for a left foot drop which required bracing for ambulation.

grasped with a large needle holder and gently pulled through maintaining countertraction on the caudal end to ensure that the wire remains tightly against the undersurface of the lamina. The wire is then pulled to one side, and both ends are bent over the lamina to prevent migration into the spinal canal during the passage of the other wires and later placement of the Luque rod implant. Some surgeons prefer single 16-gauge wires to fixate the implant. If the latter is used, then the ends of the double loop wire are cut, and one wire is pulled to each side and bent over their respective hemilamina. After all of the wires have been passed sublaminarly, an appropriately contoured implant (rectangle or C-rod) is secured

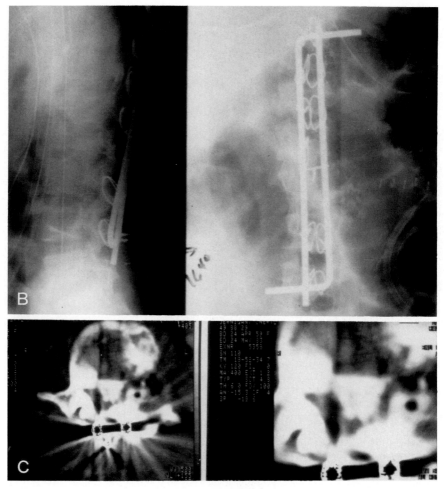

FIG. 15.6*B* and *C*

at one end of the spine, and the wires are sequentially secured over the implant, gradually correcting the spinal deformity. The contour of the implant should be designed in order to achieve optimal final correction as well as incorporate the normal kyphotic-lordotic postural curves of the thoracic and lumbar spine. Intraoperative radiographs are essential to check the reduction. The facet joints are then excised, and the spine is decorticated over the entire length of the implant and appropriately fused using autograft corticocancellous and cancellous bone. Postoperatively, the patients are nursed in bed for 2–4 days and then mobilized. We use a polyform clamshell orthosis for weight bearing for the first 3 months. Many surgeons use no postoperative immobilization, depending

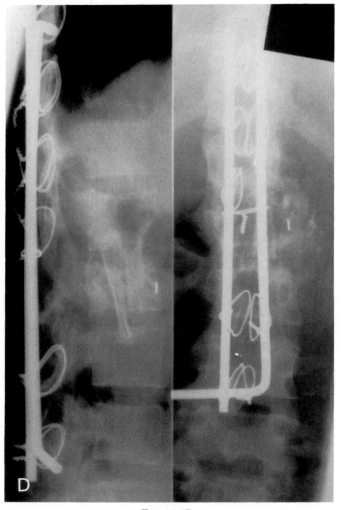

FIG. 15.6D

on the rigid fixation of the SSI implant (25). At present, the reported experience with SSI in the treatment of thoracic and lumbar spine injuries remains limited, and its role requires further clarification (1, 25, 63, 64).

Modified Weiss Springs

The Weiss spinal alloplasty spring was developed by Gruca and initially used by Weiss in the management of spinal fractures (71). Using prede- termined forces set up during spring insertion, it performs its function by dynamically stabilizing the spine with gradual correction of spinal deformities (72). However, biomechanical testing of the original implant revealed major deficiencies (37, 68). Hence, this device never received general clinical acceptance. The Weiss spring was modified to overcome some of the problems noted on biomechanical testing. An internal rod was introduced which increases the overall stiffness of the implant, yielding increased load tolerance. Moreover, the rotational deformities (68) were prevented by the internal rods and the placement of two Parham bands around the pair of springs through the interspinous ligament to transverse load the implant. The predominant action of the modified Weiss springs is compression on the fractured body and posterior elements between the laminar hooks. This force as well as 3-point bending produced by the internal rod tend to produce reduction of an angular spinal deformity (Fig. 15.1). The only extensive clinical application of the modified Weiss springs known to the author has been that of Sanford Larson and colleagues (55; and Larson, personal communication, 1986). Their technique consists of a lateral extracavitary approach to the thoracic and lumbar spine, decompressive vertebral corpectomy, anterior interbody fusion, and application of a posterior spinal device for stabilization. When Weiss springs were used, the hooks were fixed to the lamina 1–2 levels above and below the fracture and/or dislocation. The Weiss springs are applied so that a 10–30% increase in spring length was achieved consistent with a compressive force of about 10–30 lbs. Two heavy duty Parham bands (0.64 mm) passed through the interspinous ligament are used to transverse load the bilateral springs, which increases the lateral, anterior/posterior, and rotational stability of the implant. Based on a rather extensive experience with the surgical management of thoracic and lumbar spine injuries, these clinical investigators have concluded that the modified Weiss spring system is clearly superior to the Harrington rod system (6). Although the clinical results of these investigators are outstanding, their conclusions may be biased by their surgical technique which includes corpectomy and interbody fusion as well as how carefully the Harrington distraction rods were contoured to optimize correction of the deformity with maintenance of the normal spinal curvature.

Universal Instrumentation (CD)

The most recent posterior spinal instrumentation designed to correct and stabilize spinal deformities is the Universal instrumentation system or Cotrel/Dubousset (CD) system developed by Cotrel and Dubousset. This system apparently allows the 3-dimensional correction of spinal deformities. The Universal rods may be used in a distraction or compression mode (or both) as well as in 3-point bending (AP and lateral). Rotational deformities associated with congenital scoliosis may also be corrected using this system. The Universal system is potentially so versatile that it can be used to manage a wide range of thoracic and lumbar spine disorders, including spinal deformities, neoplasms, and trauma (Figs. 15.7 and 15.8). The major limitation of the Universal instrumentation system is its complexity; a substantial experience and learning curve will be required if this system is to be used appropriately and safely. The instrumentation consists of two types of rods (the Cotrel rod and a DTT or transverse loading rod) and three hooks (thoracic sublaminar hooks, lumbar sublaminar hooks, and pedicle hooks). There are also a variety of special purpose hooks and sacral staples for unique circumstances. A large number of specially designed instruments are required for insertion of the rods even in the case of a relatively simple acute traumatic spinal deformity. Although our experience with this system has been limited to date, we are very impressed with our initial clinical applications to acute traumatic thoracolumbar spine injuries. The ultimate role of the Universal Instrumentation in thoracic and lumbar spine injuries will have to await further clinical experience with this innovative spinal instrumentation (20, 50).

ANTERIOR SPINAL INSTRUMENTATION

The anterolateral approach to the thoracic and lumbar spine offers several important advantages in the surgical management of patients who suffer injuries of these regions of the spine. This approach to decompression permits direct visualization of the vertebral body injury, the most common source of neural element compression, as well as direct visual verification of anterior neural decompression. The adequacy of ventral neural decompression can be ensured. Although the efficacy of adequate neural decompression in achieving return of function in patients suffering incomplete spinal cord injuries remains a controversial subject, recent clinical data is highly suggestive that appropriate neural decompression may improve the functional outcome of such patients (8, 21, 49, 54, 58). Unfortunately, anterolateral decompressive corpectomy makes the spine even more unstable. Hence, the development of an anterior spinal implant that would span the unstable vertebral segment and restore vertebral alignment and stability would be optimal. Such a device would have the unique ability to stabilize the injured spine over only two motion segments, preserving the vital motion segments of the lumbar spine. In contrast, posterior instrumentation as presently applied to such injuries, generally requires fixation of five to seven motion segments. Recently, a variety of anterior spinal instrumentation systems

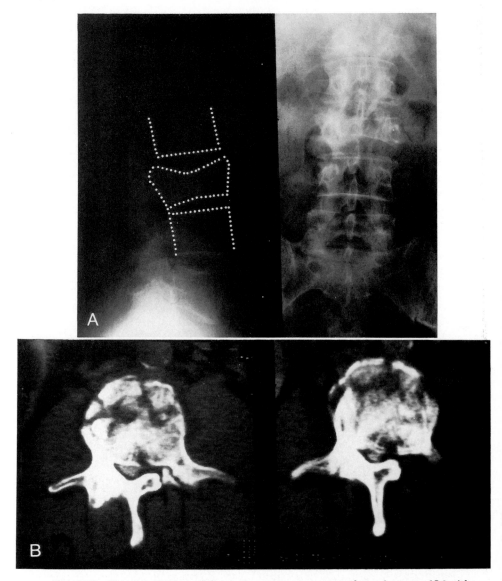

FIG. 15.7.　Use of the Universal distraction system to correct a burst fracture of L3 with retropulsed bone fragments (A) resulting in marked neural compression on CT myelography (B) in a 56-year-old male who fell 30 feet off a roof sustaining an incomplete cauda equina syndrome. During surgery, a posterolateral transpedicular approach was used to reconstruct the spinal canal. Postoperatively, the patient achieved an excellent recovery of neurological function (C) and returned to work full-time without any limitations (D). (Note excellent reconstruction of spinal canal with neural decompression).

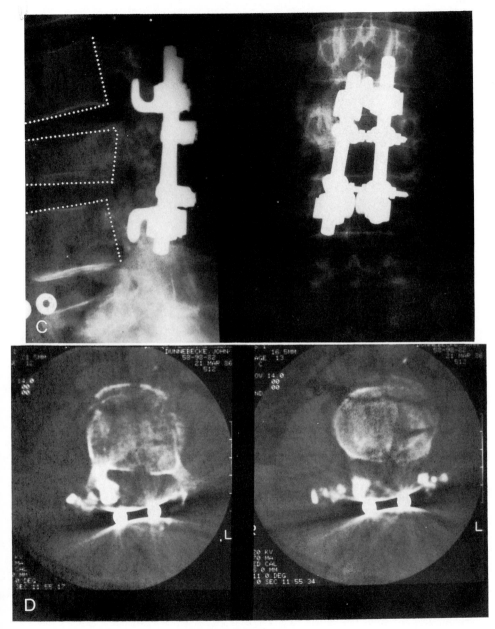

FIG. 15.7*C* and *D*

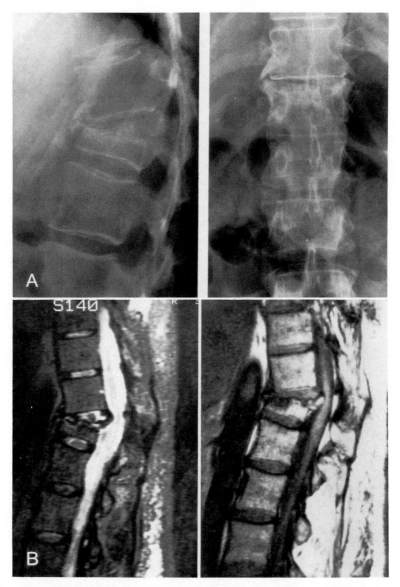

FIG. 15.8.   Use of the Universal compression system to correct a progressive posttraumatic spinal deformity of T12 (*A*) in a 48-year-old female with a progressive loss of
neurological function. The patient could not bear weight without assistance, and she was
incontinent of urine when first examined. An MRI scan demonstrated severe anterior
neural compression (*B*). A 2-stage surgical procedure was performed. The first stage was
an anterolateral microsurgical decompressive corpectomy via the 12th rib with alloimplant
femur reconstruction of the vertebral body (*C*). This was followed by application of a
posterior compression system to lock in the vertebral implant and prevent recurrent
deformity. Postoperatively, an excellent reconstruction of the spinal canal was verified by
CT scan (*D*), and the patient made a complete recovery of neurological function.

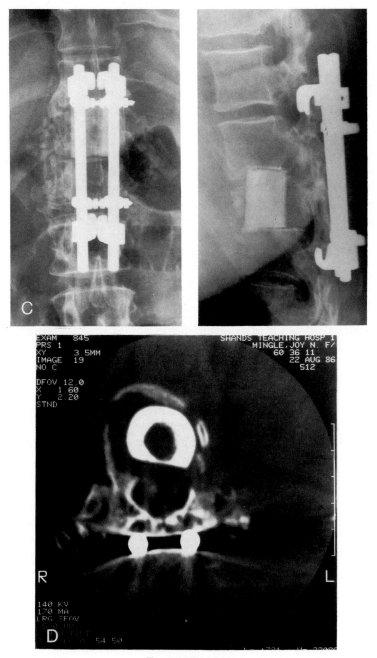

FIG. 15.8C and D

have been developed in an attempt to accomplish rigid reduction and fixation of the injured thoracic and lumbar spine. In an attempt to meet the demands that the construct must prevent axial collapse and kyphosis, rotation, and lateral bending, each of these implants consist of two rods that extend a single level above and below the injury site. These systems include the Dunn device (type III), the Kaneda implant, and the anterior Kostuik-Harrington distraction device supplemented with Dwyer screws and a solid Hall rod (21, 43, 46). None of these systems have received adequate clinical trials to date. Of these systems, the Dunn device has received the most rigorous biomechanical testing. Available evidence appears to favor the Dunn system with the most sound biomechanical principles. Although preliminary clinical trials using the Dunn system were very encouraging (21), the Dunn system is no longer commercially available. This is the result, in part, of catastrophic major vascular injuries associated with the use of the Dunn device by surgeons other than Harold Dunn. Therefore, currently available anterior implants should be thought of as struts, yielding some axial support but responding poorly to torsional and lateral bending forces such that they require either 2-stage procedures with posterior instrumentation or significant additional external support for mobilization of the patient. Research and development of a safe and biomechanically sound anterior spinal implant should be strongly encouraged as it will have great application for the treatment of various spinal disorders including trauma.

FUSION

It must be understood that spinal instrumentation used in the surgical management of spine injuries serves primarily as a temporary form of internal reduction and fixation. Long-term spinal stability depends on a solid bony union achieved by healing of the fracture or by the addition of bone grafts. Hence, every effort must be made to achieve bony arthrodesis. If the spinal implant is to remain in place throughout the patient's lifetime, then the bony fusion must encompass all of the motion segments encompassed by the implant. All artificial spinal instrumentation can be expected to eventually fail if bony arthrodesis across the instrumented motion segments does not develop or if the instrumentation is not removed when bridging unfused segments.

ORTHOSES

The need to supplement the spinal instrumentation used to correct the spinal deformity and achieve internal fixation with an external orthosis should not be considered as a failure of the spinal implant. In general, we have elected to use an external orthosis on all patients with potentially unstable thoracic and lumbar spine injuries when weight bearing despite the presence or absence of spinal instrumentation. A variety of external appliances are available to provide support and immobilization of the thoracic and lumbar spine. We have found that the removable polypropylene "clamshell" sternal-pelvic jacket (total contact orthosis) individually designed and molded by the orthotist are ideal for external immobilization of the T5 to L3 spine motion segments. If the unstable spinal injury involves the L3-S1 segments, then the orthosis includes a thigh extension to limit lumbosacral motion (modified clamshell spica). These orthotic appliances are light, reasonably comfortable, and permit the patient to be bathed on one side while lying in one-half of the shell. The orthosis is worn continuously for about 3 months. Depending upon follow-up clinical and radiographic evaluations and the patient's potential risk of a delayed spinal deformity, the device may be used for an additional 3 months when weight bearing.

COMPLICATIONS

The complications of stabilization procedures are numerous, some being very severe, and others mild. The ideal treatment for thoracic and lumbar spine injuries would, of course, exclude all such problems, but that is not realistic. Even the patients treated using a nonsurgical protocol suffer both major and minor complications related to their injury as well as the prolonged bed rest and limitation of activities associated with this therapeutic approach. However, one must always keep in mind that the surgical management of thoracic and lumbar spine injuries most certainly adds additional unique risks to the therapeutic program and that these should be weighed carefully before proceeding to operative correction and stabilization of a spinal injury. An analysis of the reported series in the literature reveals that major complications are very infrequent, which probably reflects the results of a small number of highly experienced spinal surgeons (see ref. 57). The complications of stabilization procedures may be divided into three phases: intraoperative complications, early postoperative complications, and late postoperative complications.

Intraoperative Complications

Death. Death is one of the two great complications of operative stabilization procedures; paraplegia being the other when treating patients with no neurological deficit or an incomplete myelopathy. In our experience as well as that reported in the literature, death has occurred, but rarely, and then it is due to factors that may not have been related to the surgical procedure. Our only death was due to a massive pulmonary embolus in a young adult male suffering complete paraplegia from a thoracolumbar fracture dislocation 2 weeks earlier. The event occurred during positioning of the patient immediately following satisfactory induction of general anesthesia. Additional potential causes of death include cardiac arrest related to hypoxia or hypovolemia. During surgical procedures, hypoxia appears to be the most frequent cause of intraoperative cardiac arrest. Adequate endotracheal airway and pulmonary ventilation are essential to the prevention of hypoxia. Hypovolemia is the other major cause of cardiac arrest. Spinal instrumentation surgery, even if done with great care, can result in substantial blood loss. Blood loss must be minimized with careful technique and carefully monitored. Blood replacement must be accurate. Transfused blood should be warmed before using. We have found that intraoperative autotransfusion is a safe and practical method that can be used to reduce total intraoperative blood loss by about 50%. Some spinal surgeons have advocated the use of hypotensive anesthesia. We have no experience with the latter technique, remaining somewhat fearful of lowering spinal cord blood flow by the hypotensive technique.

Neural Injury. In the 460 cases of Harrington rod instrumentation for fracture dislocations of the thoracolumbar reported in the literature and reviewed by McAfee and Bohlman (57), no cases of permanent neurological deterioration were documented. Neural injury does occur as reported by these investigators when they reviewed cases that had been referred to them. Neural injury may result from a direct injury to the spinal neural elements by surgical instruments, application of the spinal implant, or from excessive traction on the spinal cord (Fig. 15.2). These injuries should in large part be preventable in most cases by meticulous surgical technique, appropriate application of the spinal instrumentation, and the use of intraoperative radiography. Intraoperative monitoring with computer averaging evoked potential techniques may also prove useful in preventing this dreaded complication. A patient who awakens from surgery with a new severe neurological deficit should be instantly returned to the operating room, and the instrumentation should be removed and the spinal canal explored. Unfortunately, the prognosis for such patients appears to be poor for recovery of function.

Inadequate Reduction or Neural Decompression. McAfee and Bohlman (57) found that the most common complication of Harrington rod instrumentation for thoracolumbar fractures was the failure to decompress the spinal canal. When applying spinal instrumentation techniques, this complication can be reduced to a minimum by careful preoperative planning of the operative approach(es) and meticulous application of the appropriate spinal instrumentation to the spinal lesion being treated. In some cases it may be necessary to use a combination of surgical approaches including direct posterior, posterolateral extracavitary, or anterolateral approach to the spine in a single-stage procedure. For other cases, it may be appropriate to stage the spinal corrective surgery such as a posterior internal reduction-stabilization with spinal instrumentation and posterolateral decompression followed by an anterolateral decompressive corpectomy (Fig. 15.6) or vice versa (Fig. 15.8).

Pneumothorax.   Pneumothorax may arise during spinal instrumentation surgery from one of three primary problems. A tension pneumothorax may develop secondary to a respirator malfunction. The spontaneous rupture of a pulmonary bleb may also lead to a tension pneumothorax. More commonly, a nontension pneumothorax may develop from direct puncture of the pleura during some phase of the major thoracolumbar spinal corrective surgery. Whenever pneumothorax occurs, regardless of cause, chest tubes should be inserted and connected to closed underwater drainage.

Hemothorax.   Hemothorax may occur from laceration of either an intercostal artery along a rib or an intercostal branch around the vertebral bodies or transverse processes. Blood loss may go undetected until severe hypotension, cardiac arrest, or both develop. In the presence of a progressive hemothorax, the chest must be immediately opened; the bleeding artery identified and ligated or coagulated; and a chest tube inserted.

Early Postoperative Complications

Neural Injury.   All patients require careful neurological monitoring during the postoperative period. Although rare, patients can awaken from surgery without a new neurological deficit but develop neurological dysfunction during the postoperative recovery. Early recognition is essential to a successful outcome in such cases. Immediate neurodiagnostic evaluation (*e.g.,* CT myelography) should be followed by appropriate corrective surgery which may include exploration and removal of the spinal instrumentation. Based on the experience with scoliosis surgery, laminectomy would appear to be generally unnecessary unless there is specific reason to suspect the presence of a posteriorly located fragment of bone or hematoma in the spinal canal. In most cases, a posterolateral or anterolateral approach to the spinal canal is the appropriate technique to achieve adequate decompression of the spinal canal. If recognized and treated early, the prognosis is good in these patients compared to those who wake up from surgery with a severe neurological deficit.

No Neurological Improvement.   Most cases of incomplete (partial) myelopathies or cauda equina syndromes related to thoracic and lumbar spine injuries demonstrate neurological recovery following appropriate internal reduction, stabilization, and decompression (8, 49, 58, 67). Therefore, postoperative neurodiagnostic evaluation (*e.g.,* CT myelography) may be indicated in certain cases that fail to demonstrate neurological improvement.

Hypovolemia.   As mentioned, blood loss during major spinal stabilization surgery can be substantial. Moreover, substantial blood loss can occur postoperatively from the decorticated spinal column, the fracture site, and the autograft donor site. Hemothorax and retroperitoneal hemorrhage may also occur. Hypovolemia should be recognized early and treated with accurate blood replacement. In some cases of progressive hemothorax, a thoracotomy may even be necessary to control the source of hemorrhage with the insertion of a chest tube.

Pulmonary. Respiratory complications including atelectasis, pneumonia, pneumothorax, and pulmonary emboli may occur following any major spinal reconstructive procedure and require prevention, early recognition, and appropriate treatment.

Genitourinary. Urinary tract infections can almost always be prevented if catheterization can be avoided. However, we routinely prefer an indwelling urinary catheter during major thoracic and lumbar spinal surgery and the immediate postoperative period to monitor urinary output, prevent bladder overdistension, and manage a neurogenic bladder, if present. In addition, many patients find it difficult to void postoperatively due to pain, myospasm, and bed rest. Conversion to intermittent catheterization or normal voiding should be encouraged as soon as feasible to minimize urinary tract infections.

Skin. Decubitus ulceration should be prevented by frequent repositioning and turning of the patient and meticulous nursing care. Although the rotokinetic bed appears to represent a substantial advance in the postoperative management of these patients, it is not a substitute for quality nursing care.

Wound. Wound seromas are largely preventable with careful wound closure and the routine use of a closed suction-drainage system. Wound dehiscence is rare. We have not experienced this complication in our series. Wound infection is also an infrequent complication. Based on the surgical experience for scoliosis correction using spinal instrumentation and routine intravenous prophylactic antibiotics during surgery and for 48 hours following surgery, the infection rate should be less than 1%. Moreover, we have not experienced a wound infection in our series which exceeds 100 cases of adult thoracic and lumbar spine reconstruction utilizing spinal instrumentation. If an infection develops, prompt recognition and treatment are mandatory. Again, based on the scoliosis surgery experience, the treatment of choice appears to be early recognition of the wound infection, obtaining a culture via needle aspiration, and immediate surgical debridement of all devitalized tissue and irrigation after opening the entire wound. The wound is then closed meticulously over a closed suction-irrigation system. The wound is continuously irrigated with an appropriate antibiotic solution for 5–7 days. If at that time the patient is afebrile and the wound appears to be clean, the irrigation is discontinued, and suction is discontinued 24 hours later. Appropriate antibiotics are given in large doses intravenously during surgery and during the week following surgery, followed by a 6-week course of oral antibiotics. Using such a program, excellent results have been achieved for scoliosis patients.

Dislodgement or Breakage of Spinal Instrumentation. Dislodgement or breakage of the spinal stabilizing instrumentation is uncommon early and can largely be prevented by meticulous surgical technique and nursing care. When this complication occurs during the early postoperative period, the patient should be returned to the operating theater for either removal or replacement of the implant.

Late Postoperative Complications

Wound Infection. Late wound infections may become evident only a few days following discharge from the hospital or even years after spinal reconstructive surgery. It generally presents as a small draining sinus. The patient is usually afebrile. The treatment is the same as for an acute infection (see above). If the fusion mass is solid, the spinal instrumentation can be permanently removed, and the wound can be closed over suction-irrigation. A complete and thorough debridement of the entire wound is mandatory if spinal osteomyelitis and meningitis are to be prevented. The development of the latter more serious infective complications requires removal of the spinal instrumentation irrespective of the state of bony fusion.

Dislodgement or Breakage of Spinal Instrumentation. Loosening, dislodgment, or breakage of the spinal instrumentation late following insertion implies failure of fusion with the development of pseudoarthrosis. If the instrumentation dislodges and protrudes against the skin or breaks, then the device will require removal (see below). Moreover, if one rod is long and one fuse is short at the original surgery, the instrumentation should be removed as soon as a stable fusion has been achieved (generally at about 9 months postoperative).

Pseudoarthrosis and Progressive Spinal Deformity. Pseudoarthrosis is unfortunately an accepted complication of major spinal reconstructive surgery with or without instrumentation. Certainly, the correct use of spinal stabilizing instrumentation decreases the incidence of this complication. The incidence of this complication should not exceed 5%. Clinically significant pseudoarthrosis may present as: (*a*) loosening, dislodgement, or breakage of the spinal instrumentation; (*b*) intractable back and/or radicular pain at the fusion site; and (*c*) progressive spinal deformity with or without delayed progressive neurological dysfunction. The development of these latter complications may require removal of the original spinal instrumentation and partial takedown of the fusion mass and secondary autogenous fusion. If the patient develops a delayed intractable and incapacitating radicular pain syndrome or progressive neurological deterioration related to spinal deformity, an appropriate decompressive procedure should be included in any corrective spinal reconstructive surgery (8, 49, 54, 58).

SUMMARY

New concepts regarding the biomechanics of spinal instability, new technology for spinal and neurodiagnostic imaging, further evolution of the role of neurological decompression, and the development of improved systems and techniques for achieving anatomical reconstruction and fixation of the spine continue to improve the care of patients suffering injuries of the thoracic and lumbar spine. This field of medicine is in rapid evolution, and newer improved methods will be forthcoming in the near future. An understanding of all of these developments as well as their limitations and potential complications is requisite if we are to optimize the functional capability of patients suffering these catastrophic injuries.

ACKNOWLEDGMENTS

This work was supported by the Veterans Administration Medical Research Service.

REFERENCES

1. Allen, B. L., Jr., and Ferguson, R. L. The Galveston technique for L-rod instrumentation of the scoliotic spine. Spine, 7: 276, 1982.
2. Anden, U., Lake, A., and Nordwall, A. The role of the anterior longitudinal ligament in Harrington rod fixation of unstable thoracolumbar spinal fractures. Spine, 5: 23, 1980.
3. Armstrong, G. W. D., Peterson, E. W., and Adair, I. V. Harrington instrumentation for spinal fractures. Presented at the Annual Meeting of the Scoliosis Research Society, Ottawa, Ontario, September 1976.
4. Bedbrook, G. M. Treatment of thoracolumbar dislocation and fractures with paraplegia. Clin. Orthop., 112: 27–43, 1975.
5. Benzel, E. C., and Larson, S. J. Operative stabilization of the post-traumatic thoracic and lumbar spine. Surg. Forum, 33: 507–509, 1982.
6. Benzel, E. C., and Larson, S. J. Unpublished data, 1986.
7. Bohlman, H. H. Late, progressive paralysis and pain following fractures of the thoracolumbar spine. J. Bone Joint Surg. [Am.], 58A: 728, 1976.
8. Bohlman, H. H., Freehafer, A., and Dejac, J. The results of treatment of acute injuries of the upper thoracic spine with paralysis. J. Bone Joint Surg. [Am.], 67A: 360–369, 1985.
9. Bradford, D. S., Akbarnia, B. A., Winter, R. B., et al. Surgical stabilization of fractures and fracture-dislocations of the thoracic spine. Spine, 2: 185–196, 1977.
10. Brant-Zawadzki, M., Jeffrey, B., Jr., Minogi, H., et al. High resolution CT of thoracolumbar fractures. A.J.N.R., 3: 69–78, 1982.
11. Bryant, C. E., and Sullivan, J. A. Management of thoracic and lumbar spine fractures with Harrington distraction rods supplemented with segmental wiring. Spine, 8: 532–537, 1983.
12. Burke, D. C., and Murray, D. D. The management of thoracic and thoraco-lumbar injuries of the spine with neurological involvement. J. Bone Joint Surg. [Br.], 58B: 72–78, 1976.

13. Covery, F. R., Minteer, M. A., Smith, R. W., *et al.* Fracture dislocation of the dorsal-lumbar spine. Spine, *3:* 160–166, 1978.

14. Davies, W. E., Morris, J. H., and Hill, V. An analysis of conservative (non-surgical) management of thoracolumbar fractures and fracture-dislocations with neural damage. J. Bone Joint Surg. [Am.], *62A:* 1324–1328, 1980.

15. Denis, F. The three column spine and its significance in the classification of acute thoracolumbar spinal injuries. Spine, *8:* 817–831, 1983.

16. Denis, F. Spinal instability as defined by the three-column spine concept in acute spinal trauma. Clin. Orthop., *189:* 65–88, 1984.

17. Denis, F., and Armstrong, G. W. D. Compression fractures versus burst fractures in the lumbar and thoracic spine. J. Bone Joint Surg. [Br.], *63B:* 462–478, 1981.

18. Denis, F., Ruiz, H., and Searls, K. Comparison between square-ended distraction rods and standard round-ended distraction rods in the treatment of thoracolumbar spinal injuries. A statistical analysis. Clin. Orthop., *189:* 162–167, 1984.

19. Dickson, J. H., Harrington, P. R., and Erwin, W. D. Results of reduction and stabilization of the severely fractured thoracic and lumbar spine. J. Bone Joint Surg. [Am.], *60A:* 799–805, 1978.

20. Dubousset, J., Graf, H., Miladi, L., *et al.* Spinal and thoracic derotation with CD instrumentation. Scoliosis Res. Soc. Abstr., *20:* 142, 1985.

21. Dunn, H. K. Anterior spine stabilization and decompression for thoracolumbar injuries. Orthop. Clinics North Am., *17:* 113–119, 1986.

22. Edwards, C. C. The spinal rod-sleeve: Its rationale and use in thoracic and lumbar injuries. Orthop. Trans., *6:* 11–12, 1982.

23. Edwards, C. C. Early results using spinal rod-sleeves in thoracolumbar injuries. Orthop. Trans., *6:* 345–346, 1982.

24. Edwards, C. C., and Levine, A. M. Early rod-sleeve stabilization of the injured thoracic and lumbar spine. Orthop. Clin. North Am., *17:* 121–145, 1986.

24a. Erickson, D. L., Leider, L. L., and Brown, W. E. One-stage decompression-stabilization for thoracolumbar fractures. Spine, *2:* 53–56, 1977.

25. Ferguson, R. L., and Allen, B. L., Jr. An algorithm for the treatment of unstable thoracolumbar fractures. Orthop. Clin. North Am., *17:* 105–112, 1986.

26. Flesh, J. R., Leider, L. L., Erickson, D. L., *et al.* Harrington instrumentation and spine fusion for unstable fractures and fracture-dislocation of the thoracic and lumbar spine. J. Bone Joint Surg. [Am.], *59A:* 143–153, 1977.

27. Gaines, R. W., Breedlove, R. F., and Munson, G. Stabilization of thoracic and thoracolumbar fracture-dislocations with Harrington Rods and sublaminar wires. Clin. Orthop., *189:* 195–203, 1984.

28. Gaines, R. W., and Humphrey, W. G. A plea for judgement in management of thoracolumbar fractures and fracture-dislocations. Clin. Orthop., *189:* 36–42, 1984.

29. Guttman, L. Spinal deformity in traumatic paraplegics and tetraplegics following spinal procedures. Paraplegia, *7:* 38–49, 1969.

30. Harrington, P. R. Instrumentation in spine stabilization other than scoliosis. S. Afr. J. Surg., *5:* 7–12, 1967.

31. Hasday, C. A., Passoff, T. L., and Perry, J. Gait abnormalities arising from iatrogenic loss of lumbar lordosis secondary to Harrington instrumentation in lumbar fractures. Spine, *8:* 501–511, 1983.

32. Herring, J. A., and Wenger, D. R. Segmental spinal instrumentation: A preliminary report of 40 consecutive cases. Spine, *7:* 285–298, 1982.

33. Holdsworth, F. W. Fractures, dislocations and fracture-dislocations of the spine. J. Bone Joint Surg. [Br.], *45B:* 1–20, 1963.

34. Holdsworth, F. W. Fractures, dislocations, and fracture-dislocations of the spine. J. Bone Joint Surg. [Br.], *52A:* 1534–1551, 1970.

35. Jacobs, R. R., Asher, M. A., and Snider, R. K. Thoracolumbar spine injuries: A comparative study of recumbent and operative treatment of 100 patients. Spine, 5: 463–477, 1980.

36. Jacobs, R. R., and Casey, M. P. Surgical management of thoracolumbar spinal injuries. Clin. Orthop., 189: 22–35, 1984.

37. Jacobs, R. R., Nordwall, A., and Nachemson, A. Reduction, stability, and strength provided by internal fixation systems for thoracolumbar spinal injuries. Clin. Orthop., 171: 300–308, 1982.

38. Jelsma, R. K., Kirsch, P. T., Jelsma, L. F., et al. Surgical treatment of thoracolumbar fractures. Surg. Neurol., 18: 156–166, 1982.

39. Jelsma, R. K., Kirsch, P. T., Rice, J. F., et al. The radiographic description of thoracolumbar fractures. Surg. Neurol., 18: 230–236, 1982.

40. Jelsma, R. K., Rice, J. F., Jelsma, L. F., et al. The demonstration and significance of thoracolumbar fractures. Surg. Neurol., 18: 79–92, 1982.

41. Johnson, J. R., Leatherman, K. D., and Holt, R. T. Anterior decompression of the spinal cord for neurological deficit. Spine, 8: 396–405, 1983.

42. Kahanovitz, N., Bullough, P., and Jacobs, R. R. The effect of internal fixation without arthrodesis on human facet joint changes. Clin. Orthop., 189: 204–208, 1984.

43. Kaneda, K., Abumi, K., and Fujiya, M. Burst fractures of the thoracolumbar and lumbar spine with neurologic involvement—Anterior decompression and fusion with instrumentation. Orthop. Trans., 7: 16, 1983.

44. Kaufer, H., and Hayes, J. T. Lumbar fracture-dislocation. J. Bone Joint Surg. [Am.], 48A: 712–730, 1966.

45. Kelly, R. P., and Whiteside, T. E., Jr. Treatment of lumbodorsal fracture-dislocations. Ann. Surg., 167: 705–717, 1968.

46. Kostuik, J. P. Anterior fixation for fractures of the thoracic and lumbar spine with and without neurologic involvement. Clin. Orthop., 189: 103–115, 1984.

47. Laborde, J. M., Bahniuk, E., Bohlman, H. H., and Samson, B. Comparison of fixation of spinal fractures. Clin. Orthop., 152: 303–310, 1980.

48. Larson, S. J. Unstable thoracic fractures: Treatment alternatives and the role of the neurosurgeon. Clin. Neurosurg., 27: 624–640, 1980.

49. Larson, S. J., Holst, R. A., Hemmy, D. C., et al. Lateral extracavitary approach to traumatic lesions of the thoracic and lumbar spine (abstr.). J. Neurosurg., 45: 628–637, 1976.

50. Lesion, F., Mathevon, H., Villette, L., et al. Use of universal instrumentation in the dorso-lumbar spine pathology. AANS/CNS Joint Section on Spinal Disorders Abstr., 2: 13, 1986.

51. Lewis, J., and McKibbin, F. The treatment of unstable fracture-dislocations of the thoracolumbar spine accompanied by paraplegia. J. Bone Joint Surg. [Br.], 56B: 603–612, 1974.

52. Luque, E. R. The anatomic basis and development of segmental spinal instrumentation. Spine, 7: 256–259, 1982.

53. Luque, E. R., Cassis, N., and Ramirez-Wells, G. Segmental spinal instrumentation in the treatment of fractures of the thoracolumbar spine. Spine, 7: 213–217, 1982.

54. Maiman, D. J., Larson, S. J., and Benzel, E. C. Neurological improvement associated with late decompression of the thoracolumbar spinal cord. Neurosurgery, 14: 302–307, 1984.

55. Maiman, D. J., Sances, A., Jr., Larson, S. J., et al. Comparison of the failure biomechanics of spinal fixation devices. Neurosurgery, 17: 574–580, 1985.

56. Mascolm, B. W., Bradford, D. S., Winter, R. B., et al. Post-traumatic kyphosis: A

review of forty-eight surgically treated patients. J. Bone Joint Surg. [Am.], *63A:* 891–899, 1981.

57. McAfee, P. C., and Bohlman, H. H. Complications of Harrington instrumentation for fractures of the thoracolumbar spine. A ten-year experience. J. Bone Joint Surg. [Am.], *67A:* 672–686, 1985.

58. McAfee, P. C., Bohlman, H. H., and Yuan, H. A. Anterior decompression of traumatic thoracolumbar fractures with incomplete neurological deficit using a retroperitoneal approach. J. Bone Joint Surg. [Am.], *67A:* 89–104, 1985.

59. McAfee, P. C., Yuan, H. A., Fredrickson, B. E., *et al.* The value of computed tomography in thoracolumbar fractures. An analysis of one hundred consecutive cases and a new classification. J. Bone Joint Surg. [Am.], *65A:* 461–473, 1983.

60. McAfee, P. C., Yuan, H. A., and Lasda, N. A. The unstable burst fracture. Spine, *7:* 365–373, 1982.

61. Munson, G., Satterlee, C., Hammond, S., *et al.* Experimental evaluation of Harrington rod fixation supplemented with sublaminar wires in stabilizing thoracolumbar fracture-dislocations. Clin. Orthop., *189:* 97–102, 1984.

62. Murphey, M. J., Southwick, W. O., and Ogden, J. A. Treatment of the unstable thoracolumbar spine with combination Harrington distraction and compression rods. Orthop. Trans., *6:* 9, 1982.

63. Nasca, R. J. Segmental spinal instrumentation. South. Med. J., *78:* 303–309, 1985.

64. Nasca, R. J., Hollis, J. M., Lemons, J. E., *et al.* Cyclic axial loading of spinal implants. Spine, *10:* 792–798, 1985.

65. Osebold, W. R., Weinstein, S. L., and Sprague, B. L. Thoracolumbar spine fractures: Result of treatment. Spine, *6:* 13–34, 1981.

66. Paul, R. L., Michael, R. H., Dunn, J. E., *et al.* Anterior transthoracic surgical decompression of acute spinal cord injuries. J. Neurosurg., *43:* 299–307, 1975.

67. Schmidek, H. H., Gomes, F. B., Seligson, D., *et al.* Management of acute unstable thoracolumbar (T11-L1) fractures with and without neurological deficit. Neurosurgery, *7:* 30–35, 1980.

68. Stauffer, E. S., and Neil, J. L. Biomechanical analysis of structural stability of internal fixation in fractures of the thoracolumbar spine. Clin. Orthop., *112:* 159–164, 1975.

69. Sypert, G. W., unpublished data, 1986.

70. Walters, C. L., Schmidek, H. H., Krag, M. H., *et al.* The management of thoracolumbar fractures. In: *The Unstable Spine,* edited by S. B. Dunsker, H. H. Schmidek, J. Frymoyer, and A. Kahn, III, pp. 221–248. Grune & Stratton, Orlando, Fla., 1986.

71. Weiss, M. Dynamic spine alloplasty (spring-loading corrective devices) after fracture and spinal cord injury. Clin. Orthop., *112:* 150–158, 1975.

72. Weiss, M., and Bentkowski, Z. Biomechanical study in dynamic spondylodesis of the spine. Clin. Orthop., *109:* 85–96, 1975.

73. Westerborn, A., and Olsson, O. Mechanics, treatment and prognosis of fractures of the dorso-lumbar spine. Acta Chir. Scand., *102:* 59, 1951.

74. White, A. A., III, and Panjabi, M. M. *Clinical Biomechanics of the Spine.* Lippincott, Philadelphia, 1978.

74a. Whitesides, T. E., and Shah, S. G. On the management of unstable fractures of the thoracolumbar spine. Spine, *1:* 99–107, 1976.

75. Yosipovitch, Z., Robin, C. C., and Mankin, M. Open reduction of unstable thoracolumbar spinal injuries and fixation with Harrington rods. J. Bone Joint Surg. [Am.], *59A:* 1003–1015, 1977.

16

Cervical Spondylosis and Syringomyelia: Suboptimal Results, Incomplete Treatment, and the Role of Intraoperative Ultrasound

GEORGE J. DOHRMANN, M.D., PH.D., and
JONATHAN M. RUBIN, M.D., PH.D.

INTRODUCTION

All too often operative procedures for cervical spondylosis and syringomyelia have suboptimal results (1–3, 7, 9, 10, 12, 13–15). As such, cervical spondylotic myelopathy and syringomyelia represent ongoing challenges in neurosurgery. There may be multiple reasons for the above; however, one possibility is that the decompressive procedure for spondylotic myelopathy and the shunting/drainage procedure for syringomyelia may not be as complete as believed at the time of operation (4–6). The role of intraoperative ultrasound in assessing the adequacy of these procedures will be discussed.

RESULTS

In talking to patients with cervical spondylotic myelopathy or syringomyelia, the neurosurgeon frequently speaks of "stopping the progression of the disease" or "stopping the ongoing neurological dysfunction." Often it is mentioned that there may be improvement, but that is placed as the secondary goal rather than the primary one.

Decompression for Cervical Spondylotic Myelopathy (Table 16.1)

Over 300 patients with cervical spondylotic myelopathy treated by laminectomy in various series were reviewed by Haft and Shenkin (10). Forty-two percent (42%) of the patients had good to excellent results while 26% had fair results and 32% had poor results. Nurick (14) analyzed the results of cervical laminectomy for spondylotic myelopathy in 474 patients. He reported that 56% were improved; 25% were unchanged; and 19% were worse. In a 10-year follow-up of patients having had a laminectomy for cervical myelopathy, Bishara (3) noted that only 50% of the patients were improved. Fager (7) reported that 59% of the patients having a laminectomy for cervical spondylotic myelopathy improved and

32% were unchanged. After an anterior decompressive approach for myelopathy secondary to cervical spondylosis, Lunsford et al. (13) noted that 50% of the patients showed improvement. The authors said that "in many cases the symptoms of cervical spondylotic myelopathy progressed despite the intervention."

Shunting/Drainage of Syringomyelia (Table 16.2)

The results of operative treatment in syringomyelia are less good than those for cervical spondylotic myelopathy as above. In 1966, Love and Olafson (12) noted that after an operative approach to drain or shunt the syrinx, only one-third of the patients improved. Two decades later Anderson et al. (1) noted exactly the same result in that only one-third of patients operated upon for syringomyelia had improvement noted over the long-term (median follow-up: 10 years); however, they stated that when this improvement occurred, it persisted for many years. Faulhauer and Loew (9) reported that of 103 patients operated on for syringomyelia, only 34% improved while 40% were unchanged. In 1983, Peerless and Durward (15) evaluated the results of syrinx drainage procedures in 65 patients (syringosubarachnoid or syringoperitoneal shunts) and noted that although 38% improved, an even greater number (43%) continued to get worse and 19% were unchanged. Barbaro et al. (2) placed syringosubarachnoid and syringoperitoneal shunts in patients with syringomyelia and reported similar results.

TABLE 16.1
Cervical Spondylosis: Operations for Myelopathy

Author	No. of Patients	Improved (%)	Unchanged (%)	Worse (%)
Nurick ('71)	474	56	25	19
Bishara ('71)	59	50 (10-year follow-up)		
Fager ('78)	66	59	32	9
Lunsford et al. ('80)	32	50	50	

TABLE 16.2
Syringomyelia: Shunting/Drainage of Syrinx

Author	No. of Patients	Improved (%)	Unchanged (%)	Worse (%)
Faulhauer and Loew ('78)	103	34	40	26
Peerless and Durward ('83)	65	38	19	43
Barbaro et al. ('84)	34	41	27	32

DISCUSSION

Role of Intraoperative Ultrasound

CERVICAL SPONDYLOTIC MYELOPATHY

With only 50–60% of patients with cervical spondylotic myelopathy having improved following decompressive laminectomy (Table 16.1), it is clear that the reason for these results should be examined. Continued compression of the spinal cord is one of the possible reasons for such results. We have noted that when performing multilevel decompressive cervical laminectomies for spinal cord compression secondary to spondylosis that although the dura appears to pulsate well, there can be continued anterior or anterolateral compression of the spinal cord as shown by intraoperative ultrasound. If such compression continues, the dura will move rhythmically at the respiratory rate, but the spinal cord will be seen on ultrasound to be moving rhythmically at the heart rate. As we have reported previously (5, 6, 11, 17), this is probably secondary to transmitted pulsations from the anterior spinal artery from anterior compression of the spinal cord. These observations were made in such patients operated on in the prone position with the head in a pin headholder and the neck maintained in a neutral position. Following laminectomy, the wound was filled with saline and ultrasound imaging was done (Fig. 16.1) (4–6). We have noted that following multilevel laminectomy for cervical spondylosis where there was continued anterior compression noted by ultrasound (Figs. 16.1 and 16.2), the patient would improve somewhat postoperatively, then reach a plateau. Following a second operative procedure via an anterior approach to remove the anterior bony compression, further improvement would be noted.

The use of follow-up myelography has been discussed by Fager (8). Ultrasound imaging used in the operating room at the conclusion of the bony decompression is an excellent means of assessing the degree of decompression (Figs. 16.1 and 16.2). If complete decompression has not been carried out, the level of continued compression can be identified, and another decompressive procedure could be done at a later date. If the goal of the operative procedure is decompression of the spinal cord, then the use of intraoperative ultrasound is a technique for evaluating whether such decompression has been completely achieved.

Syringomyelia

The treatment of patients with syringomyelia is frequently disappointing in that only 30–40% of such patients improve (Table 16.2) even with techniques such as shunting the syrinx to the subarachnoid space or to

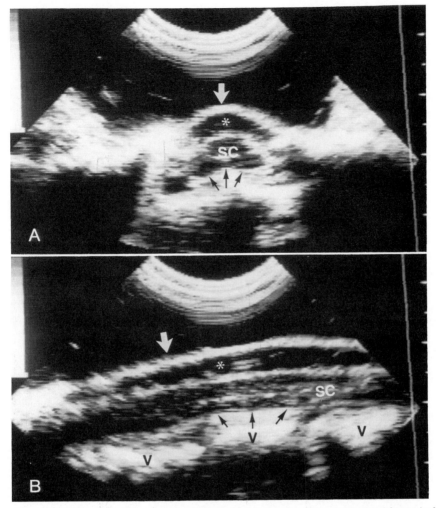

FIG. 16.1.   Intraoperative ultrasound scan of the spinal cord in a patient with cervical spondylosis with compression at multiple levels. Ultrasound scan was performed following laminectomy. Note that there is no compression of the spinal cord posteriorly; however, at one level there is continued anterior bony compression. (*A*) Ultrasound scan of spinal cord (*SC*) in cross-section. Posterior dura (*large arrow*) can be seen as well as spinal cord and posterior subarachnoid space (*). The anterior subarachnoid space is not seen because of anterior bony compression (*small arrows*) at this level. (*B*) Longitudinal ultrasound scan of spinal cord (*SC*). Posterior dura (*large arrow*); subarachnoid space (*); vertebral bodies (*V*). Note that spinal cord is still compressed at this level from anteriorly by bone (*small arrows*). Anterior subarachnoid space can be seen both superior and inferior to this bony compression. (In this patient the posterior dura "pulsated" well, and it was the assumption of the neurosurgeon at that point that the spinal cord had been well decompressed.)

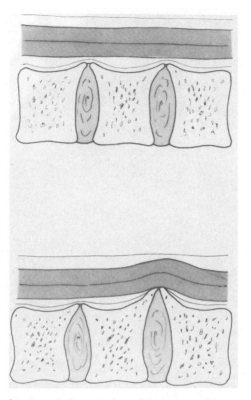

FIG. 16.2.   Line drawing of the spinal cord in a patient with cervical spondylosis
following decompressive laminectomy. (*Top*) The spinal cord was able to ride up posteriorly
and away from any bony compression anteriorly. (*Bottom*) Following the bony decompression posteriorly, the dura moved rhythmically at the respiratory rate ("pulsated"); however,
there was still bony compression of the spinal cord anteriorly. This can be seen by
intraoperative ultrasound. The spinal cord will be observed to be moving rhythmically at
the heart rate secondary to transmitted pulsations from the anterior spinal artery. (*Note*:
In both patients (*top* and *bottom*) the decompression will appear to be adequate as both
will have good "pulsations" of the dural sac. For complete decompression of the spinal cord
in the second patient (*bottom*), an anterior decompressive procedure would have to be
performed at a later time.)

the peritoneum. There are two types of syringomyelic cavities: one with
a large single syrinx (Fig. 16.3) and one with multiple syringomyelic
cavities (Fig. 16.4) extending through that portion of spinal cord. One
way of knowing for sure what type of syringomyelia is present is to do
intraoperative ultrasound. Prior to opening the dura the spinal cord can
be "explored" by ultrasound, and the position of the fluid-filled cavities
can be determined. The dura then can be opened just over the portion of
the spinal cord desired. If there is one single cavity, it is optimal for the

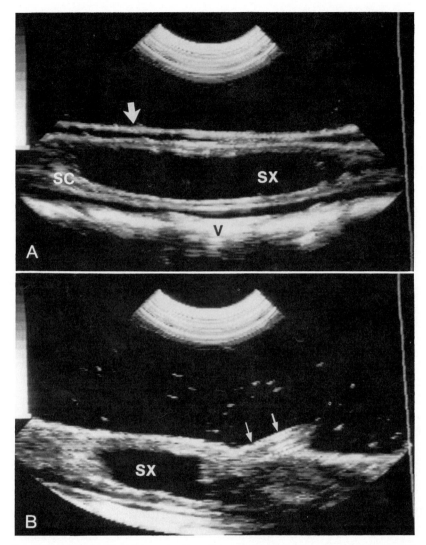

FIG. 16.3.   Longitudinal intraoperative ultrasound scans of the spinal cord in a patient
with syringomyelia. (A) This patient has a single syringomyelic cavity. Posterior dura
(*large arrow*); spinal cord (*SC*); syrinx (*SX*); vertebral body (*V*). (B) Dura has been opened,
and shunt tube (*small arrows*) is being inserted into the syrinx (*SX*). (C) Shunt tube (*small
arrows*) is advanced into the single syrinx (*SX*). (D) Shunt tube (*small arrows*) is in final
position within the syrinx. Note that the proximal end of the shunt tube is not touching
the superior wall of the syrinx.

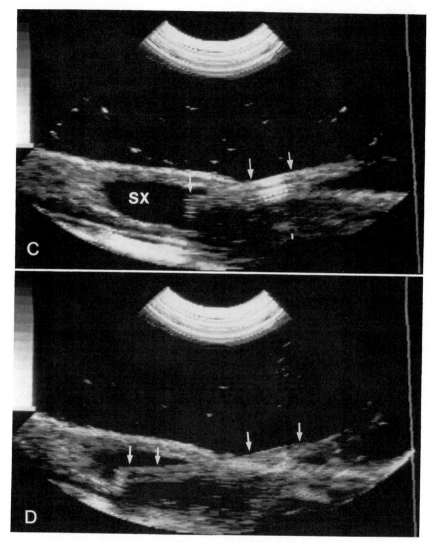

FIG. 16.3C and D

shunt tube to be placed in a more inferior location and not to extend
superiorly enough to be blocked or to be too close to the wall of the
syrinx such that the drainage of the fluid can be impeded. In patients
with a large single syrinx, intraoperative ultrasound can show the syrinx
and can be used to guide placement of the shunt tube and recheck the
position of the shunt tube within the syrinx after the shunt tube has
been secured to the pia (Fig. 16.3). One possible cause of shunt failure in

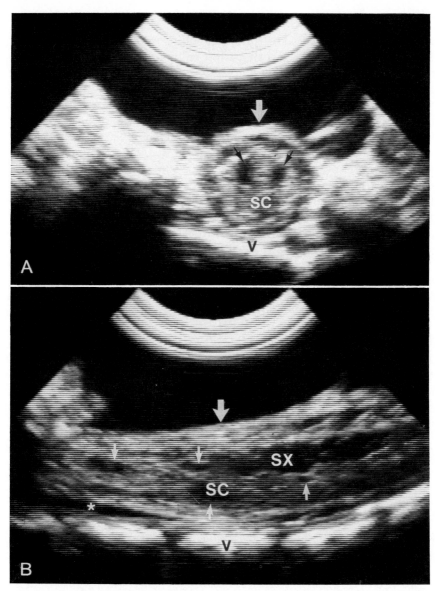

FIG. 16.4.   Ultrasound scans of a patient with syringomyelia having multiple fluid-filled cavities within the spinal cord. (*A*) Ultrasound scan of spinal cord (*SC*) in cross-section. Posterior dura (*large arrow*); multiple syrinx cavities (*small arrows*); vertebral body (*V*). (*B*) Longitudinal ultrasound scan of spinal cord (*SC*) showing the multiple branching fluid-filled cavities (*small arrows*) within the spinal cord as well as a larger syrinx cavity (*SX*). Small amount of anterior subarachnoid space (*) remaining; compare to absence of subarachnoid space at level of vertebral body (*V*) at center of scan. Posterior dura (*large arrow*). (From Dohrmann, G. J., and Rubin, J. M. Intraoperative ultrasound imaging of spinal cord: Syringomyelia, cysts and tumors. Surg. Neurol., *18:* 395–399, 1982. Reproduced with permission.)

this type of patient would be the shunt sliding into a suboptimal position. If ultrasound is used, this can be determined, and optimal positioning can be obtained. In patients with syringomyelia having multiple fluid-filled cavities throughout the involved portion of spinal cord (Fig. 16.4), the largest and most posterior of the fluid-filled cavities can be identified using ultrasound intraoperatively, and the shunt tube can be placed in that syringomyelic cavity (Fig. 16.5). In certain patients the swollen spinal cord could be seen to decrease in size immediately after the shunting, and the neurosurgeon might assume that the condition had been well shunted; however, if intraoperative ultrasound imaging is done following shunting in such patients, only one group of fluid-filled cavities would be seen to collapse, thereby indicating that all of the syringomyelic cavities did not communicate with each other and that another shunting procedure is needed (Fig. 16.5). This situation is analogous to that of patients with hydrocephalus and trapped ventricles; if only one of these ventricles is shunted, the postoperative results will be suboptimal in that the patient might improve, but only temporarily, and the progression of the dysfunction would continue. A shunt tube was placed in one of the earliest patients that we had, and the fluid-filled cavities on one side of the spinal cord were seen to collapse (Fig. 16.5); the opposite side of it was not shunted. The patient improved relative to the shunted side only. Perhaps the suboptimal results obtained in some patients having shunting procedures for syringomyelia might be related to the neurosurgeon not completely draining the fluid-filled cavities or not determining that the shunt tube has moved significantly prior to closure (4–6).

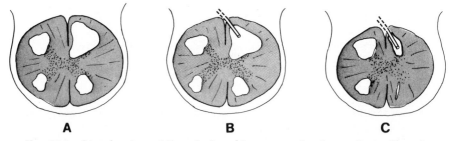

A   **B**   **C**

FIG. 16.5.   Line drawings of the spinal cord in cross-section in a patient with syringomyelia. (*A*) This patient has multiple fluid-filled cavities within the spinal cord. (*B*) With placement of a shunt tube into one of the syrinx cavities, the fluid begins to drain. (*C*) The distended spinal cord decreased in size, and it appeared to the neurosurgeon that the patient had been adequately treated. However, intraoperative ultrasound would have shown that in this patient only some of the fluid-filled cavities drained because all of the syringomyelic cavities did not communicate with each other. This would necessitate placement of another shunt tube to treat this patient completely. Without ultrasound imaging in the operating room, the neurosurgeon would not be aware of the fact that the one shunt did not effect complete treatment of the patient.

SUMMARY

The pathophysiology of cervical spondylotic myelopathy and syringomyelia is incompletely understood. Only 50–60% of the former group of patients and only 30–40% of the latter group of patients show long-term improvement. One possible cause for this might be continued anterior compression of the spinal cord in the former and incomplete drainage of the fluid-filled cavities in the latter. Intraoperative ultrasound imaging can be done in the operating room (4–6, 16–18) and can identify whether an adequate decompression has been done in patients with cervical spondylotic myelopathy and whether there has been complete drainage in shunting of patients with syringomyelia.

Intraoperative ultrasound imaging aids the neurosurgeon in checking to see if he did what he set out to do. It is useful in operative procedures for cervical spondylotic myelopathy and syringomyelia.

REFERENCES

1. Anderson, N. E., Willoughby, E. W., and Wrightson, P. The natural history and the influence of surgical treatment in syringomyelia. Acta Neurol. Scand., *71:* 472–479, 1985.
2. Barbaro, N. M., Wilson, C. B., Gutin, P. H., *et al.* Surgical treatment of syringomyelia: Favorable results with syringoperitoneal shunting. J. Neurosurg., *61:* 531–538, 1984.
3. Bishara, S. N. The posterior operation in treatment of cervical spondylosis with myelopathy: A long-term follow-up study. J. Neurol. Neurosurg. Psychiatry, *34:* 393–398, 1971.
4. Dohrmann, G. J., and Rubin, J. M. Intraoperative ultrasound imaging of spinal cord: Syringomyelia, cysts and tumors. Surg. Neurol., *18:* 395–399, 1982.
5. Dohrmann, G. J., and Rubin, J. M. Intraoperative diagnostic ultrasound. In: *Neurosurgery,* edited by R. H. Wilkins and S. S. Rengachary, pp. 457–463. McGraw-Hill, New York, 1985.
6. Dohrmann, G. J., and Rubin, J. M. Intraoperative real-time ultrasonography: Localization, characterization and instrumentation of lesions of brain and spinal cord. In: *Advanced Intraoperative Technologies in Neurosurgery,* edited by V. A. Fasano, pp. 3–19. Springer-Verlag, New York, 1985.
7. Fager, C. A. Posterior surgical tactics for the neurological syndromes of cervical disc and spondylotic lesions. Clin. Neurosurg., *25:* 218–244, 1978.
8. Fager, C. A. Evaluation of cervical spine surgery by postoperative myelography. Neurosurgery, *12:* 416–421, 1983.
9. Faulhauer, K., and Loew, K. The surgical treatment of syringomyelia. Long-term results. Acta Neurochir., *44:* 215–222, 1978.
10. Haft, H., and Shenkin, H. A. Surgical end results of cervical ridge and disc problems. J.A.M.A., *186:* 312–315, 1963.
11. Jokich, P. M., Rubin, J. M., and Dohrmann, G. J. Intraoperative ultrasonic evaluation of spinal cord motion. J. Neurosurg., *60:* 707–711, 1984.
12. Love, J. G., and Olafson, R. A. Syringomyelia: A look at surgical therapy. J. Neurosurg., *24:* 714–718, 1966.
13. Lunsford, L. D., Bissonette, D. J., and Zorub, D. S. Anterior surgery for cervical disc disease. Part 2. Treatment of cervical spondylotic myelopathy in 32 cases. J. Neurosurg., *53:* 12–19, 1980.

14. Nurick, S. The natural history and the results of surgical treatment of the spinal cord disorder associated with cervical spondylosis. Brain, *95:* 101–108, 1971.

15. Peerless, S. J., and Durward, Q. J. Management of syringomyelia: A pathophysiological approach. Clin. Neurosurg., *30:* 531–576, 1983.

16. Quencer, R. M., Morse, B. M. M., Green, B. A., *et al.* Intraoperative spinal sonography: Adjunct to metrizamide CT in the assessment and surgical decompression of post-traumatic spinal cord cysts. A.J.R., *142:* 593–601, 1984.

17. Rubin, J. M., and Dohrmann, G. J. The spine and spinal cord during neurosurgical operations: Real-time ultrasonography. Radiology, *155:* 197–200, 1985.

18. Rubin, J. M., and Dohrmann, G. J. Intraoperative sonography of the spine and spinal cord. Semin. Ultrasound CT MR *6:* 48–67, 1985.

CHAPTER

17

Anterior Approaches to Lesions of the Upper Cervical Spine

H. ALAN CROCKARD, F.R.C.S.

INTRODUCTION

Subluxations of the upper cervical spine have been recognized as a rare but dangerous complication of a variety of conditions, since Sir Charles Bell, in 1824, described the sudden death of a young man who had been admitted following a fall, to the Middlesex Hospital in London (4). He had recovered, apparently completely and, after thanking the Hospital Governors, lifted his bundle of belongings, placed them on top of his head and dropped to the floor apneic. Autopsy revealed atlantoaxial subluxation. A similar complication was described again by Bell in 1830 following syphilitic ulceration of the pharynx. Since that time, the condition has been diagnosed often at post-mortem following trauma and nasopharyngeal infections. In many instances, the first clinical suspicion of the problem has been the catastrophic terminal event. Occasionally, it was diagnosed during life, making it a problem of management. Hilton (28) in 1841 described an infant who had three transient apneic episodes, in whom the condition was suspected. The child was kept lying flat with his head between rolled towels, only to perish when the midwife, "this meddling and officious woman," ordered the child to sit up and eat breakfast.

The combination of greater clinical awareness, improved investigative procedures, and advances in anesthesia and surgery have allowed considerable progress in internal fixation and stabilization for such patients, initially by a posterior approach, but then, in selected cases, by an anterolateral approach and, more recently, by a midline anterior approach. The original posterior approaches were described by Church and Eisendrath in 1892 (10), where the spinous processes and laminae were tied together with silk.

Knowledge of the association of bony abnormalities of the upper cervical spine and neurological symptoms has gained ground since the 1840s. The early embryological work by Cunningham (18) in 1886 and Chiari pointed to the association of bony, muscle, and ligamentous abnormalities associated with abnormalities of the neural tube. List (33) illustrated how tenuous the spinal cord was in many patients at the time of their presentation with such abnormalities. Again, with improved noninvasive diagnostic techniques, the conditions are recognized more commonly, and the debate on their surgical treatment has moved from the posterior to the anterior approach.

Masses, tumorous or otherwise, involving the upper cervical vertebrae have also been recognized as causing progressive neurological complications. The disappointing results of posterior surgery have stimulated surgeons to look for another way. Anterolateral and anterior approaches have been advocated. More recently, the transoral route has been adopted.

The object of this chapter is to outline some of the more common pathological lesions of the upper cervical spine and review surgical approaches to the alleviation of the neurological problem. As my own experience is essentially based on a transoral approach to the region, a disproportionate amount of the discussion will deal with this. For the purposes of this presentation, the area under consideration will extend from the anterior rim of the foramen magnum down to the third cervical vertebra. Occasionally, because of malformation or distortion of the cervical spine, it has been possible to operate as low as the fifth cervical vertebra using the transoral approach, but this is exceptional.

SURGICAL PATHOLOGY

There is a broad spectrum of disease which can affect the craniocervical junction and the upper cervical spine. With improved visualization and experience, more and more may be amenable to surgical correction. The general principles on which decisions are based include the following: What is the abnormality? Where is it? Is there structural stability, or is the neurological condition due to movement? Will the condition be stable after surgical intervention?

Set out below are some of the commonest lesions in the area. The divisions are somewhat arbitrary, and there is obvious overlap. For instance, many degenerative conditions or developmental abnormalities present after minor trauma.

Developmental Anatomy

The area is derived from four occipital sclerotomes and the upper two cervical sclerotomes (25, 26). The fourth occipital sclerotome is responsible for the occipital condyles and the tip of the odontoid peg. From the first cervical sclerotome develop most of the first cervical vertebra and the main body of the odontoid peg, while the second cervical sclerotome produces the rest of the second cervical vertebra. There are thus many independent ossification centers in the region which would account for the wide variation in pattern which may be seen in health and disease. The axis arises from four primary ossification centers and the odontoid peg from two or perhaps three. Posterior spina bifida is quite a common abnormality in the area, being noted in 3% of all adults (32). Nonfusion during development in the odontoid peg may produce several variations, including an ossiculam terminale, os odontoideum, and nonfusion at the base of the peg (31). Fusion between the first cervical vertebra and the base of the skull (occipitalization or assimilation) of the atlas may be found in asymptomatic patients, and occasionally a third condyle may be noted anterior to the occipital condyles on the base of the skull (53). This is derived from the proatlas which is found naturally in reptiles and some rodents.

Occipitalization (assimilation) of the atlas is a well-recognized variant without neurological symptoms. It may occur in about 1% of all normal adults. It may, however, be associated with neural tube defects or signs of neuraxis compression. It is often associated with other anomalies, such as fusion of the cervical vertebrae. In those in whom there are abnormal neurological signs, the most significant is an abnormal size, position, or unusual mobility of the odontoid process.

The ligaments associated with these joints are multiple and complex. They are extremely lax until the patient reaches the age of 6, as are the neck muscles (51). The neck of the neonate and small child is, therefore, very much at risk to injury during birth or shortly after, which may lead to neurological complications at the occipitoatlantic joints. Rotation occurs around the odontoid peg as an axle, and the atlantoaxial joint allows rotation of the head but is associated with a "telescoping" effect due to the sloping atlantoaxial joint (38). The transverse ligament is extremely powerful and requires a force of 130 kg to break it (33). It holds the odontoid peg as an axle or as a button in a buttonhole. Attached to the tip of the odontoid peg are the strong alar ligaments, and behind those are the cruciate ligaments. These are taut in the midposition when the head is facing forwards (39). Menezes has shown that section of the transverse ligament will allow some displacement of the odontoid peg, up to 4 mm, but any further backward displacement is prevented by the alar ligaments (39). These also, because of their distribution, alternatively relax on one side and tighten on the other during rotation. Laxness or absence of these ligaments will allow the exaggeration of the rotation and "telescoping" effect and is considered by some to be the pathogenesis of basilar invagination due to hypermobility at the joint. Hypoplastic occipital condyles, such as would be found in Morquio's disease, or laxness of the ligaments, as in Down's syndrome, associated with an ossiculum terminale, allow excessive anterior gliding of the skull on the first joint and permit the transverse ligament to slip over the top of the incomplete odontoid peg during a forward rotatory movement, and produce fixed backward dislocation of the peg (51).

The diameters of the foramen magnum are in the region of 30 mm sagittal and coronal, and the internal diameters behind the body of the second vertebra are about 22 mm sagittal (range 16–30 mm) and 23 mm coronal (31). Correlating neurological signs, McCrae found that when the spinal canal was less than 19 mm AP, behind the odontoid peg, or when the odontoid peg was able to move more than 3 mm on flexion or extension, then there were long tract signs (36). It is generally accepted that intermittent narrowing of the spinal canal or the craniocervical junction is more likely to produce neurological signs than a fixed reduction in diameter (53).

On flexion, the cord moves anteriorly at the foramen magnum and, therefore, it is pulled against the subluxing dens. This accentuates the injury, and there was a close correlation in the series of Stevens *et al.*

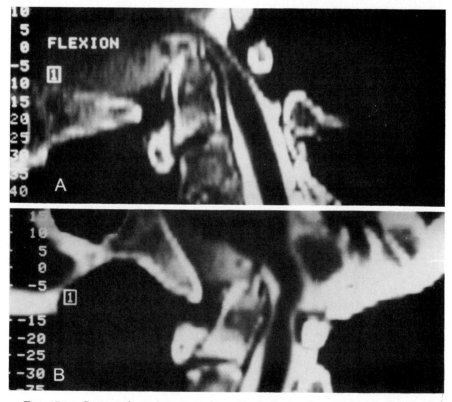

FIG. 17.1. Computed myelotomography with flexion and extension views provides maximum information on instability and cord compression. Note the cranial settling, pannus around posterior arch of C1, and approximation of odontoid peg to medulla and basilar artery in this patient with rheumatoid arthritis. (*A*) Flexion. (*B*) Extension.

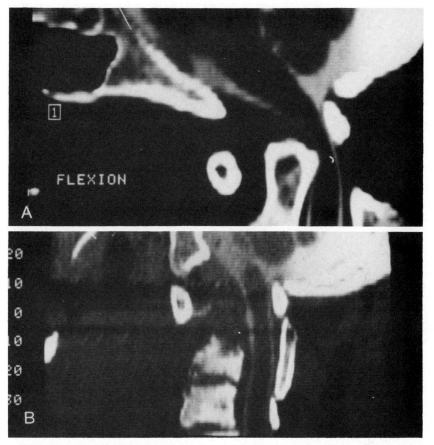

FIG. 17.2.   Computed myelotomography of a fixed subluxation of the atlantoaxial joint causing cord compression resulting from a road accident 14 years previously. (A) Preoperative view. (B) Postoperative view.

between mobility at the atlantoaxial joint, compressive deformity, and neurological signs. They consider this mobility to be more important than the absolute anteroposterior diameter in the region and believe that the cord damage is due to angulation over the subluxing dens as well as to intermittent longitudinal tensions produced in the neuraxis with head flexion (Fig. 17.1) (55).

Trauma

Either acutely or chronically, trauma at the craniocervical junction may lead to compromise of the neuroaxis of an intermittent nature, as when there is nonfusion of the odontoid peg or rupture of the ligaments, or when there is fusion, the bone unites in an abnormal fashion, reducing the AP diameter (Fig. 17.2). In the chronic situation, mild trauma

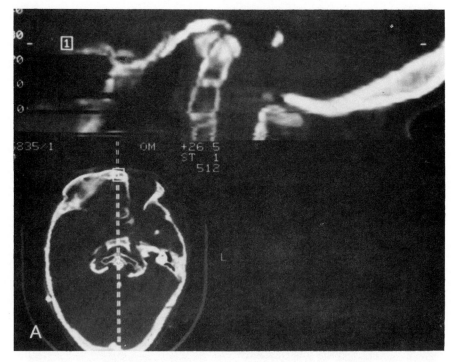

Fig. 17.3. Osteogenesis imperfecta may produce basilar invagination and medullary compression. (A) CT scan outlines bony pathology. (B) Vertebral angiogram displays extreme vascular distortion which may interfere with surgery.

associated with the previous developmental anomaly, such as assimilation of the atlas, platybasia, or the Klippel-Feil deformity, will cause long tract signs (1). As already mentioned, minor trauma will cause signs if there is a local weakness, and this is particularly true of the next three conditions.

Postinfective Condition

Following pharyngeal infection, the ligamentous apparatus at the craniocervical junction may be compromised. In the past, syphilis and tuberculosis have been common causes. Retropharyngeal abscesses and suppuration of lymph nodes in the area are perhaps more common and may be the basic pathology in the so-called hyperemic subluxations noted in young children (26). If the primary infection has settled, there will be little in the way of anterior deforming mass, and it is the ligamentous apparatus which has been compromised.

Metabolic Diseases

An inborn error of metabolism is the basis of many of these patients' problems at the craniocervical junction (29). The commonest presenta-

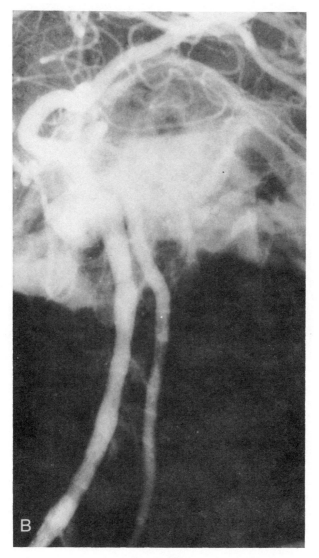

FIG. 17.3*B*

tions are in those patients with Morquio's disease, Hurler's syndrome, or other mucopolysaccharidoses. The ligaments tear or are formed inadequately; bone formation may be impeded and either "bend inwards" or deform by multiple microfractures, as in osteogenesis imperfecta (Fig. 17.3) (46). In addition, there may be ectopic soft tissue masses, as in diaphyseal eclasia, which compress and deform the neuraxis (Fig. 17.4).

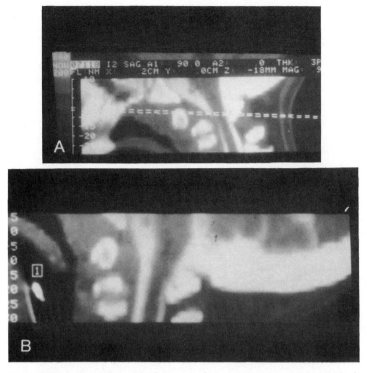

FIG. 17.4. CT myelography with flexion and extension in a patient with diaphyseal eclasia. Note agenesis of odontoid peg, and cord compression due to soft tissue, as well as instability. (A) Flexion. (B) Extension.

Inflammatory Conditions

Rheumatoid arthritis is the commonest disease in this subgroup to present with upper cervical spine problems. In the author's experience, it is the most common cause of craniocervical compression.

In a consecutive series of 104 post-mortems in patients with rheumatoid arthritis who died suddenly, 10% of the deaths were caused by atlantoaxial subluxation and, in them, the compression was by bone and pannus. All of them, whether atlantoaxial subluxation was the cause of death or not, showed an upward and backward displacement of the odontoid peg (40). "Cranial settling" (57) is estimated to be present in 5–8% of all rheumatoid arthritic patients. It was Garrod (23), in 1892, who first drew attention to the compression of the craniospinal junction in rheumatoid patients. It is of interest that he too reported extensor plantar responses in such patients 6 years before Babinski emphasized the significance of this sign. The work was largely forgotten until recently, and the condition was "rediscovered" by Davis and Markely (19) in 1951. In a recent prospective study of patients with rheumatoid arthritis,

Windfield *et al.* (60) have shown that cervical subluxation may develop in association with peripheral erosive disease within 2 years of its onset, although remaining asymptomatic. In those with longstanding disease, 25–36% have significant myelopathy (34, 54). The myelopathy is rapidly progressive in half of such cases and may cause the death of the patient within a year, despite conservative measures (43). Boyle, in his review of 325 cases from the world literature, showed that the most common joint to be affected was the atlantoaxial (49%), although all of the cervical joints could be affected, and in some cases, a "staircase" phenomenon was noted (Fig. 17.5) (6). Plain lateral radiographs of the cervical spine

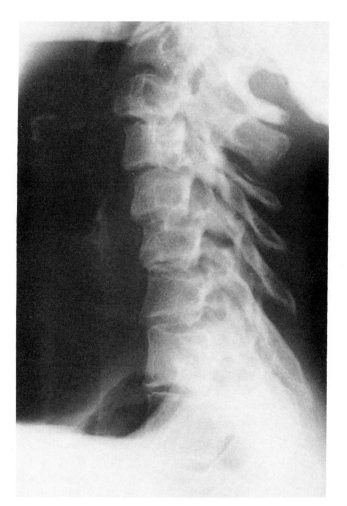

FIG. 17.5. "Staircase" phenomenon causing myelopathy in rheumatoid arthritis. Improvement with posterior stabilization.

and those in flexion and extension reveal the abnormal mobility, and it was natural that the initial operations were aimed at restoring bony alignment and inducing fixation by bone graft (8, 12, 44). From the world literature, there has been a significant mortality associated with the posterior occipitoatlantoaxial fusion and the acceptance of its inevitability which was implicit in Hamblen's contribution (27). The role of the pannus had not been taken into account, although Garrod had drawn attention to it, and Boyle had also emphasized it in his post-mortem studies. It has been the soft tissue component associated with the bony subluxation which has occupied much of our attention. The reduction in mortality associated with our surgical procedure is evidence of this aspect of the pathology (14–16).

In alkylosing spondylitis, when most of the joints are fused, there is an increase in stress on the joints that remain mobile. The atlantoaxial joint is often the last to be affected in the condition, and thus, a subluxation may occur at this joint as the last vestiges of movement in the neck disappear. A secondary phenomenon is the erosion of the occipitoatlanto and atlantoaxial joints, causing cranial settling, and thus the unfortunate patient may have significant compromise of his cervicomedullary junction (Fig. 17.6).

Extradural Tumor

These may occur in the upper cervical spine and may be primary tumors, such as aneurysmal bone cysts, osteoblastomas and, more rarely, osteoclastomas. Chordomas are commonest of these primary tumors and compose about 20% of all chordomas, the commonest sites being sacro-coccygeal (50%) and clivus (30%) (Fig. 17.7) (3).

Metastases are seen occasionally in the body of C1, the occipital condyle, or the odontoid peg and may produce unremitting occipital pain. In most, the problem can be treated by posterior fusion, followed by local radiotherapy, but in some, the metastatic mass produces significant anterior compression and, for that reason, we have debulked the tumor anteriorly by the transoral route as well as by posterior fixation followed by radiotherapy; pharyngeal spread of tumor has not been noted.

Intradural Tumor

It is very rare indeed that upper cervical tumors are inaccessible from a conventional posterior approach. Occasionally they are, and it is of considerable advantage to the surgeon to be familiar with the transoral approach to remove such tumors. It has been particularly gratifying to effect a radical and/or total removal of a schwannoma or meningioma

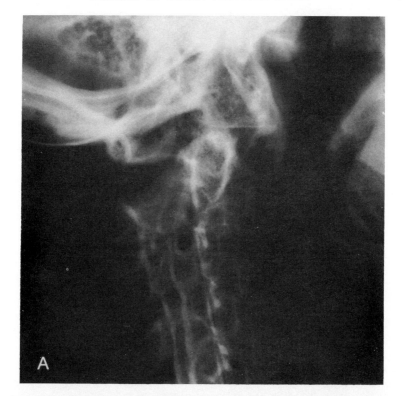

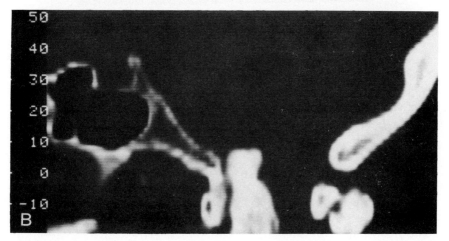

FIG. 17.6.   (A) Ankylosing spondylitis with a fixed compressive fracture dislocation of odontoid peg. (B) CT scan provides much more information and identifies "cranial settling" in some patients.

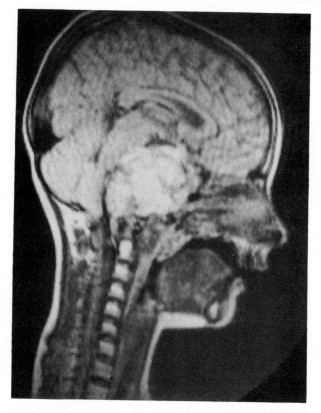

FIG. 17.7. Clival chordoma in a 12-year-old girl, extending behind odontoid and compressing base of brain. MRI provides excellent visualization of basal tumors.

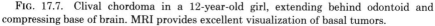

without producing neurological complications. Because the tumor lies anterior to the spinal cord, its blood supply, and the lower cranial and upper cervical nerve rootlets, there has been a good plane of cleavage between the tumor and these important structures (Fig. 17.8).

Iatrogenic Disease of the Cervical Spine

The cervical spine may develop a grotesque kyphus with a deteriorating neurological condition following radiotherapy and extensive posterior cervical laminectomy. Disruption of the interspinous ligaments and destruction of facet joints as part of a decompressive procedure may also result in later anterior angulation. Interspinous wire or plate fixation for treatment of vertebral body trauma may also result in this unpleasant complication. In such a situation, further posterior surgery would be of no advantage, and anterior removal of the "knuckle" anterior base grafting and external halo body fixation may be necessary (Fig. 17.9).

SURGICAL APPROACHES TO THE UPPER CERVICAL SPINE

At the turn of the century, an attempt was made to stabilize atlantoaxial subluxation by interlaminar wire fixation (20), and as the potential neurological problems were due to instability and not compression, this technique has been usefully developed (1). The deterioration associated with basilar invagination was recognized later, and List (32) attempted relief of the anterior compression at the craniocervical junction by posterior decompression. With the patient in the sitting position and under local anesthesia, a posterior fossa decompression and removal of the arches of C1 and C2 allowed exposure of the craniocervical junction and upper cervical spine. On occasion, the anatomy was so distorted that a band of "fibrous tissue" was divided and confirmed at post-mortem to be grossly thinned and a distorted part of still-functioning cervical spinal cord. Of the seven operative cases that he reported, three died during the operation or immediately afterwards. With improvements, the operative mortality for this approach has been reduced, but the long-term results

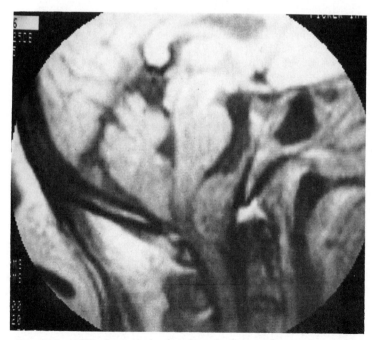

FIG. 17.8.   MRI of anteriorly placed meningioma at foramen magnum.

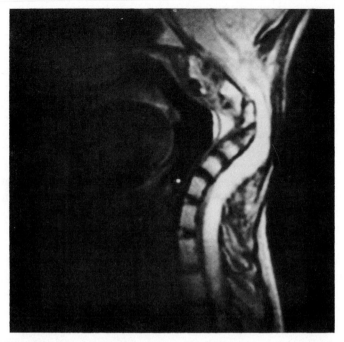

FIG. 17.9.   Decompressive laminectomy and radiotherapy produce a kyphus at C2,3,4
with bony radionecrosis and quadriplegia.

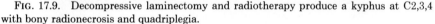

have not been entirely satisfactory. Often the neurological signs have
progressed either because the anterior compressive element had not been
relieved or because of craniocervical instability produced by the posterior
surgical decompression.

Using the anterior approach to the lower cervical spine, Cloward (11)
demonstrated that it was the anterior compressive elements in cervical
disc disease and spondylosis which most embarrassed the spinal cord and
nerve roots. These could be removed, allowed neurological recovery and,
by maintaining anatomical integrity of joints and ligaments, permitted
good postoperative movement without the complications of posterior
laminectomy, such as angulation and kyphus. The innate logic of an
anterior approach to anteriorly placed lesions in the upper cervical spine
is generally accepted, but its execution has been somewhat more taxing
because of the position of the mandible, the outflow of cranial nerves
and the position of the great vessels.

By employing an extension of Henry's exposure, Robinson (48, 49),
Cloward (11), and Verbiest (58, 59) described anterolateral approaches
to the upper cervical spine. Using an incision along the anterior border

of sternomastoid, the muscle might be disconnected at the mastoid process. The styloid process is also disconnected, and the great vessels are retracted anteriorly, which allows an approach to the tubercles and, with further retraction, to the vertebral bodies themselves. The incision may be extended to outline the anterior rim of the foramen magnum and the lower aspect of the cervical vertebral column. Verbiest and Robinson had extensive experience of bony abnormalities in the area, and Cloward describes the radical excision of a chordoma using this technique. All make the point that postoperative swelling in the surrounding tissue is a major problem.

Perforation of the pharynx with subsequent soiling was also a recognized complication. Derome (20) has approached the upper cervical spine in another way. His greatest experience has been tumor of the base of skull, and using either a rhinoseptal approach by itself or in combination with a frontal craniotomy, he has extended his exposure to the anterior margin of the foramen magnum and has excised tumors of the upper cervical vertebrae. An attempt is made to stay outside the pharynx by reflecting forward the nasopharyngeal mucosa and the superior and middle constrictors. The approach would provide excellent exposure for skull base tumors extending into the upper cervical spine but may be less useful when the lesion is located primarily at C1 and C2. Another approach involves a supraalveolar osteotomy of the maxilla with a downfracturing of the superior alveolar margin. This technique has been employed with success for a midclival procedure, including a transdural approach to midbasilar aneurysm, as well as surgery at the craniocervical junction, but may not provide an optimal view of the vertebral column.

The transoral transpharyngeal approach was described first by Kanavel in 1919 (30), who used it to extract a bullet lodged between C1 and the base of the skull. Scoville and Sherman (50) recommended it for lesions of the anterior rim of the foramen magnum, and Mullan et al. (42) used it for the removal of extradurally situated tumors. Fang and Ong (21) published the largest experience of the approach for tumors and infective conditions in the region.

The first approach to the region for rheumatoid arthritis has been attributed to Sukoff et al. (56), and since that time, there has been an increasing number of reports, describing the approach to lesions on the clivus and upper cervical spine. There have been several problems which have hindered its widespread use in the past, which include surgical exposure, lighting, access, instruments sufficiently long to operate, and the risk of infection in the soft tissue of the pharynx. Surgical progress through the dura has been limited by the fears of spinal fluid fistula and meningitis.

TRANSORAL TRANSPHARYNGEAL TECHNIQUE

There are excellent accounts in the literature describing approaches to the area (2, 5, 7, 21, 24, 42, 45). Our own has developed from these (14) and modified to allow transdural surgery anteriorly and access for a posterior occipitoatlantoaxial fusion in selected patients. The team approach is absolutely essential to the procedure's success and has evolved through the contribution of radiologist (55), anesthetist (35), orthopaedic surgeon (49), and neurosurgeon (14). This cooperative evaluation is presented below.

Radiography

Good quality plain radiographs of the skull and cervical spine with flexion and extension views are a very useful preliminary investigation. Basilar invagination or platybasia may be deduced from the plain radiographs using measurements described by McGregor (37), Chamberlain (9), and Fischgold (22). The first used a line extending from the posterior edge of the hard palate to the cordal part of the occiput. The odontoid peg should be below this line. Chamberlain's line is a modification of the former, while Fischgold's line extends through the lower part of the mastoid process, and normally this should pass through the atlantooccipital joint.

Computed Tomography (CT)

Imaging of the highest quality is the key to surgical planning and has replaced conventional multiplanar tomography. With CT reconstructions in any plane, there is information on the movement of individual joints in flexion and extension. Although some authors have recommended the procedure on its own, we have concentrated on computed myelotomography with scans in flexion and extension to provide information on the bones, the joints, the soft tissue masses, and the deformation of the spinal cord. Stevens et al. (55) emphasized the importance of cord deformity in evaluating the total neurological condition of the patient. The noncompressive deformities may be secondary to vascular events or previous injury and may not improve following surgical decompression. Compressive lesions, however, would be expected to improve following decompression. Our data would indicate that it is the intermittently applied anterior deforming force which is the most significant mechanism of injury in rheumatoid atlantoaxial subluxation. With the pannus and cranial settling, it was this information which convinced us of the correctness of the anterior surgical approach.

Angiography

Rotation of the atlas may bring the vertebral artery into the operative field. This may be anticipated by studying the CT scans but in developmental anomalies of the area, we routinely perform four vessel angiography to identify the vessels' position (Fig. 17.3B).

Magnetic Resonance Imaging (MRI)

MRI has provided excellent information, particularly in the definition of a syrinx or intradural and extradural tumors. It has been less successful in outlining the bony abnormalities of the craniocervical junction. First, the image definition is not as good as that of current CT techniques. More important, however, particularly with people in pain, is the long scanning time which, to date, has precluded flexion and extension studies. Doubtless, with the reduction of scanning time, the technique will be increasingly used.

PREOPERATIVE ASSESSMENT

General Medical Assessment

General medical assessment is obviously important. Many of the patients are on steroids and azathioprine. The skin is often thin, and degloving injuries of a limb have been described in the positioning of the rheumatoid patient on the operating table. Clotting studies may be required. The microbiological flora of the nose and throat should be examined prior to surgery.

Preoperatively, we perform somatosensory evoked potentials (52) and baseline studies of respiratory patterns. Motor evoked potentials are currently being evaluated.

The Mouth

The mouth should be inspected carefully, before a decision on transoral surgery. If the teeth do not open more than 2 cm, it is likely that a mandibular split or other technique will have to be used to approach the craniocervical junction anteriorly. Many of the rheumatoid patients have poor dentition as part of the generalized disease, and the presence of a single tooth in the upper jaw may create problems for retraction. Neck mobility should also be examined. On occasions, though the jaw opens adequately, exposure is difficult because of the deformity and marked forward flexion and may necessitate a soft and hard palate split.

ANESTHESIA FOR TRANSORAL SURGERY

Some of our early experience has been documented by Marks et al. (35), but the current protocol is that used by my colleague, Dr. Ian Calder (personal communication, 1986).

A benzodiazepine and hyoscine are administered as *premedication*, the latter to dry up nasopharyngeal secretions. Steroids are administered if there is cord compression or a "booster dose" to those who are already on steroids for their rheumatoid arthritis.

Induction of Anesthesia

The induction of anesthesia is one of the most critical parts of the procedure. Originally, we used an orotracheal airway and performed tracheostomies on most of the patients. However, with increasing experience, it is exceptional now for us to perform a tracheostomy, relying instead on an armored Mallinckrodt nasotracheal tube which is left in position for the early postoperative period. This is much better tolerated postoperatively than an orotracheal tube. A nasogastric tube is also passed and left in for 5 days, initially to empty stomach contents and later to allow feeding. Both tubes aid wound toilet, and the airway is to prevent complications from postoperative swelling in the oropharynx. The actual decision on the method of intubation depends on Cormack's formula (13). Measurements from the radiographs of the hard palate, the mandible, and the craniocervical junction allow a calculation which predicts which patient will present difficulties. In these cases, following local anesthesia in the conscious patient, the nasotracheal tube is passed with the aid of an Olympus fiberscope. If the formula predicts a relatively smooth nasotracheal intubation, the patient is anesthetized with thiopentone, is given suxamethonium, and the nasotracheal tube is passed with direct visualization, using the fiberscope. All patients are given 5–7 mg droperidol for its antiemetic properties.

Controlled ventilation with intravenous anesthetic agents is used, but in the very difficult patients, with evidence of medullary compromise prior to surgery or in whom extensive clival surgery is contemplated, we have reverted to spontaneous respiration with the patient anesthetised with halothane, as it is considered to be the least respiration-depressing of all the volatile agents. Conditions for surgery are not as good as for those whose ventilation is controlled and whose blood pressure is more easily manipulated, but the technique provides one more way of monitoring the compromised medulla during the operation by carefully observing the respiratory rate, tidal volume, and respiratory pattern during the operative procedure. This has provided a much earlier warning of medullary problems than somatosensory evoked potentials.

Transdural Procedure

For transdural procedures, a lumbar drain is inserted at this stage and left in position for 5 days to keep CSF pressure low and to remove debris; it is then converted into a permanent lumboperitoneal shunt.

Positioning

All patients' heads are held in the Mayfield skull clamp. The supine position is adopted for the transdural procedures and the extensive extradural tumors of the clivus and upper cervical spine. For the former, the supine position is particularly advantageous during the dural closure. The disadvantage of the position is that irrigating saline and blood collect in the operative site.

For this reason, and to allow posterior fixation under the same anesthetic, a lateral position has been adopted in the rheumatoid patients and those with upper cervical spine problems. The operative field is kept clear, and the surgeon may sit. The exact position of the head is determined by the deformity, by the position of least medullary or cord compression, and by any change in physiological monitoring. Ideally some extension improves surgical visibility for the transoral procedure, and slight flexion assist the passage of the interlaminar wires for the posterior fixation. The fixed head position, just as the wires are tightened to the contoured tracking loop, is one of the slight head flexion to allow the patient to scan the ground when ambulant.

Retraction and Exposure

One of the major obstacles to successful surgery in this area is exposure, particularly the pharynx behind the soft palate. Initially, the Boyle-Davis mouth gag was used with incision of the soft palate. There are problems such as breakdown of the palatal wound in the short term, and in the long term, many patients have a nasal voice and regurgitate fluids through the nose when drinking. The soft palate may be retracted up into the nasopharynx using a Jacques catheter introduced through the napes and attached to the uvular area (52). This "tenting up" provides removable midline visibility but little laterally (Fig. 17.10).

A retractor has been developed which allows cephalad and lateral visualization without splitting the soft palate. It provides protection for the nasotracheal and nasogastric tubes. In the extensive exposure requiring incisions in the soft and hard palate, that is, for tumors of the clivus, the retractor is again very useful in providing lateral exposure during the surgery. Since the development of this retractor, it is exceptional for a palatal incision to be required for any lesion below the foramen magnum (transoral retractor, Codman Ltd.)

Occasionally, the jaw will not open more than 2 cm. This usually occurs in the rheumatoid patients with affection of the temporomandibular joint by the disease. In such a situation, the transoral procedure has been used, but exposure produced by a midline mandibular osteotomy which allows lateral retraction of both parts of the mandible has also been used. The tongue and soft tissues can then be depressed downward using the retractor. At the end of the procedure, the mandible is repositioned and held with a small compression screw plate. No particular postoperative

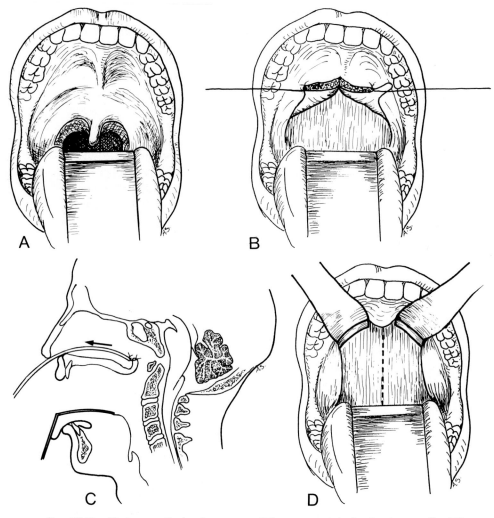

FIG. 17.10.   Various methods of exposure of the upper cervical spine transorally. (*A*) Soft palate in normal place. (*B*) Splitting soft palate. (*C*) "Tenting" using Jacques catheter. (*D*) New transoral retractor allowing cephalad and lateral exposure without palatal incision.

complications have been encountered from this more extended procedure, and the authors have been impressed by the lack of bleeding as compared to a transglottic procedure.

Surgical Exposure

The operating microscope is used for the whole of the transoral procedure. The tissue is infiltrated with Adrenalin and 1% lignocaine to reduce the bleeding. A midline pharyngeal incision is used, from the anterior rim of the foramen magnum down to the body of C2 and is extended if necessary. The incision should go through the mucosa and the muscle of the superior and middle constrictors. Lateral exposure is gained by retraction sutures. Some authors recommend a square flap in the area in an effort to reduce wound breakdown. The complication has not been a major problem in our experience; we emphasize the importance of a two-layer closure, separately suturing the constrictor muscles apart from the mucosa, and we have not had problems with wound breakdown. For that reason, a pharyngeal flap has not been considered necessary. Deep to the pharyngeal constrictor is the tubercle on the anterior arch of C1, to which is attached the anterior longitudinal ligament and the insertion of the upper fibers of the longus coli muscles. This is an important landmark, early recognition of which will greatly speed up the procedure. Very occasionally, the first or second cervical vertebrae may not only have subluxed forward, but also there may be an element of rotation as well. This is particularly true in rheumatoid patients, and in one patient, the presenting midline part was the bone over the vertebral artery canal. Careful attention to the CT reconstruction will reduce surgical anguish from this problem. Once the arch of C1 is identified, the rest of the bone in the area may be exposed in sequence. There is little difficulty in outlining the disc space between the second and third vertebra, and with angulation of the retractor, all of the third cervical vertebral body, down to the disc space, can be adequately exposed. To expose the odontoid peg, 1 cm of the anterior arch of C1 is removed using the air drill, and after removing the synovium behind it, the odontoid peg is visible. The peg is then removed using the air drill with a burr down to cortical bone and a diamond drill for final removal of the cortex. The alar and apical ligaments are often difficult structures to mobilize, but the tip of the peg may be removed without dural penetration, as the posterior longitudinal ligament should still be intact. If there has been extensive upward migration of the odontoid peg, the anterior rim of the foramen magnum may also be removed. There are usually interconnecting veins in the area between the circumferential venous sinus of the foramen magnum area and the posterior pharyngeal veins. They can be controlled with bipolar coagulation. Apart from direct injury to the vertebral artery, bleeding is not a major problem during this procedure. If the abnormality is at C2 or below, or if the odontoid peg has been eroded and replaced with soft tissue pannus, the anterior arch of C1 need not be removed. Instead, the soft tissue would be removed below and behind it, and the vertebral body of C2 may be removed with the air drill. In the rheumatoid patient, the removal of pannus is important, as it is a significant compressing factor. No attempt is made to insert bone graft anteriorly in any of the rheumatoid patients. In those with developmental or posttraumatic abnormalities, we have used cancellous bone chips rather than moulded, tight-fitting bone grafts from fibula or tibia and found good new bone formation as a result of this. In some cases, notably the hangman's fractures, a bone graft, carefully formed, has been inserted into the area. To date, we have had no rejection of bone graft and have seen good bone assimilation in all cases despite the insertion of the graft through the mouth.

For the transdural approaches, a wider bony removal has been performed, taking the lower 2 cm of the clivus, C1, and most of C2. This allows a dural exposure of up to 5 or 6 cm in length and a maximum of 14 mm in breadth (wider lateral resection into the occipital condyles may provoke massive bleeding from the veins draining into the jugular foramina). Incision of the dura will allow exposure of the tumor, which may be dealt with in the usual neurosurgical fashion. The chief advantage of the procedure for anteriorly placed meningiomas or schwannomas is that the brain stem, medulla, and upper cervical rootlets will be pushed backwards out of the operative field by the lesion (17). The vertebral arteries will also be pushed cephalad and dorsally, and only the anterior spinal artery is at risk. To date, the dissection of the lesion off the overlying neural tissue has been relatively straightforward (41). The laser has been employed, but because of the design of the handpiece, the Cavitron ultrasonic aspirator (CUSA) has not been used successfully.

Dural closure has been greatly simplified with the advent of Tisseal (Immuno, Austria), manufactured from human fibrin and thrombin. A fascia graft plus Tisseal and two layers of pharyngeal closure has produced good "waterproofing." The importance of the lumbar drain and its conversion to a lumboperitoneal shunt must be emphasized. Any rise in CSF pressure in the first 3 or 4 weeks may result in an oral CSF fistula.

Closure of the wound is by interrupted Vicryl sutures in two layers: the approximation of the muscle layer is very important. As the patient swallows, the muscles contract, and it is this mechanism which the author considers to be the cause of pharyngeal wound breakdown.

POSTERIOR FUSION

There are many stabilizing techniques which involve bone graft obtained from rib or iliac crest, but the problem is that they require a prolonged period of immobilization in a halo body jacket or in skull traction in bed. One of the major problems, particularly with sick rheumatoid patients, is that they have great difficulty in a halo body jacket; in addition, prolonged immobilization in bed results in a high incidence of complications. It was for that reason that we elected to perform a definitive one-stage procedure on such patients, performing the decompression and the posterior fixation under the same anesthetic (16). This, therefore, required firm internal stabilization as well as bony fixation. Initially, we performed bone grafts on all rheumatoid patients, as well as the internal fixation. While we had good results in terms of bone fusion in patients with basilar invagination, the incidence of firm bony union in the rheumatoid patient was so low that we have abandoned this and depend entirely on stability by a contoured tracking loop. In over 3 years now, we have had no major problems with this policy.

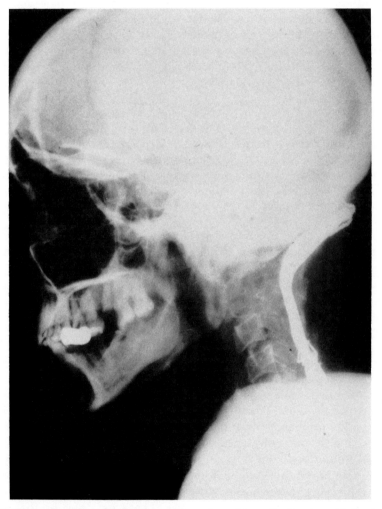

FIG. 17.11.   Posterior stabilization using contoured loop fixation is carried out under the same anesthetic in patient whose C1-2 chordoma has been excised transorally.

Initially, our posterior fixation was with interlaminar wire loops. However, the problem with this form of fixation has been the tendency of forward subluxation of the remainder of C1. For that reason, my orthopedic colleague, Andrew Ransford et al. (47) devised a tracking loop contoured to suit the occiput and the upper cervical spine (Fig. 17.11).

Having exposed the occiput and the upper cervical laminae, a flavumectomy is performed and a 20-gauge wire is passed around the laminae in the usual fashion. Initially we passed wires around the foramen magnum and through a burr hole, but this is one of the most difficult areas to pass wires around. Instead, we pass the wire through two small drill holes in the occiput along the outer margin of the tracking loop with the head fixed in the neutral or slightly flexed position.

If a bone graft is required, cancellous bone chips obtained from the iliac crest region are inserted onto the laminae and the occiput, which have been previously decorticated.

POSTOPERATIVE CARE

Our aim as far as possible is that when the patient recovers from anesthesia, the neck is stable. It is only occasionally that skull traction is used, and in the rheumatoid patients particularly, there is a considerable advantage to them waking up in a soft collar and being mobilized in 24–48 hours. Details of our postoperative regime are given elsewhere; a summary table is given here (Table 17.1).

PERSONAL EXPERIENCE

There is an increasing demand for the procedure, and the author's personal experience is given in Table 17.2. The largest experience has been with atlantoaxial subluxation in rheumatoid arthritis, and one never ceases to be amazed at the resilience of these systemically ill patients. In contrast, the young people with severe medullary compression have been very brittle and have required the most intense postoperative management.

There have been 3 deaths in 64 cases and, with hindsight, 2 of these might have been prevented. One was inadequately decompressed anteriorly; the second developed postoperative obstruction of the tracheostomy; and the third developed extensive medullary swelling. The commonest postoperative problems have been pulmonary infections which have settled with aggressive physiotherapy and appropriate antibiotics.

Palatal wound breakdown was a problem initially, but a 2-layer resuture has eliminated this complication. There have been four pharyngeal wounds which broke down, but none required resuture; all healed with delayed diversion of pharyngeal contacts. There has been no incidence of anterior bone graft rejection due to infection.

TABLE 17.1

Transoral Surgery: Postoperative Management

		Days
Airway	Until swelling subsides	$2 \to 5$
Ventilation	Depending on blood gases	$1 \to 2$
Nasogastric tube	Prevent regurgitation fluids	$1 \to 2$
	Nutrition	$2 \to 5$
Nil by mouth		5
Mouth care		$7 \to 10$
Mobilize	With soft collar	$2 \to 3$
Intravenous fluids	Avoid overload	$2 \to 3$
Analgesia	Morphine infusion (0–5 mg/hr; reduce if respiration below 10/min)	$1 \to 2$
Metoclopramide	10 mg, every 6 hr	$2 \to 3$
Cimetidine	400 mg, 12 hr	$5 \to 7$
Antibiotics	Flucloxicillin	5
	Metronidazole	5

[a] A summary of postoperative care given to medical and nursing personnel taking care of transoral patient.

TABLE 17.2

Transoral Surgery for Craniocervical Pathology (July 1983–July 1986, H.A.C.[a])

Condition	Sex		Age Span	OP Deaths	Totals
	M	F			
Developmental	5	1	$21 \to 57$	0	6
Trauma	1	2	$14 \to 46$	1	3
Metabolic	1	3	$12 \to 23$	2	4
Inflammatory	11	28	$21 \to 79$	0	39
Tumor (extradural)	2	4	$12 \to 61$	0	6
Tumor (intradural)	1	3	$47 \to 58$	0	4
Iatrogenic	2	0	$19 \to 63$	0	2
	23	41		3	64

[a] The author's transoral surgical experience is subdivided as in the surgical pathology section. The largest experience has been with rheumatoid arthritis.

CONCLUSIONS

As improved imaging techniques demonstrate more and more problems at the craniocervical junction and upper cervical spine, surgeons will be offered the opportunity to treat such patients. The transoral procedure offers another route to this area, and the base of the skull and experience to date demonstrate that it is a reliable and efficient method of surgical correction.

REFERENCES

1. Alexander, E., Forsyth, H. F., Davis, C. H., *et al.* Dislocation of the atlas on the axis: The value of early fusion of C1, C2 and C3. J. Neurosurg., *15:* 353–371, 1958.

2. Apuzzo, M. L. J., Weiss, M. H., and Heiden, J. S. Transoral exposure of the atlanto-axial region. Neurosurgery, *3:* 201–207, 1978.

3. Bell, B. A., O'Neill, P., Miller, J. D., *et al.* Fifty years of experience with chordomas in Southeast Scotland. Neurosurgery *16:* 166–170, 1985.

4. Bell, C. The nervous system of the human body, p. 93. Longman, Rees, Orme, Brown, & Green, London, 1830.

5. Bonney, G., and Williams, J. P. R. Transoral approach to the upper cervical spine. J. Bone Joint Surg. [Br.], *67B:* 691–698, 1985.

6. Boyle, A. C. The rheumatoid neck. Proc. R. Soc. Med., *64:* 1161–1165, 1971.

7. Brattstrom, H., Elner, A., and Granholm, L. Transoral surgery for myelopathy caused by rheumatoid arthritis of the cervical spine. Ann. Rheum. Dis., *32:* 578–581, 1973.

8. Brattstrom, H., and Granholm, L. Atlanto-axial fusion in rheumatoid arthritis. Acta Orthop. Scand., *47:* 619–628, 1976.

9. Chamberlain, W. E. Basilar impression (platybasia): Bizarre developmental anomaly of occipital bone and upper cervical spine with striking misleading neurologic manifestations. Yale J. Biol. Med., *11:* 487–496, 1939.

10. Church, A., and Eisendrath, D. W. A contribution to spinal cord surgery. Am. J. Med. Sci., *103:* 395–412, 1892.

11. Cloward, R. B. The anterior approach for ruptured cervical disc. J. Neurosurg., *15:* 602–614, 1958.

12. Conathy, J. P., and Mongan, E. S. Cervical fusion in rheumatoid arthritis. J. Bone Joint Surg. [Am.], *63A:* 1218–1227, 1981.

13. Cormack, R. S. Cormack's formula (letter to the editor). Anaesth *41:* 664–665, 1986.

14. Crockard, H. A. The transoral approach to the base of the brain and upper cervical cord. Ann. R. Coll. Surg. Eng., *67:* 321–325, 1985.

15. Crockard, H. A., and Bradford, R. Transoral transclival removal of a schwannoma anterior to the cranio-cervical junction. J. Neurosurg., *62:* 293–295, 1985.

16. Crockard, H. A., Essigman, W. K., Stevens, J. M., *et al.* Surgical treatment of cervical cord compression in rheumatoid arthritis. Ann. Rheum. Dis., *44:* 809–816, 1985.

17. Crockard, H. A., Pozo, J. L., Ransford, A. O., *et al.* Transoral decompression and posterior fusion for rheumatoid atlanto-axial subluxation. J. Bone Joint Surg. [Br.], *68B:* 350–356, 1986.

18. Cunningham, D. J. The development of neural tube. J. Physiol. (Lond.), *20:* 238–243, 1888.

19. Davis, F. N., and Markley, H. E. Rheumatoid arthritis with death from medullary compression. Ann. Intern. Med., *35:* 451–461, 1951.

20. Derome, P. J. The transoral approach to tumours invading the base of the skull. In: *Operative Neurosurgical Techniques,* edited by H. H. Schmidek and W. H. Sweet, p. 357–379. Grune & Stratton, New York, 1982.

21. Fang, H. S. Y., and Ong, G. B. Direct approach to the upper cervical spine. J. Bone Joint Surg. [Am.], *44A:* 1588–1604, 1962.

22. Fischgold, H., and Metzger, J. Etudes radio-tomographique de l'impression basilaire. Rev. Rheum., *19:* 261–264, 1952.

23. Garrod, A. E. A treatise on rheumatism and rheumatoid arthritis. pp. 1–342. C. Griffith, London, 1890.

24. Gilsbach, J., and Eggart, H-R. Transoral operations for cranio-spinal malformations. Neurosurg. Rev., *6:* 199–209, 1983.

25. Gladstone, R. J., and Erichsen-Powell, W. Manifestation of occipital vertebrae and fusion of the atlas with the occipital bone. J. Anat. Physiol., *49:* 190–209, 1914.

26. Greenberg, A. D. Atlanto-axial dislocations. Brain, *91:* 655–684, 1968.

27. Hamblen, D. L. Postgraduate textbook of clinical orthopaedics, pp. 487–497. Wright, Bristol, England, 1983.

28. Hilton, J. Rest and pain: A course of lectures. George Bell & Sons, London, 1892.

29. Hurwitz, L. J., and Shepherd, W. H. T. Basilar impression and disordered metabolism of bone. Brain, 89: 223–233, 1966.

30. Kanavel, A. B. Bullet located between the atlas and the base of the skull: Technique for removal through the mouth. Surg. Clin., 1: 361–366, 1919.

31. Lang, J. Cranio-cervical region: Osteology and articulations. Neuro-orthopaedics, 1: 67–92, 1986.

32. List, C. F. Neurologic syndromes accompanying developmental anomalies of occipital bone, atlas and axis. Arch. Neurol. Psychiatry, 45: 577–618, 1941.

33. MacAlister, J. Quoted in: Gray's Anatomy, Ed. 35, edited by R. Warwick and P. L. Williams, p. 1204. Longmans, London, 1958.

34. Marks, J. S. and Sharp, J. Rheumatoid cervical myelopathy. Q. J. Med., 199: 307–319, 1981.

35. Marks, R. J., Forrester, P. C., Calder, I., et al. Anaesthesia for transoral cranio-cervical surgery. Anaesthesia, 41: 1049–1052, 1986.

36. McCrae, D. L. The significance of abnormalities of the cervical spine. Ann. J Roentgenol., 84: 3–25, 1960.

37. McGregor, M. Significance of certain measurements of skull in diagnosis of basilar impression. Br. J. Radiol., 21: 171–187, 1948.

38. Menezes, A. H., Graf, G. J., and Hibri, N. Abnormalities of the cranio-vertebral junction with cervico-medullary compression. Child's Brain, 7: 15–30, 1980.

39. Menezes, A. H., Van Gilder, J. C., Clark, C. R., et al. Odontoid n rheumatoid arthritis. J. Neurosurg., 63: 500–509, 1985.

40. Mikulowski, P., Wollheim, F. A., Rotmil, P., et al. Sudden deaths in rheumatoid arthritis with atlanto-axial dislocation. Acta Med. Scand., 198: 945–951, 1975.

41. Miller, E., and Crockard, H. A. Transoral transclival removal of anteriorly placed meningiomas at the foramen magnum. Neurosurgery, 20: 683–687, 1987.

42. Mullan, S., Naunton, R., Hekmat-Panah, J., et al. The use of an anterior approach to ventrally placed tumours in the foramen magnum and vertebral column. J. Neurosurg., 24: 536–543, 1966.

43. Nakano, K. K. Neurological complications of rheumatoid arthritis. Orthop. Clin. North Am., 6: 861–881, 1975.

44. Newman, P., and Sweetnam, D. R. Posterior fusion for atlanto-axial subluxation in rheumatoid arthritis. J. Bone Joint Surg. [Br.], 51B: 423–428, 1969.

45. Pasztor, E., Vajda, J., and Piffko, P. Transoral surgery for cranio-cervical space occupying process. J. Neurosurg., 60: 276–281, 1984.

46. Pozo, J. L., Crockard, H. A., and Ransford, A. O. Basilar impression in osteogenesis imperfecta. J. Bone Joint Surg. [Br.], 66B: 233–238, 1984.

47. Ransford, A. O., Crockard, H. A., Pozo, J. L. et al. Cranio-cervical instability treated by contoured loop fixation. J. Bone Joint Surg. [Br.], 68B: 173–177, 1986.

48. Robinson, R. A. Approaches to the cervical spine C1-T1. In: Operative Neurosurgical Techniques, edited by H. H. Schmedek and W. H. Sweet. pp. 1213–1220. Grune & Stratton, New York, 1982.

49. Robinson, R. A., and Riley, L. H. Technique of exposure and fusion of the cervical spine. Clin. Orthop., 109: 78–84, 1975.

50. Scoville, W. B., and Sherman, I. J. Platybasia: Report of ten cases with comments on familial tendency, a special diagnostic sign and end result of operations. Ann. Surg., 133: 469–502, 1951.

51. Sherk, H. H., and Nicholson, J. T. Rotatory atlanto-axial dislocation associated with ossiculum terminale and mongolism. J. Bone Joint Surg. [Am.], *51A:* 957–972, 1969.
52. Spetzler, R. F., Selman, W. R., and Nash, C. L. Transoral microsurgical removal, odontoid resection and spinal cord monitoring. Spine, *4:* 506–510, 1979.
53. Spillane, J. D., Pallis, C., and Jones, A. P. I. Developmental abnormalities in the region of the foramen magnum. Brain, *80:* 11–53, 1957.
54. Stevens, J. C., Cartledge, N. E. F., Saunders, M., *et al.* Atlanto-axial subluxation and cervical myelopathy in rheumatoid arthritis. Q. J. Med., *159:* 391–408, 1971.
55. Stevens, J. M., Kendall, B. E., and Crockard, H. A. The spinal cord in rheumatoid arthritis with clinical myelopathy: A computed myelographic study. J. Neurol. Neurosurg. Psychiatry *49:* 140–151, 1986.
56. Sukoff, M. H., Kadin, M. M., and Moran, T. Transoral decompression for myelopathy caused by rheumatoid arthritis of the spine. J. Neurosurg., *37:* 492–497, 1972.
57. Van Gilder, J. C., and Menezes, A. H. Cranio-vertebral junction abnormalities. Clin. Neurosurg., *30:* 514–530, 1983.
58. Verbiest, H. A lateral approach to the cervical spine technique and indications. J. Neurosurg., *28:* 191–203, 1968.
59. Verbiest, H. Anterolateral operations for fractures and dislocations in the middle and lower parts of the cervical spine. J. Bone Joint Surg. [Am.], *51A:* 1489–1530, 1969.
60. Windfield, J., Cook, D., Brook, A. S., *et al.* A progressive study of the radiological changes in the cervical spine in early rheumatoid disease. Ann. Rheum. Dis., *40:* 109–114, 1981.

IV

Neuro-oncology

18

Neurosurgical Implications of the Acquired Immunodeficiency Syndrome (AIDS)

MARK L. ROSENBLUM, M.D., ROBERT M. LEVY, M.D., PH.D., and
DALE E. BREDESEN, M.D.

The acquired immunodeficiency syndrome (AIDS) is no longer a rare disease affecting only a small segment of the population. Today, AIDS must be considered the No. 1 public health menace in the U.S. As defined by the Centers for Disease Control (CDC), AIDS is a "reliably diagnosed disease that is at least moderately indicative of an underlying cellular immunodeficiency in a person who has no known underlying cause of cellular immunodeficiency nor any other cause of reduced resistance reported to be associated with that disease" (2). A new classification system has recently been proposed that expands the CDC surveillance criteria to include patients in high-risk groups who are confirmed to have certain neoplasms that, by themselves, could result in immunosuppression (Table 18.1) (4).

The largest groups at risk for AIDS are predominantly homosexual or bisexual men (72%) and intravenous drug abusers (17%). Table 18.2 shows the risk groups and the relative percentages of patients in those groups as defined by the CDC through their surveillance mechanisms, both for December 1985 and August 1986. Other groups at risk are recipients of blood transfusions (2%), hemophiliacs who regularly received infusions of concentrated blood products (1%), children of mothers who are infected with the AIDS virus (1–2%), and heterosexual partners of persons with AIDS (1–2%). About 2% of patients have no known risk factor other than having immigrated to the U.S. from other countries where the disease is possibly more endemic than in the U.S.; the majority of such patients have come from Haiti. Finally, about 3% of patients who have been documented to have AIDS have no known risk factors. In all but the last two categories, the number of patients diagnosed with AIDS is doubling each year (3).

According to the CDC (R Janssen: personal communication, April 1987), 13,189 new cases of AIDS were identified in 1986 (Table 18.3). An additional 7,787 patients diagnosed as having AIDS in 1985 and earlier years were alive during 1986. Therefore, approximately 20,976 patients

TABLE 18.1
Recent CDC Classification System for HIV Infections

New Classification		Common Name
Group I	Acute HIV infection (mononucleosis-like, aseptic meningitis)	Acute infection
Group II	Asymptomatic	Healthy carrier
Group III	Persistent generalized lymphadenopathy	ARC
Group IV	Other disease	
	A. Constitutional disease (fever, weight loss, diarrhea)	ARC
	B. Neurological disease (dementia, myelopathy, peripheral neuropathy)	ARC
	C. Secondary infections	
	1. CDC-defined AIDS-associated[a]	AID
	2. Other specified infections[b]	ARC
	D. Secondary cancers (CDC-defined AIDS-associated[c])	AIDS
	E. Other conditions attributed to HIV infection or immunosuppression	ARC

[a] *Pneumocystis carinii* pneumonia, toxoplasmosis, cryptococcosis, chronic cryptosporidiosis, extraintestinal strongyloidiasis, isosporiasis, candidiasis (esophageal, bronchial, or pulmonary), histoplasmosis, mycobacterial infection with *Mycobacterium avium-intracellulare* complex or *M. kansasii*, cytomegalovirus infection, chronic mucocutaneous or disseminated herpes simplex infection, and progressive multifocal leukoencephalopathy.

[b] Multidermatomal herpes zoster, oral hairy leukoplakia, nocardiosis, tuberculosis, recurrent *Salmonella* bacteremia, and oral candidiasis.

[c] Kaposi's sarcoma, non-Hodgkins high-grade lymphoma, and primary CNS lymphoma.

were treated for AIDS during 1986; 8,320 deaths from AIDS were reported during 1986. By the beginning of 1987, there will have been a cumulative total of 29,137 diagnosed cases and 16,481 deaths. AIDS is found throughout the U.S. and in almost all countries in the world. The cumulative number of cases in the U.S. averages 13/100,000 population; approximately half of all cases reside in New York City (91/100,000), San Francisco (91/100,000), and Los Angeles (32/100,000). It is anticipated that by 1991, 80% of cases will reside outside of these three population centers. Furthermore, significant changes in the epidemiology of HIV transmission are expected; for example, in 1991, 8.5% of all AIDS patients (23,000) will be heterosexuals who are not intravenous drug users. To date, the direct cost of medical care for patients with AIDS has been approximately 1 billion dollars (36), and the total economic impact of this disease is predicted to be in the billions of dollars (12). AIDS is now one of the leading causes of premature death in certain high-population areas in the U.S., such as New York City (8).

TABLE 18.2
Groups at Risk for AIDS[a]

Risk Group[b]	Percentage of AIDS Patients	
	December 1985	August 1986
Homosexual/bisexual males[c]	72.2	72.5
Intravenous drug abusers[c]	16.8	16.9
Immigrants[d]	2.5	2.1
Blood transfusion recipients	1.9	1.7
Heterosexual contact with persons with AIDS or at risk for AIDS	1.0	1.6
Children of mothers with AIDS	1.2	1.4
Hemophiliacs	0.8	0.8
No known risk	3.6	3.0

[a] Data taken from the Centers for Disease Control (3).

[b] Hierarchical ordering of risk groups. Patients with two risks factors are listed according to the more common one.

[c] 7.9% of all AIDS patients were both homosexual or bisexual and intravenous drug abusers; this dual risk group is included in the former category.

[d] Includes primarily immigrants from Haiti and Central Africa. Transmission of HIV infection in these groups is thought to be through heterosexual contact. Recent epidemiologic surveys combine these two groups with other patients who acquired AIDS through heterosexual contact.

TABLE 18.3
CDC Predictions of the Number of Patients and Their Mortality[a]

	1986[a]	1991	
		Estimate	(67% Confidence Envelope)
New cases	13,189	74,000	(46,000–91,000)
At risk	20,976	145,000	(96,000–180,000)
Deaths	8,320	54,000	(37,000–64,000)
Cumulative			
Cases	29,137	270,000	(201,000–311,000)
Deaths	16,481	179,000	(142,000–201,000)

[a] Data taken from Curran (8).

[b] Cases are deaths reported to the CDC during 1986 (R. Jahssen, personal communication, April 1987).

Investigation into the cause of AIDS has focused on a retrovirus (RNA virus) now called *human immunodeficiency virus* (HIV). This name was selected by a national panel (5) to replace the terms used for the three known variants of the virus: human T-cell lymphotropic virus type III (HTLV-III), identified by Robert Gallo and his associates at the National Institutes of Health (NIH) (11); lymphadenopathy-associated virus

(LAV), identified by Luc Montagnier and his associates in Paris (1); and AIDS-related virus (ARV), identified by Jay Levy and his associates at the University of California, San Francisco (16).

The discovery of HIV permitted the development of tests to identify and quantitate the antibodies produced by a person infected with the virus (17). Serologic testing for viral exposure has decreased the risk of AIDS transmission from blood transfusions and has fostered extensive epidemiologic studies. It is estimated that by 1986 at least 1.5 million persons had been exposed to the virus in the U.S. and that approximately 3 million people had been exposed in the world (37). A recently completed study of patients in San Francisco who had antibodies to the HIV virus at least 5 years previously suggests that the 5-year risk for development of AIDS is approximately 18% (34). An additional 54% of patients developed AIDS-related complex (ARC) within 5 years. It is not yet known what percentage of patients with ARC will develop AIDS; estimates of less than 20% are considered conservative. Therefore, it is likely that without effective treatment regimens, 25–50% of people already exposed to HIV will eventually develop AIDS.

NEUROLOGICAL MANIFESTATIONS

We first became aware of unusual nervous system pathology when an increasing number of patients with AIDS developed either dementia, aseptic meningitis, peripheral neuropathies, or intracranial space-occupying lesions. The frequency of neurological manifestations appears to be increasing in proportion to the total number of HIV-infected persons. Most of the neurological manifestations seen in patients with AIDS are common among other groups of immunosuppressed patients; however, certain diseases associated with AIDS, such as HIV encephalitis and vacuolar myelopathy, have never been identified before. Multiple intracranial processes have been observed clinically in almost 15% of all AIDS patients.

The prevalence of neurological problems in AIDS patients may be characterized by a recent review of 1286 patients with AIDS who were treated at the University of California, San Francisco (UCSF) up to April 1986 (20). Of these 1286 patients, almost all of whom were homosexual or bisexual men, 482 (37%) had a total of 556 neurological diseases: 477 diseases (86%) involved the central nervous system (CNS) and 79 (14%) involved the peripheral nervous system. Sixty-five patients (13.4%) had multiple diseases. The most commonly identified CNS diseases were HIV encephalopathy (100 cases), cryptococcal meningitis (68 cases), *Toxoplasma* abscesses (53 cases), non-HIV viral encephalitis (28 cases), and primary CNS lymphoma (25 cases) (Table 18.4).

TABLE 18.4
Central Nervous System Diseases Identified by a Review of 1286 Patients with AIDS[a]

Disease	No. of Cases	CNS Masses
Nonviral infections		
Cryptococcus	68	8
Toxoplasma	53	47
Candida	3	3
Mycobacterium	3	2
Viral infections		
HIV encephalopathy	100	0
PML	8	0
Other viral	28	5
Tumors		
Primary CNS lymphoma	25	22
Kaposi's sarcoma	2	2
Unknown		
Treated for Toxoplasmo-sis	31	22
No treatment	156	19
Total	477	130

[a] From Levy, R. M., Bredesen, D. E., and Rosenblum, M. L. Central nervous system syndromes in acquired immunodeficiency syndrome. In: *AIDS and the Nervous System*, edited by M. L. Rosenblum, R. M. Levy, and D. E. Bredesen. Raven Press, New York, in press, 1987.

Intracranial mass lesions were found in 131, or approximately 10%, of the 1286 patients. In 48 cases, the mass lesion was identified before the diagnosis of AIDS had been established. AIDS was diagnosed on the basis of the intracranial lesion in some patients and on the basis of concurrent nonneurological disease in others. The most common documented cause of intracranial mass lesions was infection with *Toxoplasma gondii* (47 cases), followed by primary CNS lymphoma (22 cases). Other space-occupying lesions included abscesses caused by *Cryptococcus neoformans* (eight cases), viruses (five cases), *Candida albicans* (three cases), and *Mycobacterium* species (two cases), and metastatic Kaposi's sarcoma (two cases). *Toxoplasma* abscesses usually respond to therapy with sulfadiazine and pyrimethamine (29, 31). Forty-two of these 89 lesions were not caused by *T. gondii*; 35 of the 42 lesions (83%) were considered possibly treatable because they were primary CNS lymphoma or metastatic Kaposi's sarcoma, which respond to radiation therapy, or abscesses due to *C. neoformans* and *C. albicans*, which may respond to drug therapy. Therefore, approximately 92% of patients (82 of 89) had intracranial space-occupying lesions that might respond, at least temporarily, to therapeutic manipulations. The mass lesions caused by mycobacterial and viral infections were not considered treatable.

SPECIFIC NEUROLOGICAL DISEASES

A detailed description of each neurological disease observed in patients with AIDS is beyond the scope of this chapter. Interested readers are referred to our recent review (19) and book, *AIDS and the Nervous System* (33), for in-depth discussions of this subject.

Nonviral Infections

Toxoplasma abscesses are the most common intracranial mass lesions in patients with AIDS. Clinical symptoms have usually been present for a few weeks when the presumptive diagnosis of a *Toxoplasma* abscess is made by computed tomography (CT) or magnetic resonance imaging (MRI) brain scans. The initial clinical findings from 150 cases cited in the literature are outlined in Table 18.5 (29). Solitary CNS mass lesions observed on MRI scans are unlikely to be toxoplasmosis. Serological studies of the blood or cerebrospinal fluid (CSF) do not reliably show whether or not an intracranial lesion is caused by *T. gondii*. Treatment consists of combination drug therapy with pyrimethamine (25–50 mg/ day) and sulfadiazine (2–4 g initially, followed by 1–1.5 g every 6 hours); leukovorin (5–25 mg/day) is given to reduce bone marrow toxicity. A dramatic resolution of the abscesses is observed in more than 75% of cases (29, 31). An example of such a case is shown in Figure 18.1. A relapse is probable in more than half of such patients if the therapy is not continued; the utility of maintenance therapy at a reduced dosage is being investigated.

Cryptococcal meningitis is the most common intracranial nonviral infection in patients with AIDS. A minimal inflammatory reaction is frequently noted on CSF examination; however, the diagnosis is readily made from India ink preparations and cryptococcal antigen studies because of the large number of cryptococcal organisms usually present.

TABLE 18.5
Initial Findings in 150 AIDS Patients with Toxoplasmosis of the Central Nervous System[a]

Findings	% of Patients
Focal symptoms	70
Headache	45
Lethargy/confusion	40
Seizures	38
Fever	35
Neck stiffness	5

[a] From Pons, V. G., Jacobs, R. A., and Hollander, H. Nonviral infections of the central nervous system in patients with acquired immunodeficiency syndrome. In: *AIDS and the Nervous System*, edited by M. L. Rosenblum, R. M. Levy, and D. E. Bredesen. Raven Press, New York, in press, 1987.

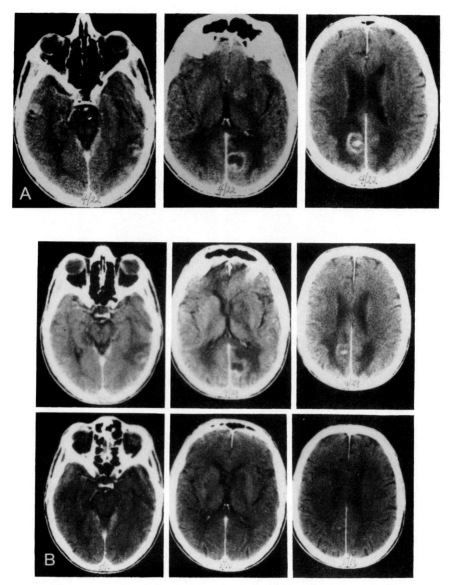

FIG. 18.1. (*A*) CT scan from a 42-year-old man with AIDS shows bilateral, contrast-enhancing lesions. (*B*) After 1 week (*upper scans*) and 4 weeks (*lower scans*) of therapy with sulfadiazine and pyrimethamine, all the lesions have disappeared. The presumptive diagnosis was cerebral toxoplasmosis. (*C*) CT scans obtained 4 weeks after successful initiation of anti-*Toxoplasma* treatment (*upper two scans*) are contrasted with CT scans of the same region obtained 6 weeks later (*lower two scans*) after the patient developed left hemiparesis and recurrent headaches. The right parietal, ring-enhancing lesion (lower right scan) was removed surgically and found to be a primary CNS lymphoma.

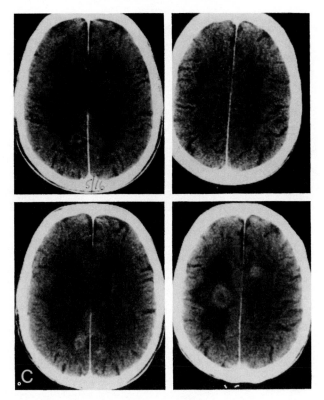

FIG. 18.1C

Cryptococcomas, which are focal intraparenchymal mass lesions caused by cryptococcal organisms, have been noted in approximately 10% of patients with cryptococcal meningitis. The treatment consists of amphotericin B (0.5 mg/kg/day IV, to a total of 2 g for a 3-month treatment) and 5-flucytosine (150 mg/kg/day). Although the survival rate among immunocompetent patients with cryptococcal meningitis is 85–100%, it is only about 15% in immunosuppressed patients. In AIDS patients it is difficult to prevent recurrence of the disease during maintenance therapy because the dosage of the drug (especially 5-flucytosine) usually must be decreased to avoid significant drug-induced toxicity (29, 31).

Other infectious organisms that involve the CNS in patients with AIDS include *Mycobacterium tuberculosis, C. albicans, Aspergillus fumigatus, Histoplasma capsulatum, Coccidioides immitis, Nocardia asteroides, Listeria monocytogenes, M. avium-intracellulare,* and *M. kansasii* (Table 18.6) (29). All but the last two organisms are potentially treatable. The

TABLE 18.6

Nonviral Infections of the Central Nervous System in Patients with Acquired Immunodeficiency Syndrome[a]

Organism	No. of Patients	Comments
Mycobacteria		
M. tuberculosis	15	Haitian or IV drug abuser; 10 brain abscess, 4 meningitis
M. avium-intracellulare	14	Most meningitis/subacute encephalitis in association with disseminated disease
M. kansasii	1	Meningitis
Fungi		
C. albicans	6	Multiple small abscesses; 2 with simultaneous CNS toxoplasmosis, 1 with *Staphylococcus epidermidis*
A. fumigatus	4	3 abscesses 1 meningitis
H. capsulatum	5	Disseminated infection
C. immitis	3	
Mucor/Zygomycetes	5	All in IV drug addicts with no other manifestations or criteria for AIDS
Bacteria		
Listeria	3	2 meningitis/encephalitis, 1 brain abscess
Nocardia + Salmonella group B	1	Brain abscess
E. coli	1	Brain abscess
Neurosyphilis	1	

[a] From Pons, V. G., Jacobs, R. A., and Hollander, H. Nonviral infections of the central nervous system in patients with acquired immunodeficiency syndrome. In: *AIDS and the Nervous System*, edited by M. L. Rosenblum, R. M. Levy, and D. E. Bredesen. Raven Press, New York, in press, 1987.

rare cases of bacterial brain abscesses and mucormycosis that have been observed are probably not AIDS-related.

Viral Infections

Primary CNS infection with the HIV is the most common neurological manifestation of AIDS. HIV is neurotropic and probably invades the CNS at a very early stage of infection. An atypical aseptic meningitis has been observed at the time of the initial viremia with HIV and in patients with ARC. HIV encephalopathy, also known as AIDS-related dementia, AIDS dementia complex, and subacute encephalitis, is a progressive subcortical encephalopathy (25, 30). The predominant symptoms are dementia and long-tract abnormalities. Atrophy is a frequent finding on CT scans. MRI brain scans occasionally reveal diffuse abnormalities of the white matter (Fig. 18.2). Autopsy studies have documented histological changes consistent with HIV encephalitis in approximately 50% of cases studied. HIV has been identified in giant cells, presumably of macrophage origin, and occasionally in cells that resemble oligodendrocytes, neurons, and astrocytes (17, 30). The clinicopathologic correlation between HIV encephalopathy and the identification of HIV in brain tissue is most readily established in the most severe cases (30); the role of other factors or infections in HIV encephalopathy has not yet been defined.

The opportunistic viral infections of the CNS in patients with AIDS include those caused by Jakob-Creutzfeldt (JC) virus (a papovavirus), cytomegalovirus (CMV), and herpes simplex virus (HSV) (10). Progressive multifocal leukoencephalopathy (PML) is caused by infection with JC virus. It has been seen in immunodepressed patients in the past but now is observed predominantly in patients with AIDS. Although PML is usually a progressive, multifocal disease of the white matter, it may present in an atypical fashion. Figure 18.3 shows the CT and MRI scans in a patient with a solitary, biopsy-proven PML lesion of the left parietal lobe. The degree of contrast enhancement is slight, and the lesion involves

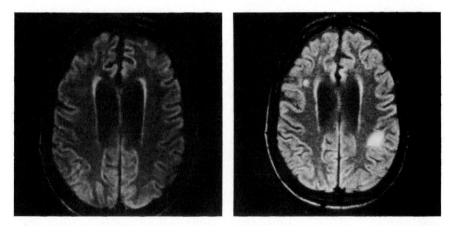

FIG. 18.2. (*Left*) MRI scan of a 32-year-old man with signs and symptoms of HIV encephalitis shows diffuse cerebral atrophy. (*Right*) A repeat MRI scan, obtained 1 month later because the patient continued to deteriorate clinically, shows regions of high signal intensity in the white matter of both cerebral hemispheres. These changes are consistent with the development of a second viral infection, most likely progressive multifocal leukoencephalopathy.

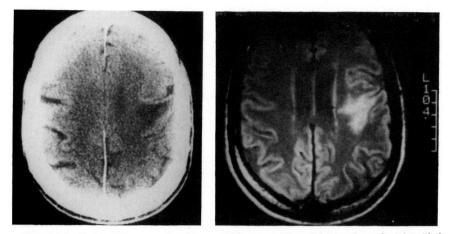

FIG. 18.3. (*Left*) CT scan of a 54-year-old man with mild speech and right-sided coordination difficulties shows a low-density lesion in the left parietal white matter. There is a slight amount of contrast enhancement and mass effect. (*Right*) The MRI scan shows a solitary left parietal lesion involving both white and gray matter. A stereotactic biopsy of the lesion was performed, and the diagnosis was progressive multifocal leukoencephalopathy.

the gray as well as the white matter of the cerebral cortex. Both CMV and HSV types I and II may cause a focal encephalitis that mimicks a mass lesion. Combined infections with CMV and HSV have been implicated in rapidly progressive cases of encephalomyelitis (10). There is no effective therapy for HIV, JC, or CMV viral infections; treatment of HSV encephalitis with acyclovir (7.5–10 mg/kg/8 hours, IV) can be effective in the early stages of the infection.

Neoplasms

Opportunistic tumors that affect patients with AIDS include Kaposi's sarcoma, systemic lymphomas of varying degrees of malignancy, and primary high-grade CNS lymphomas (38). Kaposi's sarcoma very rarely involves the brain; it has occasionally been noted to respond to radiation therapy. Systemic lymphoma may involve the CNS by infiltrating the leptomeninges, which results in lymphomatous meningitis (41). Cranial neuropathies are frequently noted, but intracerebral mass lesions are rare (38).

Primary CNS lymphomas have been rare tumors that account for only 1–2% of all primary brain neoplasms. This tumor has occurred spontaneously and in association with immune suppression in the past; it is now being observed with increasing frequency in patients with AIDS (38). In our review of AIDS cases at UCSF, 1.9% of patients developed primary lymphomas during their course; in approximately one-third of the patients, the tumor was the first manifestation of AIDS (20).

Patients with primary CNS lymphoma present most commonly with confusion, lethargy, memory loss, and focal neurological deficits (38). Seizures are eventually observed in one-third of cases. CT brain scans demonstrate space-occupying masses that are usually contrast-enhancing (Figs. 18.1C and 18.4A); this appearance is not specific for a lymphoma. Although primary CNS lymphomas have traditionally been multicentric and bilateral in 14% of cases (13, 26), CT scanning has demonstrated multicentricity in 47% of AIDS patients with these lesions and in all cases studied at autopsy (38). CSF studies are usually nonspecific and should be avoided if the CT scans show significant mass effect.

Pathological classification of AIDS-related primary CNS lymphomas has shown high-grade subtypes in most cases; large-cell, immunoblastic (30%) and small-cell, noncleaved (60%) lymphomas are the most common (38). These are the same types of primary CNS lymphomas seen before the AIDS epidemic (13, 26). About 62% of systemic lymphomas associ-

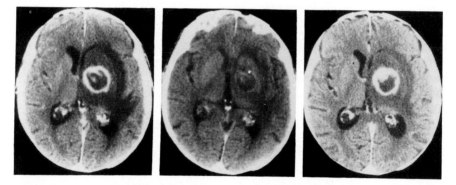

Fig. 18.4. (*Left*) Contrast-enhanced CT scan from a 54-year-old man with headaches, confusion, and mild right hemiparesis shows a large left thalamic lesion. An MRI scan showed only the same lesion demonstrated by CT. (*Middle*) CT scan obtained after 2 weeks of treatment with sulfadiazine, pyrimethamine, and high-dose corticosteroids shows a marked reduction in the amount of contrast enhancement and mass effect. A stereotactic needle biopsy was performed because a solitary mass lesion on an MRI scan is an unusual appearance for toxoplasmosis. Initial histological evaluation could not differentiate between a *Toxoplasma* abscess and a lymphoma. Because the presumptive diagnosis was toxoplasmosis, the corticosteroid dose was decreased while the antibiotics were continued at full dosage. Ten days later, analysis of a plastic-embedded biopsy specimen with lymphocyte cell-surface markers confirmed the diagnosis of a primary lymphoma of the brain. (*Right*) A repeat CT scan showed a recurrent large left thalamic lesion that showed dense contrast enhancement. The transient decrease in enhancement and mass effect documented by CT were considered to be the result of the corticosteroid therapy in a patient with primary CNS lymphoma.

ated with AIDS are high-grade tumors, compared with 17% of such lesions in the general population (41).

The established treatment for non-AIDS-related CNS lymphomas is radiation therapy, which can result in tumor response and improved patient survival (median of 15 months compared with 5 months from surgery alone) (13, 26). It has been suggested that chemotherapy may prolong patient survival modestly, but this has not been confirmed in a randomized trial. Corticosteroids alone have occasionally resulted in antitumor activity (14). Primary CNS lymphomas associated with AIDS also respond favorably to radiation therapy (38). However, a substantial increase in the duration of survival has not been observed; patients usually die of other AIDS-associated diseases (38).

The possible etiologies for primary CNS lymphomas in AIDS include impaired immune surveillance, dysregulated immunocyte proliferation, and an interaction of Epstein-Barr virus and/or HIV with cellular DNA that results in the excessive expression of oncogenes or transforming genes.

Other Diseases

Intracranial hemorrhage, usually into a neoplastic lesion, and cerebral infarctions involving the distribution of a major cortical artery have been noted in several patients with AIDS (Figs. 18.5 and 18.6). The relationship of large infarctions to AIDS has not been defined; however, evidence of smaller areas of infarction was identified in 12 of 88 CNS evaluations (14%) in an autopsy study (20). The presence of antiplatelet antibodies in patients with AIDS might be implicated in the development of such infarcts; the clinical significance of these antibodies is unknown.

Multiple intracranial pathologies are quite common in patients with AIDS. Different diseases have been identified within a single lesion and within different lesions in the same patient, both simultaneously and sequentially. Levy *et al.* (18) identified 20 homosexual or bisexual men with AIDS who had two or more diseases of the nervous system; this represented an incidence of 29% of AIDS patients with autopsy- or biopsy-proven nervous system pathology. Recent evidence for the high incidence of HIV encephalitis suggests that this may be a conservative estimate. A total of 46 pathological processes were identified in the 20 patients; these included viral infection (20 cases), primary CNS lymphoma (7 cases), metastatic Kaposi's sarcoma (1 case), cryptococcosis (5 cases), toxoplasmosis (4 cases), and one case each of infection with *C. albicans* and atypical *Mycobacterium*. Fifteen patients had two intracranial processes, and five patients had three or more. Different viral illnesses were most commonly associated (Fig. 18.2). Six patients

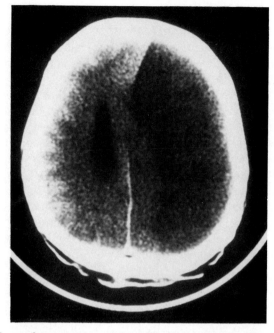

FIG. 18.5. CT scan demonstrating a left middle cerebral artery stroke in a patient with AIDS.

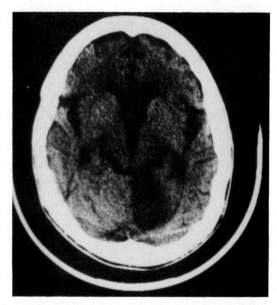

FIG. 18.6. CT scan showing a low-density lesion in the left cerebellar hemisphere in a patient with AIDS. Autopsy demonstrated a stroke in the distribution of the superior cerebellar artery.

had evidence of two nonviral pathologies. In several cases, two or more diseases were identified that could respond to distinctly different treatments. The two most commonly associated treatable lesions were toxoplasmosis and primary CNS lymphoma (Fig. 18.1).

The presence of multiple intracranial pathologies has important implications for the evaluation and treatment of CNS disease in AIDS patients. Close follow-up is critical to determine the response to therapy and to identify lesions that progress in the presence of initially effective therapy; repeat biopsy of these lesions may reveal the presence of a second intracranial process.

Occasionally, patients with AIDS will present with neurological diseases that are not a consequence of AIDS. For example, we have diagnosed malignant astrocytomas (Figs. 18.7 and 18.8), craniopharyngioma (Fig. 18.9), and a herniated lumbar disc in patients in high-risk groups with antibodies to HIV. Therefore, the clinician must remember that AIDS patients may have the same diseases as the general population.

DIAGNOSTIC STUDIES

Neuroradiology

CT and MRI brain scans are the studies of choice in evaluating AIDS patients with neurological symptoms. The CT findings in 443 AIDS

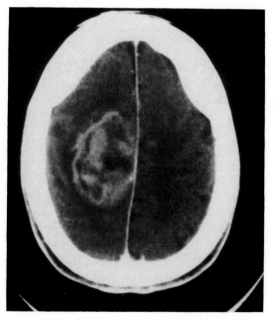

FIG. 18.7. CT scan showing a right parietal contrast-enhancing lesion in a man with AIDS-related complex. Biopsy demonstrated a glioblastoma multiforme.

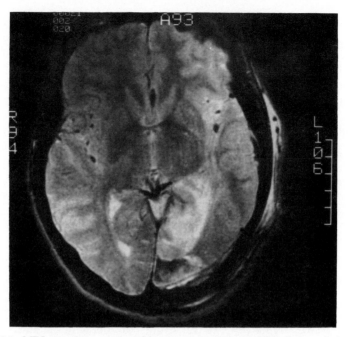

FIG. 18.8. MRI scan from a man who was seropositive for HIV shows a lesion of high signal intensity in the left occipital region. Biopsy demonstrated a moderately anaplastic astrocytoma.

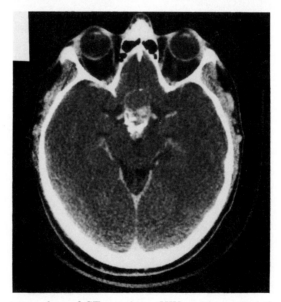

FIG. 18.9. Contrast-enhanced CT scan in an HIV-positive patient shows a suprasellar lesion. A typical craniopharyngioma was diagnosed at operation.

patients with neurological symptoms are summarized in Table 18.7; CT scans demonstrate focal lesions in about one-third of patients and atrophy in another third; the studies are normal in the remaining patients (9). The histopathological findings associated with focal and nonfocal lesions on CT are documented in Table 18.8. The most common causes of focal lesions are toxoplasmosis, primary CNS lymphoma, and PML; nonfocal lesions are most often caused by cryptococcal meningitis or CMV encephalitis. Multiple intracranial lesions have been identified by CT scan in several cases (Table 18.9) (9); toxoplasmosis and lymphoma or CMV encephalitis are the most common associations.

MRI is more sensitive than CT in detecting intracranial abnormalities

TABLE 18.7
CT Findings in 443 AIDS Patients with Neurological Symptoms[a]

Finding	No. of Patients	%	
		Range	Overall
Focal lesions	166	26–53	38
Atrophy	147	22–50	33
Normal	130	10–40	29

[a] From De La Paz, R., and Enzmann, D. Neuroradiology of acquired immunodeficiency syndrome. In: *AIDS and the Nervous System*, edited by M. L. Rosenblum, R. M. Levy, and D. E. Bredesen. Raven Press, New York, in press, 1987.

TABLE 18.8
Histopathological Diagnosis and CT Findings[a]

Pathological Findings	% of Patients
Focal lesions	
T. gondii	50–70
Primary CNS lymphoma	10–25
Progressive multifocal leukoencephalopathy	10–22
Nondiagnostic biopsy (gliosis, sterile inflammation)	10
C. albicans	3
Cryptococcoma	2
Kaposi's sarcoma	2
M. tuberculosis abscess	1
Herpes simplex virus type II	1
Nonfocal lesions	
Cryptococcal meningitis	28
Coccidioidal meningitis	1
Cytomegalovirus encephalitis	11
HIV encephalitis	3
Herpes simplex virus type I encephalitis	1
Herpes varicella zoster encephalitis	1

[a] From De La Paz, R., and Enzmann, D. Neuroradiology of acquired immunodeficiency syndrome. In: *AIDS and the Nervous System*, edited by M. L. Rosenblum, R. M. Levy, and D. E. Bredesen. Raven Press, New York, in press, 1987.

TABLE 18.9

Multiple Lesions Identified by CT Scans in 17 Patients with AIDS[a]

Lesions	No. of Patients
Toxoplasmosis and lymphoma	6
Toxoplasmosis and cytomegalovirus encephalitis	4
Toxoplasmosis and cryptococcal meningitis	1
Toxoplasmosis and tuberculous abscess	1
Toxoplasmosis and cysticercosis	1
Lymphoma and cryptococcal meningitis	1
Cryptococcal meningitis and herpes varicella zoster encephalitis	1
Cryptococcal meningitis and cytomegalovirus encephalitis	1
Herpes simplex virus type I and cytomegalovirus encephalitis	1

[a] From De La Paz, R., and Enzmann, D. Neuroradiology of acquired immunodeficiency syndrome. In: *AIDS and the Nervous System*, edited by M. L. Rosenblum, R. M. Levy, and D. E. Bredesen. Raven Press, New York, in press, 1987.

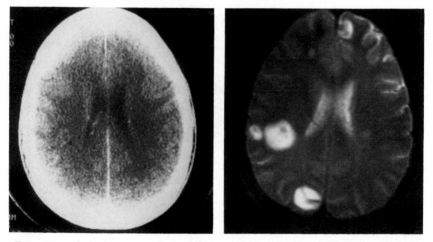

FIG. 18.10. (*Left*) Contrast-enhanced CT scan from a 30-year-old patient with multiple neurological deficits appears to be normal. (*Right*) MRI scan of the same region of the brain shows multiple areas of high signal intensity representing *Toxoplasma* abscesses.

in patients with AIDS (Fig. 18.10) (9, 22). Comparisons of CT and MRI findings according to symptoms and number of lesions are presented in Tables 18.10 and 18.11, respectively. Neither the CT nor the MRI scan can by itself definitively diagnose the cause of a lesion. Atrophy on the CT scan is a poor prognostic sign that probably reflects primary HIV infection of the brain (23). A solitary mass lesion on the MRI scan is unlikely to be a *Toxoplasma* abscess. Cryptococcal meningitis in patients with AIDS usually results in minimal basilar inflammation, and it is therefore unusual to see basilar contrast enhancement on CT scans. In general, viral infections do not cause intracerebral mass lesions that can be identified on CT scans; however, exceptions to this rule have been noted in patients with CMV and HSV infections and very rarely in those with PML.

Neuropathology

The neuropathological evaluation of brain biopsies in AIDS patients is frequently difficult because of the small specimens obtained by needle biopsy techniques and because of the unusual manifestations of the neurological diseases (28). For example, *Toxoplasma* infections frequently cause extensive necrosis and inflammatory infiltration; the degree and extent of inflammation may mimic the histological appearance of a lymphoma. Immunoperoxidase staining for *T. gondii* and lymphocyte cell-surface markers as well as electron microscopy may be needed to

TABLE 18.10
Comparison of CT and MRI Findings according to Patient Symptoms[a]

Findings	% Patients			
	Focal Symptoms		Nonfocal Symptoms	
	CT (33 patients)	MRI (49 patients)	CT (49 patients)	MRI (62 patients)
Focal lesions	70	74	22	42
Bilateral white-matter abnormality	0	8	0	13
Atrophy	12	6	31	16
Normal	18	12	47	29

[a] From De La Paz, R., and Enzmann, D. Neuroradiology of acquired immunodeficiency syndrome. In: *AIDS and the Nervous System*, edited by M. L. Rosenblum, R. M. Levy, and D. E. Bredesen. Raven Press, New York, in press, 1987.

TABLE 18.11
Comparison of CT and MRI Findings in 98 AIDS Patients[a]

Findings on Brain Scan	% Patients
MRI positive, CT negative	22
MRI more lesions than CT	22
MRI same lesions as CT	16
CT positive, MRI negative	1
CT more lesions than MRI	2
MRI and CT show atrophy	16
MRI and CT normal	21

[a] Adapted from De La Paz, R., and Enzmann, D. Neuroradiology of acquired immunodeficiency syndrome. In: *AIDS and the Nervous System*, edited by M. L. Rosenblum, R. M. Levy, and D. E. Bredesen. Raven Press, New York, in press, 1987.

make a definitive diagnosis. Occasionally, a repeat needle biopsy has been necessary; the greatest yield of diagnostic material is from specimens obtained from the edge of CT contrast-enhancing lesions.

It is recommended that brain biopsy specimens be routinely evaluated by frozen section and then fixed in formalin for embedding in paraffin or, preferably, fixed in paraformaldehyde for embedding in plastic. Plastic sections most readily permit immunoperoxidase staining for *Toxoplasma* organisms and cell-surface markers. Whenever possible, biopsies should be cultured for viruses, fungi, and bacteria, including tubercle bacillus. Touch preparations, smears, and electron microscopy may also be useful (28).

NEUROEPIDEMIOLOGY

The neuroepidemiology of AIDS was evaluated by reviewing the files of the CDC for their estimates of neurological diseases in patients with AIDS in the U.S.; diseases were segregated according to patient risk group and geographical location (21). Cerebral toxoplasmosis, cryptococcal meningitis, PML, and primary CNS lymphoma were included in the CDC surveillance forms, and their frequency as a first and reliable diagnosis could be ascertained.

Cerebral toxoplasmosis is most common in Haitians and more common in Florida than in other locations in the U.S., possibly because of the high proportion of Haitian AIDS patients in that state and the higher prevalence of toxoplasmosis in other risk groups in Florida. It is probable that the potential for exposure to *T. gondii* organisms is greater in the subtropical climate of Florida than in other regions of the country. Cryptococcal meningitis is observed more commonly in New Jersey owing to the higher prevalence in that state of blacks and intravenous drug abusers with AIDS. The prevalence of PML and primary CNS lymphoma was similar across the U.S. and in the various risk groups. This information suggests that geographical site and risk group can play a role in the frequency of specific neurological disease in the AIDS population and should be considered in the diagnosis and management of neurological syndromes in AIDS patients.

RECOMMENDED TREATMENT OF INTRACRANIAL MASSES

Because *Toxoplasma* abscesses are the most common type of CNS mass lesion, as well as the most readily treatable, we recommend a 3-week empirical trial with pyrimethamine and sulfadiazine for any patient with AIDS and intracranial masses. Corticosteroids can be administered concurrently if there is clinically significant cerebral edema; however, it must be understood that steroids can, by themselves, decrease the CT contrast enhancement induced by infectious lesions of the brain (39) and can reduce the mass produced by primary CNS lymphomas (Fig. 18.4). Therefore, once partial resolution of CT masses is documented after institution of combined anti-*Toxoplasma* therapy and corticosteroids, the steroids should be gradually withdrawn. A persistent beneficial effect from treatment with only sulfadiazine and pyrimethamine will confirm that the CNS mass lesion was caused by *T. gondii*.

Patients who are unlikely to survive the 3-week antibiotic trial or who are likely to suffer a major allergic reaction to the drugs should instead have a biopsy for definitive diagnosis. A biopsy should also be performed if all or some of the masses fail to respond to the empirical trial. Finally, since a solitary mass lesion on MRI scans is not likely to be toxoplasmosis (9), that lesion should be biopsied. The observation that the majority of mass lesions not caused by *T. gondii* are treatable suggests that this approach provides the maximum chance of benefiting such patients. A stereotactic needle biopsy guided by CT scanning or real-time ultrasound imaging is the surgical procedure of choice. This technique provides the least risk of transmitting the virus to health care workers and poses the least risk to the patient, especially when local anesthesia is used.

PREVENTION OF TRANSMISSION OF HIV INFECTION TO HEALTH CARE WORKERS

The risk of HIV transmission to health care workers is very low (6, 17, 24). Only 2 of 716 persons who had received parenteral or mucosal membrane exposure to blood or other body fluids from AIDS patients were found to have antibodies to HIV. Recommended precautions include proper disposal of syringes, needles, and other sharp instruments (6). To prevent needle-stick injuries, needles should not be recapped or otherwise manipulated by hand. When the possibility of exposure to blood or other body fluid exists, gloves and, if indicated, gowns, masks, or eye coverings are recommended. In general, the precautions usually observed to prevent transmission of hepatitis will also be effective in avoiding HIV transmission (6). HIV is readily destroyed by treatment with disinfectants such as hypochlorite (6).

PREDICTIONS: AIDS IN 1991 AND ITS IMPACT ON NEUROSURGERY

The CDC has used a polynomial mathematical model to predict the number of future cases of AIDS in the U.S. (8). These estimates are considered conservative because only confirmed AIDS cases were used in the calculations; it was assumed that there will be no changes in the epidemiology of the disease and no effective intervention. Most of the patients who will develop AIDS by 1991 have already been exposed to the virus. The yearly number of new cases, the number of AIDS patients who will be treated, the number of yearly deaths, and the cumulative number of cases and deaths are presented in Table 18.3, both for 1986 and for 1991. If these predictions come true, by 1991 AIDS will become a more frequent cause of death in the U.S. than head injury (Table 18.12).

Primary CNS lymphoma is a good example of the impact of AIDS on the incidence of a specific neurological disease. Primary CNS lymphoma accounted for 1–1.5% of all brain tumors in the pre-AIDS era (13, 26). Based on the frequency of lymphomas in our study of 1286 AIDS patients (0.6% at presentation and 1.3% after AIDS diagnosis) (20) and on CDC statistics (21), it can be predicted that in 1986, 266 cases of primary CNS lymphomas will have been associated with AIDS, as compared with approximately 225 cases reported yearly before 1979 (Table 18.13). By 1991, 1848 cases of primary CNS lymphoma might be observed annually. These predictions suggest that by 1991, the annual incidence of primary CNS lymphomas may be approaching that of meningiomas (Table 18.14) (35).

The impact of AIDS on the practice of neurosurgery can be predicted from the number of CNS mass lesions estimated from the UCSF survey combined with case predictions from the CDC. Table 18.15 shows the number of possible neurosurgical operations in 1986 and 1991 for patients known to have AIDS whose masses do not respond to empirical treatment for toxoplasmosis (3.0% of all AIDS cases) and for patients with intracranial masses who have not yet been diagnosed as having AIDS (3.7%). In 1986 and 1991, the numbers of cases that would fulfill these criteria for biopsy are 920 and 5978, respectively. Alternatively, it can be suggested that any patient in a high-risk group for AIDS who presents with multiple intracranial mass lesions be treated empirically for toxoplasmosis. This approach should not be utilized in patients with conditions

TABLE 18.12
Causes of Deaths in the USA: the Impact of AIDS based on CDC predictions

	Annual No. of Deaths	
Heart disease[a]	540,000	
Cancer[b]	385,000	AIDS
Cerebrovascular[c]	240,000 ←	1991
Head injury[c]	50,000	
Brain tumors[c]	10,000 ←	1986
CNS malformations[c]	7,000	

[a] Data taken from National Center for Health Statistics (27).

[b] Data taken from Report of the Panel on Stroke, Trauma Regeneration and Neoplasms to the National Advisory Committee to the Neurologic and Communicative Disorders and Stroke Council (32).

[c] Data taken from Kurtzke and Kurland (15).

TABLE 18.13

Prediction of the Number of Primary Central Nervous System Lymphomas in Patients with AIDS, 1986 and 1991[a]

	1986[b]	1991[c]
Alive from prior years	7,787	71,000
During year (1.3%)[d]	(101)	(923)
New cases	13,189	74,000
At presentation (0.6%)[d]	(79)	(444)
During year (0.65%)[e]	(86)	(481)
Total at risk	20,976	145,000
Total lymphomas	266	1848

[a] Numbers in parentheses in columns 1 and 2, respectively, represent the percentage and number of CNS lymphomas.

[b] Case numbers reported to the CDC during 1986 (R. Janssen, personal communication, April 1987).

[c] Data taken from Curran and Morgan (7).

[d] Data taken from Levy (20).

[e] Assuming median patient survival of 9–12 months from the diagnosis of AIDS, half of the total risk of lymphoma after AIDS is diagnosed (1.3%) is assumed during that year.

TABLE 18.14

The Possible Number of AIDS-associated Primary CNS Lymphomas Compared to the Annual Incidence of Primary Brain Tumors in the U.S.[a]

Tumor	Year Incidence	
Malignant astrocytoma	6000	
Meningioma	2250	← 1991
Astrocytoma	1500	
Pituitary tumor	1500	AIDS
Neurinoma/fibroma	750	CNS
Medulloblastoma	600	Lymphomas
Congenital	600	
Ependymoma	300	← 1986
Lymphoma	225	

[a] Incidence data taken from Schoenberg (35).

that would predispose them to bacterial brain abscesses, such as purulent sinusitis, congenital cyanotic heart disease, or recent intracranial trauma or surgery, or in patients with malignant tumors outside the nervous system. The impact of this more conservative approach is presented in Table 18.16; 656 patients in 1986 and 4498 in 1991 will fulfill these criteria for biopsy. Therefore, if either method for predicting the surgical case load is correct, the number of biopsies for AIDS-related CNS mass lesions will approach the yearly incidence of malignant astrocytomas in the U.S. (35).

These predictions for 1991 may, for a number of reasons, overestimate

CLINICAL NEUROSURGERY

TABLE 18.15

Predicted Number of Neurosurgical Operations If Biopsy Is Performed for CNS Mass Lesions in Patients Not Previously Known to Have AIDS and in AIDS Patients Who Fail to Respond to Empirical Treatment for Toxoplasmosis

	1986[a]	1991[b]
Alive from prior years	7,787	71,000
During year (3.0%)[c]	(234)[d]	(2,130)[d]
New cases	13,189	74,000
At presentation (3.7%)[c]	(488)[e]	(2,738)[e]
During year (1.5%)[f]	(198)[d]	(1110)[d]
Total at risk	20,976	145,000
Total possible operations	920	5,987

[a] Case numbers reported to the CDC during 1986 (R. Janssen personal communication, April 1987).

[b] Data taken from Curran and Morgan (7).

[c] Data taken from Levy (20). Three percent of AIDS patients will develop non-*Toxoplasma* masses after the diagnosis of AIDS is made; 3.7% of AIDS patients will present with a CNS mass from any cause before AIDS is diagnosed.

[d] Number in parentheses represents the number of non-*Toxoplasma* CNS mass lesions.

[e] Number in parentheses represents the number of CNS mass lesions from any cause.

[f] Assuming median patient survival of 9 to 12 months from the diagnosis of AIDS, half of the total risk for developing a non-*Toxoplasma* CNS mass (1.5%) is assumed during that year.

TABLE 18.16

Predicted Number of Neurosurgical Operations if Biopsy Is Performed Only in Patients with AIDS or Patients at High Risk for AIDS Who Have CNS Mass Lesions That Fail to Respond to Empirical Treatment for Toxoplasmosis

	1986[a]	1991[b]
Alive from prior years	7,787	71,000
During year (3.0%)[c]	(234)[d]	(2,130)[d]
New cases	13,189	74,000
At presentation (1.7%)[c]	(224)[e]	(1,258)[e]
During year (1.5%)[f]	(198)[d]	(1,110)[d]
Total at risk	20,976	145,000
Total possible operations	656	4,498

[a] Case numbers reported to the CDC during 1986 (R. Janssen personal communication, April 1987).

[b] Data taken from Curran and Morgan (7).

[c] Data taken from Levy (20). Approximately 4.7% of AIDS patients will develop non-*Toxoplasma* CNS mass lesions (1.7% at presentation and 3.0% after the diagnosis of AIDS).

[d] Numbers in parentheses represent the number of non-*Toxoplasma* CNS mass lesions.

[e] Numbers in parentheses represent the number of CNS mass lesions from any cause.

[f] Assuming median patient survival of 9–12 months from the diagnosis of AIDS, half of the total risk for developing a non-*Toxoplasma* CNS mass (1.5%) is assumed during that year.

the actual number of AIDS cases and the number of patients with neurological manifestations of the syndrome. Clinicians will be appropriately reluctant to suggest a brain biopsy for patients who are severely and irreversibly disabled from the systemic manifestations of AIDS. Considering the invariably fatal outcome of AIDS, patients and their families and physicians might recommend against an invasive neurosurgical procedure. The development of more effective treatments for the systemic manifestations of AIDS and an increased awareness of the low risk of stereotactic brain biopsies should influence these latter concerns. Finally, it is hoped that the future number of AIDS cases will be lower than predicted by the CDC. It has been suggested that the epidemiology of transmission of HIV has been significantly altered in the gay population in San Francisco by changes in life-style as documented by a decrease in the annual incidence of seroconversion from 18% in 1980 to 5% in 1985 (40). Furthermore, the CDC predictions are based upon the lack of effective treatment for HIV infection itself. Research both on the development of new antiviral agents and on a vaccine that will protect against the infection with HIV are proceeding rapidly. It is our fervent hope that those approaches will prove effective and will decrease both the number of patients with AIDS and the frequency of their neurological complications.

ACKNOWLEDGMENTS

Supported in part by Grants CA-31882 and CA-13525 from the National Cancer Institute, National Institutes of Health; by a gift from the Preuss Foundation; and by a grant from the UCSF AIDS Clinical Research Center.

We thank Stephen Ordway for editorial assistance.

REFERENCES

1. Barré-Sinoussi, F., Nugeyre, M., Dauguet, C., et al. Isolation of a T-lymphotropic retrovirus from a patient at risk for acquired immune deficiency syndrome. Science, 220: 868–871, 1983.
2. Centers for Disease Control: Prevention and acquired immune deficiency syndrome (AIDS): Report of interagency recommendations. M.M.W.R., 32: 101–103, 1983.
3. Centers for Disease Control: Update: Acquired immunodeficiency syndrome—United States. J.A.M.A. 255: 593–594, 1986.
4. Centers for Disease Control: Classification system for human T-lymphotropic virus type III/lymphadenopathy-associated virus infections. J.A.M.A., 256: 20–25, 1986.
5. Coffin, J., Haase, A., Levy, J. A., et al. Human immunodeficiency viruses (letter). Science, 232: 697, 1986.
6. Conte, J. E. Human immunodeficiency virus: Hospital epidemiology and infection control precautions. In: AIDS and the Nervous System, edited by M. L. Rosenblum, R. M. Levy, and D. E. Bredesen. Raven Press, New York, in press, 1987.
7. Curran, J., and Morgan, W. M. Public Health Service Plan for the Prevention and Control of AIDS and the AIDS Virus. Report of the PHS conference on Prevention

and Control of AIDS: Planning for 1991, at Coolfont in Berkeley Springs, WV, June 4–6, 1986. Science, *232:* 1589–1590, 1986.

8. Curran, J. W. The epidemiology of AIDS: Current status and future prospects. In: *Proceedings of the International Conference on AIDS*, p. 7, Paris, France, June 23–25, 1986.

9. De La Paz, R., and Enzmann, D. Neuroradiology of acquired immunodeficiency syndrome. In: *AIDS and the Nervous System*, edited by M. L. Rosenblum, R. M. Levy, and D. E. Bredesen. Raven Press, New York, in press, 1987.

10. Dix, R., and Bredesen, D. E. Opportunistic viral infections. In: *AIDS and the Nervous System*, edited by M. L. Rosenblum, R. M. Levy, and D. E. Bredesen. Raven Press, New York, in press, 1987.

11. Gallo, R. C., Salahuddin, S. Z., Popovic, M., *et al.* Frequent detection and isolation of cytopathic retroviruses (HTLV-III) from patients with AIDS and at risk for AIDS. Science, *224:* 500–503, 1984.

12. Hardy, A. M., Rauch, K., Echenberg, D., *et al.* The economic impact of the first 10,000 cases of acquired immunodeficiency syndrome in the United States. J.A.M.A., *255:* 209–211, 1986.

13. Jiddane, M., Nicoli, F., Diaz, P., *et al.* Intracranial malignant lymphoma: Report of 30 cases and review of the literature. J. Neurosurg., *65:* 592–599, 1986.

14. Kikuchi, K., *et al.* Steroid regression of primary malignant lymphoma of the brain. Surg. Neurol., *26:* 291–296, 1986.

15. Kurtzke, J. F., and Kurland, L. T. The epidemiology of neurologic disease. In: *Clinical Neurology*, Chap. 66, pp. 1–143, edited by A. B. Baker and L. H. Baker. Harper & Row, Philadelphia, 1983.

16. Levy, J., Hoffman, A., Kramer, S., *et al.* Isolation of lymphocytopathic retroviruses from San Francisco patients with AIDS. Science, *225:* 840–842, 1984.

17. Levy, J. A. The biology of human immunodeficiency virus and its role in neurological diseases. In: *AIDS and the Nervous System*, edited by M. L. Rosenblum, R. M. Levy, and D. E. Bredesen. Raven Press, New York, in press, 1987.

18. Levy, R. M., Bredesen, D. E., Davis, R. L., *et al.* Multiple intracranial pathologies in the acquired immunodeficiency syndrome: A report of 20 cases (abstr.). In: *Proceedings of the International Conference on AIDS*, Paris, France, June 23–25, 1986.

19. Levy, R. M., Bredesen, D. E., and Rosenblum, M. L. Neurological manifestations of the acquired immunodeficiency syndrome (AIDS): Experience at UCSF and review of the literature. J. Neurosurg., *62:* 475–495, 1985.

20. Levy, R. M., Bredesen, D. E., and Rosenblum, M. L. Central nervous system syndromes in acquired immunodeficiency syndrome. In: *AIDS and the Nervous System*, edited by M. L. Rosenblum, R. M. Levy, and D. E. Bredesen. Raven Press, New York, in press, 1987.

21. Levy, R. M., Janssen, R. S., Morgan, W. M., *et al.* Neuroepidemiology of acquired immunodeficiency syndrome. In: *AIDS in the Nervous System*, edited by M. L. Rosenblum, R. M. Levy, and D. E. Bredesen. Raven Press, New York, in press, 1987.

22. Levy, R. M., Mills, C. M., Posin, J. P., *et al.* The superiority of cranial magnetic resonance imaging (MRI) to computed tomographic (CT) brain scans for the diagnosis of cerebral lesions in patients with AIDS (abstr.). p. 56. In: *Proceedings of the International Conference on AIDS*, p. 56, Paris, France, June 23–25, 1986.

23. Levy, R. M., Rosenbloom, S., and Perrett, L. V. Neuroradiologic findings in AIDS: A review of 200 cases. A.J.N.R., *7:* 833–839, 1986.

24. Lifson, A. R., Castro, K. G., McCray, E., *et al.* National surveillance of health care workers. J.A.M.A., *256:* 3231–3234, 1986.

25. McArthur, J., and Johnson, R. T. Primary infection with human immunodeficiency

virus. In: *AIDS and the Nervous System*, edited by M. L. Rosenblum, R. M. Levy, and D. E. Bredesen. Raven Press, New York, in press, 1987.

26. Murray, K., Kun, L., and Cox, J. Primary malignant lymphoma of the central nervous system: Results of treatment of 11 cases and review of the literature. J. Neurosurg., *65:* 660–667, 1986.

27. National Center for Health Statistics: Births, marriages, divorces, and deaths for January 1985. Monthly Vital Statistics Rep., *34:* 1–11, 1985.

28. Nielsen, S. L., and Davis, R. L. Neuropathology of acquired immunodeficiency syndrome. In: *AIDS and the Nervous System*, edited by M. L. Rosenblum, R. M. Levy, and D. E. Bredesen. Raven Press, New York, in press, 1987.

29. Pons, V. G., Jacobs, R. A., and Hollander, H. Nonviral infections of the central nervous system in patients with acquired immunodeficiency syndrome. In: *AIDS and the Nervous System*, edited by M. L. Rosenblum, R. M. Levy, and D. E. Bredesen. Raven Press, New York, in press, 1987.

30. Price, R. W., Sidtis, J. J., Navia, B. A., *et al.* The AIDS dementia complex. In: *AIDS and the Nervous System*, edited by M. L. Rosenblum, R. M. Levy, and D. E. Bredesen. Raven Press, New York, in press, 1987.

31. Raffi, F., Leport, C., Katlama, C., *et al.* Treatment of brain toxoplasmosis with pyrimethamine and sulfadiazine in 35 AIDS patients: Efficacy of long-term continuous therapy (abstr.). In: *Proceedings of the International Conference on AIDS*, p. 38, Paris, June 23–25, 1986.

32. Report of the Panel on Stroke, Trauma, Regeneration and Neoplasms to the National Advisory Committee to the Neurological and Communicative Disorders and Stroke Council, NIH Publication No. 79–1915, 1979.

33. Rosenblum, M. L., Levy, R. M., and Bredesen, D. E. (eds.) *AIDS and the Nervous System*. Raven Press, New York, in press, 1987.

34. Rutherford, G. W., Echenberg, D. F., O'Malley, P. M., *et al.* The natural history of LAV/HTLV-III infection and viremia in homosexual and bisexual men: A 6-year followup study (abstr.). In: *Proceedings of the International Conference on AIDS*, p. 99. France, June 23–25, 1986.

35. Schoenberg, B. S. The epidemiology of CNS tumors. In: *Oncology of the Nervous System*, edited by M. D. Walker, pp. 1–29. Boston, Martinus-Nijhoff, 1983.

36. Seage, G., Landers, S., Barry, M. A., *et al.* Direct cost of medical care for patients with AIDS (abstr.). In: *Proceedings of the International Conference on AIDS*, pp. 1–29, 181. Paris, June 23–25, 1986.

37. Sivak, S. L., and Wormser, G. P. How common is HTLV-III infection in the United States? N. Engl. J. Med., *313:* 1352, 1985.

38. So, Y. T., Choucair, A., Davis, R. L., *et al.* Neoplasms of the central nervous system in acquired immunodeficiency syndrome. In: *AIDS and the Nervous System*, edited by M. L. Rosenblum, R. L., Levy, and D. E. Bredesen. Raven Press, New York, in press, 1987.

39. Whelan, M. A., and Hilal, S. K. L. Computed tomography as a guide to the diagnosis and follow-up of brain abscesses. Radiology, *135:* 663–671, 1980.

40. Winkelstein, W., Wiley, J., Lang, W., *et al.* Reduction in AIDS virus transmission: Seroconversion in San Francisco, 1982–1985 (abstr.). In: *Proceedings of the International Conference on AIDS*, p. 103. Paris, June 23–25, 1986.

41. Ziegler, J. L., Beckstead, J. A., Volberding, P. A., *et al.* Non-Hodgkins lymphoma in 90 homosexual men: Relationship to generalized lymphadenopathy and acquired immunodeficiency syndrome (AIDS). N. Engl. J. Med., *311:* 565–570, 1984.

CHAPTER

19

Monoclonal Antibodies: Their Application in the Diagnosis and Management of CNS Tumors

NICOLAS de TRIBOLET M.D., EDMUND FRANK M.D., and
JEAN-PIERRE MACH, M.D., PH.D.

INTRODUCTION

One approach to the diagnosis, localization, and treatment of brain tumors has been an attempt to identify specific antigens that allow these tumors to be differentiated from normal tissues. The initial search for tumor antigens utilized polyclonal antisera produced from either autologous sera of patients with brain tumors or heteroantisera of animals immunized with human brain tumors (6, 7, 20, 23, 24, 28, 36). Because these polyclonal antisera required exhaustive absorption to remove contaminating nontumor related antibodies, the production of these antisera was both time consuming and yielded very small quantities of specific reagent.

A major breakthrough in the search for tumor antigens occurred with the development of the technology for production of monoclonal antibodies (MABs) by Köhler and Milstein in 1975 (19). This technique utilizes the fusion of nonspecific antibody-secreting myeloma cells with naturally occurring specific antibody-secreting spleen cells. The somatic cell hybrids produced codominantly express immortality and specific antibody production so that the transient property of antibody secretion can be fixed as a permanent property of an established cell line. The resultant MAB is a pure monovalent antibody that recognizes a single specific antigenic determinant, and it can be produced in unlimited amounts (Table 19.1).

In this review we shall discuss both the novel ways in which MABs have been used in brain tumor research and the possibilities this technology presents for future investigation. Using MABs, two groups of antigens expressed by brain tumors have been identified. The first group, lymphoid differentiation antigens, are important for our understanding of immune functions within the central nervous system (CNS). The second group, tumor associated antigens (TAA), are those antigens which

446

TABLE 19.1
Steps in the Production of MAB

Immunization, fusion, screening of MAB
Radioimmunoassay
Immunohistology
Characterization of MAB, characterization of TAA,
Radioimmunolocalization
Animal models
Clinical trials

might successfully be employed for identification and therapy of brain tumors.

LYMPHOID DIFFERENTIATION ANTIGENS

Lymphoid differentiation antigens (LDA) include antigens expressed primarily by systemic circulating lymphocytes (Pan T, Thy 1), antigens expressed by malignant lymphocytic cells (CALLA), and antigens of the major histocompatibility complex (MHC) (4, 17, 29, 35). It is intriguing that some of these antigens are present within the CNS and on brain tumor cells.

Expression of the lymphoid differentiation antigen HLA-DR, a Class II MHC antigen, is necessary for a cell to function as an antigen-presenting accessory cell and therefore to stimulate helper T lymphocytes (33). It is surprising to find that activated astrocytes, fetal astrocytes, glioma cells, and endothelia of vessels within the CNS all have the ability to express HLA-DR and that this expression can in some cases be modulated by immune interferon (IFN gamma) (16, 25). The exact significance of this finding is unknown, but one is tempted to hypothesize that cells within the CNS and tumor cells have the potential to function as antigen-presenting cells when they display HLA-DR. This concept is supported by the recent finding that rat astrocytes can present myelin basic protein antigen to activate helper T lymphocytes *in vitro* (15).

The presence of LDA on cells in the CNS provides a unique perspective on immune function within the brain. This refutes the previously held view that the CNS is an immunologically privileged site and suggests that the cells comprising the central nervous system and tumor cells may function as integral parts of the cellular immune system.

TUMOR-ASSOCIATED ANTIGENS

The second group of antigens identified using MABs is tumor-associated antigens (TAA). This group comprises the neuroectodermal antigens and the glial antigens.

Neuroectodermal antigens are present on tissues derived from the neuroectoderm and the tumors that arise therefrom. *In vivo,* these antigens have been detected on melanomas, neuroblastomas, gliomas, and endothelial cells within gliomas (3, 5, 14, 18, 26, 30). Screening tissues with MABs specific for these antigens has shown that there is no one single specific neuroectodermal antigen, with universal representation on all tumors derived from the neuroectoderm, that could be used for specific identification of such tumors. Rather there is a group of antigens which may be present singly or in groups.

The use of MABs recognizing neuroectodermal antigens on the vessels within malignant gliomas may provide an important means for recognition and localization of these tumors *in vivo.*

Glial Antigens.   Much of the original investigation of tumor antigens was prompted by a search for a unique "glioma specific antigen" that would be present only on cells of a glioma. To date, no antigen solely unique to the glioma cell has been identified. In the course of this work, several glioma antigens have been recognized. These antigens are primarily expressed by glioma cells but have some other minor representation on normal tissues and reactive astrocytes (2, 11, 12).

At present investigators are attempting to characterize the exact molecule that is bound by these MABs (13). In this way similarities between various MABs recognizing glial antigens might be appreciated, and coexpression of similar antigen molecules on normal cells might be understood. An example of such investigation is the isolation of a single protein molecule by immunoprecipitation that binds with two different glioma MABs (13). This finding gives significant insight into the tremendous specificity of the immune system.

Due to the favorable specificity of the glial antigens for glial cells, MABs specific for these antigens are being carefully studied for possible use in immunodiagnosis and immunotherapy (Table 19.2).

TABLE 19.2
Potential Applications of MAB for Brain Tumors

Diagnosis
Immunopathology
Cytopathology: CSF
Scanning
Therapy
Cytotoxicity of MAB
Complement- or cell-mediated
Drug ⎫
Toxin   ⎬   Conjugation
Radionuclide ⎭
Inhibition of receptors for growth factors (EGF[a], PDGF)
Anti-idiotype MAB

[a] EGF, epidermal growth factor; PDGF, platelet-derived growth factor.

LIMITATIONS IN THE USE OF MABs

Before MABs may be safely employed *in vivo* to identify specific antigens on tumors, several important limitations in their use must be addressed. First, because MABs are produced using tissue-cultured cells, all MABs must be tested using immunohistological techniques to check their representation on human tissues *in vivo*. Second, the actual antigen that a MAB recognizes must be isolated and characterized so as to eliminate cross-reactions with similar determinants on normal tissue. Finally, cells of brain tumors have a constantly varying multiprobable antigenicity (1, 31, 35). Intrinsic and extrinsic factors such as cell age, state of the cell in its cell cycle, heterogeneity of the original clonogenic cells, and effects of attempted therapy can all modify cellular antigen expression. It is generally accepted that a given tumor-associated antigen (TAA) is usually expressed on more than one type of tumor. Neuroectodermal TAAs are good examples of this. In addition, not all tumors of a given type will express a given TAA, and not all cells within a single tumor will express this particular TAA. This concept significantly limits the probability that a MAB for a single antigen would be able to identify a critical number of tumor cells. In this case, one might consider that artificially produced polymonoclonal antibodies would be successful in recognizing enough tumor cells for useful intervention.

IMMUNOHISTOLOGICAL DIAGNOSIS OF BRAIN TUMORS WITH MABs

With the development of MABs for glial and neuroectodermal antigens, techniques for immunohistological diagnosis of brain tumors have developed rapidly. As a supplement to established histological techniques, the evaluation of tissue specimens with MABs has expanded our ability to accurately identify specific groups of cells comprising a brain tumor. By this means many CNS tumors whose diagnosis would previously have been questioned have been accurately recognized (8, 9).

Coakham and Brownell have been particularly successful using MABs for this purpose (9). Examining MAB binding to tumor antigens they established antigenic profiles for many CNS tumors, including meningiomas, gliomas, schwannomas, medulloblastomas, and neuroblastomas. Other investigators are pursuing similar investigations.

One area in which immunohistological diagnosis with MABs is of particular value is the analysis of small tissue specimens obtained by stereotactic biopsy. Careful, accurate MAB-guided diagnosis of these tumor biopsies may enhance application of appropriate specific therapy. Currently, our laboratory is analyzing stereotactic biopsies of CNS tumors using a panel of MABs for glial, neuroectodermal, and other antigens. We have found that this technique greatly assists in the diagnosis of cerebral gliomas and other brain tumors including metastases. The use of MABs to aid in the diagnosis of tumors from very small biopsies is in its infancy and promises to become an important adjunct to basic neuropathological techniques in the future.

RADIOIMMUNOLOCALIZATION OF BRAIN TUMORS USING MABs

The utilization of systemically administered labeled MABs for the immunolocalization of brain tumors is an *in vivo* extension of the use of MABs for immunohistochemical purposes. From the clinical point of view, the ability to use labeled MABs for *in vivo* diagnosis and localization of brain tumors, for evaluation of surgical tumor removal, and for early detection of metastasis and primary tumor recurrence would be extremely useful. While the concept of employing MABs for this purpose is straightforward, the translation from concept to clinical application has proven to be difficult.

The MABs used for any *in vivo* application must be very carefully evaluated. The antigen binding with the MAB must be isolated and characterized; the affinity of the MAB for this antigen must be determined, and the recognition of similar antigens on normal tissue must be known. In addition, the patient's reaction to the foreign MAB protein and the attached label must be tested. Only with this information can a MAB be chosen that will be safe for the patient and will have the highest probability of recognizing the necessary antigen.

Throughout an intracerebral tumor and in the bordering reactive brain, there is variability in the blood-tissue distribution of any protein (*i.e.*, MAB). This presents a significant problem for immunolocalization, for the success of this form of tumor localization depends upon exposing all of the tumor cells to a critical concentration of high affinity labeled MAB.

The tight junctions between the endothelial cells are considered to form the blood-brain barrier (BBB) which retards penetration of large molecular weight species into the CNS (27). Within the central necrotic areas of the tumor the BBB is abnormal either as a result of tumor-induced endothelial changes or as a result of necrosis of the vessel itself. Large molecules can easily accumulate or pool in these areas. In the case of labeled MAB this may result in nonspecific accumulation, hence, false localization of the tumor.

Conversely, at the actively growing peripheral areas of tumor, the BBB is probably near normal, as tumor growth appears to precede the development of abnormal vasculature (21). Identification of this area of tumor is of great importance for precise delineation of tumor size and/or extension. For this reason it might be necessary to utilize techniques for the disruption of the BBB to enhance entrance of labeled MAB into the peripheral areas of tumor (21, 22).

Another way to circumvent the BBB problem and to obtain better tumor localization is the use of antibody fragments. MAB fragments have been shown to be more rapidly eliminated from the circulation and to penetrate better into tumors. One has the choice between Fab fragments, the smallest, but with a single binding site, and the $F(ab^1)2$ fragments, with two binding sites. Since a relatively low affinity becomes a limiting factor when a fragment with a single binding site is used, we have chosen to work with $F(ab^1)2$ fragments.

One form of immunolocalization that is particularly attractive and presents fewer technical problems is the detection of neuroectodermal melanoma antigens on the vasculature within the tumor. Since these endothelial cells appear to express melanoma neuroectodermal antigens in response to the neighboring tumor, one might be able to identify the altered vasculature and, hence, the tumor itself using labeled MABs for these antigens. This technique would not require that the labeled MAB cross the BBB, or traverse an intercellular space before reaching the tumor cells. Our group has studied the binding characteristics of the anti-melanoma MAB Mel-14, recognizing a neuroectodermal tumor antigen of high molecular weight (250 kilodaltons glycoprotein) which, as mentioned above, is also present on glioma cells and endothelial cells within gliomas. The frozen sections of 100 intracranial tumors were studied, including 50 malignant gliomas. The antibody bound to the tumor cells and endothelial cells of more than 80% of the malignant gliomas and never to normal brain. The same MAB Mel-14 has been studied by Wikstrand for its localization *in vivo* in an athymic mouse-human glioma xenograft model (37). Paired label studies with the specific MAB and a control immunoglobulin allowed calculation of specific localization indices.

The paired-label technique permits measuring directly the intratumoral enrichment of the tumor-directed antibody due to its binding to the target cells over the nonspecific accumulation of a control immunoglobulin. It allows, by means of the specificity index, determined as the ratio of the level of MAB to that of the control immunoglobulin in a given tissue or fluid, to define specific antibody uptake, excluding factors such as BBB, vascularity, necrosis, extracellular space, binding through the F_c-portion, and uptake into the reticuloendothelial system since these factors apply equally to the control antibody and to the tumor-directed antibody. MAB Mel-14 was found to steadily accumulate into the glioma xenografts and to maintain a localization index of 2.5–5 for up to 7 days after intravenous injection.

Based on these encouraging observations we have injected four glioma patients scheduled for operation with the MAB Mel-14, having recognized a neuroectodermal tumor antigen for *in vivo* location studies of the antibody in the tumor using the paired-label technique. $F(ab^1)2$ fragments of the MAB were labeled with ^{123}I and ^{125}I and, as a control, F(ab[1])2 fragments of an irrelevant IgG were labeled with [131]I. The ^{123}I has a physical half-life of 13 hours and was used for scanning using a single photon emission computerized tomoscan (SPECT), whereas labeling with ^{125}I allowed later measurement of radioactivity of tissue specimens taken at operation. The differential counting of specifically bound radioactivity ^{125}I and nonspecifically accumulated radioactivity ^{131}I allowed the calculation of the specificity index. The patients had no history of allergy and, in order to prevent an allergic reaction, received 2 mg clemastine p.o. and 100 mg methylprednisolone i.v. before the injection of the MAB, and 400 mg perchlorate on the day of the injection. To block the thyroid, 10 drops of Lugol 5% iodine solution p.o. were given every day for 5 days, beginning on the day before the injection. Specific F(ab[1])2 fragments (1.5 mg) were labeled with 0.3 mCi ^{125}I and 10 mCi ^{123}I; the control F(ab[1])2 fragments were labeled with 0.3 mCi [131]I. The mixture was given in a 1-hour i.v. perfusion. The scans were performed 6 and 24 hours after injection and the operation 48 hours after injection. The results of this preliminary study indicate that there is a definite uptake of the antibody in the tumor due to its specificity with a specificity index of 2–3. The external detection, however, was far from optimal due to accumulation of radioactivity in the bone. In one case, for example, the activity per gram of tissue bound to the specific antibody fragment was 13.95 times higher in the tumor than in normal brain, whereas the activity bound to the control was 5.51 times higher in the tumor than in normal brain, resulting in a specificity index of localization of 2.53 as shown in Table 19.3. The same ratios for tumor and blood gave values of 2.29 for the isotope of the specific antibody fragment and 0.42 for the isotope of the control, resulting in a specificity index of 5.39. The values were obtained by taking the average of two different tumor specimens. In another case the MAB was injected by selective carotid catheterization. This procedure did not increase the specificity index in the tumor.

These preliminary results are somehow disappointing because the amount of antibody specifically binding to tumor cells *in vivo* is small. However, they show undoubtedly that specific localization does indeed take place. Our future work will concentrate on the use of combinations of different MABs to overcome antigenic heterogeneity and possibly osmotic agents to open the blood-brain barrier.

Similar human studies were performed by Coakham (10) using MAB UJ13A recognizing another neuroectodermal antigen.

A third MAB which has a very interesting potential for clinical application is 81C6 recognizing an extracellular matrix antigen (2). This MAB showed an excellent specific localization *in vivo* in the athymic

TABLE 19.3

Accumulation of Antibody Fragments in Tumor vs. Control as Compared with Normal Tissues in One Case

Comparison with Normal Tissue	Antibody Fragment Uptake[a]	Control Uptake[b]	Specificity Index[c]
Normal brain	13.95[d]	5.51	2.53
CSF	84.39	37.38	2.26
Blood	2.29	0.42	5.39
Plasma	1.46	0.26	5.61
Muscle	2.92	1.55	1.88

[a] Activity of the antibody-fragment bound isotope per gram tumor divided by the activity of the same isotope per gram normal tissue.

[b] Activity of the control-bound isotope per gram tumor divided by the activity of the same isotope per gram normal tissue.

[c] Antibody uptake divided by control uptake.

[d] All of the values refer to an average of two tumor specimens.

mouse-human glioma xenograft model (37) with localization indices up to 20 maintained at 7–9 days after injection.

IMMUNOTHERAPY UTILIZING MABs

The possibility of using a MAB as a carrier for therapeutic agents is intriguing. While this concept has been considered for many years, its realization has been obscured by many obstacles. All of the antigens recognized by the MABs produced to date have some secondary representation on normal tissues. In order for MAB therapy to be safe, the coexpression of these antigens on normal cells must be minimal as discussed above. Even if this was not a problem, there is always the possibility of an anaphylactic reaction to the foreign MAB protein, particularly if the MAB is administered repeatedly. This anaphylactic reaction can be obviated by attempts to produce human MABs or by the construction of a chimeric MAB with the specific variable binding site of mouse origin and the constant region of human origin.

Other problems that temper one's enthusiasm for this technique of therapy include the difficulty of successfully linking a MAB to a chemotherapeutic or radiotherapeutic agent without destroying either the specificity/affinity of the MAB or the toxic characteristics of the noxious agent and penetration of the MAB through the BBB.

Recently a technique has been described which allows the construction of heteroconjugates of monoclonal antibodies referred to as hybrid antibodies (32). In these hybrid antibodies, one of the component binding sites is specific for a cytotoxic T-cell receptor or any toxic substance, and the other component binding site is directed against a chosen tumor-associated antigen. The hybrid antibodies can thus focus the toxic agent on the target tumor cell.

Finally, as discussed above, there is a significant variability of antigen expression among the tumor cells. In this case using one MAB, the therapeutic agent might not be delivered to and destroy a significantly large number of cells. Again the idea of a polymonoclonal antibody might be considered in order that a critical number of cells be destroyed.

CONCLUSION

The discovery and development of techniques for the production of monoclonal antibodies has significantly aided our understanding of the immunobiology of brain tumors. This knowledge has allowed us to be more accurate in the histological diagnosis of brain tumors and has spurred investigation of possible ways in which these MABs might be used to better localize brain tumors and destroy them. At present, significant obstacles limit the practical clinical application of MABs for the above purposes. Further research and investigation both in the laboratory and *in vivo* are necessary to realize the full potential MABs may offer us. A new way might be opened by the development of MABs directed against oncogene products expressed on the surface of tumor cells in larger amounts than on normal cells. Some of these oncogene products are receptors for growth factors as, for example, the epidermal growth factor receptor encoded by the *c-erb* B oncogene, or the platelet-derived growth factor encoded by the *sis* oncogene (see ref. 34 for a review). MABs against such growth factor receptors might be used either to interfere with the action of the growth factor and its receptor on mitogenesis or to bring toxic agents in contact with the tumor cells.

ACKNOWLEDGMENT

This work was supported by Grant 3.088-0.84 of the Swiss National Science Foundation.

REFERENCES

1. Bigner, D. D. The biology of gliomas: Potential clinical implications of glioma cellular heterogeneity. Neurosurgery, 9: 320–326, 1982.
2. Bourdon, M. A., Wikstrand, C. J., Furthmayr, H., et al. Human glioma-mesenchymal extracellular matrix antigen defined by monoclonal antibody. Cancer Res., 43: 2796–2805, 1983.
3. Cairncross, J. G., Mattes, M. J., Beresford, H. R., et al. Cell surface antigens of human astrocytoma defined by mouse monoclonal antibodies: Identification of astrocytoma subsets. Proc. Natl. Acad. Sci. U.S.A., 79: 5641–5645, 1982.
4. Carrel, S., de Tribolet, N., and Gross, N. Expression of HLA-DR and common acute lymphoblastic leukemia antigens on glioma cells. Eur. J. Immunol., 12: 354–357, 1982.
5. Carrel, S., de Tribolet, N., and Mach, J. P. Expression of neuroectodermal antigens common to melanomas: Gliomas and neuroblastomas. Acta Neuropathol., 57: 158–164, 1982.
6. Coakham, H. B. Immunology of human brain tumors. Eur. J. Cancer Clin. Oncol., 20: 145–149, 1984.

7. Coakham, H. B., and Lakshmi, M. S. Tumor associated surface antigens in human astrocytomas. Oncology, *31:* 233–243, 1975.

8. Coakham, H. B., Garson, J. A., Allam, P. A., *et al.* Immunohistological diagnosis of central nervous system tumors using a monoclonal antibody panel. J. Clin. Pathol., *38:* 165–173, 1985.

9. Coakham, H. B., Garson, J. A., Brownell, B., *et al.* Monoclonal antibodies as reagents for brain tumor diagnosis: A review. J. R. Soc. Med. *77:* 780–787, 1984.

10. Coakham, H. B., Kemshead, J. T., Davies, R. B., *et al.* Clinical experience with antiglioma monoclonal antibodies. J. Neurooncol., *4:* 101, 1986.

11. de Muralt, B., de Tribolet, N., Diserens, A. C., *et al.* Reactivity of antiglioma monoclonal antibodies for a large panel of cultured gliomas and other neuroectodermal derived tumors. Anticancer Res., *3:* 1–6, 1983.

12. de Tribolet, N., and Carrel, S. Human glioma associated antigens. Cancer Immun. Immunother., *9:* 207, 1980.

13. de Tribolet, N., Carrel, S., and Mach, J. P. Brain tumor associated antigens. Prog. Exp. Tumor Res., *27:* 118–131, 1984.

14. Dickinson, J. G., Flanigan, T. P., Kemshead, J. T., *et al.* Identification of cell surface antigens present exclusively on a sub-population of astrocytes in human foetal brain cultures. J. Neuroimmunol., *5:* 111–123, 1983.

15. Fontana, A., Fierz, W., and Wekerle, H. Astrocytes present myelin basic protein to encephalitogenic T cell lines. Nature, *307:* 273–276, 1984.

16. Gerosa, M., Chilosi, M., Iannucci, A., *et al.* Immunohistochemical characterization of Ia-DR positive cells in normal brain and gliomas. J. Neurooncol., *2:* 272, 1984.

17. Kemshead, J. T., Ritter, M. A., Cotmore, S. F., *et al.* Human Thy-1 expression on cell surfaces of neuronal and glial cells. Brain Res., *236:* 451–461, 1982.

18. Kennett, R. H., and Gilbert, F. M. Hybrid myelomas producing antibodies against human neuroblastoma antigen present on foetal brain. Science, *203:* 1120–1121, 1978.

19. Köhler, G., and Milstein, C. Continuous cultures of fused cells secreting antibody of predefined specificity. Nature, *256:* 495–497, 1975.

20. Mahaley, M. S. Jr. Experiences with antibody production for human glioma tissue. Prog. Exp. Tumor Res., *17:* 31–39, 1972.

21. Neuwelt, E. A. Therapeutic potential for blood brain barrier modification in malignant brain tumors. Prog. Exp. Tumor Res., *28:* 51–66, 1984.

22. Neuwelt, E. A., Specht, H. D., and Hill, S. A. Permeability of human brain tumor to 99 m Tc-glucoheptonate and 99 m Tc-albumin: Implications for monoclonal antibody therapy. J. Neurosurg., *65:* 194–198, 1986.

23. Pfreundschuh, M., Röhrich, M., Piotroski, W., *et al.* Natural antibodies to cell surface antigens of human astrocytoma. Int. J. Cancer, *29:* 517–521, 1982.

24. Pfreundschuh, M., Shiku, H., Takahashi, R., *et al.* Serologic analysis of cell surface antigens of malignant human brain tumor. Proc. Natl. Acad. Sci. U.S.A., *75:* 5122–5126, 1978.

25. Piguet, V., Carrel, S., Diserens, A. C., *et al.* Heterogeneity of the induction of HLA-DR expression by human immune interferon on glioma cell lines and their clones. J. Natl. Cancer Inst., *76:* 223–228, 1986.

26. Piguet, V., Diserens, A. C., Carrel, S., *et al.* The immunology of human gliomas. Springer Semin. Immunopathol., *8:* 111–127, 1985.

27. Rapoport, S. I. *Blood Brain Barrier in Physiology and Medicine.* Raven Press, New York, 1976.

28. Schnegg, J. F., de Tribolet, N., Diserens, A. C., *et al.* Characterization of a rabbit antihuman malignant glioma antiserum. Int. J. Cancer., *28:* 265–269, 1981.

29. Seeger, R. C., Damon, Y. L., Rayner, S. A., *et al.* Definition of Thy 1 determinant on

human neuroblastoma, glioma, sarcoma and teratoma cells with monoclonal antibody. J. Immunol., *128:* 983–989, 1982.

30. Seeger, R. C., Rosenblatt, H. M., Imai, K., *et al.* Common antigenic determinants on human melanoma, glioma, neuroblastoma and sarcoma cells defined by monoclonal antibodies. Cancer Res., *41:* 2712–2717, 1981.
31. Shapiro, J. R., Yung, W. A., and Shapiro, W. R. Isolation, karyotype and clonal growth of heterogeneous subpopulations of human malignant gliomas. Cancer Res., *41:* 23–59, 1981.
32. Staerz, U. D., Kanagawa, O., and Bevan, M. J. Hybrid antibodies can target sites for attack by T cells. Nature, *314:* 628–631, 1985.
33. Unanue, E. R., Beller, D. I., Lu, C. Y., *et al.* Antigen presentation: Comments on its regulation and mechanism. J. Immunol., *132:* 1–14, 1984.
34. Westermark, B., Nister, M., and Heldin, C. H. Growth factors and oncogenesis in human malignant glioma. Neurol. Clin., *3:* 785–799, 1985.
35. Wikstrand, C. J., Bigner, S. H., and Bigner, D. D. Demonstration of complex antigenic heterogeneity in a human glioma cell line and eight derived clones by specific monoclonal antibodies. Cancer Res., *43:* 3327–3340, 1983.
36. Wikstrand, C. J., Mahaley, M. S., and Bigner, D. D. Surface antigenic characteristics of human glial brain tumors. Cancer Res., *37:* 4267–4275, 1977.
37. Wikstrand, C. J., McLendon, R. E., Carrel, S., *et al.* Comparative localization of glioma-reactive monoclonal antibodies *in vivo* in an athymic mouse human glioma xenograft model. J. Neuroimmunol., in press, 1987.

20

Tumors of the Cerebellopontine Angle: Combined Management by Neurological and Otological Surgeons

STEVEN L. GIANNOTTA, M.D., and JACK L. PULEC, M.D.

INTRODUCTION

The trend toward superspecialization in the surgical subspecialties has spawned two counteractive tendencies affecting interspecialty relationships. As anatomic regionalization begins to focus the surgeon on an ever-decreasing frame of reference, the inevitable border dispute flares up involving a specialist from a different discipline who innocently "trespasses" onto that same territory. Examples are legion, but the thyroid gland, carotid artery, and intervertebral disc are intermittently plundered during surgical turf battles.

"If you can't beat 'em, join 'em" characterizes the opposing and perhaps more productive trend, namely, the alliance of two or more surgical subspecialists in attacking a common problem. It is precisely the collaboration between neurosurgeons and otologists in dealing with cerebellopontine (CP) angle tumors which will serve as the focal point of this discussion. Excellent examples of the synergy possible in this type of relationship can be appreciated from the writing of House and Hitselberger, Harner and Laws, Ojemann and Montgomery, among others (5–9, 11, 13, 14). Although each of these associations is unique in terms of its interpersonal dynamics, their success is based on mutual respect, and parity of skill and innovation. The following provides simply another example of how one neurosurgeon-otologist team approaches the problem of CP angle lesions.

DIAGNOSIS

Gone are the days when a patient staggers into a neurosurgeon's office with a 5-year history of hearing loss, tinnitus, headache, and ataxia preliminary to a workup which will ultimately identify a 5-cm acoustic neuroma. Most acoustic tumors are diagnosed in the office of an otolaryngologist, as the ever-more medically sophisticated American populace begins to take their ear problems to an "ear doctor." The increasing availability of otologists with supporting audiologists, combined with the advances in electrophysiological monitoring equipment, has produced two phenomena. First, tumors are being identified at earlier stages. Second, otologists are increasingly in "control" of these patients. Our personal experience bears out the latter fact, since between 85 and 90% of CP angle tumor patients are referred to or discovered by the otologist member of the team. Referral patterns, seniority, and other factors may modify this ratio. Currently, two-thirds of our patients have hearing loss as their only physical finding, and this overall trend will likely continue.

Since abnormalities in vestibulocochlear function are the earliest manifestation of CP angle lesions, audiometry and vestibular testing play a major roll in the screening and diagnosis. When the complaint of unilateral hearing loss is confirmed by routine testing, special testing is indicated. Pure tone audiometry for air and bone conduction, speech reception threshold, and speech discrimination scores are basic to the evaluation. If these suggest a retrocochlear pathologic process, or if localization of the hearing abnormality is insufficient to establish a diagnosis, brainstem-evoked responses are performed (BAERs). An abnormality of the early latencies of the auditory brainstem response (0–8 milliseconds) reflects involvement of the cochlear nerve and brainstem. Abnormal middle latency responses (8–50 milliseconds) suggest a problem in the primary auditory projection pathway (thalamus to auditory cortex). An acoustic tumor within the internal auditory canal or CP angle not touching the brainstem produces changes in early waveform morphology, increasing wave I-V interwave latency. A delay in the wave I-V interval of 0.2 millisecond strongly suggests the presence of a tumor. When both auditory brainstem response and middle latency response are abnormal, an acoustic tumor can be expected to be pressing on the brainstem and be in excess of 2.5 cm in diameter. Should the opposite side have abnormal waveform morphology, a very large tumor (4–5 cm) can be expected with the brainstem displacement toward the normal side. We have accumulated several examples wherein routine audiometry has failed to define the cause of the hearing abnormality, and evoked response testing identified a retrocochlear pattern leading to the demonstration of an acoustic neuroma.

Of critical importance in the use of BAERs for detection of CP angle lesions is the presentation of stimuli (short square-wave clicks) at various intensities above threshold. Figure 20.1 shows the deterioration of waveform morphology and an increase in interpeak latencies when progressively weaker stimuli (90, 70, or 50 dB above threshold) are presented to the ear harboring an intracanalicular acoustic neuroma.

Audiometry testing provides additional valuable information relative to patient management. Patients with small acoustic neuromas with

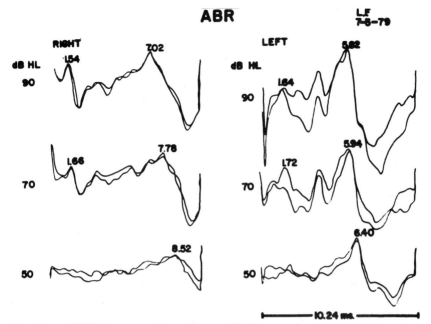

FIG. 20.1.   BAERs from a patient with a small right acoustic neuroma showing progressive increase in interpeak latencies and deterioration in wave form morphology with weaker stimuli. *ABR*, auditory brain stem (evoked) response; *HL*, hearing level.

preserved hearing and 50% or greater speech discrimination are candidates for operative approaches in which cochlear nerve function can be preserved. In this circumstance, the combined experience of neurosurgeon and otologist working as a team will be valuable in selecting the appropriate surgical approach. Our practice has been to remove intracanalicular tumors with preserved hearing through a middle fossa route (6). However, we have recently had experience with preserving cochlear nerve function using the retrosigmoid approach.

Appropriate audiologic testing has been helpful in planning our approach to other lesions in the CP angle. For example, we have found the translabyrinthine operation to be useful in certain cases of large CP angle meningiomas wherein hearing has been lost.

APPROACHES

Although the presence of two conflicting opinions can complicate the decision-making process, in general we have found that the added breadth of experience, background, and skills inherent in a multidisciplinary approach improves outcome. Also, bringing together the skills of the neurosurgeon and otologist has resulted in an expansion of the kinds of approaches used for CP angle tumors. Our experience has caused us to employ the translabyrinthine approach for most CP angle lesions in which hearing preservation is not an issue. A description of the operative technique will serve as an example of the cooperation between otologist and neurosurgeon.

Translabyrinthine Approach

Traditional thinking dictates that the translabyrinthine approach to CP angle lesions is the otological approach while the retromastoid or suboccipital approach is the neurosurgical one. With the advent of neurosurgical-otological collaboration, these approaches now can be prescribed for a given situation based on their own relative merits and drawbacks. We have chosen to use the translabyrinthine approach for all but the smallest or very large acoustic neuromas (1). Our perception of the advantages includes: (a) shorter distance between the surface and the neoplasm; (b) absence of brainstem or cerebellum retraction; (c) avoidance of the sitting position; (d) improved surgeon comfort; (e) identification of the facial nerve early in the procedure at a constant bony landmark; (f) increased preservation of the functional and anatomical integrity of the facial nerve. Drawbacks include: (a) sacrifice hearing; (b) unfamiliar anatomy; and (c) increased risk of cerebrospinal fluid (CSF) leak.

The procedure is carried out in the supine position with the head turned to the side opposite the tumor and resting on a soft pad. The surgeon is seated at the side of the table facing the mastoid area. Although convention may dictate each surgeon's role in the operative procedure, we have found it expedient that both be comfortable with all aspects of the procedure. This may necessitate some added training or experience in either surgeon's case. Especially with large and difficult tumors, the luxury of having an associate take over the procedure at any juncture is advantageous.

The mastoid is removed, skeletonizing the facial nerve and removing the entire lip of the internal auditory canal. Upon opening the dura, one is faced immediately with the tumor surface. Intracapsular removal commences following identification of the appropriate arachnoid plane. Gentle dissection around the tumor capsule is used to affect an infolding of the tumor surface toward the surgeon. This allows for appropriate bipolar coagulation of feeding vessels under direct vision. These maneuvers are always followed by further intracapsular decompression until the capsule can be infolded to the point at which brainstem and cranial nerves can be viewed along the medial aspect of the mass. Judicious resection of the tumor can then be accomplished to the point at which the tumor is maneuverable enough to allow further facial nerve dissection. The nerve is reidentified at the vertical crest in the internal canal. Fine arachnoid investments are incised sharply. The nerve is continuously bathed in CSF or saline, and traction on the nerve is minimized as much as possible. Once the tumor is removed, autologous fat is packed into the mastoid cavity, occluding the dural opening.

We have utilized this approach for 50 acoustic neuromas. Anatomical preservation of the facial nerve was accomplished in 96%, with functional preservation in 92%. Only one patient experienced prolonged neurological morbidity other than hearing loss.

Transotic Approach

For CP angle tumors with marked medial or middle fossa extension, such as large acoustic neuromas or petrous apex meningiomas, the transotic approach provides certain benefits. It is a natural extension of the translabyrinthine approach since hearing preservation is not an issue. The translabyrinthine approach is accomplished in the usual fashion. In order to get further exposure in an anteromedial direction, the greater superficial petrosal nerve is divided at its junction with the geniculate ganglion (Fig. 20.2). This allows the facial nerve to be removed from the Fallopian canal and mobilized inferiorly. The cochlea and surrounding

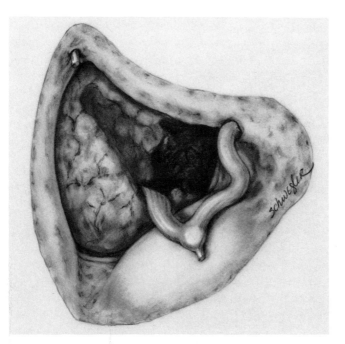

FIG. 20.2.   Partial resection of right CP angle tumor through a transotic approach. The greater superficial petrosal nerve has been divided to mobilize the facial nerve.

bone is removed with the drill, providing exposure all the way to the petrous apex. An example of a petrous meningioma removed through this approach can be seen in Figure 20.3.

Combined Approaches

In those unfortunate circumstances where CP angle tumors have grown so large that they defy removal through one of the more traditional portals, the skills of the otologist and neurosurgeon can be combined to design alternative strategies. King and Morrison have championed the translabyrinthine transtentorial approach for lesions which extend into the middle fossa (7). Tator and Nedzelski added their modifications, claiming improved facial nerve preservation in conjunction with enhanced exposure (12).

Following the standard translabyrinthine dissection, a temporal bone flap is removed. The remaining bone of the middle fossa plate is drilled away. The dura over the temporal lobe, floor of the middle fossa, and posterior fossa is opened in conjunction with the tentorium to the incisura. Temporal lobe retraction remains a necessity with this approach.

Tumors with extensive involvement inferiorly may best be handled with a combined retromastoid-translabyrinthine approach. An example

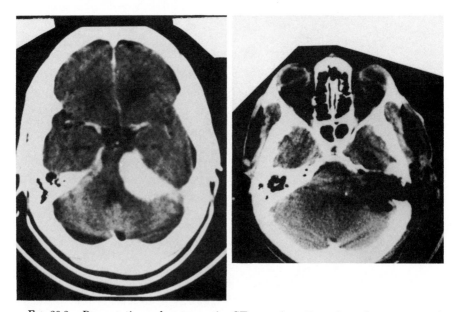

FIG. 20.3.   Preoperative and postoperative CT scan of a patient who underwent transotic removal of petrous ridge meningioma.

of a tumor removed through this approach in which the sigmoid sinus impeded exposure to the posterior extent of the mass is shown in Figure 20.4. To be able to resect a lesion of this magnitude without resecting or retracting the cerebellar hemisphere was felt to be a distinct advantage. Our experience has been that with continued familiarity with the translabyrinthine approach, larger tumors can be removed through this portal alone.

INSTRUMENTATION

One of the byproducts of a close affiliation with another surgical specialty is the exposure to a variety of instrumentation. Over the years, our favorite tools have been combined to the point at which the operating room setup is a hybrid between that of a neurosurgeon and an otolaryngologist. Mayo stands and back tables supplant the traditional "overhead" apparatus. A powerful foot-controlled, well-balanced drill with suction irrigation sits side-by-side with Malis bipolar electrocautery. For microdissection, a dizzying array of raspatories, spatulas, nerve hooks, canal knives, and curets provides added versatility. Tumors of virtually any consistency will yield to the House-Urban rotodissector, argon or CO_2 laser, or Cavitron. Microneedle holders and tying forceps appropriated

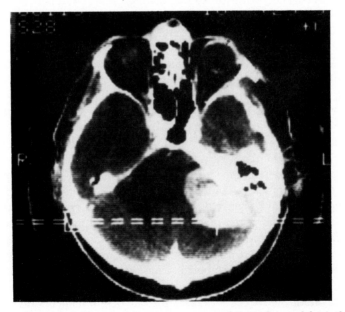

FIG. 20.4. Large recurrent acoustic neuroma removed through translabyrinthine-transigmoid approach.

from the bypass tray are available for facial nerve anastomosis at the termination of a successful facial neuroma removal.

Neurosurgery has never hesitated to borrow freely from head and neck instrumentation. Woodson, Sheehy, Freer, and House are some of the notable contributors to "neurosurgical" instrumentation.

COMPLICATIONS

CSF Leak

One of the more frustrating complications of an otherwise successful removal of a CP angle tumor is CSF otorhinorrhea. Contemporary series of acoustic neuroma resection using various techniques place the incidence of CSF leak at 6–30% (3, 4). Innovations resulting from the joint efforts of neurosurgeons and otologists have made the management and avoidance of this problem more successful.

Historically, the translabyrinthine approach to the CP angle has the higher incidence of otorhinorrhea in comparison to the retromastoid approach. Our early experience with this complication approached a 20% incidence of leakage either through the nose or the skin incision with a 10% chance of clinical or laboratory evidence of meningitis. Attempts at obtaining a watertight dural closure, even utilizing tissue adhesives, proved futile. Despite a large autologous fat graft in the mastoid, leaks would still occur. Our solution to this problem involves opening the facial recess at the end of each procedure using a small diamond drill. This, of course, puts the facial nerve at greater risk; however, a skillful otologist should have no difficulty with this technique. The tubotympanum is entered, and its mucosa and the Eustachian tube are roughened using a ring curet. An autologous temporalis muscle graft is packed into the orifice so as not to compress the facial nerve. The fat graft taken from the lower abdomen is carefully packed into the antrum to provide a temporary barrier until the regenerating arachnoid can form a proper seal. This technique in our hands has virtually eliminated rhinorrhea as a complication of the translabyrinthine approach.

Occasionally CSF leakage through the skin incision will mar an otherwise successful operation. If local measures are unsuccessful at stopping the drainage, we have eschewed the use of lumbar spinal drainage, and gone directly to revising the operative site. This is performed under local anesthesia by either one of the cosurgeons. The incision is reopened, and the fat graft is examined under the operating microscope. Frequently a rearrangement of the graft to better occlude the dural opening and tight reclosure of the skin are all that is necessary. If the adipose graft is deemed too small, more fat is taken from the original specimen harvested during the first procedure and kept refrigerated for this eventuality. This procedure has invariably been effective at stopping the leak and does not unduly prolong the hospital stay.

Harner and Laws have recommended the translabyrinthine approach for repair of CSF fistula resulting from a retromastoid removal of acoustic neuromas (4). They emphasized the greater likelihood of identification of the site of leakage as well as the ability to seal off the Eustachian tube as benefits of this procedure.

Facial Nerve Injury

On three occasions (one facial neuroma, two acoustic neuromas) we have been faced with either partial or total transection of the facial nerve. In one instance 80% of the diameter of the nerve was transected. The transected portions were repaired primarily with 10-0 nylon without disrupting the intact portion. For the total transections, a cable graft was fashioned. The otologist harvests an appropriate-sized segment of greater auricular nerve from the ipsilateral neck while the neurosurgeon prepares the instrumentation and facial nerve ends to accept the graft (10). Using 20-cm bayonet microforceps and needle holders, a 10-0 nylon suture is used to create the anastomosis. Eighty to 85% return with minimal synkinesis resulted from one such repair, while insufficient time has elapsed to assess the other.

CONCLUSION

Many positive benefits can occur from a successful alliance among surgical subspecialties. In our own practices, the inevitable cross-fertilization of ideas has spawned innovative procedures useful for conditions other than those subject to the original collaboration. We are convinced that our surgical results have measurably improved as a result. It is important that for a lasting and successful relationship of this sort, the principals be of reasonably similar skill levels and work to maintain cooperative attitudes.

REFERENCES

1. Giannotta, S. L., Pulec, J. L. Translabyrinthine approach for cerebellopontine angle lesions. Contemp. Neurosurg., 8: 1–5, 1986.
2. Giannotta, S. L., Pulec, J. L., and Goodkin, R. Translabyrinthine removal of cerebellopontine angle meningiomas. Neurosurgery, 17: 620–625, 1985.
3. Harner, S. G., and Ebersold, M. J. Management of acoustic neuromas. J. Neurosurg., 63: 175–179, 1985.
4. Harner, S. G., and Laws, E. R., Jr. Translabyrinthine repair for cerebrospinal fluid otorhinorrhea. J. Neurosurg., 57: 258–261, 1982.
5. Harner, S. G., and Laws, E. R., Jr. Clinical findings in patients with acoustic neurinoma. Mayo Clin. Proc., 58: 721–728, 1983.
6. House, F., and Hitselberger, W. E. The middle fossa approach for removal of small acoustic tumors. Acta Otolaryngol. [Stockh.], 67: 413–427, 1969.

7. King, T. T., and Morrison, A. W. Translabyrinthine and transtentorial removal of acoustic nerve tumors: Results in 150 cases. J. Neurosurg., *52:* 210–216, 1980.

8. Moller, A. R., and Jannetta, P. J. Preservation of facial function during removal of acoustic neuromas. J. Neurosurg., *61:* 757–760, 1984.

9. Ojemann, R. G., Levine, R. A., Montgomery, W. M., and McGaffigan, P. Use of intraoperative auditory evoked potentials to preserve hearing in unilateral acoustic neuroma removal. J. Neurosurg., *61:* 938–948, 1984.

10. Pulec, J. L. Symposium on ear surgery. II. Facial nerve neuroma. Laryngoscope, *82*(7): 1160–1176, 1972.

11. Sterkers, J-M., Desgeorges, M., Sterkers, O., *et al.* Our present approach to acoustic neuroma surgery. In *Neuro-Otology and Skull Base Surgery*, edited by P. van den Brock, C. Cremers, G. Hoogland, and J. Manni, pp. 160–164. Karger, Basel, 1984.

12. Tator, C. H., and Nedzelski, J. M. Facial nerve preservation in patients with large acoustic neuromas treated by a combined middle fossa transtentorial translabyrinthine approach. J. Neurosurg., *57:* 1–7, 1982.

13. Tator, C. H., and Nedzelski, J. M. Preservation of hearing in patients undergoing excision of acoustic neuromas and other cerebellopontine angle tumors. J. Neurosurg., *63:* 168–174, 1985.

14. Tew, J. M., Yeh, H-S., Miller, G. W., *et al.* Intratemporal schwannoma of the facial nerve. Neurosurgery, *13*(2): 186–188, 1983.

CHAPTER

21

Spectrum of Exposures for Skull Base Tumors

CLARENCE T. SASAKI, M.D.

INTRODUCTION

For years otolaryngologists have treated the paranasal sinuses and mastoids, structures anatomically constituting the skull base. However, contemporary skull base surgery traverses the cranial base, tending to be more complex and often implying the combination of multiple surgical disciplines in a truly team effort.

Of course, the team concept is not a new one.

Historically, surgery began outside the more learned profession of medicine as the art of practitioners who were able to treat injury and disease by cutting, fulgurating, or realigning tissues. Since the turn of the century, subspecialization of surgery developed on the basis of the need for knowledge of specific body systems, special diagnostic tools and tests, distinctive surgical skills and instruments, and the prevention and treatment of complications of surgical procedures. These bases defined surgical subspecialty areas and patients, medicine, and surgery benefited.

However, a liability of this development arose by the very same aspects that originally delineated the specialist and advanced his science and art. Territorial limitations prevented the subspecialist from readily engaging in surgery of diseases that overlapped his area of subspecialization. Thus, any one subspecialty was inadequate to treat all conditions and especially those conditions for which a territorial claim had not yet been clearly defined. Surgery of the skull base is precisely where such a cooperative need arises and where Neurosurgery and Otolaryngology may be necessary to treat a patient's disease adequately and safely (2).

With this realization, surgery of the skull base flourishes, and patients rightfully benefit.

On a parallel level, advances in skull base surgery have heavily depended on recent technological improvements. The capability of sophisticated diagnostic imaging, laser hemostasis, surgical illumination, and magnification collectively have exerted unprecedented impact on a form of regional surgery previously hampered by great anatomic complexity. Furthermore, improved understanding of brain protection and primary closure of wounds with well-vascularized local and regional skin flaps now greatly diminish the incidence of exposure-necrosis and life-threatening infection, thus further reducing the morbidity and mortality of surgical intervention.

Thus the recent growth of surgery related to the cranial base rests on two major factors: (a) recent technological advances; and, (b) the spirit of cooperative effort across disciplines.

The spectrum of modern skull base surgery now safely includes transethmoid and transseptal exposures of the pituitary fossa, transpalatal routes to the basisphenoid, infratemporal exposure of the clivus, and translabyrinthine or transcochlear routes to the cerebellopontine angle. This chapter is based upon two procedures that best exemplify the impact of technological advances and the spirit of cooperative effort between the subspecialties.

TUMORS OF THE ANTERIOR SKULL BASE

Malignancies involving the anterior skull base constitute a unique group of neoplasms posing one of the most formidable problems in oncologic management. Such cancers, biologically no different from other histologic types found in the head and neck, produce a significant therapeutic dilemma due to the proximity of the eye, brain, major dural sinuses, carotid artery, and cranial nerves (Figs. 21.1–21.3). Any or all of these structures may be invaded by cancer, and their vital functions can be greatly disturbed by either the disease itself or by subsequent therapy. Whereas the same histologic tumor, arising elsewhere in the head and neck, is aggressively attacked and, as a result, often successfully eradicated, tumor surgery of the cranial base is often compromised for technical reasons related to anatomic complexity. For this reason, malignancies involving the anterior skull base have historically carried a dismal, if not altogether hopeless, outlook.

The recent use of combined craniofacial resection has improved curability for many patients once considered hopeless, effectively changing our therapeutic outlook for disease in this location. Dandy (4) in 1941 first described a transcranial approach to resect orbital tumors. A decade later, others (6, 9, 13) reported successes in resecting frontoethmoid cancers by this technique. While the benefits of this surgery were high, so were the initially reported complications: 7% mortality, 80% morbid-

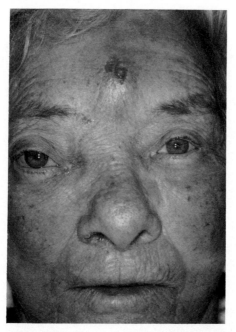

FIG. 21.1. Preoperative examination reveals tumor at the midline of the forehead also producing proptosis and lateral displacement of the right eye. Note purulent right nasal discharge.

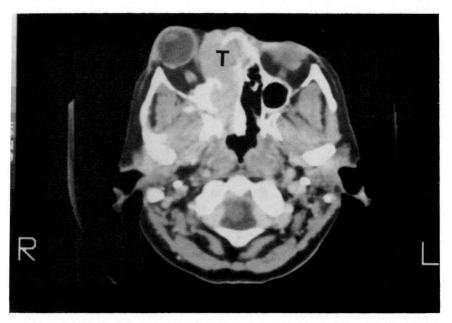

FIG. 21.2. Computed tomography indicates tumor (*T*) has eroded the right ethmoids and extends into the right orbit.

469

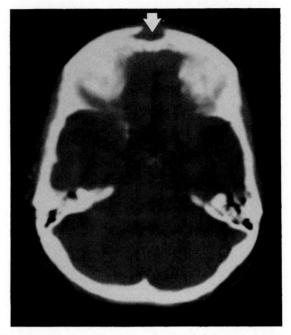

Fig. 21.3.   Tumor within the frontal sinus has eroded through its anterior wall in the midline (*arrow*).

ity. Since then, Sisson *et al.* (12) and Schramm and Myers (10) have reported useful reconstructive techniques to minimize the expected morbidity of otherwise heroic surgery, resulting in further surgical acceptability.

Nevertheless, potentially life-threatening complications continue to threaten otherwise successful oncologic resections with exposed bone and cerebrospinal fluid (CSF) leaks in half the patients and as reported by others infection in almost all of them (6). Such morbidity may be related to inadequate intracranial protection by split-thickness skin grafts that may not take completely in all areas of repair following curative radiation therapy. Furthermore, we may anticipate that the use of vascularized flaps would not only better seal against CSF leaks, but also would afford improved protection against bacterial invasion at the operative site. Upon these anticipated benefits, we will report on 10 cases using the pectoralis major myocutaneous flap in the reconstruction of anterior skull base defects following major oncologic resections.

Operative Procedure

The combined intracranial-extracranial approach for *en bloc* resection is worth a brief description:

1. Perioperative antibiotics, based upon a recent nasal culture, are begun the night before surgery and are continued every 4 hours through surgery. Antibiotics are directed against the *predominant* bacterial organism obtained from the nose. If a CSF leak occurs during surgery, antibiotics are continued for 5 days postoperatively. If no leakage has occurred, only two additional doses are administered postoperatively.

2. To prevent secondary injury to the brain following intraoperative retraction, dexamethasone is administered the day prior to surgery at a dose of 4 mg every 6 hours. This dose is continued intravenously through surgery and is rapidly tapered in 3–4 days postoperatively.

3. Following the administration of general anesthesia, a lumbar subarachnoid catheter is inserted. Slow, gentle suction or gravity drainage is used to remove 100–120 ml of CSF. Brain relaxation will minimize the need for prolonged brain retraction and compression, reducing direct injury to the frontal cortex.

4. Controlled hyperventilation is used to lower the pCO_2 to approximately 25 torr. This accomplishes an additional decrease in brain volume by cerebral vasoconstriction.

5. To further minimize brain retraction, mannitol (500 ml) is administered as a 20% solution to dehydrate and shrink the brain. It is given intravenously when the scalp incision is made.

6. A frontal craniotomy is performed through a large bicoronal flap. The dura of the frontal lobe is retracted to expose the floor of the anterior cranial fossa, the degree of retraction depending upon the extent of resection planned (Fig. 21.4).

7. The tumor with its surgical margin is mobilized from below through facial incisions using standard otolaryngologic techniques (Fig. 21.5).

8. Anterior bone cuts at the cranial base are made transfacially with direct visualization of these cuts as the brain is retracted posteriorly from the cranial side. However, the posterior bone cuts into the sphenoid and along the optic nerves are made transcranially as the brain is sufficiently retracted for adequate exposure below (Fig. 21.6).

9. Bone margins are smoothed with bone rongeurs, and all remaining and exposed sinus mucosa is removed.

10. Because olfactory nerves must be transected in this operation, CSF leaks are inevitable. Meticulous dural repair is mandatory, using pericranial or fascial grafting techniques.

11. Using a posteriorly based mucoperichondrial flap from the nasal septum, the nasopharynx is partitioned from the operative cavity

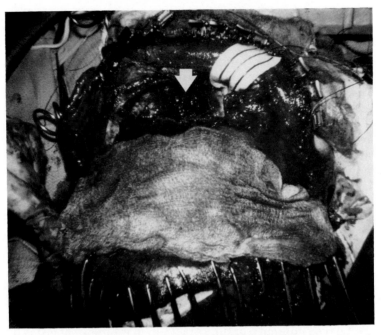

FIG. 21.4. A frontal craniotomy provides wide exposure of the floor (*arrow*) of the anterior cranial fossa.

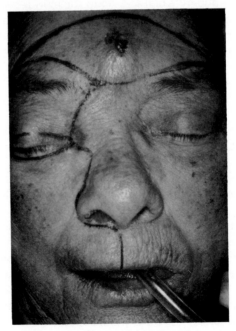

FIG. 21.5. Proposed facial incisions.

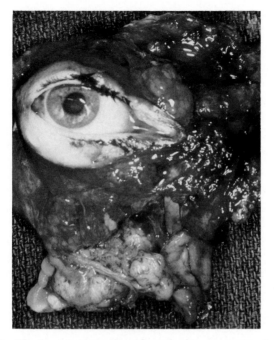

FIG. 21.6.   The frontal sinus, ethmoids, and orbit are exentered *en bloc.*

in preparation for further reconstruction using the pectoralis major myocutaneous flap. This is a key step in providing effective separation of the skull base defect from the nasal cavity (Figs. 21.7–21.9).

12. Bone grafts, used to support the brain, are rarely necessary in our experience. When used, however, wire sutures are avoided to prevent scatter of postoperative radiation therapy. Embedded hardware may also interfere with subsequent computed tomography (CT) or magnetic resonance imaging (MRI) and is thus to be avoided.

13. A pectoralis major myocutaneous flap is elevated the full length across the chest and should be as wide as the diameter of the skull base defect (Figs. 21.10 and 21.11).

14. Skin is removed from the distal 4–6 cm of the flap. The distal muscle and subcutaneous tissue are used to fill the facial cavity. The edges of the skin flap are then sutured to the wound edges, and the chest donor site is closed by advancement of skin.

15. In these cases, the flap is brought up over the neck and face as an external pedicle to avoid tunneling the pedicle under the neck and facial skin. Since the undersurface of the pedicle is raw, care should be taken to prevent desiccation of the tissue that would result in

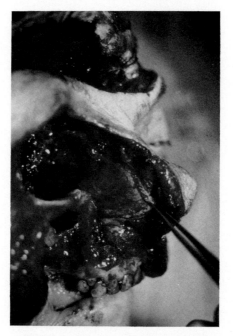

FIG. 21.7.   A posteriorly based mucoperichondral flap of the nasal septum is prepared.

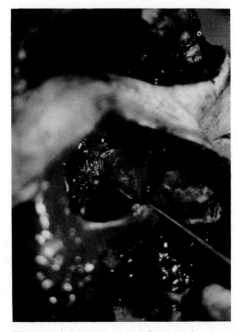

FIG. 21.8.   The septal flap is transposed across the posterior choana.

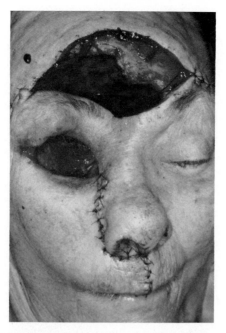

FIG. 21.9. The facial incision is closed after watertight dural repair has been accomplished. A large, common frontoorbital defect remains.

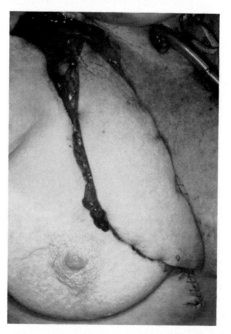

FIG. 21.10. A pectoralis major myocutaneous flap is elevated the full length of the chest.

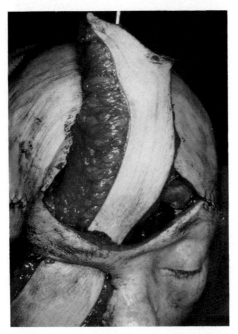

FIG. 21.11.   The pectoralis flap is positioned to fill the frontoorbital defect.

thrombosis of vessels and necrosis of the flap. The topical application of antibacterial cream (such as silvadiazine) is used for this purpose. The pedicle is also covered by petrolatum gauze that is changed daily (Fig. 21.12).

16. The pedicle can be divided and inset at the end of 2 weeks. The excess pedicle may be discarded (Fig. 21.13).
17. Prior to the patient's hospital discharge, a baseline CT scan is obtained, against which follow-up CT scans can be compared.

RESULTS

Ten patients with an average age of 62 years (ranging from 33 to 82 years in age) underwent anterior skull base resections repaired with pectoralis myocutaneous flaps. The predominant tumor histology was squamous carcinoma, although one patient, age 33, presented with osteosarcoma and two others with adenocarcinoma. Four patients had received previous high dose radiation therapy. The remaining patients underwent planned postoperative radiation. There were no operative mortalities, and no patient suffered an operation-related brain injury. None developed CSF leaks, while two patients suffered perioperative meningitis that responded to revised antibiotic coverage. No patients experienced significant wound separation or infection, and none developed exposure necro-

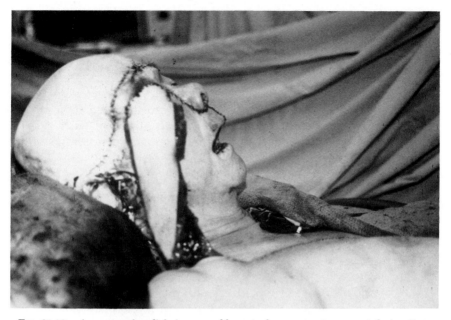

FIG. 21.12.   An external pedicle is covered by petroleum gauze to prevent desiccation.

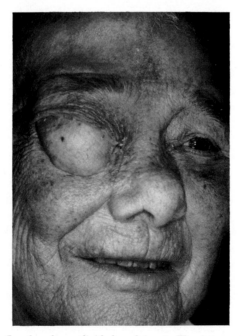

FIG. 21.13.   The flap has been divided and inset. The late postoperative result is satisfactory.

sis of bone. Postoperative hospital stay ranged from 14 to 32 days with an average of 21 days.

The development of *regional* myocutaneous flaps has indeed opened a new era in reconstructive surgery. The impact of this new concept in surgical technique is reflected in the volumes of recent literature. Patients with problems in tissue coverage for which no solutions were readily available or for which multiple operations were required may now be managed in one reliable operation. The advantages of such surgical reconstruction are especially valued following massive resections at the skull base for the following reasons:

1. Wound separation and infection with exposure necrosis of bone and dura are avoided by the reliable vascularity and viability of the pectoralis major flap.
2. A negligible incidence of operative-related CSF leaks and meningitis reduces surgical morbidity and potentially diminishes postoperative mortality.
3. An early and reliable repair avoids lengthy delays in postoperative recovery, favoring early institution of postoperative radiation therapy when indicated. For those patients in whom histologic margins are of questionable adequacy, early radiation may be of critical value in control of locoregional disease.
4. The avoidance of traditional open cavities decreases local infection and reduces the burden of difficult postoperative hygiene.
5. In most patients postoperative cosmesis is satisfactorily restored, providing early social rehabilitation as well.

While we recognize the virtues of other techniques, we are of the opinion that myocutaneous flap reconstruction of the anterior skull base is an acceptable if not preferred method of reconstruction with numerous advantages, not the least of which may be lifesaving. For this purpose the pectoralis major myocutaneous flap may be especially well suited.

TUMORS OF THE POSTERIOR SKULL BASE

The histologic diagnosis of mastoid or middle ear carcinoma is made by biopsy in patients who exhibit changes in symptomatology previously considered to be inflammatory rather than neoplastic. Unremitting pain should raise the spectre of underlying malignancy rather than chronic infection. Bleeding, deafness, vertigo, or facial paralysis are usually late manifestations of this disease. Routine x-rays of the skull and petrous bone generally precede CT evaluation. Angiography and MRI also assist in delineating the precise extent of disease. We feel the most important role of imaging is to determine whether disease has extended into vital areas which would render any operative intervention inadvisable. Our criteria of "inoperatibility," therefore, include the invasion of the carotid artery, invasion of the temporal lobe dura medial to the entry of the middle meningeal artery, or invasion of the posterior fossa dura medial to the internal auditory meatus.

Historically, both surgery and radiation have been advocated for cancer involving the temporal bone. Whereas radiation therapy alone effects a 5-year survival rate of 14% in the report of Sinha and Aziz (11), surgery alone produces a comparable 16% in the series of Conley and Novack (3). Radical mastoidectomy and postoperative radiation are described by Boland and Paterson (1), who observed that an open mastoid cavity increases the incidence of painful osteoradionecrosis and life-threatening meningitis. A 5-year survival rate of only 8% is reported from Memorial Hospital using this once prevalent treatment (8). Needless to say, treatment of temporal bone cancer was historically not very good.

Nevertheless, from these early experiences have emerged principles of management that nearly double curability and greatly improve functional preservation. Five-year cure rates for mastoid cancer now approach 30% in a report by Lewis (7) and over 40% in a report by Gacek and Goodman (5). In the past, principal causes of therapeutic failure and unacceptable morbidity have resulted from (a) subtotal, piecemeal removal of tumor; (b) irradiation of exposed and infected bone; and (c) intracranial complications caused by impaired healing and sepsis. Recognizing such pitfalls, we therefore advocate (a) *en bloc* resection when possible; (b) coverage of exposed bone by vascularized skin-muscle flaps; and (c) postoperative rather than preoperative radiation.

Operative Procedure

A combined intracranial-extracranial approach for en-bloc resection represents a rather massive if not heroic exercise and is for this reason worth a brief description (Fig. 21.14).

A temporal craniotomy is first accomplished in order to evaluate the medial extent of tumor involvement (Fig. 21.15A). Recognizing that extradural extension of tumor is at best difficult to assess by noninvasive means, we have come to rely on wide craniotomy for this definitive decision. In general, the tumor is considered unresectable when dura is invaded medial to the foramen spinosum. If dura is necessarily resected medial to this foramen, watertight closure of the subarachnoid space is difficult to achieve using fascial grafting techniques. Because the probability of CSF leak and subsequent meningitis represents too great a risk for resection of tumor located so medially, we would generally consider the operation terminated at this point.

On the other hand, if the tumor is considered to be resectable, the

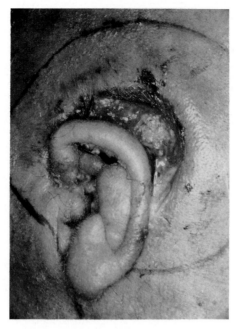

FIG. 21.14.   An ulcerating tumor of the external auditory canal has invaded the temporal bone.

craniotomy is extended into the posterior fossa, allowing the sigmoid sinus and jugular bulb to be mobilized from their attachments to bone (Fig. 21.15B). In order to control the great vessels at the skull base, a total parotidectomy with facial nerve dissection is first accomplished. The mandibular condyle is resected for exposure of the internal carotid artery and jugular vein (Fig. 21.15C). Through the tempromandibular joint, the intratemporal carotid is identified and with use of an air drill, is mobilized from its attachment to the temporal bone (Fig. 21.16). Needless to say, this represents the single most important step in allowing the temporal bone to be removed without harm to the intracranial circulation.

A partial or subtotal resection of the temporal bone may now be accomplished by creating a controlled fracture line across the axis of the petrous bone with an orthopaedic chisel (Fig. 21.17). Depending on the location of the tumor, the temporal bone may be resected lateral to the eardrum for tumor localized to the external auditory meatus. It may be resected lateral to the cochlea for tumor localized to the external auditory canal, or it may be resected lateral to the internal auditory meatus for tumor localized to the middle ear and mastoid. It is worth noting that

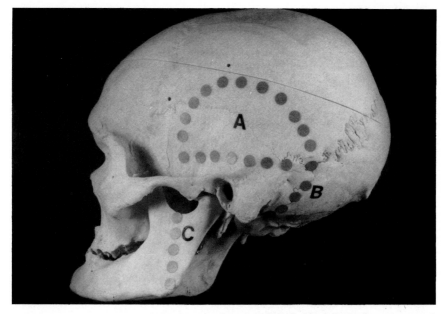

FIG. 21.15. (A) A temporal craniectomy is accomplished. (B) A limited craniectomy is extended into the posterior cranial fossa. (C) The mandibular condyle is resected in order to gain exposure of the carotid artery as it courses through the petrous bone.

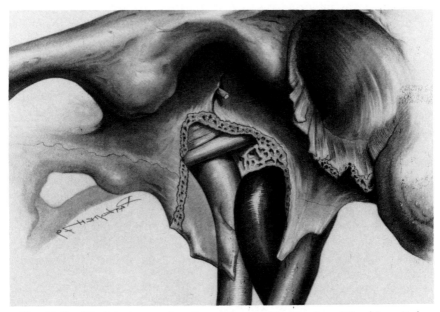

FIG. 21.16. The intratemporal portion of the carotid artery is mobilized from its bony attachments by an approach through the temporomandibular joint.

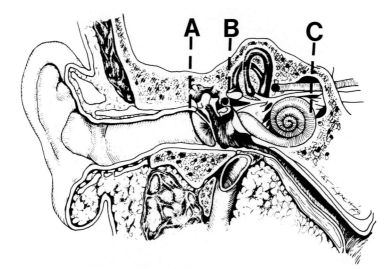

FIG. 21.17. (*A*) A limited partial resection of the temporal bone is indicated when tumor is localized to the meatus. (*B*) An extended partial resection is necessary when tumor invades the bony external auditory canal. (*C*) A subtotal resection of the temporal bone is indicated when tumor invades the mastoid or middle ear.

any resection medial to the cochlea results in division of the facial nerve and cochlear-vestibular nerves. A 7–12 anastomosis may be accomplished for facial rehabilitation. The wound is then closed with a skin-muscle flap obtained from the chest (Fig. 21.18). The patient is now ready to receive radiation therapy.

RESULTS

In our institution over the past several years, roughly 20 patients have been treated by *en bloc* resection and postoperative radiation. Seven have died from recurrent tumor. Thirteen patients are alive without recurrent disease. There has been no operative mortality. We have had no radionecrosis of bone.

Although the number of our patients is small and the follow-up too short to formulate statistically significant conclusions, we can make some important observations:

(*a*) Although the degree of surgical complexity is great, morbidity and mortality are surprisingly low, an observation shared by Gacek and Lewis.

(*b*) Total gross removal of tumor can be accomplished without undue sacrifice of vital intracranial structures.

(*c*) The final decision for resectability is made intraoperatively, only after the medial extent of the disease is determined by subtemporal craniotomy.

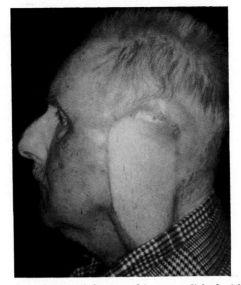

FIG. 21.18.   In this case, closure of the wound is accomplished with a pectoralis major myocutaneous flap.

(*d*) Radiation therapy delivered postoperatively eradicates residual microscopic tumor in high risk areas determined at the time of surgical exposure. Such practice limits the radiated field, thereby avoiding unnecessary exposure of vital intracranial structures, including the brainstem and spinal cord. This cannot be accomplished with planned preoperative radiation.

(*e*) In addition, the use of postoperative radiation does not compromise or impair the healing wound, thereby avoiding life-threatening cerebrospinal fluid leaks and meningitis.

(*f*) Osteoradionecrosis is prevented by the avoidance of open mastoid cavities which heal by secondary intent. Open mastoids are contaminated wounds harboring high levels of aerobic and anaerobic microorganisms and for this reason tolerate radiation less well. By covering the surgical defect with vascularized skin-muscle flaps, we believe that early wound stabilization is achieved without risk of subsequent infection and necrosis.

CONCLUSION

Cancers of the skull base are not hopeless. A system of management which evolves through the cooperation of the otolaryngologist, neurosurgeon, and radiotherapist uniquely reduces morbidity. Curability is determined by early diagnosis and the completion of high risk surgery and radiation by an experienced team of specialists.

REFERENCES

1. Boland, J., and Paterson, R. Cancer of the middle ear and external auditory meatus. J. Laryngol., *69:* 468, 1955.
2. Collins, W. J., Jr. Foreword. In: *Surgery of the Skull Base*, edited by C. T. Sasaki, B. F. McCabe, and J. A. Kirchner. Lippincott, Philadelphia, 1984.
3. Conley, J. J., and Novack, A. J. The surgical treatment of malignant tumors of the ear and temporal bone. Arch. Otolaryngol., *71:* 46, 1960.
4. Dandy, W. E. Orbital tumor: Results following the transcranial operative attack. Oskar, New York, 1941.
5. Gacek, R. R., and Goodman, M. Management of malignancy of the temporal bone. Laryngoscope, *87:* 1622, 1977.
6. Ketcham, A. S., Hoye, R. C., VanBuren, J. M., *et al.* Complications of intracranial facial resection of tumors of the paranasal sinuses. Am. J. Surg., *112:* 591, 1966.
7. Lewis, J. S. Cancer of the ear: A report of 150 cases. Laryngoscope, *70:* 551, 1960.
8. Lewis, J. S., and Page, R. Radical surgery for malignant tumors of the ear. Arch. Otolaryngol., *83:* 114, 1966.
9. Malecki, J. New trends in frontal sinus surgery. Acta Otolaryngol., *50:* 137, 1959.
10. Schramm, V. L., Myers, E. N., and Maroon, J. L. Anterior skull base surgery for benign and malignant disease. Laryngoscope, *89:* 1077, 1979.
11. Sinha, P. P., and Aziz, H. I. Treatment of carcinoma of the middle ear. Radiology, *126:* 485, 1978.
12. Sisson, G. A., Bytell, E. D., Becker, S. P., *et al.* Carcinoma of the paranasal sinuses and craniofacial resection. J. Laryngol. Otol., *90:* 59, 1976.
13. VanBuren, J. M., Ommaya, A. K., and Ketcham, A. S. Ten years' experience with radical combined craniofacial resection of malignant tumors of the paranasal sinuses. J. Neurosurg., *28:* 341, 1968.

22

The Diagnosis and Treatment of Orbital Tumors

JOSEPH C. MAROON, M.D., JOHN S. KENNERDELL, M.D., and
ADNAN ABLA, M.D.

For the last 12 years, we have worked as a Neurosurgical-Ophthalmic team in the diagnosis and treatment of orbital tumors. As a result, we have evaluated approximately 500 patients with orbital tumors and have performed surgical procedures in approximately 400 of them (Table 22.1). The purpose of this report is to summarize our diagnostic and therapeutic approaches to patients with intraorbital tumors.

DIAGNOSIS

The diagnostic "decision tree" attempts to classify orbital tumors according to symptoms and signs and also to simplify diagnostic workup and therapeutic options (Fig. 22.1). Approximately 75% of our patients are first seen for evaluation of painless proptosis. Dermoid, hemangioma, lymphangioma, neurofibroma, optic glioma, and meningioma account for the majority of neoplasms with this symptom. After a thorough history and physical examination, which includes an evaluation of visual acuity, color vision, visual fields, extraocular mobility, Hertel measurements, fundus examination, and ultrasonography, a computed tomographic (CT) scan and/or magnetic resonance (MRI) scan is obtained. The majority of these tumors can be diagnosed preoperatively with an 80–90% reliability with this series of tests.

Painful proptosis or proptosis associated with some discomfort suggests lesions such as nonspecific orbital inflammatory process, infection, metastatic lesion, primary orbital malignancy, lymphoma, and rhabdomyosarcoma. After these diagnostic procedures, appropriate hematologic studies, as well as fine needle aspiration biopsy, may be considered.

Decreased visual acuity and/or impaired visual field function without proptosis suggests small lesion that may be circumferential and constricting the optic nerve such as meningiomas, hemangiomas, neurofibromas, or tumors located deep in the orbital apex or in the optic canal. CT and MRI scans are indispensable in evaluating patients with these complaints.

TABLE 22.1
Orbital Tumors and Pseudotumors between 1975–1986

1. Adenoid cystic carcinoma	8
2. Benign mixed lacrimal gland tumor	8
3. Dermoid	45
4. Hemangioma	33
5. Hemangiopericytoma	11
6. Lymphangioma	15
7. Meningioma	51
8. Metastatic tumor	105
9. Nonspecific orbital inflammation	95
10. Neurofibroma	10
11. Optic nerve glioma	18
12. Rhabdomyosarcoma	8
13. Fibrous histiocytoma	3
14. Cholesteatoma	1
15. Venous varices	3
Total	414

A lesion that causes much confusion and at times false-negative surgical explorations includes those associated with nonspecific orbital inflammatory processes, and these are commonly called pseudotumor. These lesions may or may not be associated with pain and/or proptosis; they appear as an orbital mass on CT and MRI studies as well as ultrasonography. They may develop acutely or have a chronic indolent course. Ultrasonography, duction tests, CT scanning, and MRI usually are diagnostic and result in a trial of cortocosteroids which may prove dramatic therapeutically. Other patients may require a brief course of radiation therapy after confirmation with fine needle aspiration biopsy.

Once it is determined that a surgical lesion exists, it is essential to further determine the precise relationship of the tumor to the optic nerve. This will then determine the least traumatic surgical approach for removal.

TRANSCRANIAL APPROACH

The transcranial approach is used for all tumors with intracranial extension, for those located in the apex and/or optic canal, and for tumors in the apex medial to the optic nerve. This surgical approach may be performed in the standard way described by Housepian (7). We utilize this craniotomy when dissection is not required deep in the apex or when the optic canal does not need to be unroofed.

If it is necessary to dissect deep in the orbital apex, particularly medial to the optic nerve, and to unroof the optic canal, then we prefer a transcranial frontoorbital temporal approach. With this method we remove the orbital rim and orbital roof with the bone flap *en bloc*. This

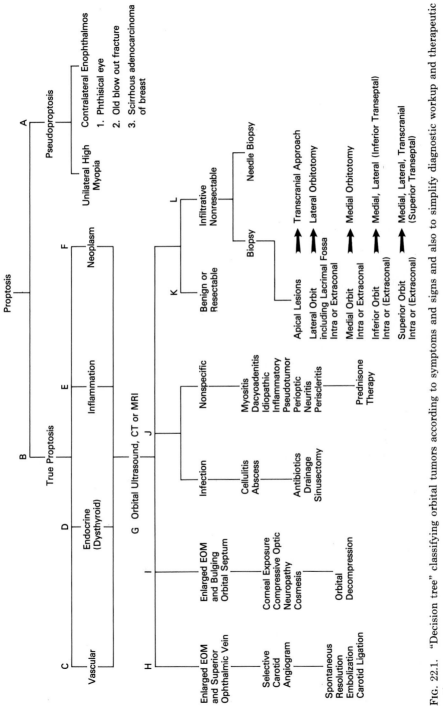

FIG. 22.1. "Decision tree" classifying orbital tumors according to symptoms and signs and also to simplify diagnostic workup and therapeutic options.

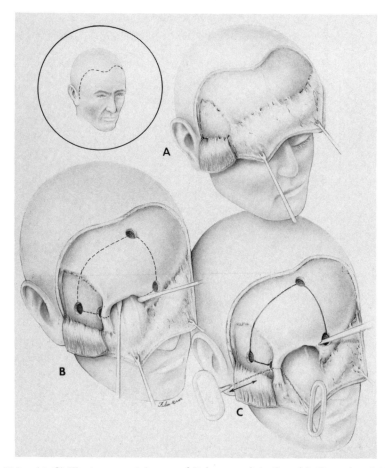

FIG. 22.2.   (A–G) The transcranial supraorbital approach to the orbit. For a description of the technique see text.

permits the best possible visualization of the orbital contents with the least amount of brain retraction.

We have described the technique previously (11, 14, 16, 17), and a brief description follows. A bicoronal skin incision is made a few millimeters behind the hairline just anterior to the tragus of the ear on the affected side extending approximately to the superior temporal line on the opposite side. This anterior incision with minimal shaving has resulted in excellent cosmetic appearance with no wound infections to date. Subperiosteal dissection is used to elevate the entire frontal flap and the temporalis muscle (Fig. 22.2A). The supraorbital nerve is identified and, if encircled in the supraorbital foramen by bone, a small osteotome is

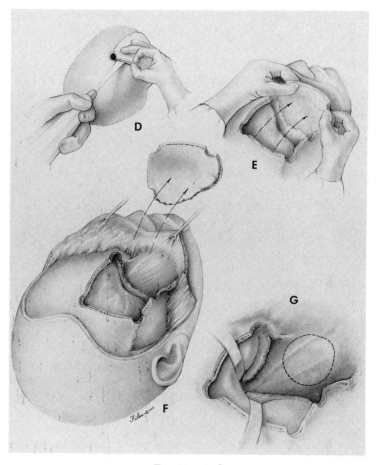

FIG. 22.2. A–G

used to free it. Often the nerve is not bound in the notch and is elevated with subperiosteal dissection.

With a blunt dissector, the subperiosteal dissection proceeds into the orbit so that the periorbital tissue, which is continuous with the pericranium, is displaced from the superior orbital roof. This dissection is continued laterally so that the lateral periorbita is separated from the frontal portion of the zygomatic bone. The temporalis muscle is dissected from the anteriormost portion of the temporal fossa down to the zygomaticotemporal suture line (Fig. 22.2B).

A 3- to 5-holed bone flap is then prepared. The first hole is in the temporal fossa anteriorly so that the lateral wall of the orbit, as well as the intracranial compartment, is exposed. A second hole is placed immediately above and lateral to the glabella. This usually perforates the frontal sinus. Two to three additional holes are used at the surgeon's preference.

The orbital rim above the dissected periorbital fascia, and the zygomatic arch, are transected (Fig. 22.2C). Standard saw cuts are then made to connect the remaining burr holes. An osteotome is used to transect the anteromedial orbital ridge.

With these bone cuts made, the bone flap is elevated in the standard way; the only bone remaining untransected is the thin superior orbital roof. This usually breaks posteriorly so that the entire supraorbital ridge, superior orbital roof, and frontal bone are removed in one piece (Fig. 22.2D and E). With minimal retraction on the dura and using small bone-biting rongeurs, it is a simple matter to remove the remaining portion of the orbital roof, including the bone over the optic canal (Fig. 22.2F and G). The periorbita is often opened during the elevation of the bone flap with subsequent pouching out of orbital fat. This is of little consequence. Standard precautions are taken with the frontal sinus and the ethmoid sinus if these are transgressed by the elevation of the bone flap.

At this point, if the lesion extends intracranially, it is convenient to look at the optic nerve and the chiasm for possible involvement. If one is confronted with an optic nerve meningioma, then surgical decisions are made relative to complete removal with optic nerve transection or decompressive palliative surgery. If the tumor is in the orbital apex, but not intracranially, it may best be approached extradurally by retracting the levator and superior rectus muscles laterally.

We have found that intraorbital exploration is greatly facilitated by microdissection techniques and by self-retaining intraorbital retraction provided by the Greenberg retractor (Codman Company, Randolph, Mass.). Three to four retractor blades may be used to retract brain as well as the intraorbital contents. In this manner, one may utilize the laser, ultrasonic aspirator, or some other tumor-extirpating devices with good control.

In drilling off remnants of the optic canal either from the intradural or extradural routes, a fine diamond, high speed air drill is used. The anatomical relationship of the ethmoid sinuses medially and the pneumatized anterior clinoid process laterally must be kept in mind, or persistent CSF leaks may occur. Intraoperative monitoring of visual evoked responses is helpful when it is necessary to manipulate the optic nerve.

Closure of the wound requires a watertight dural repair. The frontal, ethmoid, and sphenoid sinuses are closed by impacting them with muscle and then oversewing with pericranium and dura. The bone, with its intact roof, is replaced, so an orbital roof prosthesis is unnecessary and avoids late complications (1). The bone flap is fixed into place with fine-gauge wire or 0 silk, and the skin is closed in the usual fashion. A subgaleal drain is routinely used for 24 hours. A tarsorrhaphy is not usually required. Methyl methacrylate cranioplastic plugs are placed in all of the burr holes except those under the temporal muscle.

The cosmetic results with this procedure are excellent. Enophthalmos may be seen, but this has not resulted in diplopia, and within a week or two is unnoticeable. We have had no cases of pulsating proptosis in over 100 cases of transcranial orbital explorations without roof replacement. We have had no CSF leaks and no extraocular disturbances or corneal infections secondary to the surgical approach.

LATERAL MICROSURGICAL APPROACH

The lateral microsurgical approach is used for tumors located in the superior temporal or inferior compartment of the orbit and those in the lateral apex (15). The more anterior the lesion, the more easily accessible it is with this technique. Those tumors deep in the apex, even though lateral, may require removal of a portion of the greater wing of the sphenoid for optimal exposure.

The skin incision for this approach is 35–40 mm long and begins superiorly and laterally in the eyebrow and is carried posteriorly along a line that would be covered by the temples of a pair of eyeglasses (Fig. 22.3). We initially advocated transecting the lateral canthal ligament, but complications of reapproximation occurred.

After the skin incision is made, the temporalis fascia (but not the muscle) is incised, beginning at the midportion of the frontozygomatic bone and extending posteriorly the length of the skin incision. A curved incision is then made through the periosteum of the frontozygomatic bone. With a periosteal elevator, the periorbital fascia is removed from the inner surface of the lateral wall of the orbit, using a malleable brain retractor to depress the periorbita as dissection is carried posteriorly. The muscle in the temporal fossa is then dissected subperiosteally and retracted posteriorly to expose the external lateral orbital bone. Bleeding is reduced by the injection of 1:200,000 units of epinephrine into the muscle and temporal subperiosteal area prior to the skin incision. The zygomatic artery and the meningeal branch of the lacrimal artery, which may be encountered during the subperiosteal dissection, are easily controlled with electrocautery or bone wax.

A reciprocating saw is used to incise the lateral rim of the orbit just above the zygomaticofrontal suture line and to make another cut approximately 1 cm below this. These two cuts are made while an assistant

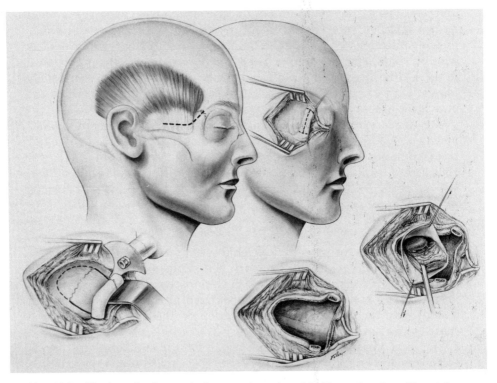

FIG. 22.3.   The lateral microsurgical approach to the orbit illustrating the self-retaining lateral orbital retractor. For a description of the technique see text.

protects the intraorbital contents with a malleable brain retractor inserted between the inner surface of the lateral wall of the orbit and the periorbital fascia. After these cuts are made, a rongeur is used to grasp the orbital rim and break the bone posteriorly at this attachment to the greater wing of the sphenoid. Additional bone is then rongeured away from the greater wing of the sphenoid.

If it is necessary to obtain proximal exposure of the optic nerve or to gain access to the deep lateral portion of the muscle cone, additional bone is removed from the sphenoid bone with a high-speed air drill and small angled rongeurs. We have frequently exposed the anterior temporal dura as well as the frontal dura through this approach for excellent visualization deep in the orbital apex. This bone may be quite vascular, and frequent applications of bone wax are required.

With the bone thus removed, the periorbital fascia and retrobulbar contents become visible. A traction suture through the lateral rectus muscle at its globe attachment allows identification of the muscle through the periorbital fascia. With gentle palpation, tumors can frequently be felt at this point. An incision can then be made in the fascia parallel to and above or below the lateral rectus muscle to gain access to the intraconal compartment. The orbital self-retaining retractor is then inserted with one blade retracting the temporalis muscle. Another two blades are used for superior and inferior retraction of the orbital fat. With one assistant aspirating any blood and holding a fourth retractor blade gently on the globe, the primary surgeon identifies the optic nerve or tumor, using microdissecting techniques. The fine neural vascular structures in the lateral compartment of the orbit are carefully preserved. Tumors in the lateral intraconal compartment, such as hemangiomas or neurofibromas, may be grasped with an ophthalmic cryoprobe of the kind generally used for detached retinas or for removing cataracts. The tip of this instrument is "frozen" to the tumor capsule and allows retraction without perforating the capsule.

If the purpose is to remove a tumor attached to the optic nerve, proximal and distal exposure of the nerve is obtained. Exophytic or extradural tumors such as meningioma are found by palpation and subsequent dissection. If the mass is large, bulk tumor reduction is accomplished either with the Cavitron ultrasonic aspirator (CUSA) or a laser. Depending on the vascularity of the tumor, we occasionally employ both instruments in the orbit as in the intracranial compartment. In our recent experience, the laser appears to provide a delicate controlled method for reducing the mass of such a tumor.

Once the mass is reduced in size, a plane may be seen between the normal dura and the tumor. This plane is exploited, and the tumor is removed from its dural attachment with microdissecting techniques. If no plane is seen, the dura of the optic nerve is incised, and an attempt is made at removal from the intradural compartment. This is done provided the CT scan does not show axial intracranial extension of the tumor.

ANTERIOR MEDIAL MICROORBITOTOMY

Tumors located anterior in the orbit and medial to the optic nerve lying within the muscle cone can be conveniently removed through a medial microorbitotomy. Although the operative space is limited, additional exposure can be obtained by concurrently performing a lateral orbitotomy to obtain increased lateral retraction on the globe. A specially designed medial-orbitotomy self-retaining retractor has been used to facilitate this procedure.

After the usual ophthalmic preparation of the orbit and periorbital area, a small eyelid speculum is inserted to begin the operation (Fig. 22.4, *upper left*). A 360° periectomy is performed around the cornea. Conjunctival relaxing incisions are made superior and inferior to the medial

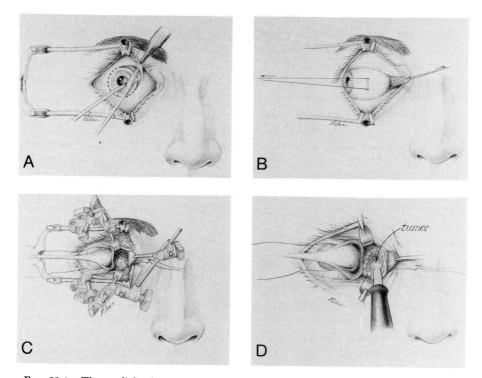

FIG. 22.4. The medial microsurgical approach to the orbit illustrating use of the self-retaining medial orbital retractor. For a description of the technique see text.

rectus muscle and angled away from the muscle. A muscle hook is placed under the medial rectus muscle, which is freed from its intermuscular septa and check-ligaments distally. The muscle is imbricated near its insertion site with 6-0 double-armed Vicryl suture, doubly locked at both borders. The muscle is then severed from the insertion site. A hemostat is placed on the suture, and the muscle is retracted medially (Fig. 22.4, *upper right*). At this point, the standard lid retractor is removed, and the specially designed medial orbital self-retaining retractor is inserted (Fig. 22.4, *lower left*). This retractor has an enucleation spoon which is placed into the medial orbital compartment. The teeth of the retractor are inserted superiorly and inferiorly under the conjunctiva. The handle of the retractor is angled so that it rests on the temporalis muscle lateral to the eye. The enucleation spoon is placed over the globe in a medial position so that retraction from medial to lateral is carried out. Next, the dissecting blades, similar to those used on the lateral orbital retractor, are inserted and used to dissect the intraorbital fat and identify the tumor. With this retractor in place, the operating microscope with a 300-

mm objective is brought into use. As dissection proceeds deeper in the intraconal compartment, the orbital fat is retracted superiorly and inferiorly with cottonoids, and additional malleable retractors are attached to the base of the self-retaining retractors as needed (Fig. 22.4, *lower right*).

If additional exposure is required, a lateral orbitotomy may be carried out so that the globe can be retracted even further laterally for excellent visualization. When the intraconal dissection is completed, complete hemostasis is obtained, and the medial rectus muscle is reattached to the globe with a double-armed 6-0 absorbable suture. The conjunctiva is closed with purse-string sutures, which are inserted through the conjunctiva near the limbus at the area of the superior and inferior conjunctival relaxing incisions. An antibiotic ointment is applied, and the eye is firmly patched. Morbidity during this procedure is minimal and can be compared with that of extraocular muscle surgery, provided that surgical manipulation was not excessive.

FINE NEEDLE ASPIRATION BIOPSY

This technique, initially introduced in the U.S. by one of the authors (J.S.K.) (10), is used in patients in whom the histology of an orbital tumor is in doubt and wherein treatment might change, depending on the cytology. Such suspected lesions include metastatic tumor, pseudotumor, and intrinsic tumors of the optic nerve.

The procedure is performed usually on an outpatient basis using a pistol-grip syringe connected to a No. 22 3.75-cm long needle. Axial and coronal CT views are used to localize the tumor. A needle is then introduced into the lesion. CT guidance is used for optic nerve tumors. Strong negative suction is applied to obtain the specimen, and cytological slide preparations are made immediately following withdrawal of the needle with the slides fixed in 95% alcohol. The slides are then stained with a Papanicolaou and hematoxin and eosin stain, and are read by a cytologist.

In approximately 175 cases thus treated, complications have included 12 minor intraorbital hemorrhages and two inadvertent perforated lobes. We have heard of one case in which death occurred due to inadvertent penetration of the internal carotid artery and subsequent intracranial hemorrhage. With CT scan guidance, this type of complication should be avoidable.

DISCUSSION

A wide variety of new diagnostic modalities have been introduced for the workup of patients with orbital lesions. The advent of high resolution CT scanning made it possible to evaluate lesions of the optic nerve, orbit, and extraocular muscles in both the axial and coronal planes (5, 10, 19, 21, 22). The CT appearance of orbital lesions is usually indicative of the underlying pathology (8, 20). It also demonstrates the exact boundaries of the lesion and its relationship to the optic nerve, orbit, extraocular muscle, and extraorbital extension, thus providing all the elements necessary to the surgeon for planning the operative approach. In situations where the CT appearance is not highly diagnostic, the lesion may be nonresectable or inflammatory in nature, and a fine needle aspiration biopsy can be very helpful (2, 13). MRI imaging of the optic nerve and chiasm is becoming more useful in determining the location and the extent of the lesion and its suitability for surgical resection or other forms of therapy (4, 6).

The treatment of orbital tumors requires attention to the same surgical principles used in intracranial surgery for vascular lesions or neoplasms around sensitive neural structures. This includes the smallest exposure of normal tissue, precise and delicate retraction, and meticulous dissecting techniques with magnification and optimal illumination.

Adjuncts such as ultrasonic aspirators and carbon dioxide lasers are also very helpful. We have found the milliwatt CO_2 laser particularly useful in reducing the size of large lymphangiomas (Fig. 22.5) (12) and debulking large tumors in the orbital apex prior to microsurgical removal with an ophthalmic cryoprobe.

Despite technical advances, we remain stymied by deep orbital apex lesions such as meningiomas that involve the superior orbital fissure and the optic canal and nerve. In the rare case of an exophytic meningioma of the optic nerve anteriorly located, a lateral microorbitotomy may be used with good results. However, most tumors deep in the apex are still associated with a high incidence of neural dysfunction with complete removal.

We have, subsequently, evolved to recommending radiation therapy more frequently for lesions located circumferentially around the optic nerve and deep in the apex if abnormal visual acuity and visual fields are observed and after fine needle biopsy confirms the tissue diagnosis. Anecdotally, we have had three patients with preoperative third nerve dysfunction and one with optic nerve impairment improve following radiation therapy. All patients had optic nerve meningiomas. Contrariwise, in one patient in whom removal of a subdural optic nerve meningioma was carried out, recurrence with intracranial spread developed 4 years later and necessitated a craniotomy and complete removal of the optic nerve. The precise place of radiation therapy in these lesions is unknown, but Smith, as well as others, has reported beneficial results, and additional long-term studies are necessary.

In 1924, Walter Dandy stated the only reliable approach to intraorbital tumors was transcranial (3). At that time, there was no way to determine preoperatively whether a tumor involved the intracranial compartment. In 1948, Naffziger observed that the diagnosis and treatment of intraorbital tumors was lacking in a systematic approach (18). With the introduction of CT and MRI scanning, ultrasonography, and fine needle aspiration biopsy techniques, not only the diagnosis, but also the precise relationship of tumors to the optic nerve can now be determined preoperatively. Combining this knowledge with microsurgical advances, we have attempted to outline a systematic approach to orbital tumors. Surely, the morbidity has been greatly reduced with intraorbital surgery, and most benign lesions can be removed safely. The malignant and deep apical tumors, however, remain a challenge and await further advances and help from other disciplines.

REFERENCES

1. Abla, A. A., Maroon, J. C., Kennerdell, J. S., et al. Fibrosis surrounding a silicone implant simulating recurrent orbital meningioma. J. Neurosurg., 63: 467–469, 1985.
2. Czerniak, B., Woyke, S., Daniel, B., et al. Diagnosis of orbital tumors by aspiration biopsy guided by computerized tomography. Cancer, 54: 2385–2389, 1984.
3. Dandy, W. E. Orbital Tumors: Results following the Transcranial Operative Attach, pp. 161–164. Oskar Piest, New York, 1941.
4. Daniels, D. L., Kneeland, J. B., Shimakawa, A., et al. MR imaging of the optic nerve and sheath. AJNR, 7: 249–253, 1986.
5. Forbes, G. S., Earnest, F., and Walter, R. R. Computed tomography of orbital tumors, including late-generation scanning techniques. Radiology, 142: 387–394, 1982.
6. Holman, R. E., Grimson, B. S., Drayer, B. P., et al. Magnetic resonnance imaging of optic gliomas. Am. J. Ophthalmol. 100: 596–601, 1985.
7. Housepian, E. M. Intraorbital tumors. In: Operative Neurosurgical Techniques, edited by H. H. Schmidek and W. H. Sweet. Grune & Stratton, New York, 1982.
8. Jackobiec, F. A., Depot, M. J., and Kennerdell, J. S., et al. Combined clinical and computed tomographic diagnosis of orbital glioma and meningioma. Ophthalmology, 91: 137–144, 1984.
9. Kennerdell, J. S., Dubois, P. J., Dekker, A., et al. CT-guided fine needle aspiration biopsy of orbital optic nerve tumors. Ophthalmology, 87: 491–496, 1980.
10. Kennerdell, J. S., and Ghoshhajra, K. Computed tomographic scanning of orbital tumors. Int. Ophthalmol. Clin., 22(4): 99–131, 1982.
11. Kennerdell, J. S., and Maroon, J. C. Microsurgical approach to intraorbital tumors: Technique and instrumentation. Arch. Ophthalmol., 94: 1333–1336, 1976.
12. Kennerdell, J. S., Maroon, J. C., Garrity, J. A., et al. Surgical management of orbital lymphangioma with the carbon dioxide laser. Ophthalmology, 102: 308–314, 1986.
13. Kennerdell, J. S., Slamorits, T. L., Dekker, A., et al. Orbital fine-needle aspiration biopsy. Am. J. Ophthalmol., 99: 547–551, 1985.
14. Mark, L. E., Kennerdell, J. S., Maroon, J. C., et al. Mircosurgical removal of a primary intraorbital meningioma. Am. J. Ophthalmol., 86: 704–709, 1978.
15. Maroon, J. C., and Kennerdell, J. S. Lateral microsurgical approach to intraorbital tumors. J. Neurosurg., 44: 556–561, 1976.

16. Maroon, J. C., and Kennerdell, J. S. Surgical approaches to the orbit. Indications and techniques. J. Neurosurg., *60:* 1226–1223, 1984.
17. Maroon J.C., and Kennerdell J.S. Tumors of the orbit. Neurosurgery, *1:* 964–976, 1985.
18. Naffziger H.C. Progressive exophthalmos following thyroidectomy: Its pathology and treatment. Ann. Surg., *94:* 582–586, 1948.
19. Peyster, R. G., Hoover, E. D., Hershey B. L., *et al.* High-resolution CT of lesions of the optic nerve. AJR, *140:* 869–874, 1983.
20. Rothfus, W. E. Orbital masses. In *Computed Tomography of the Head, Neck, and Spine,* edited by R. E. Latchaw, pp. 379–411. Year Book Medical Publishers, Chicago, 1985.
21. Rothfus, W. E., and Curtin, H. D. Extraocular muscle enlargement: A CT review. Radiology, *151:* 677–681, 1984.
22. Rothfus, W. E., Curtin, H. D., Slamovits, T. L., *et al.* Optic nerve/sheath enlargement. A differential approach based on high-resolution CT morphology. Radiology, *150:* 409–415, 1984.

23

Surgery of Masses Affecting the Third Ventricular Chamber: Techniques and Strategies

MICHAEL L. J. APUZZO, M.D.

INTRODUCTION

A wide spectrum of pathological lesions affects the anterior and mid third ventricular chamber (30). From the surgical perspective each presents both an intellectual and technical challenge (29, 61). This discussion will direct attention to the definition of major presenting groups of structural substrates which may then serve as a directive toward selection of either certain open surgical corridors or indirect surgical methodologies. It will focus upon technical maneuvers attendant to the superior operative approaches and surgical options at the foramen of Monro to gain exposure of the chamber. It will discuss the impact of image directed stereotaxy on the evaluation and management of disease processes in this most challenging region. Finally, comments will be made related to the current management of colloid cysts, the prototype of "classical" tumors of the third ventricular chamber.

THE STRUCTURAL SUBSTRATE

In consideration of structure, it is of value to initially identify three major groups (Fig. 23.1) by computed tomography (CT) and magnetic resonance imaging (MRI) (5, 13, 40). These are termed: (*a*) extraaxial intraventricular; (*b*) intraaxial with ventricular component; and (*c*) basal.

Extraaxial intraventricular are histologically benign masses with minimal areas of origin and adherence to the elements of the ventricular wall. The colloid cyst is the primary example of this group; however, a variety of developmental neoplastic, vascular, and infectious processes may account for this structural presentation (Figs. 23.2–23.4) (10, 25).

Intraaxial lesions may directly expand into the chamber, metastasize, or secondarily deform the wall. Intrinsic tumors of the glial spectrum are the most common initiators of such a structural presentation (Figs. 23.5–23.7).

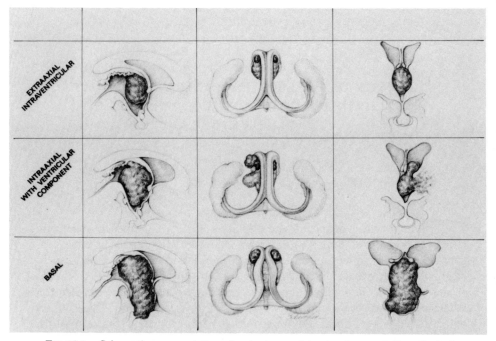

FIG. 23.1.   Schematic representation of major types of structural presentation of anterior and mid-third ventricular masses.

Basal masses may have developmental, neoplastic, vascular, or infectious etiologies. However, they share a common region of origin in the sella, skull, or brain base, subsequently expanding rostrally to involve the third ventricular cavity (Fig. 23.8). Occasionally in their expansion the hypothalamic floor will be disrupted, and the lesion will present at the foramen of Monro (Fig. 23.9).

OPERATIVE OBJECTIVES AND APPROACHES IN RELATION TO STRUCTURE

With recognition and imaging definition of such a structural process the surgeon must direct his efforts toward achieving four major goals (10, 51): (*a*) definition of the nature of the process; (*b*) maximum feasible excision of the lesion; (*c*) relief of alteration in cerebral spinal fluid dynamics; (*d*) relief of local signs and symptoms attendant to the regional mass.

For purposes of description of operative corridors two major groups may be considered (13). These are the *basal*, which include all extraaxial approaches to the brain base (*i.e.*, transsphenoidal, subfrontal, frontotem-

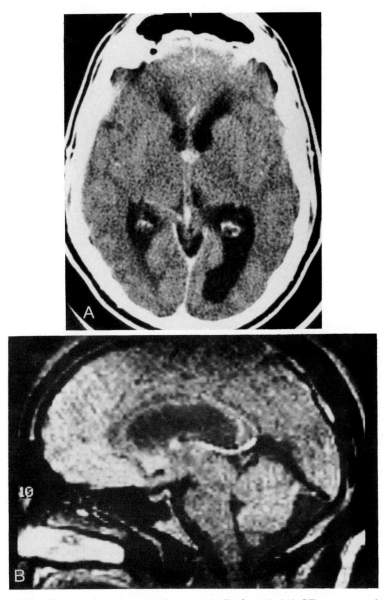

FIG. 23.2.   Extraaxial intraventricular mass (colloid cyst). (*A*) CT contrast-enhanced axial slice of 1-cm mass with element of ventriculomegaly in 23-year-old male. (*B*) Sagittal MRI of same patient managed by transcallosal, transforaminal excision.

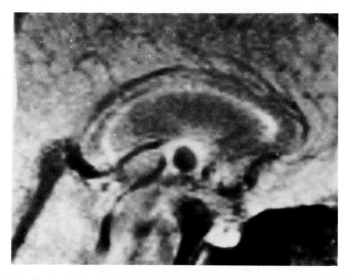

FIG. 23.3.   Extraaxial intraventricular mass (craniopharyngioma) sagittal MRI managed by transcallosal interforniceal excision.

poral, pterional, and subtemporal), and the *superior*, which include the intraaxial transfrontal and transcallosal routes.

In consideration of the structural substrates, tumors with basal origin are generally best approaches by a basal corridor (1, 2, 23, 45, 46, 52, 56–58, 60), the particular angle of access and desired exposure being dictated by the location and extent of basal origin and direction of mass extention. Occasionally, a basal exposure *combined* with a superior corridor should be considered either in a single or staged procedure (62).

For purposes of this discussion, focus will be directed toward superior approaches as they provide the major capability for entry to and visualization of the third ventricular chamber (7).

Superior Operative Approaches

These corridors afford exposure of the foramen of Monro and diencephalic roof via entry through the middle frontal gyrus or trunk of the corpus callosum (5, 6). The exposures provide an initiation for excision of intraventricular lesions or intraventricular components of lesions that are not accessible by basal exposures. They are applied to extraaxial intraventricular lesions and may be considered for intraventricular components of the axial processes (Fig. 23.5) in the event that (7): (*a*) The histological nature as defined by imaging directed biopsy is not manageable by indirect methods, *i.e.*, radiotherapy, chemotherapy, antibiotics. (*b*) The lesion is not highly malignant. (*c*) The intraventricular compo-

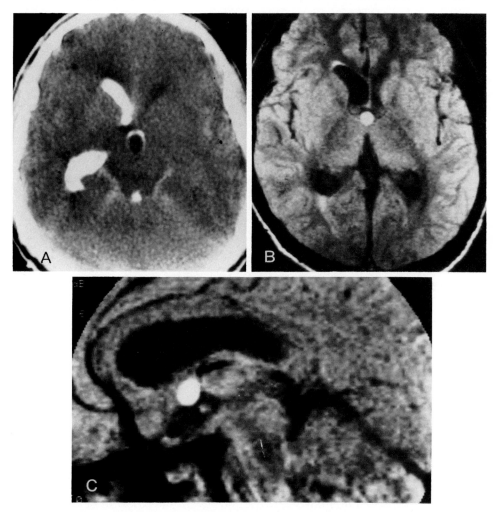

FIG. 23.4.   Extraaxial intraventricular mass (cysticercosis cyst). (A) CT water-soluble contrast ventriculogram demonstrating mass and unilateral ventriculomegaly. Axial (B) and sagittal (C) MRI views of same lesion managed by CT-guided ventriculoscopic excision.

nent is the major component of mass presentation. (d) Signs and symptoms related to the mass presence (exclusive of hydrocephalus) exist.

Certain basal masses with superior extension may be managed entirely by this corridor (7, 9). These are cylindrical lesions with a base in the midline and are no greater than 2.5 cm in width, with associated disruption of the diencephalic floor and presentation at the foramen of Monro (Fig. 23.9).

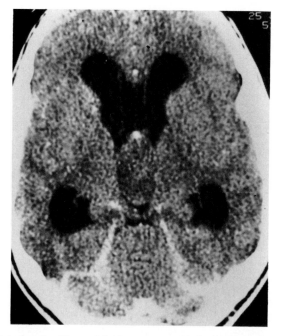

Fig. 23.5. Intraaxial with ventricular component (astrocytoma) axial contrast-enhanced CT slice of thalamic lesion with intraventricular component in a 9 year old girl. Evaluated by CT-guided stereotactic biopsy prior to subtotal excision by means of transcallosal transforaminal corridor.

The *transcortical* approach is undertaken through the right middle frontal gyrus in the presence of ventriculomegaly. It offers excellent visualization of the foramen of Munro with satisfactory visual alignment for lesions of the mid- and anterior component of the third ventricular chamber. It provides optimum angulation for employment of the subchoroidal transvelum interpositum exposure (31, 35, 41, 42). It offers less satisfactory visual alignment for the interforniceal exposure or appreciation of the contralateral foramen. Its limitations for flexibility of intraoperative options and sacrifice of cortical tissue make it a less desirable corridor.

The *transcallosal* corridor fashioned by interhemispheric exposure of the body of the corpus callosum in the pericoronal region with 2-cm incision of the trunk offers major advantages of constant anatomy, shorter transit to the diencephalic roof, and ability to easily develop exposure of the entire third ventricular cavity (7, 9, 11, 53). There is no disruption of the hemispheric tissue, and ventricular size is irrelevant. For these reasons, this approach has been used nearly exclusively in cases requiring exposure of the third ventricular region in our hands.

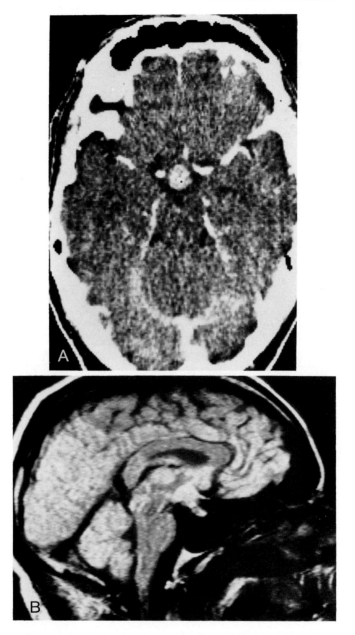

FIG. 23.6.   Intraaxial with ventricular component (metastatic germinoma). (*A*) Axial
CT contrast-enhanced slice in 20-year-old male. (*B*) Sagittal MRI managed by CT-guided
stereotactic biopsy with 2° radiotherapy (Markers, negative).

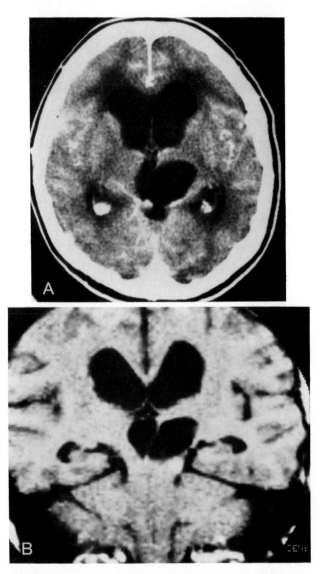

FIG. 23.7. Intraaxial with ventricular component (cystic ganglioglioma). (*A*) Axial
contrast-enhanced CT. (*B*) Coronal MRI managed by CT-guided stereotactic biopsy,
placement of drainage conduit (Rickham reservoir), and regional teleradiography with
secondary intracystic brachytherapy.

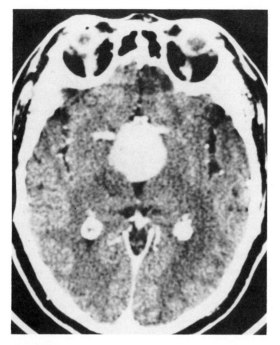

FIG. 23.8.   Basal (diaphragma sella meningioma) contrast-enhanced axial CT slice. Excision by basal approach (frontotemporal).

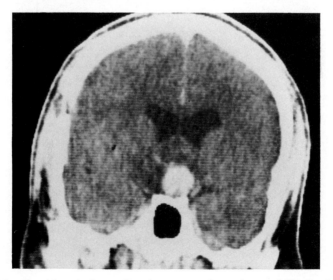

FIG. 23.9.   Basal (craniopharyngioma) contrast-enhanced coronal CT slice. Note narrow (<2.5 cm) solid and superior cystic component. Lesion had disrupted hypothalamic floor and presented at foramen of Monro. Total excision by transcallosal interforniceal approach.

The approach is not only facilitated, but its safety is enhanced by attention to cortical venous anatomy during the preoperative evaluation of the patient (9). We have recommended evaluation of the venous phase of cerebral angiography in planning of bone flap placement and more recently have used MRI images which will provide elements of detail in parasagittal venous anatomy in the pericoronal region (Fig. 23.10). Attention to this detail, preservation of regional venous structures (55), and minimization of retraction will assure minimum occurrence of postoperative cortical deficit. The deformation of midline should not exceed 5 cm, and retraction of the medial hemisphere from the falx should not exceed 2 cm at the surface of the corridor (11).

Midcallosal section is accomplished with apparently minimal physiological cost as presently assessable (9, 17, 36). However, certain *possible* exceptions to this generalization exist (17): (*a*) mutism, (*b*) auditory effects, and (*c*) tactile transfer deficits.

Transient mutism may be observed after either bilateral cingulate retraction or thalamic injury in association with midcallosal section. Auditory suppression may be detected in one ear if dichotically tested in the occasional patient. Dependent on the difficulty of the task, deficits in somesthetic transfer may be observed in some patients; however, our experience with test batteries designed to elicit such deficits failed to

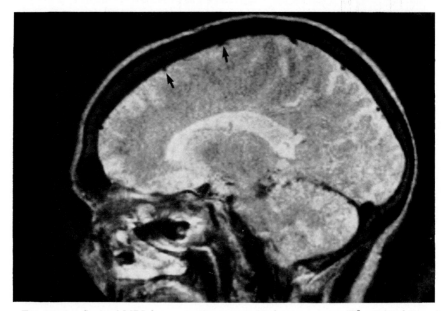

FIG. 23.10.   Sagittal MRI demonstrating parasagittal venous entry (T^2 weighted image) which may be employed in planning bone flap and entry corridor.

disclose any. Detailed further evaluation of individuals undergoing trunk section is indicated and required to afford an absolute statement regarding these issues; however, the observed costs of transcallosal entry would appear to be within acceptable limits and minimal generally requiring specialized testing to elicit.

Chamber Entry

Following exposure of the lateral ventricle in the region of the foramen of Monro a number of options (Fig. 23.11) are available for third ventricular entry. These include (7, 32): (*a*) transforaminal entry (unilateral or bilateral); (*b*) transforaminal entry expanded by ipsilateral forniceal column section; (*c*) subchoroidal entry; (*d*) interforniceal entry.

These maneuvers afford options to the surgeon as he attempts to maximize excision with a balance of minimal trauma to adjacent neural tissues. The amount of exposure required will vary with the type of

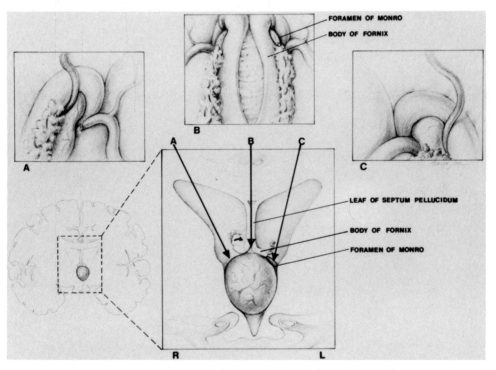

FIG. 23.11.   Major options for chamber entry following lateral ventricular access. (*A*) Subchoroidal exposure via velum interpositum viewed at right foramen with sacrifice of thalamostriate vein to expand entry area over tumor. (*B*) Interforniceal exposure. (*C*) Transforaminal exposure (viewed at left foramen).

disease process and the experience of the operator. Requirements for exposure are variable, but familiarity with each method of exposure increases the options and hence the potential for positive accomplishment in each operative procedure.

Transforaminal entry is facilitated by the presence of a large lesion which distends foramen. This is not a dependable feature of third ventricular masses. In addition, the *angle of exposure* and access to the foramen are critical, as the surgeon's ability to satisfactorily deal with a mass within the chamber through the limitation of foraminal exposure may be compounded by the visual angle of the surgical corridor (Fig. 23.12). The *consistency of the lesion* and its resistance to methods of microexcision are another important factor in both achievement of lesion excision and avoidance of a neural injury.

Section of a column of the fornix is not recommended, as other maneuvers permit the realization of adequate exposure without sacrifice of neural elements.

Subchoroidal exposure exploits a natural plane at the lateral margin of

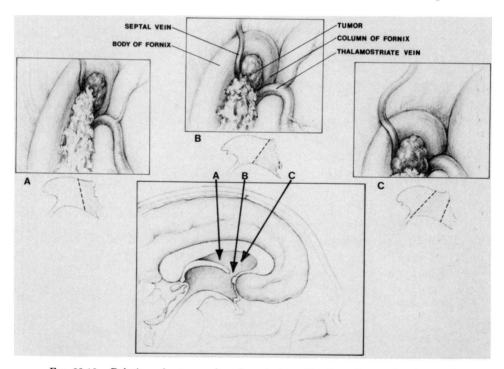

Fig. 23.12. Relation of entry angles of surgical corridor in pericoronal region to view of foramen of Monro and transforaminal exposure of chamber. Posterior (*A*), coronal (*B*), and anterior (*C*) views within chamber will vary additionally in relation to size of foramen.

the choroid plexus which allows mobilization of the choroid and forniceal complex away from the side of dissection (31, 35, 41, 42, 59). The method provides access to the central portion of the chamber via the velum interpositum. The exposure may be further enlarged by sacrifice of the *thalamostriate vein* at the foramen. This method appears to be safe and would appear to confirm the ability of collateral connections to shunt from deep medullary to subependymal venous systems (24, 35, 42). Lines of visualization are optimized by the transcortical approach. In the presence of a small lesion, retraction of the thalamus may be required to achieve adequate visualization (42).

The *interforniceal maneuver* (9, 11) develops a natural division (forniceal raphe) between the columns and body of the fornix, which opens through the diencephalic roof (Fig. 23.13). This division is easily appreciated with the presence of the cavum septum or may be developed by separating the septum leaves. Occasionally, it is partially initiated by distension of the dorsal forniceal complex by a mass. The line of septal attachment to the fornix defines its origin. *This exposure combined with the transcallosal corridor affords complete access to the third ventricular chamber and basal midline structures.* Mass presence generally negates the requirement for active retraction in the region. The internal cerebral veins are displaced laterally by the mass and easily moved from the active operative field.

This exposure may be used with biforaminal visualization and simultaneous mass manipulation in the event that it is required. Development of the raphe should be initiated at the foramen of Monro and should not

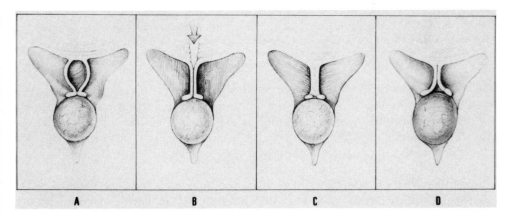

A	B	C	D

FIG. 23.13. Anatomical variations encountered in region of septum pellucidum in relation to surgical development of forniceal raphe. (*A*) Cavum septum pellucidum. (*B*) Separate leafs of septum pellucidum. (*C*) Fusion of leafs. (*D*) Raphe opened by mass presence.

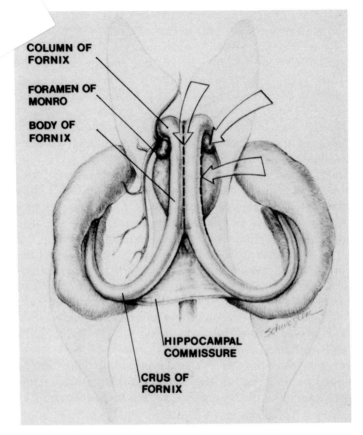

FIG. 23.14. Schematic representation of anatomy of fornix (dorsal view) with extent of raphe development for interforniceal corridor. Hippocampal commissure (A) to be preserved is shown, as well as transforaminal transforamenal (B) and (C) subchoroidal entry regions.

exceed 2 cm in extent to preserve the hippocampal commissure (Fig. 23.14). It should be stressed that although this has been our primary method of attaining extensive midline exposure, *it is undertaken only if transforaminal exposure is inadequate or manipulating seems excessive.*

The technique may be employed safely without natural corridors enhanced by ventriculomegaly or regional mass.

Our recent experience with 30 cases operated via a transcallosal interforniceal corridor is presented in Table 23.1. Exposure proved to be adequate for total excision of 22/25 (88%) lesions which were potentially excisable (*i.e.*, extraaxial intraventricular or components of basal masses). There were no mortalities, and major morbidity included only transient short-term memory loss, in 10/30 (33%) of patients. This

TABLE 23.1

Interforniceal Exposure (30 Cases)[a]

Location	Pathology
1. Ant. III	Colloid cyst (1.5 cm) (V, *, T)[b]
2. Ant. III	Colloid cyst (2 cm) (V, T)
3. Ant. III	Colloid cyst (1 cm) (T)
4. Ant. III	Colloid cyst (1.5 cm) (T)
5. III	Colloid cyst (2.5 cm) (V, *, T)
6. Ant. III	Colloid cyst (1.5 cm) (V, T)
7. III	Craniopharyngioma (3 cm) (V)
8. III	Craniopharyngioma (2.5 cm) (V, T)
9. III	Craniopharyngioma (2.0 cm) (V, *, T)
10. III	Craniopharyngioma (2.5 cm) (V, T)
11. III	Craniopharyngioma (4 cm) (V, *)
12. III	Craniopharyngioma (3.0 cm) (V, *, T)
13. III	Craniopharyngioma (2.5 cm) (V, *)
14. Mid & Post III	Cysticercosis (2 cm) (V, T)
15. FM Ant. III	Cysticercosis (1.8 cm) (V, T)
16. FM Ant. III	Cysticercosis (1.7 cm) (V, T)
17. FM Ant. III	Cysticercosis (2 cm) (V, T)
18. FM Ant. III	Cysticercosis (2 cm) (V, T)
19. FM Ant. III	Cysticercosis (2 cm) (V, T)
20. Ant. III	Cysticercosis (2 cm) (V, *, T)
21. III	Cysticercosis (2.5 cm) (V, T)
22. III	Cysticercosis (2 cm) (V, T)
23. Post III	Cysticercosis (1.5 cm) (*, T)
24. III	Glioma (V, *)
25. III	Glioma (V)
26. III	Glioma (V)
27. III	Glioma (V)
28. III	Glioma (V)
29. FM III	AVM (*, T)
30. Post III	Bullet (22 Cal)

[a] Thirty consecutive cases of transcallosal interforniceal exposure of the third ventricular chamber. Note range of size, consistency, and texture of lesions in relation to transient postoperative disturbance in mentation.

[b] V, ventriculomegaly; *, transient memory loss; T, total excision (CT); FM, foramen of Monro.

problem resolved in one week in 70% of cases, and no patient exhibited alteration in retention 3 months postoperatively.

In consideration of this complication, it is apparent that soft, easily decompressed lesions carried the least risk of complication (*i.e.*, cysticercosis cysts, 20%), while firm lesions, which required more extensive regional trauma for excision, carried a much higher risk (*i.e.*, craniopharyngioma, 57%). This data would imply the relative safety of the corridor, but the inherent difficulty of microexcision of firm lesions in this region without some temporary cost of neurological impairment.

MEMORY

As noted, although a number of complications have developed in the hands of experienced microsurgeons (9, 22, 40, 43, 47, 54), the most frequent postoperative problem associated with manipulation of the midline basal cerebral structures is a transient amnestic syndrome. The alteration in mentation is observed in the immediate postoperative period and usually resolves in days to several weeks (9).

The fornix by "tradition" rather than fact has received primary focus as the structure of injury in such cases. The literature fails to provide substantive evidence that integrity of the fornix is required for normal memory (9, 13, 28). Although this structure represents a major limbic pathway, significant comparable fiber bundles would remain intact following isolated forniceal injury. Almost all hippocampal connections with the associated cortices would be preserved.

It is becoming apparent that diffuse, multifocal midline injury is required with additive and collective impact on regions concerned with the memory process (28, 32, 33). These include: (a) basal forebrain nuclei; (b) thalamic nuclei; and (c) inferior thalamic peduncle.

The *basal nucleus* of Meynert lies in the substantia innominata, adjacent to the midline and millimeters from the third ventricle. Major cortical cholinergic input is derived from this region. Forniceal injury could alter cholinergic input to the hippocampal formication, which could compound basal nuclei injury and alter all cortical cholinergic innervation.

The *nuclei reuniens* and *paraventricular nuclei of the thalamus* are situated between the anterior reticular and the dorsal medial thalamic nucleus. They provide major input to the entorhinal cortex. The nucleus reuniens projects to the hippocampus. In the event of forniceal injury, associated injury to these nuclear groups would alter hippocampal afferent and efferent activities.

The *inferior thalamic peduncle* carried a major component of amygdaloid output and provides a major connection with the dorsal medial thalamic nucleus, both considered primary structural components of the memory process. Its proximity to the third ventricle places this vital component of memory structure at risk.

IMAGING GUIDANCE STEREOTAXY

The combination of principles of stereotaxy, radiographic imaging techniques, and microinstrumentation has added a new and vital dimension to the management of intracranial mass lesions (12, 16, 19, 34, 37–

39). The deep midline structures of the third ventricular region are particularly accessible by this approach with a precision and inherent safety that has not been available in the past.

A number of stereotactic devices that provide capability for translation of imaging data in a rapid and useful fashion to the operating room are currently commercially available. Our experience with the Brown-Roberts-Wells System (BRW) at the University of Southern California Medical Center Hospitals in over 750 cases attests to the value, safety, and flexibility of such a system with appropriate support that is a resource in major medical centers.

Access to the target point is achieved readily, rapidly, and safely with local anesthesia and an anesthesiologist standing by in all but selected pediatric patients for whom general anesthesia is required (6, 8). Access to the target point is usually attained within 60 minutes from the time of initiation of the procedure with all trajectory settings and target locales verified extracranially on a phantom simulator (8).

Multiple microinstrumentation capabilities at the target point allow for: (a) histological and microbiological assay; (b) cyst and abscess aspiration; (c) installation of permanent or temporary drainage conduits; (d) point source or colloid-based brachytherapy (or other methods of intralesional therapy); (e) cerebroscopy and ventriculoscopy with biopsy, aspiration, or excision.

Ventriculoscopy (7, 8) is performed with local anesthesia and standby (Fig. 23.15). A *target* is selected at the right foramen of Monro for cystic lesions presenting in the anterior component of the chamber. An *entry point* is centered at or slightly anterior to the coronal suture in the pupillary line. An 18-mm burr hole is prepared, and after cruciate opening of the dura a 1-cm cortical window is designed at the point of entry of the ventriculoscope sheath. We have employed a 6.2-mm endoscope sheath with a blunt obturator which is introduced to the target. With removal of the obturator an angled ventriculoscope is introduced which allows for capabilities of visualization, irrigation (Ringer's lactate solution), aspiration, and introduction of instrumentation for biopsy, cyst perforation, and aspiration, or quartz fiber for conduction of argon laser energy. The sheath is introduced through a rigid bushing directed by the arc guidance component of the BRW system with precise placement to the foramen. Minor adjustments and changes in angulation may be made by adjustment of four angulation settings on the arc which allow infinite degrees of motion.

Targeting for 150 lesions of the third ventricular region at the University of Southern California Medical Center Hospitals is presented in Figure 23.16. Histological verification of a process was attained in 95% of cases, and realization of objectives of a procedure was achieved in

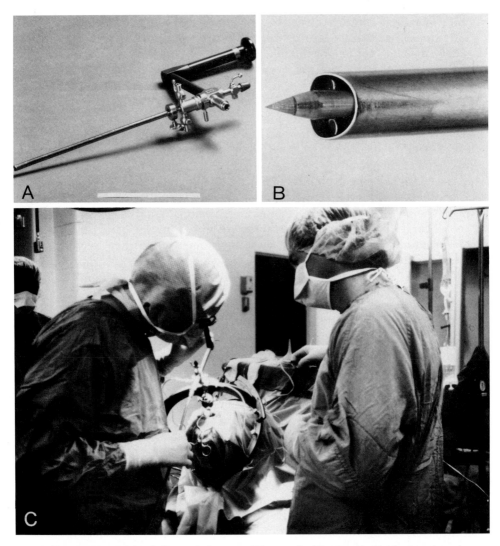

FIG. 23.15. (*A*) Angled ventriculoscope. (*B*) cannula (13-gauge) with sharp stylette for cyst puncture prior to entry. Shown emerging from the tip of ventriculoscope. (*C*) Instrument used in conjunction with stereotactic frame.

97%. These objectives included biopsy, biopsy with culture, biopsy with aspiration, biopsy with installation of Rickham drainage systems, point source or colloid brachytherapy, endoscopic visualization with biopsy, and endoscopic excision. Operative morbidity was less than 1%, while only one death occurred in this series. Craniotomy was indicated or ultimately required in less than 20% of those undergoing the initial stereotactic procedure.

These methods are particularly valuable in the assessment, management, and logical development of treatment plans in the individuals with lesions affecting the third ventricular chamber. They should be considered part of the management armamentarium for the following reasons.

The histological nature of the intraaxial lesions may be rapidly and safely assessed, often circumventing the need for craniotomy.

Cystic lesions of basal or intraaxial origin may be drained with precise control with permanent conduits placed for later treatment with colloid brachytherapy or other intralesional methods.

Intraventricular cystic lesions may be aspirated under endoscopic visualization (colloid cyst) or totally excised (cysticercosis cyst).

Basal lesions with superior extension, to or above the foramen of Monro, may be evaluated by ventriculoscopy to assess disruption of the hypothalamic floor prior to developing a primary surgical strategy.

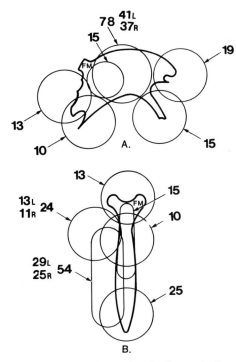

FIG. 23.16. Targeting for 150 lesions in the third ventricular region by CT-guided stereotactic techniques. Lateral (A) and superior (B) third ventricular silhouettes with *circles* indicating lesion location. *Numbers* indicate number of cases. *FM*, foramen of Monro.

Third ventriculostomy may be performed in cases of aqueductal or fourth ventricular outlet atresia or stenosis.

COLLOID (NEUROEPITHELIAL) CYST

Colloid cysts represent the classical prototype of the benign tumor of the third ventricular chamber (3). Most commonly, these lesions arise in the anterior part of the third ventricle immediately posterior to the foramen of Monro (30). They usually project inferiorly into the third ventricle and vary in extent superiorly and rostrally. Attachments of various dimensions are present with the tela choroidea of the third ventricular roof. Occasionally, the forniceal columns superior to the anterior commissure will be separated by the mass presence and involve the septum pellucidum (28). The cyst is well circumscribed, smooth, and spherical with dimensions that have been reported to vary from 0.3 to 9 ml. They are filled with homogeneous material of varying viscosity containing cellular debris. This variability is related to multiple factors including desquamated epithelial cells, leukocytes, red cells, gitter cells, and cholesterol pigment.

These lesions may occur posterior to the foramen of Monro and be attended by various degrees of aqueductal stenosis (20).

Presentation may be in the form of: (a) acute and intermittent increases in intracranial pressure; (b) chronically increased intracranial pressure; (c) local pressure effects; and (d) truly "incidental" findings on imaging studies.

CT scanning demonstrates an anterior third ventricular mass usually with attendant ventriculomegaly. The lesion is commonly slightly hyperdense with enhancement with contrast. Isodense, nonenhancing lesions or ring enhancement may be encountered (22). "Incidental" lesions generally present as a small (less than 1 cm) mass posterior to the foramen of Monro without ventriculomegaly.

Because of their location and mechanical propensities, these lesions represent a menace to life (26, 50). Although the absolute risk of demise in the individual patient has not been accurately determined, the location of the lesion and repeated documentation of rapid and fatal neurological deterioration dictate a need to initiate definitive management to either reduce cyst mass and/or maintain normal CSF dynamics.

Arguments exist for the following management options: (a) biventricular shunting; (b) stereotactic aspiration; and (c) direct excision. Options 2 and 3 do not necessarily obviate the need for some form of CSF diversion as approximately 30% of these lesions are associated with aqueductal stenosis or atresia (20).

Stereotactic aspiration is best accomplished under direct vision. We have employed a 6.2-mm endoscope in association with a 13-gauge cannula with blunt and sharp (for capsule penetration) stylettes for this purpose. Our modest experience (six cases), personal communications (E-O. Backlund, April 1986; T. Rahn, June 1986), and review of available literature would indicate that cyst aspiration is possible in 50–60% of cases by current techniques. It is our experience that difficulty is encountered with lesions of less than 1 cm in diameter. Although a large body of data is not available, it would appear that at least in certain cases this method will offer feasible therapy and should be pursued to ultimate refinement, including laser reduction of the cyst capsule.

Our current method of management of these lesions is to attempt endoscopic aspiration in all cases if the cyst is greater than 1 cm in diameter (5, 7). If unsuccessful, primary excision is offered to individuals less than 50 years old and biventricular CSF diversion to those declining surgical excision or more than 50 years old. Craniotomy is undertaken with a transcallosal corridor with foraminal exposure alone or augmented by the interforniceal approach.

CONCLUSION AND SUMMARY

Surgery of lesions affecting the third ventricular chamber is a technical and intellectual challenge. It requires lucid comprehension of normal (44, 48, 51) and pathological alterations of anatomy on the part of the managing surgeon. Multiple options are available, and familiarity with these as well as thoughtful experience in the management of problems involving the region will enhance the opportunity for satisfactory results and minimize complications.

REFERENCES

1. Al-Mefty, O., Hassounah, M., Weaver, P., et al. Microsurgery for giant craniopharyngiomas in children. Neurosurgery, 17: 585–595, 1985.
2. Al-Mefty, O., Holoubi, A., Rifai, A., et al. Microsurgical removal of suprasellar meningiomas. Neurosurgery, 16: 364–372, 1985.
3. Antunes, J., L., Kenneth, M. L., and Ganti, S. R. Colloid cysts of the third ventricle. Neurosurgery, 7: 450–455, 1980.
4. Apuzzo, M. L. J. CT guidance stereotaxis in the management of 94 lesions of the third ventricular region. In: Surgery in and around the Brain Stem and the Third Ventricle, edited by M. Samii. Springer-Verlag, Berlin, 1985.
5. Apuzzo, M. L. J. Strategies of anterior third ventricular surgery. In: Decision Making in Neurological Surgery, edited by K. R. Smith and R. Bucholz. B. C. Decker, Philadelphia, 1987.
6. Apuzzo, M. L. J., Chandrasoma, P. T., Cohen, D., et al. Computed imaging stereotaxy: Experience and perspective related to 500 procedures applied to brain masses. Neurosurgery, in press, June 1986.
7. Apuzzo, M. L. J., Chandrasoma, P. T., Zelman, V., et al. Computed tomographic guidance stereotaxis in the management of lesions of the third ventricular region. Neurosurgery, 15: 502–508, 1984.
8. Apuzzo, M. L. J., Chandrasoma, P., Zelman, V., et al. Application of computerized

tomographic guidance stereotaxis. In: *Surgery of the Third Ventricle*, edited by M. L. J. Apuzzo. Williams & Wilkins, Baltimore, 1987.

9. Apuzzo, M. L. J., Chikovani, O. K., Gott, P. S., *et al.* Transcallosal, interfornicial approaches for lesions affecting the third ventricle: Surgical considerations and consequences. Neurosurgery, *10:* 547–554, 1982.

10. Apuzzo, M. L. J., Dobkin, W. R., Zee, C. S., *et al.* Surgical considerations in treatment of intraventricular cysticercosis. An analysis of 45 cases. J. Neurosurg., *60:* 400–407, 1984.

11. Apuzzo, M. L. J., and Giannotta, S. Interforniceal approach. In: *Surgery of the Third Ventricle*, edited by M. L. J. Apuzzo. Williams & Wilkins, Baltimore, 1987.

12. Apuzzo, M. L. J., and Sabshin, J. K. Computed tomographic guidance stereotaxis in the management of intracranial mass lesions. Neurosurgery, *12:* 277–285, 1983.

13. Apuzzo, M. L. J., Zee, C. S., and Breeze, R. E. Anterior and midventricular lesions: Surgical overview. *In: Surgery of the Third Ventricle*, Williams & Wilkins, in press, 1987.

14. Backlund, E-O. Studies on craniopharyngiomas. III. Stereotaxic treatment with intra-cystic yttrium-90. Acta Chir. Scand., *139:* 237–247, 1973.

15. Backlund, E-O. Studies on craniopharyngiomas. Stereotaxic treatment with radiosurgery. Acta Chir. Scand., *139:*344–351, 1973.

16. Backlund, E-O. Role of stereotaxis in the management of midline cerebral lesions. In: *Surgery of the Third Ventricle*, edited by M. L. J. Apuzzo, Williams & Wilkins, Baltimore, 1987.

17. Bogen, J. E. Physiologic consequences of complete or partial commissural section. In: *Surgery of the Third Ventricle*, edited by M. L. J. Apuzzo. Williams & Wilkins, Baltimore, 1987.

18. Bosch, D. A., Rahn, T., Backlund, E. O. Treatment of colloid cysts of the third ventricle by stereotactic aspiration. Surg. Neurol., *9:* 15–18, 1978.

19. Bosch, D. A. Indications for stereotactic biopsy in brain tumours. Acta Neurochir. (Wien), *54:* 167–179, 1980.

20. Brun, A., Egund, N. The pathogenesis of cerebral symptoms in colloid cysts of the third ventricle: A clinical and pathoanatomical study. Acta Neurol. Scand., *49:* 525–535, 1973.

21. Bullard, D. E., Osborne, D., Cook, W. A. Colloid cyst of the third ventricle presenting as a ring-enhancing lesion on computed tomography. Neurosurgery, *11:* 790–791, 1982.

22. Carmel, P. W. Surgical syndromes of the hypothalamus. Clin. Neurosurg., *27:* 133–159, 1980.

23. Carmel, P. W. Craniopharyngiomas. In: *Neurosurgery*, edited by: R. H. Wilkins and S. R. Sett, pp. 905–916. McGraw-Hill, New York, 1985.

24. Caron, J. P., Nick, J., Contamin, F., *et al.* Tolerance de la ligature et de la thrombose aseptique des veines cerebrales profondes chez l'homme. Ann. Med. Intern., *128:* 899–906, 1977.

25. Cashion, E. L., Young, J. M. Intraventricular craniopharyngioma. J.Neurosurg., *34:* 84–87, 1971.

26. Chan, R. C., and Thompson, G. B. Third ventricular colloid cysts presenting with acute neurological deterioration. Surg. Neurol., *19:* 358–362, 1983.

27. Ciric, I., and Zivin, I. Neuroepithelial (colloid) cysts of the septum pellucidum. J. Neurosurg., *43:* 69–73, 1975.

28. Damasio, A., and Van Hoesen, G. Anatomy and physiology of memory. In: *Surgery of the Third Ventricle*, edited by M. L. J. Apuzzo. Williams & Wilkins, Baltimore, 1987.

29. Dandy, W. E. *Benign Tumors in the Third Ventricle of the Brain: Diagnosis and Treatment.* Charles C Thomas, Springfield, Ill., 1933.
30. Davis, R. Pathological lesions of the third ventricular region. In: *Surgery of the Third Ventricle,* edited by M. L. J. Apuzzo. Williams & Wilkins, Baltimore, 1987.
31. Delandsheer, J. M., Guyot, J. F., Jomin, M. *et al.* Acces autroisieme ventricule par voie interthalamo-trigonale. Neurochirurgie, *24:* 419–422, 1978.
32. Ehni, G., and Ehni, B. Considerations in transforaminal entry. In: *Surgery of the Third Ventricle,* edited by M. L. J. Apuzzo. Williams & Wilkins, Baltimore, 1986.
33. Garretson, H. Memory in man: A neurosurgeon's perspective. In: *Surgery of the Third Ventricle,* edited by M. L. J. Apuzzo. Williams & Wilkins, Baltimore, 1986.
34. Heilbrun, M. P., Roberts, T. S., Apuzzo, M. L. J., *et al.* Preliminary experience with Brown-Roberts-Wells computerized tomographic stereotaxic guidance system. J. Neurosurg., *59:* 217–222, 1983.
35. Hirsch, J. F., Zouaoui, A., Renier, D., *et al.* A new surgical approach to the third ventricle with interruption of the striothalamic vein. Acta Neurochir., *47:* 135–147, 1979.
36. Jeeves, M. A., Simpson, D. A., And Geffen, G. Functional consequences of the transcallosal removal of intraventricular tumours. J. Neurol. Neurosurg. Psychiatry, *42:* 134–142, 1979.
37. Kelly, P. J. Computer-assisted laser microsurgery. In: *Surgery of the Third Ventricle,* edited by M. L. J. Apuzzo. Williams & Wilkins, Baltimore, 1987.
38. Kelly, P. J., Alker, G. J., and Goerss, S. Computer-assisted stereotactic laser microsurgery for the treatment of intracranial neoplasms. Neurosurgery, *10:* 324–331, 1982.
39. Kelly, P. J., Goerss, S., Kall, B. A. *et al.* Computed tomography-based stereotactic third ventriculostomy: Technical note. Neurosurgery, *18:* 791–794, 1986.
40. Konovalov, A. N. Technique and strategies of direct surgical management of craniopharyngioma. In: *Surgery of the Third Ventricle,* edited by M. L. J. Apuzzo. Williams & Wilkins, Baltimore, 1987.
41. Lavyne, M. H., and Patterson, R. H. Subchoroidal trans-velum interpositum approach to mid-third ventricular tumors. Neurosurgery, *12:* 86–94, 1983.
42. Lavyne, M. H., and Patterson, R. H. Subchoroidal Approach. In: *Surgery of the Third Ventricle,* edited by M. L. J. Apuzzo. Williams & Wilkins, Baltimore, 1987.
43. Long, D. M., and Leibrock, L. The transcallosal approach to the anterior ventricular system and its application in the therapy of craniopharyngioma. Clin. Neurosurg., *27:* 160–168, 1980.
44. Ono, M., Rhoton, A. L., Jr., Peace, D., *et al.* Microsurgical anatomy of the deep venous system of the brain. Neurosurgery, *15:* 621–657, 1984.
45. Patterson, R. H. Subfrontal translamina terminalis approach. In: *Surgery of the Third Ventricle,* edited by M. L. J. Apuzzo. Williams & Wilkins, Baltimore, 1987.
46. Patterson, R. H., and Danylevich, A. Surgical removal of craniopharyngiomas by a transcranial approach through the lamina terminalis and sphenoid sinus. Neurosurgery, *7:* 111–117, 1980.
47. Posner, J. Anatomy and physiology of consciousness: Syndromes of altered consciousness related to third ventricle lesions. In: *Surgery of the Third Ventricle,* edited by M. L. J. Apuzzo. Williams & Wilkins, Baltimore, 1987.
48. Rhoton, A. Surgical anatomy of the third ventricular region. In: *Surgery of the Third Ventricle,* edited by M. L. J. Apuzzo. Williams & Wilkins, Baltimore, 1987.
49. Rivas, J. J., Lobato, R. D. CT-assisted stereotaxic aspiration of colloid cysts of the third ventricle. J. Neurosurg., *62:* 238–242, 1985.
50. Ryder, J. W., Kleinschmidt-DeMaster, B. K., Keller, T. S. Sudden deterioration and

death in patient with benign tumors of the third ventricle area. J. Neurosurg., *64:* 216–223, 1986.

51. Seeger, W. (ed.): *Mircosurgery of the Brain, Vols. 1 and 2.* Springer Verlag, Wien, 1980.
52. Shillito, J. Craniopharyngiomas: The subfrontal approach, or none at all? Clin. Neurosurg.
53. Shucart, W. Anterior transcallosal *versus* transcortical approaches. In: *Surgery of the Third Ventricle*, edited by M. L. J. Apuzzo. Williams & Wilkins, Baltimore, 1987.
54. Shucart, W. A., and Stein, B. M. Transcallosal approach to the anterior ventricular system. Neurosurgery, *3:* 339–343, 1978.
55. Sugita, K., Kobayashi, S., Yokoo, A. Preservation of large bridging veins during brain retraction. J. Neurosurg., *57:* 856–858, 1982.
56. Suzuki, J. Anterior interhemispheric approach. In: *Surgery of the Third Ventricle*, edited by M. L. J. Apuzzo. Williams & Wilkins, Baltimore, 1987.
57. Sweet, W. H. Recurrent craniopharyngiomas: Therapeutic alternatives. Clin. Neurosurg., *27:* 206–229, 1980.
58. Tindall, G. T., Tindall, S. C. Pterional approach to the third ventricular region. In: *Surgery of the Third Ventricle*, edited by M. L. J. Apuzzo. Williams & Wilkins, Baltimore, 1987.
59. Viale, G. L., and Turtas, S. The subchoroid approach to the third ventricle. Surg. Neurol., *14:* 71–76, 1980.
60. Weiss, M. H. Transsphenoidal approach. In: *Surgery of the Third Ventricle*, edited by M. L. J. Apuzzo. Williams & Wilkins, Baltimore, 1987.
61. Wilkins, R. H. The history of surgery of the third ventricular region. In: *Surgery of the Third Ventricle*, Williams & Wilkins, Baltimore, 1987.
62. Yasargil, G. M. Combined approaches to the anterior third ventricular regions. In: *Surgery of the Third Ventricle*, edited by M. L. J. Apuzzo. Williams & Wilkins, Baltimore, 1987.

24

Tumors of the Fourth Ventricle: Technical Considerations in Tumor Surgery

HAROLD J. HOFFMAN, M.D., F.R.C.S.(C.)

INTRODUCTION

Tumors of the fourth ventricle can be grouped into those arising from the lining membrane, which are the ependymomas; those arising from the contents, which are the choroid plexus papillomas; and those which encroach on the walls of the fourth ventricle. The common tumors in this latter group consist of dermoids, cerebellar astrocytomas, brainstem gliomas, and medulloblastomas. The most frequent tumors in and about the fourth ventricle seen in our institution are the ependymomas, the cerebellar astrocytomas, the brainstem gliomas, and the medulloblastomas (Table 24.1).

INVESTIGATION

Modern imaging with magnetic resonance imaging (MRI) and computed tomography (CT) provides superb anatomical detail of the posterior fossa tumors of childhood. Because of the ready availability of these imaging facilities, children are now presenting at an earlier stage in their disease and not in the critically ill condition seen in earlier times.

Furthermore, modern imaging has done away with invasive tests such as ventriculography, pneumoencephalography, and angiography. In the past, following a ventriculogram the child was frequently too ill from the manipulative efforts required for this study to withstand a major craniotomy. For this reason we resorted to a temporizing ventriculoperitoneal (VP) shunt (4). Such shunts, however, had many disadvantages. Shunts can malfunction and become infected. With rapid decompression of the ventricles, subdural hematomas can occur. Furthermore, shift of the tumor in the posterior fossa produced by a sudden change in hydrodynamics supratentorially can lead to upward herniation of the posterior fossa contents with brainstem compression and, frequently, hemorrhage within the tumor (2, 3, 10, 11). Furthermore, the malignant tumors can metastasize down the shunt into the peritoneal cavity, from whence they can disseminate widely (Fig. 24.1) (4).

Instead of a diversionary VP shunt, we therefore prefer to catheterize

TABLE 24.1
Fourth Ventricle Tumors: Hospital for Sick Children, Toronto 1970–1985

	%
Tumors of lining membrane	
Ependymoma	14
Tumors of contents	
Choroid plexus papilloma	0.4
Tumors encroaching on fourth ventricle	
Dermoid tumor	2.7
Cerebellar astrocytoma	27
Brainstem glioma	29
Medulloblastoma	26.9
Total	100%

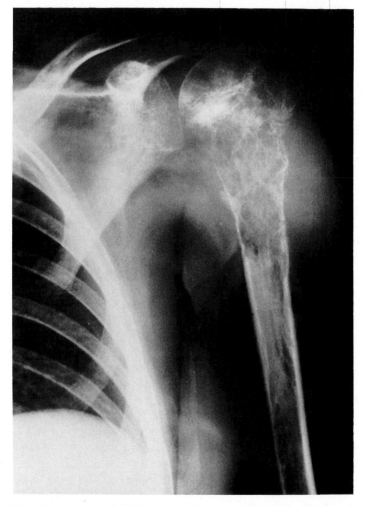

FIG. 24.1. Metastatic medulloblastoma in humerus of a child with diversionary VP shunt.

the aqueduct of Sylvius with a Silastic catheter in those cases in which there is risk that normal pathways of CSF circulation will not open up (Fig. 24.2). On removing a fourth ventricle tumor the aqueduct is always in clear view and can easily be cannulated under direct vision (Fig. 24.3).

At the present time, we do not carry out angiography on a child with a posterior fossa tumor except in the most unusual of circumstances. We do not use a preoperative shunt unless the patient is in desperate straits. The patient is placed on steroids, on a dose of 0.5 mg/kg/day administered in four doses, and is prepared for surgery.

MRI is especially helpful for evaluation of posterior fossa lesions. The problems of partial volume averaging seen with CT are not seen with MRI because MRI does not image bone, and thus the definition of studies of the posterior fossa is frequently better with MRI than CT. Furthermore, MRI can scan both in the coronal and sagittal plane without reformatting, and it is therefore much easier to anatomically define the lesion in the posterior fossa.

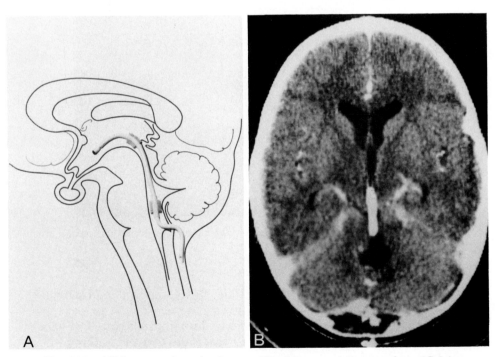

FIG. 24.2. (A) Lapras catheter in place as utilized for cannulating aqueduct of Sylvius. (B) CT scan after resection of fourth ventricular ependymoma showing Lapras catheter in position.

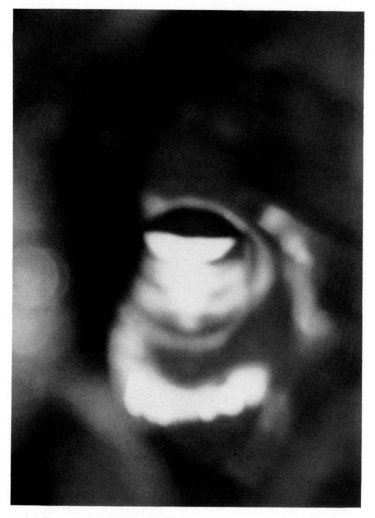

FIG. 24.3. Patent aqueduct of Sylvius as seen through operating microscope after resection of fourth ventricular tumor.

ANESTHESIA

Anesthesia is induced with thiopentone, muscle relaxant, and atropine. Lidocaine in a dose of 1.5 mg/kg is given intravenously to prevent any precipitous rise in pressure intracranially during intubation. The endotracheal tube is introduced through a nasal route to avoid kinking when the neck is flexed.

Anesthesia is maintained with isoflurane and muscle relaxant, with the addition of narcotic. The patient is given mannitol in a dose of 2 gm/kg as the operation begins.

Isoflurane or nitrous oxide combined with a narcotic and muscle relaxants is used for maintenance of anesthesia. Hyperventilation is used to keep the arterial $PaCO_2$ between 28 and 30 torr.

ESSENTIAL MONITORING EQUIPMENT

A Foley catheter is placed in position to deal with the diuresis produced by the mannitol. An arterial line is inserted to monitor pressure accurately. A precordial Doppler is utilized to help detect air embolism. In addition, end tidal CO_2 is measured in order to help with the detection of air embolism. Air in the pulmonary vessels interferes with gaseous exchange and causes retention of CO_2, giving rise to a rapid fall in end tidal CO_2 (7).

An esophageal stethoscope is introduced to monitor heart rate and also to help in detecting air embolism. ECG leads are fixed to the patient. A rectal temperature probe is introduced and connected to a monitor. Maintenance of normal body temperature is essential in the infant and small child. A large bore intravenous line is placed in the saphenous vein percutaneously. Central venous lines are usually not placed because they tend to kink during the flexed prone position that is utilized in our institution.

OPERATIVE POSITIONING

For over 25 years at the Hospital for Sick Children in Toronto, all surgical procedures on the posterior fossa have been carried out with the patient in the prone position (Fig. 24.4). The arguments for the sitting position for posterior fossa surgery include the effectiveness of this position in draining blood and CSF away from the operative field as well as maintaining a lower venous pressure in the head. However, the sitting position has many pitfalls, including the risk of air embolism, systemic hypotension, and the difficulty in maneuvering the patient into the sitting position.

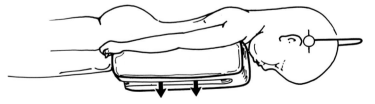

FIG. 24.4.   Position of patient for posterior fossa craniotomy for tumor.

The prone position is easily maintained. The operating table can be tilted to improve venous drainage. The microscope can be easily used in the prone position. There is not the same tiring effect on the arms of the surgeon as there is in the patient who is sitting.

The risk of air embolism in the sitting position varies between 2 and 33% (2, 5). During the past 10 years, in well over 450 operative procedures on the posterior fossa in the prone position in our institution, we have encountered no case of air embolism.

OPERATIVE TECHNIQUE

Ventriculostomy is rarely used. With hyperventilation and mannitol, one can expect a slack posterior fossa in all patients with a posterior fossa tumor. If, however, there is concern that these techniques may not adequately decompress the posterior fossa, plans for an occipital burr hole should be made to allow for operative aspiration of CSF from the ventricles.

The patient's skin is adequately prepared, the skin incisions are marked with sterile pen, and the entire area is covered with an adhesive transparent drape.

Patients under 2½ years of age are placed face down in a well-padded horseshoe head-holder. For patients between the ages of 2½ and 8, infant pins and the Mayfield head-holder are used to position the head, and above the age of 8, adult pins are used.

The head is flexed in the head-holder to open up the space between the arch of C1 and the foramen magnum. The operative site is injected with a solution of 1:200,000 epinephrine.

A midline skin incision is made from inion to midcervical region. Care must be taken once the skin is incised not to immediately insert a self-

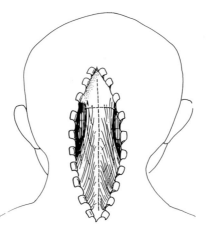

FIG. 24.5.   Outline of muscle incision for posterior fossa craniotomy.

retaining retractor since this may distort anatomical landmarks and take one down a paramedian course into muscle which can produce brisk bleeding. The retractor is therefore not inserted until the midline ligamentum nuchae have been incised down to the spinous processes. Once this is done, self-retaining retractors are placed. A horizontal incision is placed in the paraspinal muscles in the midoccipital region, which will help in the eventual suturing of the musculature (Fig. 24.5). The muscle is then taken off of the occipital bone, and any bleeding occipital emissary veins are coagulated and the orifices filled with wax. Using sharp dissection, the periosteum is cut over the arch of C1 on either side of the midline. With the index finger covered with gauze, the periosteum is stripped off the arch of C1, thus avoiding injury to the vertebral artery (Fig. 24.6). With the power craniotome, a burr hole is placed on either side of the midline just below the inion. The occipital bone is then rongeured between the burr holes across the midline and then downwards on either side towards the foramen magnum. With this done, the occipital bone is grasped with the rongeur and taken off the underlying dura, leaving the remaining attachment of the atlantooccipital membrane intact (Fig. 24.7). This membrane which extends from the lip of the foramen magnum to the arch of C1 is sharply divided at its attachment to the arch of C1, and the occipital bone is removed in one piece. The arch of C1 is then removed.

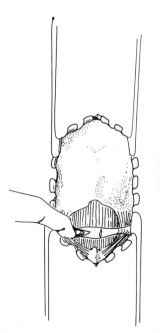

FIG. 24.6.   Method of stripping periosteum from arch of C1 using finger.

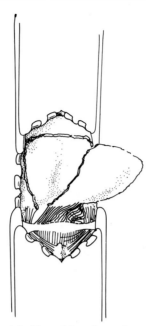

FIG. 24.7.   Freed up occipital bone hinged on atlantooccipital membrane.

The dura is now divided running from a superolateral position inferiorly and creating a "V"-shaped incision in dura with the bottom of the "V" just below the foramen magnum.

If one V's the dural incision just below the foramen magnum, one should avoid brisk bleeding from the annular sinus. Occasionally in childhood, there may be a midline falx cerebrelli and, again, dividing the dura with a "V"-shaped incision which extends to just below the lip of the foramen magnum will carry one below the falx cerebelli and avoid the difficulty of cutting across the falx.

The dura is then hinged upward by a ligature placed around the occipital sinus at its inferior extent. The dural incision is now extended into a "Y" by dividing the dura over the cervical region (Fig. 24.8). The dural edges must all be coagulated to avoid continuous venous ooze. The cisterna magna is then opened. This allows one to view the cerebellar tonsils, the upper cervical cord, and tumor. Early in the operation on a fourth ventricular tumor the floor of the fourth ventricle should be identified and protected by a cotton patty (Fig. 24.9).

EPENDYMOMA

Ependymomas make up some 14% of fourth ventricular tumors in our institution. In childhood, these tumors frequently take up the entire configuration of the fourth ventricle, insinuating themselves into the

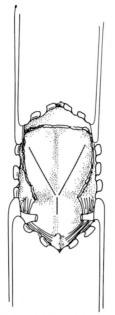

FIG. 24.8.   Outline of dural incision.

foramina of Luschka as well as out through the foramen of Magendie onto the dorsal aspect of the cord (Fig. 24.10). It was for this reason that Courville referred to them as plastic ependymomas (1).

Modern imaging techniques will typically show the tumor extending onto the dorsal aspect of the spinal cord, below the level of the foramen magnum. The tumor can also frequently be seen to extend into the cerebellopontine angle through a distended foramen of Luschka (Fig. 24.11). The tumor as it spills out into the basal cisterns can mingle with the lower cranial nerves.

About one-third of ependymomas in childhood have a malignant appearance histologically with mitotic figures, pleomorphism, and necrosis. Such tumors are extremely vascular and tend to infiltrate surrounding structures and can almost never be totally removed. In dealing with these tumors one must ensure careful hemostasis since the residual tumor with its vascularity may ooze and lead to a postoperative clot.

Although two-thirds of the ependymomas in the posterior fossa have a benign histologic appearance, many of them have a poor outcome. If the tumors are free of the floor of the fourth ventricle, they can be totally excised, leaving no residual tumor. However, many of the "so-called" benign ependymomas of the fourth ventricle invade the floor of the fourth ventricle, making it necessary to leave residual tumor. It is in such situations that existing hydrocephalus may continue, and it is therefore

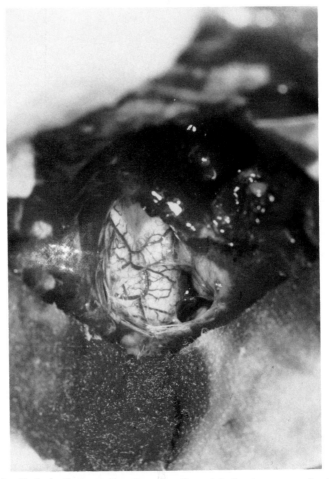

Fig. 24.9.   Early in the operation for a fourth ventricular tumor one should obtain a
good view of the floor of the fourth ventricle and insert a cotton patty on the floor of the
fourth ventricle, separating overlying tumor from the fourth ventricle floor.

important to catheterize the aqueduct of Sylvius to maintain a patent
CSF channel and avoid the need for a diversionary ventriculoperitoneal
shunt.

Ependymomas can readily metastasize through CSF pathways, and for
this reason our practice at the Hospital for Sick Children is to give these
children postoperative craniospinal radiation.

CHOROID PLEXUS PAPILLOMAS

Choroid plexus papillomas of the fourth ventricle are rare in childhood,
and make up only 0.4% of tumors in and about the fourth ventricle in

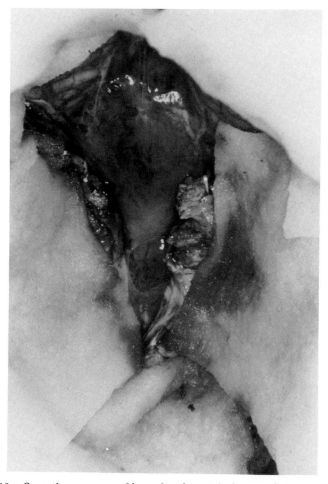

FIG. 24.10.   Operative exposure of large fourth ventricular ependymoma which is seen extending over dorsal aspect of closed medulla and upper cervical cord.

our institution. These tumors typically fill the fourth ventricle and do not invade the walls of the fourth ventricle (Fig. 24.12). They are richly supplied with blood, usually through the posterior inferior cerebellar arteries, and they brightly contrast enhance on CT scan. Because the tumor effectively blocks the fourth ventricle, obstructive hydrocephalus is common. Once the blood supply of the tumor is secured, it is relatively easy to totally resect it.

DERMOID TUMORS

Dermoid tumors are typically midline tumors which in the posterior fossa occupy the vermis and encroach on the fourth ventricle. They

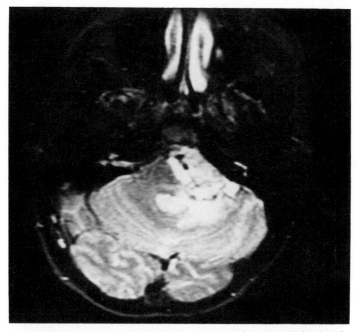

FIG. 24.11. MRI scan of posterior fossa showing ependymoma of the fourth ventricle passing out into cerebellopontine angle.

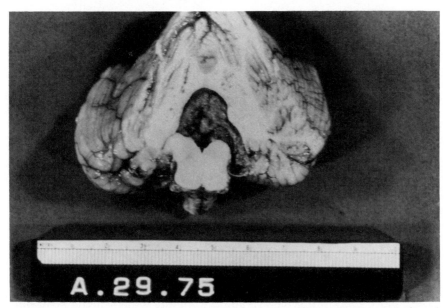

FIG. 24.12. Post-mortem specimen of choroid plexus papilloma showing tumor free of walls of fourth ventricle.

comprise 2.7% of the tumors in and about the fourth ventricle at the Hospital for Sick Children. They are usually associated with a dermal sinus which typically runs in a caudal direction from a skin dimple near the inion (Fig. 24.13). Rarely, the dermal sinus may run cephalad from a dimple in the neck.

Ideally if one visualizes a dimple in a child's occipital region, neuroimaging should be carried out to rule out an intracranial dermoid tumor. However, these dimples are usually covered with hair and are therefore frequently undetected until the children present with a septic meningitis or precipitous enlargement of the tumor due to abscess formation within the tumor.

These tumors should be removed under the cover of antibiotics. The dermal sinus should be traced to its termination. Typically it will pierce the dura in the midoccipital region and end in a firmly encapsulated

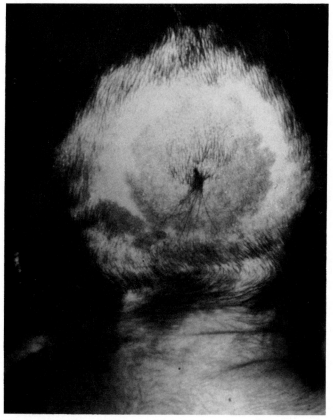

FIG. 24.13.   Occipital dermal sinus which led into a dermoid tumor in the cerebellar vermis.

dermoid tumor in the cerebellar vermis. The encapsulated tumor can be readily dissected free of surrounding cerebellum and removed.

CEREBELLAR ASTROCYTOMAS

Cerebellar astrocytomas are common tumors encroaching on the fourth ventricle. They comprise 27% of the tumors in and about the fourth ventricle at the Hospital for Sick Children. They are typically benign tumors. In our institution, the commonest histologic type of cerebellar astrocytoma is the pilocytic tumor. Occasionally the tumor may be fibrillary or gemistocytic or, rarely, mixed with oligodendroglial components.

Modern imaging has allowed for accurate assessment of these tumors. About 40% of cerebellar astrocytomas are solid, but may contain small intratumoral cysts (Fig. 24.14). Twenty-seven percent are the typical cystic astrocytomas which contain a mural nodule and are associated with a cyst lined by gliosed cerebellum (Fig. 24.15). Thirty-three percent

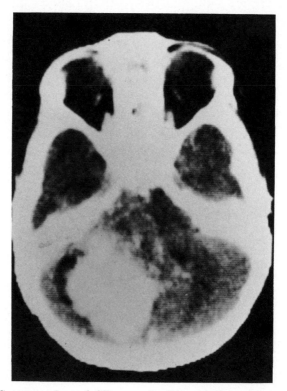

FIG. 24.14. Contrast-enhanced CT scan of solid cerebellar astrocytoma with small tumoral cyst.

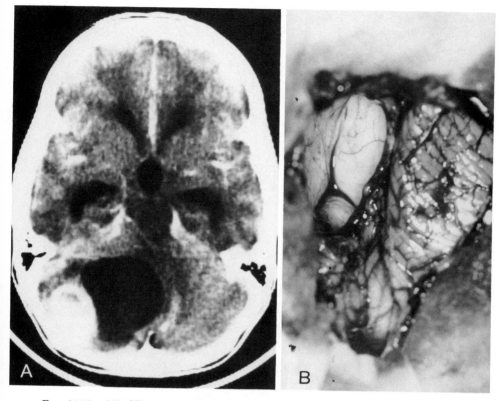

FIG. 24.15. (A) CT scan of typical cystic cerebellar astrocytoma showing contrast-enhancing mural nodule and nonenhancing cyst wall. (B) The cyst wall at operation of patient whose CT scan is seen in A. Note the gliotic nontumoral cyst wall in this patient.

are the false cystic astrocytomas in which the cyst wall consists of tumor. In these patients the cyst wall may be thick or very thin and may contain a mural nodule (Fig. 24.16).

If one totally resects a cerebellar astrocytoma, there is no risk of recurrence. Recurrences occur when false cystic astrocytomas are mistaken for typical cystic astrocytomas and part of the tumor cyst wall is left behind, which allows for reaccumulation of the cyst and reformation of the tumor. The ultrasonic aspirator is a very efficient tool for removing the cyst wall of the false cystic astrocytoma.

On opening the dura in the case of a cerebellar astrocytoma, one typically sees a larger cerebellar hemisphere on the side of the tumor with distended cerebellar folia and a tonsil which is pushed lower on the side of the tumor (Fig. 24.17). If the astrocytoma is in the vermis, then the cerebellar vermis is enlarged.

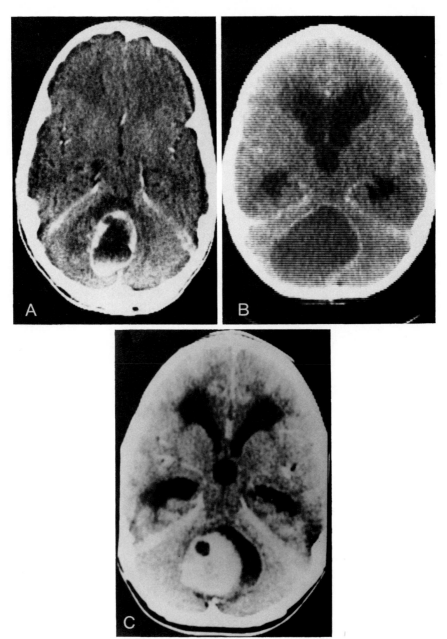

Fig. 24.16. (A) Contrast-enhanced CT scan of thick-walled false cystic cerebellar astrocytoma. Note enhancing cyst wall. (B) Enhanced CT scan of thin-walled false cystic cerebellar astrocytoma. (C) Enhanced CT scan of mural nodule and enhancing cyst wall of patient with false cystic cerebellar astrocytoma.

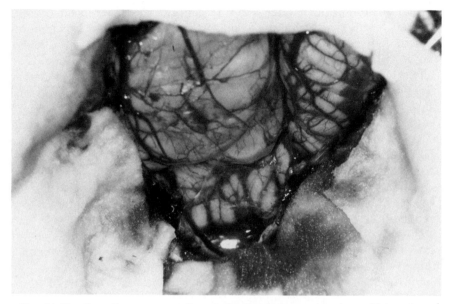

FIG. 24.17. Operative exposure of cerebellar hemisphere astrocytoma. Note enlarged folia of enlarged cerebellar hemisphere.

Operative ultrasound will display the presence of cystic and solid portions of the tumor and localize the tumor prior to any incision in cerebellum.

In the case of solid tumors, it is essential to remove all of the tumor, and again the ultrasonic aspirator is valuable in carrying this out. In the case of typical cystic astrocytomas, it is only necessary to remove the mural nodule. Frequently the mural nodule is quite small. With the mural nodule removed, the gliosed cyst rapidly collapses. In the case of false cystic astrocytomas, the entire cyst wall, including any mural nodule if present, must be removed to prevent tumor recurrence.

BRAINSTEM GLIOMAS

These tumors comprise 29% of tumors about the fourth ventricle. In the past, brainstem gliomas were regarded as inoperable tumors which were malignant by virtue of their location. Modern neuroimaging has allowed us to categorize these tumors and demonstrate that a significant proportion of them behave in a benign fashion.

We have divided our brainstem tumors into four groups (9). Group 1 consists of tumors which are dorsally exophytic into the fourth ventricle. These tumors tend to be low grade astrocytomas and gangliogliomas. Cranial nerve deficits and long tract signs are relatively uncommon, and the patients tend to be young. On CT scan, the tumors are isodense and enhance brightly with contrast (Fig. 24.18). Hydrocephalus is commonly present. With subtotal resection of the tumor, the patients have a benign course.

The Group 2 tumors are the diffuse intrinsic tumors of brainstem. These tumors typically extend from midbrain to medulla and may extend upwards into thalamus (Fig. 24.19). The vast majority of these tumors, on presentation on CT scan, are hypodense and nonenhancing. In time, however, various portions of the tumor begin to enhance, and the tumor shows exophytic components anteriorly and into the cerebellopontine angle. These tumors have a variable pathologic appearance and can be mistakenly diagnosed as a low grade astrocytoma on the basis of a small biopsy. At post-mortem, however, they all have the appearance of a malignant astrocytoma or a frank glioblastoma multiforme.

These patients have a short history and present with cranial nerve palsies and long tract signs. If neuroimaging shows a diffuse intrinsic tumor of brainstem, biopsy is not indicated, and surgery has no role to play. Unfortunately, modern techniques of radiotherapy and chemotherapy have had little impact on these tumors.

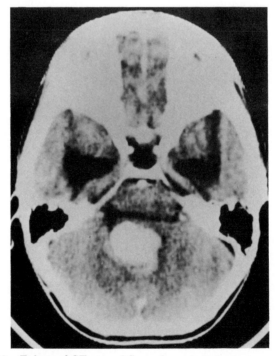

FIG. 24.18.   Enhanced CT scan of Group I exophytic brainstem tumor.

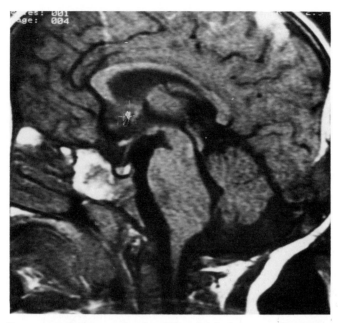

FIG. 24.19. MRI scan showing diffuse intrinsic tumor of brainstem.

The Group 3 tumors are focal cystic tumors intrinsic in brainstem. These tumors can be either low grade or high grade in nature. They may have a mural nodule or consist entirely of a tumor cyst. We advocate marsupializing these cysts either into the basal cisterns or into the fourth ventricle and obtaining a biopsy of the cyst wall. If the cystic portion of the tumor extends high into the midbrain, we have used a subtemporal route with incision of the tentorium cerebelli as our operative approach to the tumor. Postoperative radiotherapy is indicated in these tumors.

The fourth group of tumors in the brainstem consists of focal, solid intrinsic tumors. These tumors tend to occur at the cervicomedullary junction, but can occur in any part of the brainstem. They typically contrast enhance on CT and frequently are low grade astrocytomas. These tumors can be partially resected, and the patients should receive postoperative radiotherapy.

MEDULLOBLASTOMAS

Medulloblastomas are common tumors encroaching on the fourth ventricle and comprise 26.9% of tumors in and about the fourth ventricle in our institution.

These tumors are frequently not visible on opening dura until the cerebellar tonsils are spread apart, revealing the inferior vermis and

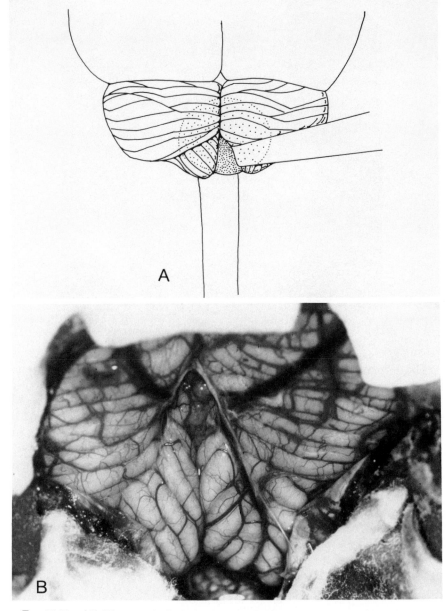

FIG. 24.20.   (A) Diagramatic depiction of position of medulloblastoma. (B) Exposure of posterior fossa which harbors a medulloblastoma. (C) Medulloblastoma is exposed in the same patient as in Figure 24.20B, after separating cerebellar tonsils.

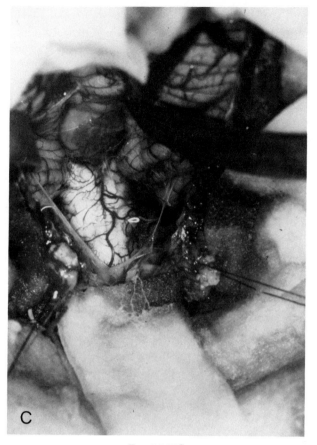

FIG. 24.20C

exposing the tumor (Fig. 24.20). It is important to protect the floor of the fourth ventricle by inserting a patty between tumor and floor of fourth ventricle. The cerebellar vermis is split using bipolar cautery, laser, and ultrasonic aspirator. The tumors lie in the roof of the fourth ventricle and under magnification can be removed, frequently totally. Unfortunately in 30% of cases, the tumor infiltrates the floor of the fourth ventricle, and in such situations one is forced to leave tumor in the floor of the fourth ventricle (8). The tumor can bulge into the aqueduct of Sylvius but rarely invades the walls of the aqueduct and typically can be pulled down from the aqueduct. In such cases and in cases in which tumor is left in the floor of the fourth ventricle, insertion of a Lapras catheter from third ventricle to cisterna magna is of value (Fig. 24.2).

OPERATIVE MANEUVERS

After removal of a tumor of the fourth ventricle, it is essential that hemostasis be secured. Those venous oozers which can not be closed off with bipolar cautery will frequently seal off utilizing hemostatic agents. A piece of rubber dam on top of the hemostatic agent ensures that it will not float off with irrigation. Gentle pressure on the pack of hemostatic agents is applied by inserting a piece of cotton soaked in 3% hydrogen peroxide. This is left in place for 3–5 minutes. The cotton and rubber dam are then irrigated out, leaving the hemostatic agent adherent to any bleeding points.

Prior to closing the dura, one should ask the anesthetist to raise the intracranial venous pressure to ensure that there are no venous bleeders. The dural opening is frequently shrunk at this point due to coagulation of the dural edges. I feel that a watertight dural closure is necessary in patients who have had a fourth ventricle tumor removed. Securing a good dural closure prevents blood and debris, from the soft tissues of the neck, from entering the CSF space and giving rise to an aseptic meningitis. We therefore use a patch of cadaver freeze-dried dura to secure a watertight closure of the dura after removal of a fourth ventricle tumor (Fig. 24.21).

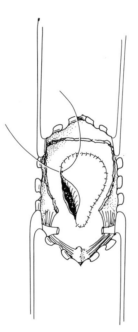

FIG. 24.21. Suturing of dural graft in order to achieve watertight closure of posterior fossa dura after resection of fourth ventricular tumor.

Postoperatively, if a Lapras catheter has been left in place, we perform a lumbar puncture on the patient 24 hours after surgery to encourage circulation of CSF. A follow-up CT scan is done 24 hours postoperatively to see if there is residual tumor and to estimate the size of residual tumor. Artifact is minimized during the first 2 or 3 days after surgery.

CONCLUSIONS

Over one-third of patients with fourth ventricular tumors have a perfectly benign course and can be managed without adjuvant radiotherapy or chemotherapy. Over half of the malignant tumors of the fourth ventricle are curable with modern techniques of radiotherapy and chemotherapy. Modern neuroimaging has led to earlier diagnosis and better understanding of the anatomy of the lesion by the neurosurgeon, and modern surgical tools have allowed the neurosurgeon to safely excise fourth ventricular tumors in a manner not possible in the past.

REFERENCES

1. Courville, C. B., and Broussalian, S. L. Plastic ependymomas of the lateral recess. Report of eight verified cases. J. Neurosurg., 18: 792–799, 1961.
2. Cucchiara, R. F., and Bowers, B. Air embolism in children undergoing suboccipital craniotomy. Anesthesiology, 57: 338–339, 1982.
3. Epstein, F., and Murali, R. Pediatric posterior fossa tumors: Hazards of the "preoperative" shunt. Neurosurgery, 3: 348–350, 1978.
4. Hoffman, H. J., Hendrick, E. B., and Humphreys, R. P. Metastasis via ventriculoperitoneal shunt in patients with medulloblastoma. J. Neurosurg., 44: 562–566, 1976.
5. Hurter, D., and Sebel, P. S. Detection of venous air embolism. Anaesthesia, 34: 578–582, 1979.
6. Lapras, C., Patel, J. D., Derex, M. C., et al. Astrocytoma du cervelet chez l'enfant. A propos de 57 observations. Neurochirurgie, 29: 241–246, 1983.
7. Matijasko, J., Petrozza, P., and MacKenzsie, C. F.: Sensitivity of end-tidal nitrogen in venous air embolism detection in dogs. Anesthesiology, 63: 418–423, 1985.
8. Park, T. S., Hoffman, H. J., Hendrick, E. B., et al. Medulloblastoma. Clinical presentation and management. Experience at HSC 1950–1980. J. Neurosurg., 58: 543–552, 1983.
9. Stroink, A., Hoffman, H. J., Hendrick, E. B., et al. Diagnosis and management of pediatric brainstem gliomas. J. Neurosurg., 65: 745–750, 1986.
10. Vaquero, J., Cabezudo, J. M., DeSola, R. G., et al. Intratumoral hemorrhage in posterior fossa tumors after ventricular drainage. J. Neurosurg., 54: 406, 1981.
11. Waga, S., Shimuzu, T., Shumosaka, S., et al. Intratumoral hemorrhage after ventriculoperitoneal shunting procedure. Neurosurgery, 9: 249–252, 1981.

V

Trauma

25

The Role of Aggressive Therapy for Head Injury: Does It Matter?

LAWRENCE F. MARSHALL, M.D.

INTRODUCTION

The modern era of clinical head injury research can be directly attributed to the pioneering efforts of Jennett and his colleagues in Glasgow (8). Certainly, the development of the Glasgow Coma Scale (15) and a systematic approach to the prospective evaluation of patients made available for the first time a vehicle which would permit a reasonable comparison of patients cared for in different hospitals. Of course, the initial motive of the Glasgow group was to study the prediction of outcome and to determine when firm outcome predictions could be made for patients suffering severe closed head injury. Thus, they chose the period 6 hours following injury as the time at which the first predictions could be made and also as the time when comparisons would be made between centers. The 6-hour rule, while appropriate for the comparisons which they were interested in, namely, in permitting firm predictions, has major disadvantages if one is interested not only in the natural history of severe head injury, but also in the effects of intervention. This is because many patients who are operated on will have their clot removed prior to the 6-hour period and may (*a*) never lapse into coma or (*b*) have their coma reversed and, thus, not be included using the 6-hour criterion.

If one is interested in studying the efficacy of therapy, and not primarily the development of predictive indices, then a 6-hour rule is inappropriate. The National Head Injury Data Bank, which had as its mandate the study of traumatic coma, chose to define severe head injuries as those patients who had a Glasgow Coma Scale score of 8 or less following nonsurgical resuscitation. This was defined as adequate volume repletion and the correction of ventilatory failure, a common accompaniment of severe head injury. Given the fact that approximately one-half of patients suffering severe head injury in the U.S. have multisystem injuries, this attention to the immediate sequelae of head injury and early resolution in order to define those patients with severe head injuries was appropriate.

One additional caveat regarding the initial Glasgow data is the fact that patients who are considered to be brain dead or who were thought to be likely to reach that status within the 6-hour period following admission were excluded, an exclusion criterion that was not generally known at the time that the initial multinational study was published. Again, this is an appropriate step when one is looking at prediction, but this practice should be taken into account when comparisons between institutions are made, particularly if such exclusions are not universally applied.

PROSPECTIVE STUDIES OF HEAD INJURY

Following the publication of the multinational study, Becker and Miller published the results of a series of prospectively collected patients in Richmond (1). This landmark paper demonstrated a substantially improved mortality and morbidity following severe head injury, but there were differences between patient entry criteria between the two series. In an attempt to reconcile these, Miller and Becker reanalyzed their data and attempted to apply the multinational data bank entry criteria to their patient set (12). They continued to find a reduced mortality and morbidity, although the differences had been reduced from approximately 17% to approximately 12%. Miller concluded that there was a substantial difference in outcome, but it was approximately a 20% reduction in mortality and not 35%. There was also no increase in the number of poor outcomes in the Richmond series. The Richmond series pointed out the necessity for making such comparisons based on comparability of patients, a position Jennett had previously espoused when he said that one must be certain that the patients are matched properly, that the data is collected prospectively, and that the conclusion is an actual product of the data.

These concerns are appropriate because the influence of age, mechanism of injury, type of intracranial lesion, and the clinical status of the patient, either at 6 hours or following resuscitation, are major factors in determining whether one is comparing similar patients or patients who are remarkably dissimilar. Many have demonstrated the adverse influence of age, and Jane, in an analysis of the National Head Injury Data Bank, showed that much of this is a product of the fact that in older patients subdural hematoma becomes more frequent and all recognize that this lesion is associated with a higher mortality than, for example, diffuse axonal injury (6).

In 1979, the San Diego group published their experience in 100 consecutive prospectively studied head-injured patients using the 6-hour rule and in whom very aggressive therapy for moderate elevations of intracranial pressure (ICP) was used (10). The mortality reported in that report was approximately 35%, similar to the data reported from Richmond, and was a seeming improvement over the data reported by the multinational study. However, there were substantial differences in the patient population. The number of patients with mass lesions was relatively low in the San Diego experience, a reflection of the high number of motor vehicle accidents, which more frequently caused diffuse axonal injury. Furthermore, the population was a bit younger, although not significantly so. Nevertheless, the influence of small differences in age has not been well studied, and this may also have been a factor.

As a follow-up to the San Diego study, Bowers and Marshall reported on a prospectively studied group of patients in whom care was rendered both at the University of California Medical Center and in three community hospitals in San Diego County (3). This data reported a mortality rate of less than 40%, and a serious attempt was made to match these patients with the multinational data bank (8). The Bowers and Marshall study, which to date is the only study involving community hospitals studied in a prospective fashion, reported results which, if one looks at the data in more detail, are of considerable interest. There was a small but consistent difference in the outcome of patients with diffuse injuries and elevated pressure between those patients cared for in a university setting and those cared for in a community hospital. This difference was significant, but there was no overall significant difference because the outcome in patients with mass lesions was identical. This, perhaps, indicates that in patients with surgical lesions, if surgical therapy is rendered quickly, the outcome will be about the same if care is well organized in a region, but that experience with aggressive therapy for intracranial hypertension may make a difference in patients with specific types of lesions. The multicenter barbiturate trial apparently demonstrates the same conclusion.

Moreover, there were some interesting differences between community hospitals themselves. While the outcome for patients with mass lesions was not materially different, in those patients with diffuse injuries patient outcome was improved when ICP was monitored and, thus, presumably treated. This difference was sharpest for patients who did not have abnormal motor movements, suggesting at least that there may be a specific group of patients in whom outcome differences are a product of progressive therapy. This issue must also be taken into account when comparing outcome.

MORBIDITY, MORTALITY, AND INTRACRANIAL HEMATOMA

It is appropriate to note the fact that the mortality rate from traumatic intracranial hematomas has dropped substantially in Glasgow since their initial publication. These patients would not have shown up in the initial

Data Bank nor in a subsequent study because many of them were individuals who did not lapse into coma in the second series. What does this reflect? It reflects, as Teasdale and his colleagues reported in the *British Medical Journal* (14), a change in policy regarding where patients are hospitalized and how rapidly computed tomographic (CT) scanning is undertaken. In the Glasgow unit, in the first 4 years before the change in policy, there was a 38% mortality in patients with intracranial hematomas, but this decreased to 29% later. This study of 683 patients indicates, in my view, that the 6-hour rule is flawed when making patient intercenter comparisons, and that it is likely to mask important differences of treatment because of the homogenization that occurs if someone has been operated on and remains decerebrate 6 hours thereafter. Moreover, the Glasgow group demonstrated a reduction in the number of patients who talked and then died from 31% before the change in policy to 16% thereafter. This is also an indication of an improvement in triage, and brings the Glasgow experience more into line with the experience in American regions where triage systems have been in place for some time and where overall incidence of "talk and die" patients is 10–15%, as it was in the National Head Injury Data Bank.

Thus, if one then views the Glasgow experience as a whole over the last 15 years, one sees that while they have been skeptical regarding an improvement in mortality in the most severely injured, they have themselves demonstrated that in patients who would have died had therapy not been instituted earlier, a change in management philosophy influenced outcome.

A PREDICTIVE MODEL OF HEAD INJURY

In an attempt to develop a more rational mechanism for comparing both patients and institutions, Klauber et al., working on an extremely large data set, in collaboration with the three Comprehensive Central Nervous System Injury Centers for Defined Geographic Regions of the United States, developed a predictive model for making interpatient comparisons (M. R. Klauber, L. F. Marshall, R. Frankowski, *et al.* Determinants of head injury: Importance of the low risk patient, unpublished manuscript). This model utilized a large number of variables which were immediately available to the neurosurgeon caring for the patient, such as the neurological examination and the vital signs. By applying this model and the variables which are shown in Table 25.1, Klauber was able to make comparisons between three regions of the U.S.: the greater metropolitan area for Houston, Texas; the Bronx, New York; and San Diego, California. In that study patients at moderate risk, that is, patients with a Glasgow Coma Scale score of 7 or greater, were those who were most at risk from dying if the level of surveillance in the hospital was

TABLE 25.1.

Logistic Regression Coefficients by Factor Obtained Using Backward Stepping

Order of Importance	Factor Level	Coefficient
Constant		0.1491
1 Motor score		
	1	−1.7029
	2	−1.1875
	3	−0.5977
	4	0.0798
	5	0.4732
	6	2.9351
2 No reactive eyes		
	0	−1.0540
	1	−0.4244
	2	0.7244
	Unknown	0.7540
3 Systolic blood pressure (mm Hg)		
	0–84	−0.5646
	85–174	0.6006
	175+	
4 Abdominal injury		
	Yes	−0.3142
	No	0.3142
5 Age (yr)		
	0–4	1.0043
	5–9	1.0988
	10–19	1.1644
	20–29	0.3832
	30–39	0.2555
	40–49	−0.0650
	50–59	−0.4149
	60–69	−0.2980
	70–79	−1.7619
	80+	−1.3667
6 Hospital unit (not in model to estimate risk)		
7 Chest injury		
	Yes	−0.1995
	No	0.1995

Example: A patient with motor score 2, one nonreactive eye, systolic blood pressure 0–85 mm Hg, age 25, with no abdominal or chest injury:

Y = Sum of corresponding coefficients

= 0.1491 −1.875 −0.4244 −0.5646 +0.3832 +0.3142 +0.1995

= 1.130

Estimated probability of survival = $100/(1 + Exp(-Y))$

= 24%

not optimal. This indicates that the role of aggressive therapy or early attention to the likelihood of deterioration is going to have its biggest payoff in the care of patients who are most likely to make a useful recovery following moderate or severe head injury. Thus, it appears appropriate to emphasize that the definition of aggressive therapy needs to be broadened to include early surveillance, which should, just as the introduction of CT scanning did, reduce the number of patients, particularly those with intracranial hematomas, who die or are left severely damaged because of a failure to establish the diagnosis quickly.

THE ROLE OF CRITICAL CARE

If, however, one leaves the emphasis on the aggressive therapy only at the level of prehospital care and the early detection of intracranial hematomas and ignores the influence of critical care, the story is left unfinished. The therapy of intracranial hypertension and the role of continuous recording of intracranial pressure (ICP) is discussed in detail elsewhere. But it is important to note that the beginning of neurosurgical intensive care really commenced with the recognition that brain swelling played a substantive role in the deterioration of patients with a variety of intracranial lesions, and particularly in patients with head injury. The addition of systematic and organized protocols for the therapy of brain-injured patients took as its fundamental precept the expectant treatment of intracranial hypertension (11). Many, including the Glasgow group, have questioned the role of what has been termed the "superaggressive approach" taken by neurosurgical units in the U.S., particularly our own, in the treatment of intracranial hypertension.

In an attempt to determine whether such criticism had merit, the Comprehensive Central Nervous System Injury Centers for Defined Geographic Regions of the United States embarked on a collaborative trial to determine the role of high dose barbiturate therapy in the treatment of uncontrolled intracranial hypertension. The introduction of barbiturates in this study was the last step in an extremely aggressive approach towards the treatment of ICP in which all sustained elevations above 20 mm Hg were treated and wherein stringent management guidelines for the treatment of intracranial mass lesions as well as of ICP for the maintenance of the patient's physiologic status were strictly delineated. This study demonstrated that patients without cardiac compromise in whom barbiturates were utilized fared significantly better than those in the control population, indicating that the aggressive treatment of intracranial hypertension will not only increase the number of survivals, but also will yield an improved survival (4).

This series of patients, which represents a landmark in neurosurgical clinical investigation, certainly does demonstrate that the treatment of intracranial hypertension does matter and that many of the concepts underlying the rational therapy of the head-injured patient have been affirmed. It will be extremely difficult for someone to argue that monitoring ICP is of little consequence, given this unequivocal demonstration that the treatment of elevations of ICP above 25 mm Hg, which are sustained, can be effectively carried out with an improved outcome. This study did not address the role of treating even lower ICPs, a subject which is now open to further discussion.

The recognition that ICPs under 20 mm Hg can be associated with brain stem compression has altered our view of what level of ICP can produce further brain damage. There have been studies from others which have provided circumstantial evidence that the earlier treatment of more elevations of intracranial hypertension is associated with a better outcome. But these studies, particularly that of Saul and Ducker, have been criticized because of their sequential rather than concurrent nature (13). Nevertheless, their observations, and the observation that the incidence of uncontrolled ICP has declined dramatically in all centers participating in the National Collaborative Study on the use of barbiturates, suggest at least that aggressive early therapy of intracranial hypertension reduces the incidence of uncontrollable episodes, which should certainly be seen as beneficial to the patients.

Our own experience, particularly our association of pupillary abnormalities such as the oval pupil with ICPs of less than 20 mm Hg, indicates that transtentorial herniation, depending on the location of the mass, can occur at quite low ICPs (9). This would seem to indicate that a small improvement in the outcome of head injury in those units that are already quite sophisticated in the care of such patients might be expected if patients with posterior frontal and temporal lobe lesions, as shown in Figure 25.1, are operated on earlier rather than later.

It is important to point out that for a significant number of head-injured patients the die is cast from the moment of injury. In some that means that death or a very severely damaged state is inevitable while for others, even if no intervention were carried out, survival with a high quality of recovery would be the rule. Thus, the neurosurgeon can only influence the outcome in a limited number of patients who reach the hospital alive, perhaps a group no greater than 50%. Such influence, however, will not only impact mortality, which is easy to measure, but also morbidity, which is much more difficult to measure and, therefore, to quantify.

A perusal of recent outcome studies would indicate that a mortality of approximately 35–40% in patients studied prospectively and well matched is achievable. Variations from such an overall percentage of mortality are acceptable provided there are an excess number of either

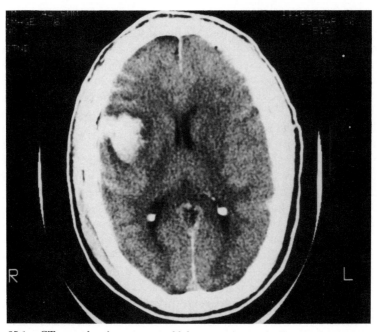

FIG. 25.1.   CT scan showing a temporal lobe contusion typically associated with an oval pupil.

aged patients; more severely injured patients, *i.e.*, those with brain stem signs at the time of admission; or unusual mechanisms of injury. The comparison paper by Genarelli summarized the experiences in a number of centers and served to emphasize the point that a mortality rate of approximately 40% should be achievable (5). Thus, this is the outcome number in terms of mortality that we must improve on. Bergman and Rockswold's recent study in Minnesota serves to emphasize, as it reports an experience almost a decade later than the original Richmond or San Diego papers, how difficult it is likely to be to do substantially better because of the severity of injury (Fig. 25.2) (2). The number of patients who are entered into any one study on the high end of the severe injury scale is likely to decline as prehospital care and the rapid evacuation of hematomas becomes the national standard. What it behooves us to do now is to develop better measures of the influence of therapy on morbidity. In fact, one of the major objectives for the last half of this decade should be not only the development of better therapies for the morbid effects of brain injury, but also of better measures in the acute state of the morbidity, perhaps based on imaging techniques, so that the early effectiveness of such therapies might potentially be measured. Given the

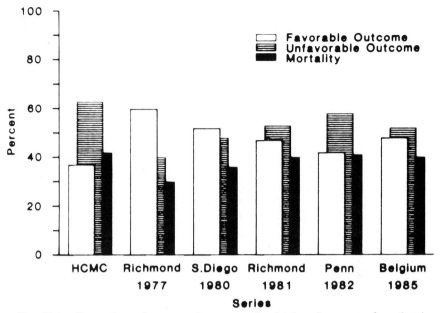

FIG. 25.2.   Comparison of outcome from severe head injury from a number of series. (From Bergman, T. A., Rockswold, G. L., Haines, S. J., *et al.* Outcome of severe closed head injury in the Midwest: A review and comparison with other major head trauma studies. *Neurosurgery*, 1987, with permission).

fact that in laboratory models of head injury that mild hypoxia and hypotension significantly exacerbate an otherwise completely recoverable brain injury, is it not likely that morbidity is likely to be substantially improved by aggressive therapy, not only for secondary insults, but also for the primary insult to the brain?

CONCLUSIONS

As one who has cared for head injuries for approximately 15 years, the improvement in outcome recently reported by several centers appears to be substantial. Not only are more patients surviving, but fewer are deteriorating to the point where their survival is ever in question. Thus, if one uses a broad definition of aggressive therapy so that it includes a well-organized and rapidly responsive prehospital system and also includes in such a definition a high standard of operative and intensive care, there appears to be little question that aggressive therapy plays a substantive role in the outcome of head injuries. The recent demonstration of the National Collaborative Barbiturate Trial indicates beyond a reasonable doubt that aggressive therapy of intracranial hypertension is worthwhile and is not simply a medical and laboratory exercise.

No one can doubt that we need better therapies for tissue injuries to the brain and a much better understanding of the molecular nature of both diffuse axonal and neuronal injuries which are not completely irreversible. The concept that hippocampal damage in ischemic brain injury is a dynamic process which might be reversed by pharmacologic means is an exciting possibility. The need for region-specific therapies for brain injury rather than for global treatment is also obvious, but our ability to determine the regions at risk in most instances is still poor. Nevertheless, a substantial impact on the mortality and, perhaps even more important, on the morbidity of head injury has been made in much of Western society. Who can deny that the rapid evacuation of hematomas has resulted in improved mortality and morbidity? Who can argue that a reduction in the number of patients who talk and then deteriorate in the National Head Injury Data Bank is not a substantive accomplishment, as has recently been demonstrated? Who can deny that we need better therapies for brain injury? Certainly, no one can, but given the fact that a consensus has emerged regarding the systematic therapy of these patients there has been real progress over the last 15 years. Further refinements in head injury care await a better understanding of the neurobiology of such injuries and the imaginative application of therapies by young investigators.

REFERENCES

1. Becker, D. P., Miller, J. D., Ward, J. D., et al. The outcome from severe head injury with early diagnosis and intensive treatment. J. Neurosurg., 47: 491–502, 1977.
2. Bergman, T. A., Rockswold, G. L., Haines, S. J., et al. Outcome of severe closed head injury in the Midwest: A review and comparison with other major head trauma studies. Neurosurgery, in press, 1987.
3. Bowers, S. A., and Marshall, L. F. Outcome in 200 cases of severe head injury treated in San Diego County: A prospective analysis. Neurosurgery, 6: 237–242, 1980.
4. Eisenberg, H. The National Collaborative Trial of High Dose Barbiturate Therapy for Uncontrolled Intracranial Hypertension, 1986.
5. Gennarelli, T. A., Spielman, G. M., Langfitt, T. W. et al. Influence of the type of intracranial lesion on outcome from severe head injury: A multicenter study using a new classification system. J. Neurosurg., 56: 26–32, 1982.
6. Jane, J. A. Age and outcome from head injury. Transactions of the World Federation Neurotrauma Society. Motevideo, Uruguay, November 1984.
7. Jenkins, L. W., Marmarou, A., Lewelt, W., et al. Increased vulnerability of the traumatized brain to early ischemia. In: Mechanisms of Secondary Brain Injury, edited by A. Boethmann. NATO Advanced Research Workshop. in press, 1985.
8. Jennett, B., Teasdale, G., Galbraith, S., et al. Severe head injury in three countries. J. Neurol. Neurosurg. Psychiatry, 40: 291–298, 1977.
9. Marshall, L. F., Barba, D., Toole, B. M., et al. The oval pupil: Clinical significance and relationship to intracranial hypertension. J. Neurosurg., 58: 566–568, 1983.
10. Marshall, L. F., Becker, D. P., Bowers, S. A., et al. The National Traumatic Coma Data Bank. Part 1. Design, purpose, goals, and results. J. Neurosurg., 59: 276–284, 1983.

11. Marshall, L. F., and Bowers, S. B. Medical management of intracranial pressure. In: *Head Injury*, Ed. 2, Chap. 11, edited by P. Cooper. Williams & Wilkins, Baltimore, 1986.
12. Miller, J. D., Butterworth, J. F., Gudeman, S. K., *et al.* Further experience in the management of severe head injury. J. Neurosurg., *54:* 289–299, 1981.
13. Saul, T. G., and Ducker, T. B. Effect of intracranial pressure monitoring and aggressive treatment on mortality in severe head injury. J. Neurosurg., *56*(4): 498–503, 1982.
14. Teasdale, G., Galbraith, S., Murray, L., *et al.* Management of traumatic intracranial haematoma. Br. Med. J., *285:* 1695–1697, 1982.
15. Teasdale, G., and Jennett, B. Assessment of coma and impaired consciousness: A practical scale. Lancet, *2:* 81–83, 1974.

26

Is ICP Monitoring Worthwhile?

THOMAS G. SAUL, M.D., F.A.C.S.

INTRODUCTION

In 1965, Nils Lundberg *et al.* published their experience of intracranial pressure (ICP) monitoring of head-injured patients. He concluded that "continuous recording of the ventricular fluid pressure in cases of severe traumatic injury of the head facilitates the evaluation of intracranial dynamics and offers a more rational basis for treatment than do conventional measures" (5).

Two decades later we are contemplating the question: "Is ICP monitoring worthwhile?" In order to do this we must first define "worthwhile." Specifically, we mean does ICP monitoring enhance the clinical management of the head-injured patient in such a way that: (*a*) morbidity and mortality are decreased; (*b*) therapy is facilitated; (*c*) prognostication is improved; and (*d*) the risks do not exceed the benefit. With that in mind, let's examine the facts regarding this question. Neurotrauma research has proved that increased intracranial pressure kills! Normal intracranial pressure is 15 mm mercury (mm Hg) or less, and the literature documents that the "kiss of death" is somewhere between 20 and 25 mm Hg. Therefore, there is not a large margin of safety. A review of the literature that documents this fact is important in reaching the ultimate conclusions on this issue.

ICP, MORBIDITY AND MORTALITY

In 1979, Marshall and others reported on a series of 100 patients with severe head injuries (6). In a review of 75 patients in that series with nonsurgical lesions, we see the effect that elevated ICP has on the outcome (Table 26.1). Thirty-five patients had ICP less than 15 mm Hg. Twenty-seven of those 35 patients made good or moderately disabled recoveries, and only 8 of them were severely disabled, vegetative, or dead. However, in the 40 patients whose ICPs were above 15 mm Hg, 23 patients were severely disabled, vegetative, or dead, and only 17 made a good or moderately disabled recovery.

Miller *et al.*, in 1981, published a study of a series of 225 patients with severe head injury (7). Table 26.2 shows the ICP data on 196 of those patients. Patients in whom ICP was never over 20 mm Hg had a good or moderately disabled recovery 74% of the time, and 18% died. Those patients whose ICPs went above 20 mm Hg *but were reducible* with aggressive treatment had a mortality rate of 26% and a good or moderately disabled outcome of 55%. However, if the ICP went above 20 mm Hg and *was not reducible*, the mortality rate was 92%, and the good or moderately disabled outcome was only 3%. They concluded that "virtually all patients in whom ICP cannot be controlled died."

In 1982, Saul and Decker reported on 106 patients with Glasgow Coma Scores (GCS) of 7 or less (10). In this series there was an unacceptable mortality rate of 69% of the patients in whom ICP was 25 mm Hg or greater. This was compared to a mortality rate of 15% if the ICP remained less than 25 mm Hg (Table 26.3).

TABLE 26.1

Effect of Elevated ICP on Outcome as Reported by Marshall et al. (6)[a]

ICP	GD[b]/MD	SD/V/D
<15 mm Hg ($N = 35$)	27	8
>15 mm Hg ($N = 40$)	17	23
		($p < 0.01$)

[a] From Marshall, L. F., Smith, R. W., and Shapiro, H. M. The outcome with aggressive treatment in severe head injuries. J. Neurosurg., *50:* 20–25, 1979.

[b] GD, good; MD, moderately disabled; SD, severely disabled; D, dead.

TABLE 26.2

The Effect of Elevated ICP on Outcome as Reported by Miller et al. (7)[a]

ICP	GR[b]/MD (%)	SD/V (%)	Dead (%)
<20 mm Hg ($N = 91$)	74	9	18
>20 mm Hg (but reducible) ($N = 75$)	55	19	26
>20 mm Hg (not reducible) ($N = 31$)	3	3	92

[a] From Miller, R. D., Butterworth, J. F., et al. Further experience in the management of severe head injury. J. Neurosurg., *54:* 289–299, 1981.

[b] GR, good recovery; MD, moderately disabled; SD, severely disabled; V, vegetative.

TABLE 26.3

Effect of Elevated ICP on Mortality as Reported by Saul and Ducker (10)[a]

ICP	Mortality
<25 mm Hg ($N = 80$)	12 (15%)
≥25 mm Hg ($N = 26$)	18 (69%)

[a] From Saul, T. G., and Ducker, T. B. Effect of intracranial pressure monitoring and aggressive treatment on mortality in severe head injury. J. Neurosurg., *56:* 498–503, 1982.

Finally, Bellegarrigue and Ducker published another study confirming the same (1). In a series of 97 patients (GCS equal to or less than 7) there was a mortality rate of 75% in patients with ICPs greater than 25 mm Hg and a mortality rate of 22% in the patients with intracranial pressures of 25 mm Hg or less.

In addition to documenting that elevated ICP results in a worse outcome, there is mounting evidence that aggressive therapy improves outcome. Marshall *et al.*, in 1979, (6) concluded that there was better outcome due to early diagnosis and intervention and aggressive neurosurgical intensive care, *including ICP measurements*. They also concluded that aggressive treatment did not yield a higher percentage of vegetative survivors. The 100 patients they reported on demonstrated no verbal response and inability to follow commands within 48 hours of admission. Their treatment was based on direct ICP readings. There was a 28% mortality rate and a good or moderately disabled recovery rate of 60%. Marshall's group compared their results to the multi-institutional severe head injury study commonly referred to as the International Data Bank Group (3). This was the three-center head injury study by the groups in Glasgow, the Netherlands, and Los Angeles. Marshall's series had a 28% mortality rate compared to 50% in the International Data Bank Group. The good recovery and moderately disabled rate was 60% compared to 39% in the International Data Bank Group.

It should be noted, however, that the multi-institutional study was not put together to assess specific aggressive treatment protocols. Nor did they specifically examine the ICP monitoring question. It was simply a reference group of patients with similar neurological conditions to which subsequent aggressively treated groups can be compared. It should also be noted that the incidence of surgical mass lesions in Marshall's study was only 25% compared to 46% in the multi-institutional study. This may account for the difference in mortality rates. The presence of intracranial surgical mass lesions generally results in a higher mortality rate. However, Marshall explained the difference in the incidence of surgical lesions as being primarily due to the difference in indications for surgical treatment rather than to the difference in the actual clinical status of the patient.

Bowers and Marshall reported an expanded series from San Diego of 200 patients with severe head injury (2). This reconfirmed that the good and moderately disabled recovery is again in the range of 52% with aggressive treatment. In that same publication, Bowers and Marshall also looked at the effect that monitoring intracranial pressure had on mortality rate. They reviewed a subgroup of 86 patients with GCS equal to or less than 5. Forty-nine of these 86 patients had their ICP monitored and had a mortality rate of 39% compared to a mortality of 62% in the

37 patients who did not have their ICP monitored (Table 26.4). Although this is not statistically significant, it strongly suggests that the ICP monitoring influenced the outcome.

Miller *et al.*, from Richmond, Va., published a study of a series of 225 patients with severe head injuries (7). These patients were not uttering recognizable words and not following commands at the time resuscitation was completed. They received an aggressive treatment protocol based on the data from ICP monitoring. Fifty-six percent of the patients made a good or moderately disabled recovery, and there was a mortality rate of only 34%. In the review of their 225 cases, they found 158 that were compatible with the International Data Bank Group as described by Jennett *et al.* (3). This entry criteria required that the patient not open his eyes, not speak, and not follow commands for 6 hours postinjury or that he subsequently deteriorated to that status. They compared these 158 patients to those in the International Data Bank. Table 26.5 shows the statistically significant difference in the mortality rate. There was a

TABLE 26.4

Outcome as Related to the Use of ICP Monitoring in Patients with GCS $\gtrless$ 5 as Reported by Bowers and Marshall (2)[a]

	GR	MD	SD	V	D[b]	Total
ICP monitor	18 (37%)	6 (12%)	2 (4%)	4 (8%)	19 (39%)	49
No ICP monitor	9 (24%)	2 (6%)	2 (6%)	1 (3%)	23 (62%)	37

[a] From Bowers, S. A., and Marshall, L. F. Outcome in 200 consecutive cases of severe head injury treated in San Diego County: A prospective analysis. Neurosurgery, *6:* 237–242, 1980.

[b] ($p < 0.05$).

TABLE 26.5

Comparison of Outcomes of Richmond Series to the Outcomes of the International Data Bank Group (3, 7)[a]

	Richmond IDB	Glasgow	Netherlands	L.A.
N	158	593	239	168
Avg age	31	35	32	35
Surgical lesions	44%	54%	28%	56%
GR[b]/MD	47%	41%	41%	31%
SD/V	12%	12%	9%	19%
D[c]	40%	48%	50%	50%
		49%		

[a] From Jennett, B., Teasdale, S., *et al.* Severe head injuries in three countries. J. Neurol. Neurosurg. Psychiatry, *40:* 291–298, 1977; Miller, R. D., Butterworth, J. F., *et al.* Further experience in the management of severe head injury. J. Neurosurg., *54:* 289–299, 1981.

[b] GR, good recovery; MD, moderately disabled; SD, severely disabled; D, dead.

[c] ($p < 0.001$).

lower mortality rate of 40% in the Richmond series compared to 49% overall in the International Data Bank Group. The results of their study encouraged the Richmond Group in the belief that a real although modest reduction in the mortality of severe head injury had been obtained by their treatment protocol and ICP monitoring. They felt that they could safely conclude that ICP monitoring is "an important variable to measure in the head injured patient."

COMPARING RESULTS OF LARGE SERIES

Certainly there are definite problems comparing series from one center to another. There are questions about the entry criteria of patients. That is to say: What specifically constitutes severe head injury? What role does eye opening play? At what point in time do you enter a patient into a severe head injury study? Certainly, any significant difference in the number of surgical lesions (especially acute subdural hematomas) makes comparing results difficult. One should look at age differences, not just average age difference but the difference in the distribution of the age throughout the decades. A study of predominantly teenagers and 20 year olds will have a different outcome than that with patients who are predominantly 40 years old and older. One should also pay attention to GCS and distributions in the various GCS. When a series states that all patients had GCS of 8 or less, it is important to know how many were GCS of 3–5, and how many patients had scores that were GCS of 6–8. Finally, difference in timing of neurosurgical referral to definitive treatment may indeed impact markedly on mortality rates.

In 1982, Saul and Ducker published a report in which the problems of comparison were minimized (10). They were able to compare two series of patients who were: clinically similar; from the same catchment area; had the same prehospital care; and were treated at the same center with the same protocol *except* that the first series was treated without strict ICP management protocol and the second series was treated with strict ICP management protocol, based on the level of ICP. In the first series (Series 1), the treatment for ICP was instituted at various levels between 20 and 40 mm Hg. The dosing regimen was not uniform. In the second series (Series 2), all patients were begun on mannitol and Lasix and were continued on hyperventilation as soon as the ICP was 16 mm Hg or higher for 10 minutes. Cerebrospinal fluid drainage was also employed. If the patient's ICP went to 25 mm Hg, it was randomized into a high-dose intravenous barbiturate therapy protocol. Series 1 compared very closely to Series 2 in the number of patients, average age, incidence of life-threatening-associated injuries, and the incidence of intracranial surgical mass lesions (Table 26.6). More importantly, the age distributions in both series were very similar, with the ages being distributed

TABLE 26.6

Comparison of Clinical Features of Both Treatment Groups as Reported by Saul and Ducker (10)[a]

	No. of patients	Male:Female	Avg. Age	Polytrauma		Intracranial Surgery (%)
				1 System (%)	2 + System (%)	
Series 1 (1977–1978)	127	96:31	29	60	25	32
Series 2 (1979–1980)	106	80:26	29	56	25	31

[a] From Saul, T. G., and Ducker, T. B. Effect of intracranial pressure monitoring and aggressive treatment on mortality in severe head injury. J. Neurosurg., 56: 498–503, 1982.

equitably throughout the various decades of life. Finally, there was similar distribution of GCS within each series. This demographic information has been reported previously (10).

In comparing the results, there were two significant findings (Table 26.7). The number of patients whose intracranial pressures reached life-threatening levels (equal to or greater than 25 mm Hg) was reduced. In Series 1 34% of the patients had ICP of 25 mm Hg or greater, but in Series 2 (the aggressively and early treated group), only 25% of the patients had ICP equal to or greater than 25 mm Hg. More importantly, the overall mortality rate dropped from 46% in Series 1 to 28% in Series 2. The 6-month outcome demonstrated a good and moderately disabled group of 54%. There was a total mortality rate at 6 months of 33%, and only 13% were severely disabled and vegetative. Saul and Ducker concluded that early aggressive treatment of increased ICP based on the monitoring data reduces the incidence of life-threatening levels of ICP, which in turn significantly reduces mortality rate. At the same time it does not result in a disproportionate number of severely disabled or vegetative patients. Their final conclusion was that aggressive treatment based on intracranial pressure monitoring data is beneficial in the treatment of severe head injury.

In 1983 at the annual meeting of the American Association of Neurological Surgeons (AANS), Smith et al., from Winston-Salem, N.C., presented an interesting study of a series of patients (11). They prospectively randomized 80 patients with GCS of 8 or less into two mannitol treatment groups. In the first group (I) the mannitol treatment was based on data from ICP monitoring. They began mannitol whenever the ICP was 25 mm Hg or greater. The second group (II), although they had monitors in place, were treated with mannitol empirically. Therefore this study was designed to examine the mannitol regimen, not ICP monitoring efficacy. The interesting thing was that in both groups the outcomes were similar (Table 26.8). At first one might conclude that ICP monitoring does not

TABLE 26.7

Comparison of Results in Both Series as Reported by Saul and Ducker (10)[a,b]

	No. of Patients	ICP < 25 mm Hg	ICP ≥ 25 mm Hg	Overall Mortality
Series 1 (1977–1978)	127	84 (66%)	43 (34%)	58 (45%)
Series 2 (1979–1980)	106	80 (75%)	26 (25%) ($p < 0.05$)	30 (28%) ($p < 0.0005$)

[a] From Saul, T. G., and Ducker, T. B. Effect of intracranial pressure monitoring and aggressive treatment on mortality in severe head injury. J. Neurosurg., 56: 498–503, 1982.

[b] Note the significant decrease in the number of patients with ICP > 25 and in the mortality rate in Series 2 compared to that in Series 1.

TABLE 26.8

Comparison of Outcomes of Empirically Treated Patients (II) vs. Those Treated Based on ICP Readiness (I) as Reported by Smith et al. (11)

	GR[b]/MD	SD/V	Dead	Total
I	20 (54%)	4 (11%)	13 (35%)	37
II	19 (47.5%)	4 (10%)	17 (42.5%)	40

[a] From Smith, H. P., Kelly, D. L., *et al.* Comparison of mannitol regimens in patients with severe head injury undergoing intracranial monitoring. J. Neurosurg., in press, 1987.

[b] GR, good recovery; MD, moderately disabled; SD, severely disabled; V, vegetative.

make any difference in outcome based on a small series of patients. However, it should be noted that the empirically treated patients had a lower mean ICP than those treated based on the ICP data. It should be noted that in this latter group treatment was withheld until ICP reached 25 mm Hg. It was Smith's conclusion that the empirically treated patients were probably having their ICP treated at lower levels, thus keeping intracranial pressure from reaching life-threatening levels. In this way the results support the findings of Saul and Ducker. They concluded that the results following ICP monitoring might well be significantly better if the patients are treated at the lower level of 15 mm Hg. They further concluded that subsets of patients will significantly benefit from monitoring.

This concept of early monitoring of ICP has also been proposed by Klauber *et al.* in San Diego (4). In 1984 they published some findings in the patients who "talk and die." They showed evidence that suggested that ICP as low as 18–20 mm Hg may indeed result in deterioration of a patient and a poor outcome, particularly in those patients with temporal lobe lesions.

In spite of the fact that comparisons from center to center are difficult, evidence is available in the 1980s that early aggressive management and treatment of intracranial pressure does benefit the patient.

It is not unusual in medicine that when evidence seems to be mounting in support of a particular contention, something comes along and completely reverses some people's thinking and steeps the issue once again in controversy. In 1983, Stuart *et al.* of the Royal Brisbane Hospital in Queensland, Australia, published data suggesting that ICP monitoring has no therapeutic advantage if used routinely in cases of severe head injuries (12). They presented 100 consecutive patients with GCS of 8 or less within 48 hours after injury. None of these patients underwent ICP monitoring. The treatment regimen described in their article for these patients was not uniform. Only 43 of the 100 patients were treated with assisted ventilation in order to "provide optimal oxygenation for neurons." There were 52 patients requiring hematoma evacuation, some of which were done at country hospitals prior to their transfer to Brisbane. Their medical treatment varied widely. Fifty-six of the patients received steroids, and only 21 patients received mannitol, mostly for dilated pupils and/or if they underwent a craniotomy. They compared their results to the Richmond, Glasgow, and San Diego series. Brisbane had a 34% mortality rate compared to 40% in Richmond, 48% in Glasgow, and 28% in San Diego. Good and moderately disabled outcomes totalled 49% for Brisbane and 47%, 41%, and 60% for the other centers, respectively. Severely disabled and vegetative outcomes were 17% in Brisbane and 12% in all of the other series. Certainly according to these statistics, Brisbane's series with no ICP monitoring compared similarly to Richmond and Glasgow. They were not quite as good as the outcomes seen in the San Diego group. It should be pointed out once again that the number of surgical lesions in San Diego was only 25% compared to 52% in the Brisbane group. That might partially explain the difference in the mortality rates and in the good and moderately disabled outcomes.

What does this mean? Just as there were difficulties in comparing various series that were previously mentioned, this author is compelled to also point out a few problems with the Brisbane study.

Overall it was difficult to gain a good concept of how severely injured and sick the patients in this study really were. Only 43% of these patients required ventilatory assistance. This is not similar to the experience in other centers of patients with GCS equal to or less than 8. In addition, no mention was made of the incidence of life-threatening associated injuries, the complications of which are known to alter outcome. We also were given no information on the distribution of the GCS on the 100 patients. In the series, 12% of the patients were children under 10 years of age. This certainly might skew the results, especially when compared to series which are composed predominantly of adult populations. The reason for the 52% incidence of surgical lesions is unclear to this author because of the policy of surgical intervention. Specifically they state: "When a patient in the country hospital is deteriorating too rapidly, their policy was to advise exploratory burr holes and evacuation of surface hematomas prior to transfer." Their statistics show that at least six patients received their craniotomies under such conditions before admission to Brisbane. This raises the question as to the criteria upon which a craniotomy was performed, who is making those decisions, and under what adverse conditions out in the country. This raises the ultimate question: Did the performance of the craniotomy necessarily mean there was a definitive surgical lesion present?

The most serious problem with the Brisbane study is that there was a process of natural and medical selection in the entry of these patients into the study. Over half of the patients were from areas distant to

Brisbane. The farther from Brisbane the patient was transferred, the lower the mortality rate. This implied that the patients most likely to survive were being transferred and thus entered into the study. The authors also note this fact themselves in their publication. Therefore, a close analysis of the Brisbane publication leads this author to the opinion that *one should not* base a decision *not to monitor* ICP on the data from this series.

ICP AND EXTRACRANIAL FACTORS

Since lower levels of intracranial pressure are helpful to the patient, then one should know when the ICP gets above those levels. For it is only with this information that one knows when to start and stop the various treatment modalities designed to decrease elevated ICP. Logical analogies would certainly be the use of arterial pressure monitoring in patients with subarachnoid hemorrhage. By continuously measuring the systemic pressure, one knows when to start antihypertensives to prevent rebleed and, likewise, one knows when to start pressure agents to avoid ischemia when vasospasm is present. Taking a basic example from our medical colleagues, it would seem futile to treat someone in a diabetic coma without sequential blood sugar determinations to assess efficacy of that treatment.

There are many extracranial factors that can elevate ICP: motor posturing; the use of positive end expiratory pressure (PEEP); intrinsic pulmonary pathology; any type of jugular compression (iatrogenic or pathologic); metabolic abnormalities such as hyponatremia; and various therapeutic endeavors. Having an ICP monitor in place, one can assess the consequences of these extracranial conditions and the various forms of treatment inflicted on a multiple trauma patient.

COMPLICATIONS OF ICP MONITORING

Like any endeavor, ICP monitoring is not without its adverse side affects. This perhaps has been one of the major points of contention on the part of ICP monitoring opponents. However, it behooves us to put this into proper perspective (Table 26.9). Although Dr. Lundberg did not look closely at the complication factor, he did conclude that "there was no excessive risk in intraventricular catheter monitoring" (5). Rosner and Becker, in 1976, reported a minimal infection rate of 4.7% in a combined series of intraventricular catheters and bolts (9). Winn et al. reported 650 patients monitored with a subarachnoid bolt with an incidence of 0.7% central nervous system infection; 1.4% superficial skin infection; and an 8% failure rate of the subarachnoid bolt (14). Finally, Narayan et al. reported on over 200 monitored patients, with 91% using an intraventricular catheter and the other 9% using a subarachnoid bolt

TABLE 26.9

Summary of Reports of Complications due to ICP Monitoring (5, 8, 9, 14)

Lundberg (1965)—No excessive risk
Rosner and Becker (1976)—Minimal infection = 4.7%
                                          IVC and Bolt
Winn, Dacey, Jane (1977)—0.7% CNS infection
                                   —1.4% Skin infection
                                   —Bolt
                                   —8% Failure
Narayan *et al.* (1982)—6.3% Infection
                              —1.4% Hemorrhage
                              —91% IVC
                              —9% Bolt

 a Modified from Lundberg, N., Troupp, H., and Lorin, H. Continuous recording of the ventricular-fluid pressure in patients with severe acute traumatic brain injury. J. Neurosurg., *22:* 581–590, 1965; Narayan, R. K., Kishore, P. R., *et al.* Intracranial pressure: To monitor or not to monitor. J. Neurosurg., *56:* 650–659, 1982; Rosner, M. J., and Becker, D. P. ICP monitoring: Complications and associated factors. Clin. Neurosurg., *23:* 494–517, 1976; Winn, H. R., Dacey, R. G., Jane, *et al.* Intracranial subarachnoid pressure recording: Experience with 650 patients. Surg. Neurol., *8:* 41–47, 1977.

(8). The infection rate was 6.3%, and there was an intracerebral hemorrhage rate of 1.4% that was directly attributed to the passing of the catheter through the brain. Although one must take into consideration these rates of infection and other complications, it would not deter this author from employing ICP monitoring in order to gain the beneficial effect expressed earlier in this chapter.

CONCLUSIONS

What are *your* conclusions today? They would certainly have to be based on your own personal evaluation of the data presented here and your own clinical practice environment. It would be advisable, however, that if one did not monitor ICP in a patient who was comatose and not purposefully, one should be committed: (*a*) to repeating a CT scan at regular intervals; (*b*) to treating empirically with hyperventilation and osmotherapy if allowed by the patient's hemodynamic status; and (*c*) to being vigilant of all the other extracranial factors that can increase ICP during the patient's management.

What are *my* conclusions today?

Interestingly enough, Tindall expressed them nicely at the 1971 meeting of the Congress of Neurological Surgeons (CNS), when he stated that "continuous ICP measurement in a head injured patient serves not only to indicate need to institute therapy to reduce elevated ICP, but also monitors effectiveness of therapy" (13). In other words, YES! ICP monitoring of patients with severe head injury is worthwhile!

We should remember that ICP monitors themselves do not save lives. The people who judiciously use the data from ICP monitoring can save lives and alter the outcome of a significant portion of patients with severe head injury.

REFERENCES

1. Bellegarrigue, R., and Ducker, T. B. Control of Intracranial Pressure in Severe Head Injury. In: *Intracranial Pressure V*. Springer-Verlag, Berlin, 1983.
2. Bowers, S. A., and Marshall, L. F. Outcome in 200 consecutive cases of severe head injury treated in San Diego County: A prospective analysis. Neurosurgery, *6:* 237–242, 1980.
3. Jennett, B., Teasdale, S., Galbraith, S. Severe head injuries in three countries. J. Neurol. Neurosurg. Psychiatry, *40:* 291–298, 1977.
4. Klauber, M. R., Toutant, S. M., and Marshall, L. F. A model for predicting delayed intracranial hypertension following severe head injury. J. Neurosurg., *61:* 695–699, 1984.
5. Lundberg, N., Troupp, H., and Lorin, H. Continuous recording of the ventricular-fluid pressure in patients with severe acute traumatic brain injury. J. Neurosurg., *22:* 581–590, 1965.
6. Marshall, L. F., Smith, R. W., and Shapiro, H. M. The outcome with aggressive treatment in severe head injuries. J. Neurosurg., *50:* 20–25, 1979.
7. Miller, R. D., Butterworth, J. F., Gudeman, S. K., Becker, D. P. Further experience in the management of severe head injury. J. Neurosurg., *54:* 289–299, 1981.
8. Narayan, R. K., Kishore, P. R., McWhorter, J. M. Intracranial pressure: To monitor or not to monitor. J. Neurosurg., *56:* 650–659, 1982.
9. Rosner, M. J., and Becker, D. P. ICP monitoring: Complications and associated factors. Clin. Neurosurg., *23:* 494–517, 1976.
10. Saul, T. G., and Ducker, T. B. Effect of intracranial pressure monitoring and aggressive treatment on mortality in severe head injury. J. Neurosurg., *56:* 498–503, 1982.
11. Smith, H. P., Kelly, D. L., Smith, J. A. Comparison of mannitol regimens in patients with severe head injury undergoing intracranial monitoring. J. Neurosurg., in press, 1987.
12. Stuart, G. G., Merry, G. S., Dunion J. J. Severe head injury managed without intracranial pressure monitoring. J. Neurosurg., *59:* 601–605, 1983.
13. Tindall, G. T., Patton, J. M., *et al.* Monitoring of patients with head injuries. Clin. Neurosurg., *19:* 332–360, 1971.
14. Winn, H. R., Dacey, R. G., Jane, J. A. Intracranial subarachnoid pressure recording: Experience with 650 patients. Surg. Neurol., *8:* 41–47, 1977.

27

The Devastated Head Injury Patient

HOWARD M. EISENBERG, M.D., and HARVEY S. LEVIN, PH.D.

INTRODUCTION

The most depressing aspect of the care of patients with severe head injury is not having to contend with patients who die, but dealing with those who survive yet don't make a meaningful recovery to the extent that they can interact socially or that their interaction is so limited or aberrant that they cannot live away from highly sheltered environments. These are the patients whom we would consider devastated. Others no doubt would even extend their definitions to include those patients who are less limited, yet still dependent. Obviously, a universally accepted definition of "devastated" as would be used in the context of this chapter is not at hand, and in the beginning of this discussion we will provide at least an operational definition, one that can be applied to data available from recent studies. Other issues to be addressed include prediction of this outcome; what parameters might be the most potent predictors and when, how soon after injury could they be reliably employed. Lastly, we will consider therapy, particularly attempts to develop methods of cognitive rehabilitation.

AN OPERATIONAL DEFINITION OF "DEVASTATED" AND THE FREQUENCY OF THIS OUTCOME

Almost all recent large prospective studies have assessed global outcome using the Glasgow Outcome Scale (GOS) (16). This outcome scale, like the Glasgow Coma Scale (GCS) (36), attempts to utilize easily applied and exclusive definitions. Both scales have sacrificed detail for simplicity and presumed reliability. Unfortunately, interobserver reliability for the Outcome Scale may not be as good as for the Coma Scale (25). Nonetheless, the Outcome Scale has practicality and is widely used. Five categories of outcome are defined: good recovery, moderate disability, severe disability, the persistent vegetative state, and death. There is no category provided for persistent coma, presumably an extremely rare event. Patients classified as moderately disabled are distinguished from those who are severely disabled by their ability to participate in activities beyond dressing and minimal self-care. For example, the moderately disabled can travel alone using public transportation and can be employed at least in a sheltered environment. The persistent vegetative state (PVS) is a term devised by Jennett and Plum (17) to describe patients who never regain any degree of higher cortical function while regaining the alerting mechanism and sleep-wake cycling. These patients are inaccessible, neither speaking nor following even the simplest commands. For the purposes of this discussion, we will define those patients whose ultimate outcome is severe disability (SD) or PVS as devastated.

We recognize that SD probably covers a wide range of outcomes. However, all are dependent as defined above and, further, no body of data is available for discussion of the incidence of the subcategories. However, Jennett and his colleagues (18) reported on the results of neurological and neuropsychological examinations performed at least one year after head injury in 150 conscious survivors who were studied as part of the International Coma Data Bank. Of the total series, 30 cases (20%) were classified as SD; they needed the assistance of another person to perform some daily activities due to a combination of physical handicap and neurobehavioral impairments. On neurological examination, the SD patients were distinguished from the moderately disabled (MD) and good recovery (GR) groups primarily by severe residual hemiparesis (40% vs. 0% of the GR group and 20% of the MD group), severe aphasic deficit (30% vs. 0% in GR and 12% in MD), and the concurrent manifestation of both of these deficits (Table 27.1). Neuropsychological results obtained in a subgroup of each outcome category confirmed severe impairment of intellectual function, defective memory, and marked alteration of personality in nearly all SD patients, whereas the results were more variable in the GR and MD groups. The panel of examiners determined that neurobehavioral deficit was equally or more limiting than physical hand-

TABLE 27.1

Frequency of Physical Sequelae in Each Outcome Category[a]

	GR (N = 60)	MD (N = 60)	SD (N = 30)
Hemiparesis			
Mild	25%	40%	37%
Severe	0	20%	40%
Dysphasia			
Mild	10%	32%	17%
Severe	0	12%	30%
Both (either severe)	0	27%	60%
Epilepsy	17%	10%	30%

[a] From Jennett, B., Snoek, J., Bond, M. R., et al. Disability after severe head injury: observations on the use of the Glasgow Outcome Scale. J. Neurol. Neurosurg. Psychiatry, 44: 285–293, 1981.

TABLE 27.2

Contribution of Mental and Physical Features to Overall Disability in Each Outcome Category[a]

	GR (%)	MD (%)	SD (%)
Mental, worse	56	48	63
Physical, worse	27	30	23
Equal	17	22	13
(Mental ≥ physical)	(73)	(70)	(76)

[a] From Jennett, B., Snoek, J., Bond, M. R., *et al.* Disability after severe head injury: Observations on the use of the Glasgow Outcome Scale. J. Neurol. Neurosurg. Psychiatry, *44:* 285–293, 1981.

icap in 72% of the total series and that the disproportionate contribution of cognitive and behavioral problems was similar across all three levels of outcome (Table 27.2). Interviews with the families disclosed that behavioral disturbances such as outbursts of temper, irritability, overtalkativeness, and lack of insight posed far greater burdens than the physical limitations, such as decreased mobility.

While SD and the PVS then constitute our devastated group, we hypothesize that they are not a continuum. The pathology of the PVS as it applies to etiologies other than traumatic head injury is assumed to be diffuse involving primarily cortex (cortical laminae necrosis) with sparing of the brain stem (10, 30). The mechanism in those cases is generally attributed to severe, generalized ischemia or hypoxia. This also may be the case in patients with severe head injury in which the ischemia or hypoxia could result from multiple injuries or secondary intracranial events. The pathology of the SD is almost certainly similar to that of severely injured patients with other outcomes differing only in degree, a heterogeneous pattern of focal and diffuse white matter injury.

How common are these two outcomes? Recently, we reviewed nine large published series of patients that included only patients with severe head injury, either Glasgow Coma Score (GCS) ≤8 or ≤7; all had at least 100 patients. The outcomes according to the GOS are shown in Table 27.3. The Seven Center Study included patients who were also accounted for in some of the other cited studies. When the relative rates of outcome were calculated for the remaining eight studies, the relative frequency for the PVS ranged from 1–6%, and 57 of the 2049 patients (3%) were so classified 3–12 months after injury. For SD, the percentages ranged from 4 to 14, 174 of the 2049 (8%). Only 11% of this large group of patients would then be considered devastated by our criteria in comparison to 731 of the 2049 who died (36%). If these data are representative, and we believe they are, these two outcomes, SD and PVS combined, are relatively infrequent. They nonetheless represent an important social

TABLE 27.3

Outcome According to Glasgow Outcome Score

	GR (%)	MD (%)	SD (%)	V[a] (%)	D (%)
Glasgow (N = 593)					
Jennett et al. (20)					
Mean age 35 yr					
GCS ≤ 8 at ≥ 6 hr					
Outcome at 6 mos	23	18	10	2	48
The Netherlands (N = 305)					
Braakman et al. (3)					
Combined data from two centers					
Mean age 32 yr					
GCS ≤ 8 at ≥ 6 hr					
Outcome at 6 mos	27	16	7	2	49
Los Angeles (N = 168)					
Jennett et al. (20)					
Mean age 35 yr					
GCS ≤ 8 at ≥ 6 hr					
Outcome at 6 mos	12	19	14	5	50
Seven Center USA Study (N = 1107)					
Gennarelli et al. (12)					
GCS ≤ 8 at ≥ 6 hr					
Outcome at 3 mos	26	16	13	4	41
Milan (N = 288)					
Levati et al. (22)					
GCS ≤ 8 at ≥ 6 hr	36	11	4	1	40
Philadelphia (N = 164)					
Langfitt and Gennarelli (21)					
Mean age 20 yr					
GCS ≤ 8 at ≥ 6 hr					
Outcome at 3 mos	34	12	10	6	38
Richmond (N = 225)					
Miller et al. (27)					
Mean age 31 yr					
GCS ≤ 9					
Outcome at 3–12 mos	45	11	7	3	34
San Diego (N = 200)					
Bowers and Marshall (2)					
Mean age 25–29 yr					
GCS ≤ 7 at ≥ 6 hr	42	10	8	4	36
Maryland (N = 106)					
Saul and Ducker (33)					
Mean age 29 yr					
GCS ≤ 7	48	6	10	3	33

[a] V, vegetative; D, dead.

and economic problem. If we estimate that the incidence of severe head injury for those surviving to reach a hospital (a requirement for inclusion in the cited studies), the incidence of devastated outcomes is approximately 5 per 100,000 or about 11,000 new cases per year in the U.S. Considering the mean age of head-injured patients, the prevalence must be considerable (even recognizing that the life span of the PVS patient is limited (15)).

PREDICTION OF THE "DEVASTATED" OUTCOME

There is little in the way of specific information that can be directly applied to prediction of PVS or SD. If, however, we assume that the predictors of dying can also be used to predict SD, a reasonable possibility, we can list the potentially most important factors. Of these, GCS and the presence of a mass lesion, particularly a subdural hematoma, are among the most reliable.

Age is also a potent predictor of dying. Mortality rates of patients over 60 years of age are considerably higher (70–88%) compared with those of younger patients. Even those 40–60 are higher (1, 14, 20, 22, 28, 29). An observation pertinent to this discussion is that mortality in the older age groups can be accounted for by extracranial causes while cerebral deaths are age independent (1, 5). If this is correct, it indicates that increasing age is not as potent a predictor of SD as it is of death.

What about the opposite end of the age spectrum? Here, the information we have is even less direct. Again with respect to the risk of dying, children in general seem at less risk even than young adults, although the mechanisms of injury and perhaps the significance of a low GCS are not the same in these groups of patients. There is evidence suggesting that the youngest patients, 0–5 years of age, are at greater risk for dying than older children (20). However, it is generally believed that young children have a greater capacity to recover than do adults. If this is correct, the effect of age, even early age, might be canceled out. That is, the infant's risk of dying would be greater but the risk for a SD outcome would be less. In contrast is the idea that when considering the effects of diffuse injury, the youngest group (0–5 years of age) may be relatively less spared; increased plasticity generally applies to recovery from focal lesions (23).

When we looked at this question comparing the recovery of memory after severe injury in a group of adolescents and younger children, we found no evidence for sparing in the younger group; if anything, the younger children as a group made lesser recoveries (24). It is possible then that injury at a very young age is a predictor of SD.

Other parameters have been used for prediction. Important among these are pupillary and eye signs, intracranial pressure, and information about evoked potentials. Some investigators have used data from their patients to rank these factors alone or in combination: examples are shown in Tables 27.4 and 27.5.

If the PVS in head-injured patients represents a separate entity, with its own pathology, then specific parameters might be useful for prediction. Probable candidates would include those patients suffering hypoxia and shock. We looked at the relationship between the presence of these complications and outcome in the pilot phase of the National Coma Data Bank (11). In this study, hypoxia was defined as an initial PaO_2 ≤60 mm Hg or in patients ventilated before the measurement of blood gases a clear history of apnea. Shock was defined as a systolic blood pressure ≤90 mm Hg prior to admission. The association between these complications and outcome are shown in Figure 27.1. In this study, death and the PVS were, unfortunately for our present purposes, combined. However, as more patients are added to the data bank, we will be able to analyze for the PVS separately. A final consideration regarding the PVS is whether intensity of therapy is related to this outcome. Is, for example, highly intensive management associated with fewer deaths, but a greater number of patients in the PVS? Clearly, there is no evidence that allows study of this question directly. However, one can compare the relative risk of death and PVS in two centers that were different with regard to intensity of their management, San Diego and Glasgow. The San Diego

TABLE 27.4

Statistical Importance of 12 Variables[a, b]

Ranking of Factors in Order of Prognostic Importance	Regression Coefficients (Mean ± SE)	Asymptotic Z-Test
1. Requirement for surgical decompression	−2.55 ± 0.98	−2.60
2. Age	−0.06 ± 0.02	−2.56
3. PO_2, ≤65; PCO, >45; systolic blood pressure, ≤90; hematocrit, ≤30	−2.72 ± 1.18	−2.32
4. Motor response	−3.57 ± 1.59	−2.24
5. Pupil light response	−2.59 ± 1.31	−1.97
6. Interaction between motor response and presence of mass lesion	3.23 ± 1.71	1.89
7. Mass lesion presence on CT scan	−1.81 ± 1.01	−1.80
8. Eye opening to pain	−1.63 ± 1.01	−1.62
9. Pupil size	−1.75 ± 1.24	−1.41
10. Sex	1.18 ± 0.91	1.29
11. Oculocephalic response	1.46 ± 1.26	1.16
12. Verbal response	0.785 ± 0.99	0.80

[a] From Stablein, D. M., Miller, J. D., Choi, S. C., *et al.* Statistical methods for determining prognosis in severe head injury. Neurosurgery, 6(3): 243–248, 1980.

[b] The regression coefficient for the intercept term is $a = 6.23 ± 1.54$.

TABLE 27.5

Accuracy and Confidence of Outcome Predictions Using Different Indicants (%)[a]

Confidence Levels (Data Used)	Correct Predictions				Wrong Predictions			Modified Prediction Rate[b]
	Total	>90%	70-90%	50-70%	Total	Falsely Optimistic	Falsely Pessimistic	
All six clinical data[c]	82	43	23	16	18	9	9	91
GCS alone	80	25	34	21	20	13	7	93
CT data alone	64	0	37	27	36	7	29	71
ICP data alone	75	0	52	23	25	11	14	86
MEP data alone	91	25	66	0	9	9	0	100
Clinical + CT data	77	52	14	11	23	14	9	91
Clinical + ICP data	80	55	18	7	20	11	9	91
Clinical + MEP data	89	64	14	11	11	7	4	96
Best five indicants	86	64	18	4	14	7	7	93
All nine indicants	86	61	18	7	14	7	7	93

[a] From Narayan, R. K., Greenberg, R. P., Miller, J. D., et al. Improved confidence of outcome in severe head injury. J. Neurosurg., 54: 751-762, 1981.

[b] Modified prediction rate = percent correct predictions with falsely optimistic errors eliminated.

[c] Age, GCS, pupillary response, eye movements, surgery, and motor posturing. Best five indicants in order of significance: MEP data, age, ICP data, GCS, and pupillary response. All nine indicants, all six clinical indicants + CT data + ICP data + MEP data.

group have been advocates of aggressive care, particularly with regard to use of ventilation and expectant removal of hematomas. The risk of death was less in the San Diego center, but the relative frequency of PVS or, for that matter, SD was not proportionately increased (see Table 27.3).

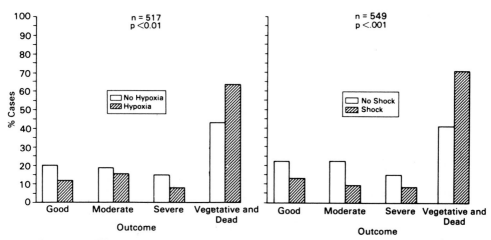

FIG. 27.1. The relationship between outcome and hypoxia or shock (hypoxia: $\chi^2 = 14.62$, $df = 3$), (shock: $\chi^2 = 47.31$, $df = 3$). (From Eisenberg, H. M., Cayard, C., Papanicolaou, A. C., *et al.* The effects of three potentially preventable complications on outcome after severe closed head injury. In: *The Vth International Symposium on Intracranial Pressure*, Chap. 93, pp. 549–553. Springer-Verlag, Berlin, 1983.)

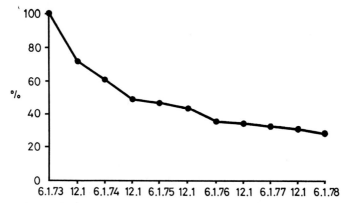

FIG. 27.2. Survival rates of vegetative patients (all etiologies) at intervals of 6 months over the 5 years from June 1973 to June 1978. (From Higashi, K., Hatano, M., Abiko, S., *et al.* Five-year follow-up study of patients with persistent vegetative state. J. Neurol. Neurosurg. Psychiatry, *44:* 552–554, 1981.)

An issue even more important than refinement of prediction by assessing multiple parameters alone or in combination is this question: "When can prediction be reliably made?" Based on recovery curves, Jennett and Teasdale and their co-workers (19, 37) suggest that prediction based on the GOS at 6 months postinjury is reliable for comparison of groups of patients. They showed that assessment at longer intervals did not uncover improvement of a sufficient degree to result in change in classification in very many cases. Of patients who were assigned to either the good recovery or the moderately disabled group at 1 year, two-thirds had recovered to that level at 3 months and 90% at 6 months (20). Small changes in the relative frequency of outcome between 6 and 12 months could be attributed primarily to deaths in the SD and PVS groups. While a 6-month interval may be adequate for global comparison among groups, the recovery curves for specific behavioral deficits may be different in the SD group, and classification of SD at 6 months should not be used as the sole factor for decisions regarding continuation of specific therapies.

The emergence of the PVS was the subject of a study by Bricolo and his colleagues (4). In this study of 135 patients with severe head injury who were in prolonged coma (>2 weeks) half began to follow commands during the first 3 months after injury, and 13% did so after the third month, but only 1.5% after 6 months. This contrasted with the first appearance of eye opening, which occurred by 1 month in 78% of cases and by 3 months in 93%. In this series, only 11 patients were ultimately classified as PVS, and the authors felt that this classification could be made with virtual certainty only by 1 year. In a 5-year follow-up study of 110 patients in PVS related to various etiologies, Higashi and his co-workers (15) found that the overall mortality was 73% (65% by 3 years), whereas the attrition was slightly lower in the 38 patients who were rendered vegetative by head injury (55% by 3 years, 66% by 5 years). Of the total series, only five survivors at the end of the study interval were "responsive" to commands (but not necessarily obeying them), and two of these cases (neither of whom was head-injured) unequivocally regained expressive and receptive language function to a level which permitted them to communicate with others and perform many activities of daily living. Based on the brief description of these two patients provided by the authors, it is clear that the 5-year outcome in both of these cases was at least at the level of severe disability. In summary, it appears that the prognosis for recovery in a head-injured patient who is still vegetative at 1 year is grim (Fig. 27.2).

REHABILITATION OF THE DEVASTATED HEAD-INJURED PATIENT

Programs specializing in the rehabilitation of head-injured patients have proliferated in North America and the United Kingdom during the past decade. Efforts to develop rehabilitation programs for head-injured patients which incorporate principles of cognitive training and neuropsychology have recently emerged amid growing recognition that disturbances of attention, memory, and behavior overshadow the contribution of focal motor deficits to chronic dependency in these young patients (18). The pattern of neuropsychological and behavioral disturbances exhibited by patients sustaining severe closed head injury requires a different approach as compared to that used in the rehabilitation of older patients following cerebrovascular insults and in whom focal neurologic deficits and aphasia are the most prominent problems. Although occupational therapy, physical therapy, and speech therapy contribute to the rehabilitation of head-injured patients, these conventional treatments are integrated into specialized programs utilizing a team approach to address the core neurobehavioral problems. While the optimal time for transferring patients from a neurosurgery service to a rehabilitation unit varies according to the presence of medical complications and the resources available at each center for treatment, Cope and Hall (7) reported that early referral to rehabilitation was associated with a shorter duration of total hospitalization.

The strategy developed at the Institute of Rehabilitation Medicine at New York University (9) for rehabilitating the head-injured patient has served as a prototype for other programs directed towards this population. The NYU program uses an individualized, graduated approach in which the head-injured patient progresses through successive "modules" (interactive computer programs). Designed primarily for patients sustaining severe head injury whose recovery has reached an apparent plateau, the program begins with computer-assisted training in attention, perception, and orientation as a prerequisite for more complex modules which involve problem solving, memory, and social skills. Depending on the individual's progress, later stages of the program include occupational training, vocational trials, and job placement. Preliminary outcome data from the NYU program indicate that this strategy can raise the quality of long-term outcome in severely head-injured patients who are disabled primarily by cognitive deficit and behavioral disturbance. However, the selection criteria utilized in the NYU program (and many other rehabilitation programs for head-injured patients) include an intellectual quotient of at least 80 and tractable behavior (i.e., excluding markedly aggressive patients).

Other techniques employed in cognitive rehabilitation include group exercises in which the therapist and group members provide individual patients with consensual validation of their interpretations of events and interpersonal situations. In this setting, paranoid concerns, unrealistic plans, and inaccurate self-appraisal are subjected to public scrutiny in an effort to improve the patient's acceptance of disability and motivation

for treatment. Initially, group techniques may focus on reality orientation, including orientation to person, place, and time; adherence to a
calendar of scheduled activities; and reporting on recent events (8).
Following reality orientation, group treatment includes tasks such as
composing telegrams to concisely convey messages about hypothetical
situations presented by the therapist (usually a psychologist). Inefficient
filtering of irrelevant material frequently obscures the communications
of severely injured patients during the early stages of their rehabilitation.
Repeated feedback provided by the therapist and the group assists the
patient in developing skills to monitor communications to more clearly
and succinctly convey the essential points.

WHAT CAN THE DEVASTATED HEAD-INJURED PATIENT LEARN?

Impairment of learning and memory is one of the most persistent and
disabling sequelae of severe head injury, affecting approximately one-
fourth of these patients (32). Although conventional therapies have been
ineffective in treating memory disorders secondary to head injury (or any
other etiology), recent studies have shown that the capacity to learn and
retain motor skills is relatively preserved in many patients. Miller (26)
showed that severely head-injured patients could benefit from practice
on a spatial formboard task and display positive transfer of skills to
slightly different formboards presented on successive days. Although
limited to a small series of head-injured cases, Miller's demonstration
supports the postulation that these patients may be capable of impressive
acquisition of visual motor skills despite persistent impairment in learning and memory of material (e.g., word lists) which requires conceptual
organization, rehearsal strategies, active association of the elements to
be remembered, and utilization of cues at the time of retrieval.

More recently, Schacter and his associates (34) have reported that
patients with marked memory impairment secondary to head injury can
be trained to utilize equipment such as a microcomputer that may enable
them to attain greater independence and eventually obtain gainful employment. Schacter et al. also found that incidental exposure to key words
would facilitate retention of these words on a later test, a phenomenon
referred to as the "repetition priming" effect. The relative preservation
of this phenomenon in survivors of severe head injury suggests that
further investigation of techniques to exploit residual skills may yield
fruitful results. However, Schacter and his co-workers have cautioned
clinicians about developing expectations that memory capacity can be
retrained in a manner analogous to muscle strength in physical therapy.
Rote repetition by computer games (or any other modality) is unlikely
to produce reproducible improvement on standard recall measures of
memory. Consistent with the studies by Miller and Schacter, Cohen and
Squire (6) found that amnesic patients were capable of acquiring skills

such as mirror reading with practice despite persistently impaired recall of word lists.

Extrapolation from these recent investigations of amnesic disorder would suggest that disabled head-injured patients are frequently capable of learning relatively nonverbal, procedural skills which may enhance their quality of life. In contrast, there is no convincing evidence that extensive training can improve memory skills on tasks such as recall of word lists, paragraphs, specific designs, or other discrete items.

CONTROLLED STUDIES ON OUTCOME OF REHABILITATION

There is a dearth of controlled studies concerning the effects of rehabilitation on neuropsychological recovery from head injury. Research is complicated by heterogeneity in the type and severity of injury, variation in selection criteria for rehabilitation programs, individual differences in preinjury ability, and difficulty in serially studying a control group matched to the rehabilitation group on relevant variables. Other methodological points include definition of the target problem (*e.g.*, memory deficit), appropriate tasks and follow-up intervals to assess improvement, specification of the training procedure employed, and defining the criteria for a satisfactory outcome (9). Apparent gains in specific skills following introduction of a training procedure in rehabilitation may be misleading unless improvements are observed to generalize across various situations and persist after the patient is discharged from the program.

Although no investigation of head injury rehabilitation has yet fully satisfied the criteria for a randomized controlled study, Prigatano and his associates (31) were the first investigators to approximate this goal. They found that long-term survivors of severe head injury exhibited gains in neuropsychological functioning following 6 months of intensive, outpatient treatment which focused on cognitive, emotional, and motivational disturbances and development of independence and vocational skills. The control group recruited by Prigatano *et al.* consisted of patients with injuries which less frequently produced hemiparesis; they were studied somewhat earlier after injury than the treated patients and for various reasons had failed to comply with recommendations for participation in neuropsychological rehabilitation. The findings reported by Prigatano *et al.* provided at least preliminary support for the efficacy of rehabilitation in chronic survivors of severe head injury.

NEUROPHARMACOLOGIC INTERVENTION

In view of recent studies implicating the cholinergic pathways of the brain in memory, investigators have recently explored the possibility of augmenting cognitive recovery by cholinergic treatment. Two studies have provided preliminary evidence that the combined treatment of head-injured patients with lecithin (a dietary source of the acetylcholine) and physostigmine (a cholinesterase inhibitor) enhances the memory of head-injured patients (13, 38). These preliminary findings are encouraging with respect to further development of pharmacologic approaches to posttraumatic memory disorder.

FUTURE DIRECTIONS IN REHABILITATION

Specialists in the rehabilitation of head-injured patients widely acknowledge that long-term goals must be individualized for devastated patients who are permanently disabled with respect to gainful employment. Consequently, long-term placement in a setting which provides some independence and a reasonable quality of life for permanently disabled individuals is a pressing need. At some point, many survivors of severe head injury exhibit diminishing gains in programs providing intensive rehabilitation services which may be better utilized by other patients. Residential communities incorporating day treatment, part-time supervised employment, and other activities provide long-term living arrangements and an opportunity for the residents to attain a level of independence commensurate with their abilities. Further investigation is warranted to develop criteria for determining the point at which severely head-injured patients are unlikely to benefit from further intensive rehabilitation and are clearly incapable of competitive employment.

A second emerging trend in the rehabilitation of brain-injured patients is the educational model which has been most fully developed in California. Designed primarily for patients functioning in the moderately disabled range, courses are offered in a community college setting which prepare patients for reintegration into the family and community and future employment. The educational model holds considerable promise because it is compatible with the concept that long-term rehabilitation is essentially a learning process.

REFERENCES

1. Becker, D. P., Miller, J. D., and Greenberg, R. P. Prognosis after head injury. In: *Neurological Surgery*, edited by J. R. Youmans, Chap. 60, pp. 21–42. Saunders, Philadelphia, 1982.
2. Bowers, S. A., and Marshall, L. F. Outcome in 200 consecutive cases of severe head injury treated in San Diego county: A prospective analysis. Neurosurgery, 6: 237–242, 1980.
3. Braakman, R., Gelpke, G. J., Habbema, J. D. F., *et al.* Systematic selection of prognostic features in patients with severe head injury. Neurosurgery, 6: 362–370, 1980.
4. Bricolo, A., Turazzi, S., and Feriotti, G. Prolonged posttraumatic unconsciousness. J. Neurosurg., 52: 625–634, 1980.
5. Carlsson, C. A., von Essen, C., and Lofgren, J. Factors affecting the clinical course of patients with severe head injuries. Part 1. Influence of biological factors. Part 2. Significance of posttraumatic coma. J. Neurosurg., 29: 242–251, 1968.

6. Cohen, N. J., and Squire, L. R. Preserved learning and retention of pattern-analyzing skill in amnesia: Dissociation of knowing how and knowing that. Science, *210:* 207–209, 1980.

7. Cope, D. N., and Hall, K. Head injury rehabilitation: Benefit of early intervention. Arch. Phys. Med. Rehabil., *63:* 433–437, 1982.

8. Corrigan, J.D., Arnett, J.A., Houck, L. J., et al. Reality orientation for brain injured patients: Group treatment and monitoring of recovery. Arch. Phys. Med. Rehabil., *66:* 626–630, 1985.

9. Diller, L., and Gordon, W. A. Interventions for cognitive deficits in brain-injured adults. J. Consult. Clin. Psychol., *49:* 822–834, 1981.

10. Dougherty, Jr., J. H., Rawlinson, D., Levy, D. E., et al. Hypoxic-ischemic brain injury and the vegetative state: Clinical and neuropathological correlation. Neurology, *29:* 591, 1979.

11. Eisenberg, H. M., Cayard, C., Papanicolaou, A. C., et al. The effects of three potentially preventable complications on outcome after severe closed head injury: In: *The Vth International Symposium on Intracranial Pressure,* Chap. 93, pp. 549–553. Springer-Verlag, Berlin, 1983.

12. Gennarelli, T. A., Spielman, G. M., Langfitt, T. W., et al. Influence of the type of intracranial lesion on outcome from severe head injury. J. Neurosurg., *56:* 26–33, 1982.

13. Goldberg, E., Gerstman, L. J., Mattis, S., et al. Effects of cholinergic treatment on posttraumatic anterograde amnesia. Arch. Neurol., *39:* 581, 1982.

14. Heiskanen, O., and Sipponen, P. Prognosis of severe brain injury. Neurol. Scand., *46:* 343–348, 1970.

15. Higashi, K., Hatano, M., Abiko, S., et al. Five-year follow-up study of patients with persistent vegetative state. J. Neurol. Neurosurg. Psychiatry, *44:* 552–554, 1981.

16. Jennett, B., and Bond M.: Assessment of outcome after severe brain damage. Lancet, *1:* 480–484, 1975.

17. Jennett, B., and Plum, F. Persistent vegetative state after severe brain damage. Lancet, *1:* 734–737, 1972.

18. Jennett, B., Snoek, J., Bond, M. R., et al. Disability after severe head injury: Observations on the use of the Glasgow Outcome Scale. J. Neurol. Neurosurg. Psychiatry, *44:* 285–293, 1981.

19. Jennett, B., Teasdale, G., Braakman, R., et al. Predicting outcome in individual patients after severe head injury. Lancet, *2:* 1031–1035, 1976.

20. Jennett, B., Teasdale, G., Braakman, R., et al. Prognosis of patients with severe head injury. Neurosurgery *4:* 283–289, 1979.

21. Langfitt, T. W., and Gennarelli, T. A. Can the outcome from head injury be improved? J. Neurosurg., *56:* 19–25, 1982.

22. Levati, A., Farina, M. L., Vecchi, G., et al. Prognosis of severe head injuries. J. Neurosurg., *57:* 779–783, 1982.

23. LeVere, T. E. Neural stability, sparing, and behavioral recovery following brain damage. Psychol. Rev., *82:* 344–358, 1975.

24. Levin, H. S., Eisenberg, H. M., Wigg, N. R., et al. Memory and intellectual ability after head injury in children and adolescents. Neurosurgery, *11:* 668–673, 1982.

25. Maas, A. I. R., Braakman, R., Schouten, H. J. A., et al. Agreement between physicians on assessment of outcome following severe head injury. J. Neurosurg., *58:* 321–325, 1983.

26. Miller, E. The training characteristics of severely head-injured patients: A preliminary study. J. Neurol. Neurosurg. Psychiatry, *43:* 525–528, 1980.

27. Miller, J. D., Sweet, R. C., Narayan, R. K., et al. Early insults to the injured brain. J.A.M.A., *240:* 439–442, 1978.

28. Narayan, R. K., Greenberg, R. P., Miller, J. D., *et al.* Improved confidence of outcome in severe head injury. J. Neurosurg., *54:* 751–762, 1981.
29. Pazzaglia, P., Frank, G., Frank, F., *et al.* Clinical course and prognosis of acute posttraumatic coma. J. Neurol. Neurosurg. Psychiatry, *38:* 149–154, 1975.
30. Plum, F., and Posner, J. *The Diagnosis of Stupor and Coma*, Ed. 3. F. A. Davis, Philadelphia, 1980.
31. Prigatano, G. P., Fordyce, D. J., Zeiner, H. K., *et al.* Neuropsychological rehabilitation after closed head injury in young adults. J. Neurol. Neurosurg. Psychiatry, *47:* 505–513, 1984.
32. Russell, W. R. *The Traumatic Amnesias.* Oxford University Press, New York, 1971.
33. Saul, T. G., and Ducker, T. B. Effect of intracranial pressure monitoring and aggressive treatment on mortality in severe head injury. J. Neurosurg., *56:* 498–503, 1982.
34. Schacter, D. L., Rich, S. A., and Stampp, M. S. Remediation of memory disorders: Experimental evaluation of the spaced-retrieval technique. J. Clin. Exp. Neuropsychol., *7:* 79–96, 1985.
35. Stablein, D. M., Miller, J. D., Choi, S. C., *et al.* Statistical methods for determining prognosis in severe head injury. Neurosurgery, *6:* 243–248, 1980.
36. Teasdale, G., and Jennett, B. Assessment of coma and impaired consciousness. A practical scale. Lancet, *1:* 81–83, 1974.
37. Teasdale, G., and Jennett, B. Assessment and prognosis of coma after head injury. Acta Neurochir., *34:* 45–55, 1976.
38. Walton, R. G. Lecithin and physostigmine for posttraumatic memory and cognitive deficits. Psychosomatics, *23:* 435–436, 1982.

28

Controversies in Medical Management of Head Injury

GUY L. CLIFTON, M.D.

INTRODUCTION

The clinical use of three well-investigated therapies in comatose, head-injured patients will be discussed: nutritional replacement, barbiturate coma, and steroid therapy. The contribution of each to neurologic outcome is to varying degrees unproven from clinical series, and each have potentially deleterious systemic side effects.

NUTRITIONAL REPLACEMENT

Energy Requirements after Neurological Injury

A number of recent publications have dealt with energy requirements after head injury (7–9, 13, 21, 25, 30, 39, 41, 42, 54). The technique of measurement is indirect calorimetry which measures the rate of oxygen utilization and gives energy expenditure by the known caloric yield of 1 liter of oxygen. The metabolic expenditure of a rested, young, 70-kg male of 1.83 M^2 surface area is 1700 kcal/24 hour or 24 kcal/kg/day. Since caloric expenditure varies with age, sex, and body surface area, metabolic expenditure is expressed as a percent of normal at rest for a given patient. This value for each patient can be found in standard tables. Data from all investigators have yielded a mean increase in metabolic expenditure in rested, comatose patients with isolated head injury of approximately 140% of the expected value at rest with variations in metabolic expenditure of 120–250% of that expected among patients. Importantly, only the data of Young et al. (54) and Deutschman et al. (13) are in nonsteroid-treated patients, and it is in agreement with other calorimetric data in steroid-treated, head-injured patients.

The duration of this hypermetabolic response and the cause of the wide variation in intensity have been the subject of recent investigation to enable more accurate estimation of caloric needs. Metabolic expenditure using indirect calorimetry was measured in 57 patients 312 times during the first 2 weeks after severe head injury without other major injuries (9). Data was taken when patients were lying still in bed or slightly moving, were not paralyzed with pancuronium bromide and, if sedated, were only lightly so with morphine. At the time of measurement, heart rate, temperature, blood pressure, and Glasgow Coma Score (GCS) were recorded. By multiple regression analysis, a significant relationship in patients who were comatose (GCS ≤ 7) between heart rate, day after injury, and Glasgow Coma Score was found according to this relationship:

$$\%RME = 152 - 14\,(GCS) + 0.4\,(HR) + 7\,(DSI)\ (n = 111, r = 0.7, p < 0.0001)$$

where $\%RME$ = resting metabolic expenditure as a percent of normal, GCS = Glasgow Coma Score; HR = heart rate, and DSI = day since injury. Application of this mathematical relationship to patient care is illustrated in the Figure 28.1. This formula allows prediction of metabolic expenditure for a comatose, head-injured patient in the first 2 weeks after injury.

The duration of this response and the contribution of muscle tone and activity to it have been investigated. That the severity of injury alone does not determine metabolic expenditure is clear from the relationship of heart rate and time after injury with it. That a major part of the response is related to muscle tone is proven by the finding in head-

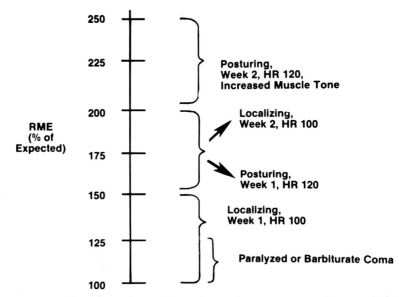

FIG. 28.1. This nomogram can be used to estimate energy requirements (caloric expenditure) in comatose patients during the first 2 weeks after injury. The nomogram is based on an equation which relates Glasgow Coma Score, heart rate, and day since injury to metabolic expenditure.

injured patients that paralysis with pancuronium bromide or barbiturate coma decreased metabolic expenditure from a mean of 160% of that expected to 100–120%. Even with paralysis, energy expenditure remained 20–30% elevated in some patients (7).

In the first 2 weeks, energy expenditure seems to rise regardless of neurological course. The duration of hypermetabolism beyond the first 2 weeks is not known. At some point, the pathologically increased caloric requirements fueled by increased muscle tone and an altered hormonal milieu are replaced by the increased requirements which would normally accompany increased activity as the patient improves.

Nitrogen Metabolism

Nitrogen balance is defined as the difference between nitrogen intake and nitrogen excretion. Nitrogen excretion is measured by analyzing urinary nitrogen or urea and adding a factor of 2–3 g for fecal and cutaneous nitrogen loss. Urinary urea can be readily measured in any hospital's clinical laboratory and comprises on the average 85% of total urinary nitrogen. Because urea can vary from 60 to 95% of urinary nitrogen, it is only an estimate of total nitrogen excretion. In metabolic studies, urinary nitrogen is measured by either the Kjehldahl technique (in which nitrogen-containing components are enzymatically digested) or by the chemiluminescent technique (in which very high temperatures reduce all nitrogen-containing components to elemental nitrogen). In nutritional management, the term nitrogen is used interchangeably with protein since measured nitrogen has a constant relationship to protein taken in or catabolized:

$$\frac{1 \text{ g of protein}}{6.25} = 1 \text{ g nitrogen}$$

For each gram of nitrogen measured in the urine (plus fecal loss) 6.25 g of protein have been catabolized.

In normal and injured man, optimal protein utilization has been found to be heavily dependent upon the adequacy of caloric intake. Catabolism of protein, which yields only 4 kcal/g (as opposed to fat, which yields 8 kcal/g), makes up 10% or less of consumed calories in normal man (15). The minimal nitrogen requirement for active adults with full replacement of expended calories has been found to be 3–5 g/day or 20–30 g of protein (5, 6). At this level of nitrogen intake, nitrogen equilibrium is just maintained if sufficient calories accompany the dietary protein. With full caloric intake, a sharp increase in nitrogen balance occurs with each added gram of nitrogen intake per day up to 7–8 g nitrogen intake per day. At this point, the improvement in nitrogen balance per gram nitrogen intake diminishes sharply, that is, nitrogen is catabolized (16).

This physiology becomes important in head injury management when nitrogen balance is used as an end point of nutritional therapy.

After severe head injury, not only do energy requirements rise greatly, but also so does nitrogen excretion. The contribution of protein to consumed calories after head injury rises to levels as high as 30% (given 10 g/day nitrogen intake and full caloric replacement) (9). The elevated urinary nitrogen reflects catabolism of amino acids derived primarily from muscle tissue.

Unlike metabolic expenditure, nitrogen balance is profoundly affected by both the level of caloric intake and the level of nitrogen intake, so that comparison of nitrogen balance data among patient groups is only possible with the same protein intakes and full caloric replacement. Recall that the minimal level of nitrogen (N) intake and excretion in moderately active normal man is 3–5 g N/day or 0.04–0.07 g N/kg/day with usual levels of 14–16 g N/day or 0.20 g N/kg/day. In 10 comatose, head-injured patients studied within the first 2 weeks after head injury with steroid treatment (16 mg/day of dexamethasone), nitrogen excretion was 26.8 g/day (0.39 g N/kg/day) with 18 g/day nitrogen intake (7). In fasted patients with severe head injury, levels of nitrogen excretion of 0.199 g N/kg/day have been found (21). Nitrogen excretion in normal, fasted man falls 2–3 times below this level. In severe head injury at levels of nitrogen intake of 10 g N/day, values of 0.28 g N/kg/day and 0.214 g N/kg/day have been found (7, 54). The metabolic defect in head injury, as in most major trauma, is in elevation of nitrogen excretion during fasting and the inability to achieve nitrogen balance with protein administration. The peak in nitrogen excretion appears to occur in the second week with improvement in nitrogen retention by the third week. It is only after the third week that achievement of nitrogen balance becomes possible.

The question of steroid effect on nitrogen excretion has been addressed in two publications. Robertson *et al.* compared nitrogen balance in two matched groups of 10 comatose patients fasted for 3 days and then fed at full caloric replacement with 15 g N/day. Steroids resulted in a 30% increase in nitrogen excretion during fasting, but the difference was lost during feeding (42). Young *et al.* in a series of head-injured patients in coma in the first week after injury who were fed 15 g N/day found nitrogen excretion of 0.24 g N/kg/day consistent with previously published data in steroid-treated patients (54). The increased nitrogen excretion of neurological injury cannot then be attributed to steroids. Some degree of nitrogen wasting is probably due to immobilization. The classic studies of Deitrick *et al.* have shown a marked rise in nitrogen excretion occurring several days after immobilization of normal young men (11).

Levels of nitrogen excretion of 25 g N/day were found with 15 g N/day intake.

Some feeling for the potential sequelae of these levels of nitrogen loss may be gained from the following facts. A 30% preoperative weight loss increased the morbidity and mortality of gastric surgery by 10-fold (49). It is, therefore, generally assumed that a 10–15% weight loss in a bedfast patient is of little consequence, but that a 30% weight loss is potentially very deleterious. The average nitrogen loss of the fasted head-injured patient is 0.2 g N/kg/day (14 g N), about double or triple the normal loss, with values of fasted nitrogen loss of up to 25 g N/day being frequently seen. This level of nitrogen loss will produce a 10% decrease in lean mass in 7 days, hence, underfeeding for a 2- to 3-week period could result in a 30% weight loss in 3 weeks or less.

Caloric Replacement

Full replacement of expended calories is the objective of nutritional management since, without it, protein is wasted. Greatly exceeding metabolic expenditure is possible but can result in 1} hyperglycemia and 2} fat synthesis with increased CO_2 production. While not attempted in head injury, feeding 2 times metabolic expenditure has not achieved nitrogen balance in burned patients (53). In normal man and probably injured man, the relative nitrogen retention resulting from increased caloric administration sharply falls beyond 75% caloric replacement, so that beyond full caloric replacement there is a diminishing return in terms of improving nitrogen balance. In one study of head-injured patients which attempted to achieve nitrogen balance by enteral hyperalimentation, levels of 40% over measured metabolic expenditure (average value of 3500 kcal/day) were administered with increased carbon dioxide production as the only systemic complication (8). Hyperglycemia (>150 mg/dl) was found only in a few aged patients, and elevation of blood urea nitrogen (BUN) was not found. Table 28.1 lists the recommended range of caloric intake based on measured metabolic expenditure for different categories of patients. There is neither experimental nor clinical data to support exceeding this range, which represents 100% of measured metabolic expenditure.

Nitrogen Balance

Whereas replacement of expended calories as accurately as possible is a clear goal of nutritional management, the desired level of reduction of nitrogen loss is less well quantified. The rise in nitrogen excretion which occurs with feeding in head-injured patients demonstrates a defect in utilization of nitrogen. The relative gains in nitrogen balance achieved

TABLE 28.1

Caloric Replacement of Patients with Acute Neurological Injury Based on Metabolic Expenditure

Patient	Caloric Replacement (kcal/kg)
Resting 70-kg male (normal)	26
Postoperative craniotomy (best estimate)	26
Posturing (GCS 4–5), 1st week	40–50
Posturing (GCS 4–5), 2nd week	50–60
Localizing or flexor withdrawal (GCS 6–7), 1st week	30–40
Localizing or flexor withdrawal (GCS 6–7), 2nd week	40–50
GCS 8–12	30–35
Paraplegia	27
Quadriplegia	23

with high protein feeding can be illustrated. Two matched groups of comatose head-injured patients were treated with intakes of 17.6 ± 3.6 g N/day and 29.0 ± 5.3 g N/day, respectively, at 140% replacement of expended calories (8). Data is from 7-day balance periods within the first 2 weeks after injury. A nitrogen balance of −9.2 ± 6.7 g/day was found in the lower protein group and a balance of −5.3 ± 5.0 g/day in the higher protein group. These data suggest that at a high range of nitrogen intake (>17 g/day), less than 50% of administered nitrogen is retained after head injury. This nitrogen loss and balance data is summarized in Table 28.2. The level of nitrogen intake which generally results in <10 g nitrogen loss per day is 15–17 g N/day or 0.3–0.5 g N/kg/day. As it turns out, this value is about 20% of the caloric composition of a 50-kcal/kg/day feeding protocol. Twenty percent is the maximal protein content of most enteral feedings designed for the hypermetabolic patient (Ensure, Sustacal) and is the maximal amino acid content of most parenteral formulations. The level of protein and caloric intake desirable, then, is not really in question. Controversy in nutritional replacement lies in two areas: (*a*) enteral feeding *vs.* parenteral; and (*b*) Should this level of feeding be reached early after injury and, if so, how soon?

Nutritional support may be administered either enterally or parenterally. There are advantages to enteral alimentation if it can be used. The major one is avoidance of a central venous catheter and its associated septic complications. There is no evidence in any patient group that superior nutrition is achieved by enteral alimentation as compared to intravenous alimentation or the reverse. There are some important points which must be understood if enteral alimentation is to be used. First, most marketed formulas contain insufficient water for the hypermeta-

TABLE 28.2

Levels of Nitrogen Loss in Head Injury (70-kg Man)

	Nitrogen Excretion (g N/day)	Nitrogen Balance (g N/day)
Normal man (fasted)	2 g	−2 g
Normal man (fed 10 g N/day)	10–13 g	0
Immobilized man (fed 15 g N/day)	18 g	−3 g
Comatose (fasted)	14 g	−14 g
Comatose (fed 15 g N/day)	25 g	−10 g
Comatose (fed 30 g N/day)	35 g	−5 g

bolic patient and, if 30–60 ml/hour of water are not given orally or intravenously, hypernatremia is very common. Second, rapid administration of enteral feedings will almost always result in diarrhea, which is not only a problem in care, but also indicates malabsorption. Experience has shown that by slow advancement of feeding over several days, enteral alimentation will be tolerated in many patients. A recommended schedule is to use a continuous infusion beginning at 25 ml/hour of full strength formula and advancing it by 25 ml every 12 hours until full intake is achieved, usually at infusion rates of 100–150 ml/hour. Others prefer to use diluted formulas as a method of advancing intake. By either method, at least 3 days is taken to achieve full replacement. The gastric contents are aspirated every 4 hours and feedings decreased for residual volumes of >200 ml. Metamucil can be placed down a nasogastric tube and will increase stool bulk.

Experience has shown that some patients after acute neural injury will not tolerate enteral feedings. The author has found that about 80% of patients will tolerate feedings by 3–5 days after injury, allowing full caloric replacement by 7–10 days after injury. Patients treated with morphine will have impaired gastric emptying. Patients treated with broad spectrum antibiotics will often develop diarrhea which does not respond to slowing feedings. One concern about enteral feeding is the risk of aspiration. In the intubated patient, this is less of a concern. In the patient with a tracheostomy, which is uncuffed, or in the extubated patient, aspiration can occur. Since aspiration of the stomach is necessary periodically initially to determine if feedings are tolerated, a nasogastric tube is used at first. If feedings are well tolerated, a smaller feeding tube may be later inserted. Early placement of a gastrostomy is helpful in patients who are likely to require prolonged support. These measures decrease the likelihood of aspiration.

In many respects, with the sophisticated nutritional support available in most hospitals, it is simpler to administer parenteral than enteral formulas. There is no question of tolerance; fewer adjustments of rate are necessary; and higher rates of intake are achieved earlier in many patients. Nursing personnel are more tolerant of intravenous solutions than enteral feeding. Standard formulations are available through the hospital pharmacy. Failure of delivery of full caloric requirements enterally by the seventh day after neurological injury in a patient who will require prolonged nutritional support constitutes, in the author's experience, a definite indication for parenteral hyperalimentation. Initial failure of tolerance of enteral formulas due to gastric retention usually indicates that the patient will not tolerate enteral formula for a long period of time, and this also constitutes an indication for parenteral alimentation. No study in any group of hypermetabolic patients has established any detrimental effects of a brief fast (3 days) after injury, but to achieve full caloric replacement by day 7 with either enteral or parenteral therapy, feeding must be begun by the third or fourth day after injury by either enteral or parenteral means.

There is one potential contraindication to parenteral therapy: cerebral edema. Waters *et al.* have shown aggravation of edema in a cold lesion model with parenteral alimentation (52). In the very acute phase of neurological injury with increased intracranial pressure (ICP) where mannitol is required, the use of parenteral therapy is possible but requires great attention to detail in management and in patients requiring maximal therapy for intracranial hypertension can complicate management. No aggravation of ICP has been noted clinically with parenteral therapy but, because of the complexity of management, it seems reasonable to withhold parenteral therapy until ICP is normal or mannitol is not required.

What evidence supports the goal of achievement of full caloric replacement by the seventh day after injury? Despite many studies, no clear relationship of the extent of nutritional support to outcome has been documented in any patient group except at the extremes. It was for this reason that aggressive attempts to achieve nitrogen equilibrium were largely abandoned in most hypermetabolic patients. One comparative study has been done in neurosurgical patients by Rapp *et al.* (39). Eighteen head-injured patients were treated with parenteral nutrition and 17 with enteral nutrition. Analysis of this data shows that this was a study of what has probably been common neurosurgical management: severe undernutrition *vs.* nutritional replacement. Unreplaced nitrogen losses of 14–22 g N/day occurred for 2 weeks in the enterally alimented group with caloric intakes of only 200–1000 kcal/day. In the parenterally alimented group, nitrogen losses due to greater nitrogen intake (i.e., caloric intake 1800–3000 kcal/day) were 10–12 g N/day. A significant improvement in mortality and morbidity was found in the parenterally alimented group. This study documented the consequence of one extreme of management, failure of nutritional support, and is important in verifying the need to replace expended calories and to provide a level of nitrogen intake likely to reduce daily nitrogen losses to below 10 g.

BARBITURATES

Interest in barbiturate use in head injury began with the observation by Shapiro et al. in 1973 and 1974 that anesthetic doses of thiopental and pentobarbital rapidly decreased intracranial pressure intraoperatively and in five comatose patients in the intensive care unit (46, 47). The metabolic effects of barbiturates included decreased cerebral blood flow and a 50% reduction in cerebral metabolic rate (34). These effects were likened to those of hypothermia to 27°C, and it was hoped that barbiturates would offer similar cerebral protection. Profound hypothermia to 8–10°C had been shown to significantly extend ischemic time in some models. The hope of significant ischemic protection by barbiturates persisted, and a considerable literature developed in the ensuing years examining barbiturate use in experimental ischemia models.

Rockoff et al. first reported their experiences with high dose barbiturate therapy in 45 patients with head injury and a small mixed group of other comatose patients in 1979 (43). These investigators found a rapid decrease in intracranial pressure in 29 patients allowing a reduction in mannitol dosage. Neurologic outcome was significantly better in those patients who responded to barbiturates, compared with a 90% mortality rate in those who did not. This finding was consistent with the findings of Miller et al., who showed in 1977 in a series of 160 comatose, head-injured patients, that uncontrollable elevated ICP was uniformly fatal and that even a moderate increase in ICP (>20 mm Hg) was associated with a higher morbidity (35).

Marshall et al., in 1979, reported a consecutive series of 100 comatose, head-injured patients, of whom 25 had ICP uncontrolled by conventional management (ICP >40 mm Hg for 15 minutes) (32). This group received pentobarbital in a loading dose of 3–5 mg/kg followed by a continuous infusion resulting in blood levels of 2.5–3.5 mg%. Intracranial pressure was normalized in 13 patients (<15 mm Hg), reduced in 6, and unaffected in 6. All of the barbiturate nonresponders died or were vegetative, and 10 of the 19 barbiturate responders made a good outcome. Miller et al., as noted, had reported 100% mortality in 23 patients who had ICP uncontrolled by mannitol and hyperventilation and 50% poor outcome (severe disability, vegetative, or dead) in 41 patients who had ICP >20 mm Hg which was controlled by mannitol and hyperventilation. This rather striking difference in the two series in the outcome of patients who did not respond to conventional management suggested (a) that barbiturates exerted a powerful effect in controlling ICP unmanageable conventionally with a marked improvement in outcome; or, (b) that different levels of intensity of management were used to define patients who were nonresponders to conventional therapy. Use of mannitol, ventricular drainage, and hyperventilation in both studies was not quantified in a way that definite comparisons of management could be made. Other publications followed, modeled after the management protocol detailed by Miller (40, 44). These showed that barbiturates did decrease intracranial pressure and, that if ICP was uncontrolled by conventional or barbiturate management, mortality was almost certain. The same problems of potential variation in what was termed conventional management and variations in definition of increased ICP prevented conclusions as to the ability of barbiturates when used to control increased ICP to reduce mortality and morbidity. All investigators agreed that barbiturates effectively reduce ICP. No evidence from these publications suggested that morbidity or mortality was increased by this therapy.

Light has been shed on the subject by one randomized, prospective study of barbiturate coma in severe head injury. Ward et al. in 1985 reported the results of a trial of barbiturate coma given prophylactically to patients in coma from a mass lesion or with flexor posturing or extension and no mass lesion (51). This group of patients in previous series had a mortality rate of 60% and a prevalence of intracranial hypertension of over 70%. Fifty-three patients were randomized, 26 to control and 27 to pentobarbital treatment. Pentobarbital was given within 24 hours of injury regardless of ICP. Electroencephalography (EEG) and blood levels of barbiturates confirmed anesthetic levels in the treatment group. No difference in ICP levels, mortality, or neurologic outcome was found in the two comparable groups. Hypotension was more common in the pentobarbital-treated group, but no other systemic complications were related to barbiturate administration. This work has conclusively shown the lack of efficacy of barbiturates given prophylactically in either preventing increased ICP or improving outcome. Whether the use of barbiturates to further decrease intracranial pressure when conventional management has failed reduces mortality and improves outcome remains unanswered. A randomized, multicenter trial, which is soon to be reported, should definitively answer this question.

STEROIDS

Steroids were first used in neurologic patients in 1960 when French attempted treatment of a patient with a glioblastoma by intracarotid injection of Hypaque to open the blood-brain barrier followed by intracarotid cortisone (20). He attempted to deliver high doses of steroids into the tumor as an antineoplastic agent. This lethargic patient became alert the following day. Similar studies in comparable patients resulted in "the same pleasant result" (20). Subsequent work in animals and man demonstrated the ability of corticosteroids to diminish extracellular fluid microscopically around tumors or growing mass lesions. The drug became standard in treatment of tumors, its efficacy so clear that randomized studies were quite unnecessary. Subsequent studies of edema formation in animals with cold lesion injuries showed conflicting effects of dexamethasone in doses used clinically for treatment of cerebral edema from tumors, 0.25–2.5 mg/kg/day (14, 33). Limited studies of edema from trauma in animals have shown a slight effect in decreasing edema (29, 50). Recent work stimulated by the protective effect of very high dose steroids in hemorrhagic shock has examined neurologic outcome in spinal cord injury and head injury but not edema formation. A striking effect of methylprednisolone and of dexamethasone in improving experimental spinal cord injury given in doses of 15–30 mg/kg and 3–5 mg/kg, respectively, within 1 hour of injury, has been found by several investigators (1, 17, 55). Lower doses or later administration have not been effective in experimental spinal cord injury. In the single study of the effect of steroids on experimental head injury Hall found that a dose of 30 mg/kg significantly improved outcome (26). Extensive investigation of the pharmacology of steroids in these doses has shown enhancement of (Na^+ + K^+) ATPase activity and attenuation of lipid peroxide formation, effects not found at lower doses (12, 27). Not only does this dose improve outcome, but also spinal cord blood flow and evoked potentials are improved by pretreatment or posttreatment within 1 hour of spinal cord injury (55). The experimental data and pharmacology have been recently reviewed by Braughler and Hall (4).

It seems very likely that the effect of steroids in decreasing peritumoral edema is quite different pharmacologically from its effect on improving spinal cord injury. Higher doses given much sooner are effective in spinal cord injury but have little effect on cord edema. Little work has been done in head injury models with steroid treatment. It is instructive to review the clinical series of steroids in head injury with this experimental background. Table 28.3 summarizes these series.

The first randomized series of steroids in head injury was reported by Ransohoff in 1972. Methylprednisolone (125 mg q 6 h × 4 days) was given within 24 hours of admission (38). A trend toward improved survival was found but without statistical significance. By present standards, insufficient clinical data to compare groups is available. Gobiet *et al.* in 1976 treated three groups of 30 head-injured patients, each with dexamethasone: (*a*) 48 mg, then 8 mg q 2 h; (*b*) 16 mg, then 4 mg q 6 h; and (*c*) no steroids (23). The high dose group was found to have a 20% mortality rate compared to 40% in the other two groups with lower ICP

TABLE 28.3
Summary of Clinical Series Comparing Steroids in Head Injury

Investigators	Design	Year	Patients	Time of Steroid Administration After Injury (hr)	Dose	Conclusion
Sparacio et al. (48)	Anecdotal	1965	36	24	M[a], 40 mg	+
Ransohoff (38)	Randomized	1972	35	24	M, 25 mg	−
Gobiet et al. (23)	Randomized	1976	93	24	D, 48 mg 16 mg	+
Cooper et al. (10)	Randomized	1979	76	24	D, 96 mg 16 mg	−
Miller (35)	Measurement of ICP	1977	20	24	M, 40 mg	−
Pitts and Katkis (37)	Randomized; end point was ICP	1980	76	24	D, 16 mg 24 mg	−
Saul et al. (45)	Randomized	1981	100	24	M, 250 mg	−
Braakman et al. (2)	Randomized	1983	161	6	D, 100 mg	−
Giannotta et al. (22)	Randomized	1983	88	6–12	M, 30 mg/kg 1.5 mg/g	−

[a]M, methylprednisolone; D, dexamethasone.

and fewer systemic complications. Insufficient data to ensure comparability of groups is included in this publication, but patients were comparable by pathologic diagnoses. Cooper *et al.* in a well-designed study of 76 patients compared placebo, low dose dexamethasone (16 mg/day), and high dose dexamethasone (96 mg/day) (10). He found no improvement in outcome and no increase in complications with steroids, except hyperglycemia. Incidence of increased ICP was not different. Gudeman and Miller, who had previously documented an improvement in intracranial pressure and pressure volume index in patients with tumors treated with steroids, found no effect of increasing methylprednisolone from 40 mg to 2000 mg in 20 comatose, head-injured patients (24, 36). Pitts *et al.*, in a similar study of placebo, (16 mg/day and 24 mg/day of dexamethasone), found no difference in ICP characteristics (37). Subsequent randomized studies within single institutions, using groups comparable by age, sex, primary diagnosis, and Glasgow Coma Score, tested doses of dexamethasone of 50–100 mg/day and doses of methylprednisolone of up to 750 mg/day. These all failed to show any advantage or adverse effect of steroids as compared to placebo (2, 31, 45). Giannotta *et al.* in a study of 80 patients tested methylprednisolone 30 mg/kg q 6 h × 2, then 250 mg q 6 hr; methylprednisolone 1.5 mg/kg q 6 h × 2, then 25 mg q 6 h; and placebo. Significant differences in morbidity, mortality, and ICP between groups were not found (22). When low dose and placebo groups were combined and compared to the high dose group, a reduction in mortality of patients under 40 years of age was found in the high dose group. While this statistical maneuver would preclude any firm conclusions and was not claimed to, it is at least of interest that the only reported positive findings are in the series of Giannotta *et al.*, Gobiet *et al.*, and Faupel *et al.* In these studies, patients were treated with 30 mg/kg of methylprednisolone or doses of dexamethasone of 1.4 mg/kg, at least approaching the levels effective in spinal cord injury (19, 22, 23). Examination of this large mass of data leaves little doubt that doses of dexamethasone of 50–100 mg/day and of methylprednisolone of 1000 mg/day given within 24 hours of head injury have no significant effect either positive or negative on head injury outcome. Since each series numbered less than 200 patients and was usually divided into three groups, it cannot be conclusively stated that some subgroup might not benefit. Probably a clinically significant improvement would have been detected in such a group even in these comparatively small randomized studies.

No rational basis for steroid usage in the doses given has emerged in head injury. It should be noted that the use of steroids in these studies is fundamentally different from that of the experimental studies in spinal cord and head injury which show CNS protection. In experimental studies, doses of 15–30 mg/kg of methylprednisolone and doses of 3–6 mg/kg of dexamethasone are used and are given within 1 hour of injury. In the clinical series reviewed here, steroids have usually been administered within 24 hours of injury and, at the earliest, within 6 hours. The high dose range in these trials is one-third or less of the effective loading dose in spinal cord injury in a 24-hour period. Hall has advised repeated dosing at levels of 15 mg/kg q 2 h in experimental spinal cord injury to maintain high CNS levels (28). To perform a clinical protocol pharmacologically consistent with the effects found in the laboratory, patients would require randomization at the roadside or at the latest in the emergency department. Loading doses of methylprednisolone of 2000 g followed by a dose of 1000 mg every 2 hours for the duration of therapy would be required to maintain effective CNS levels. The only randomized trial of high dose steroids in spinal cord injury done to date used a dose of 1000 mg methylprednisolone initially, then 250 mg q 6 h for 10 days (3). Braughler and Hall have pointed out that this dose (14 mg/kg in a 70-kg person) is just at the level of effectiveness found experimentally and that the maintenance doses are far below those necessary to maintain high CNS levels (4). A further limitation of this study, which reported no effect, is that rarely was the drug given within 6–8 hours of injury. It is likely that a short course of very high dose steroids would have few adverse effects. Administration of the drug within 1 hour of injury entails randomization of a comatose patient in the field. This has prevented a proper clinical trial of steroids in CNS injury. Until such a study is done, the question remains unanswered.

CONCLUSIONS

The current usage of nutritional therapy, barbiturates, and steroids in head injury has been detailed. In each area, there is fertile ground for clinical and basic investigation. In nutritional therapy, the most important unanswered question is the effect of the abnormal systemic metabolic profile on the injured brain. In addition to elevated oxygen consumption and nitrogen wasting, a profile of elevations in plasma levels of some classes of amino acids and decreases in others, such as the branched chain amino acids, have been found. Glucose and lactate are systemically elevated. There is strong evidence that the arterial blood levels of amino acids drive the net brain uptake or excretion of those amino acids. Low-branched chain amino acids could result in a net loss of brain structural proteins. Elevations of tyrosine or phenylalanine could result in creation of toxic false neurotransmitters, as found in hepatic encephalopathy. Hyperglycemia and increased lactate are both deleterious in stroke and may, also, be so in head injury. Hence, future nutritional management will probably be directed toward creation of an optimal metabolic milieu for brain recovery rather than achieving nitrogen and caloric balance, as such. The failure of anesthetic doses of barbiturates, given irrespective of intracranial pressure, to alter head injury outcome closes a chapter on the idea of cerebral metabolic inhibition as a therapy in head injury. A similar lack of positive clinical results diminished enthusiasm for barbiturate usage in stroke. Barbiturates do decrease intracranial pressure in patients refractory to other methods. The question remaining to be answered in regard to intracranial pressure control with barbiturates when other methods have failed is whether mortality is decreased and, if so, whether neurologic outcome of the survivors is better than vegetative. The question of dose and time of administration of steroids in head injury therapy was fully covered. In discovering the answers to what is the optimal metabolic management of head injury and what is the proper use of steroid therapy, a major impediment is a lack of animal models of head injury which will permit therapeutic testing. Sufficient basic data to justify costly and potentially risky clinical trials in these areas has not yet been generated. Further progress in these areas awaits data from the laboratory.

REFERENCES

1. Anderson, D. K., Means, E. D., and Waters, T. R. Microvascular perfusion and metabolism in injured spinal cord after methylprednisolone treatment. J. Neurosurg., 56: 106–113, 1982.
2. Braakman, R., Schouten, H. J. A., Blaauw-Van Dishoeck, M., et al. Megadose steroids in severe head injury. Results of a prospective double-blind clinical trial. J. Neurosurg., 58: 326–330, 1983.
3. Bracken, M. B., Collins, W. F., Freeman, D. F., et al. Efficacy of methylprednisolone in acute spinal cord injury. J.A.M.A., 251: 45–52, 1984.
4. Braughler, J. M., and Hall, E. D. Current application of "high dose" steroid therapy for CNS injury. J. Neurosurg., 62: 806–810, 1985.
5. Calloway, D. H., and Margen, S. Variation in endogenous nitrogen excretion and dietary nitrogen utilization as determinants of human protein requirement. J. Nutr., 101: 205–216, 1971.
6. Calloway, D. H., and Spector, H. Nitrogen balance as related to caloric and protein intake in active young men. Am. J. Clin. Nutr., 2: 405–412, 1954.
7. Clifton, G. L., Robertson, C. S., and Choi, S. C. Assessment of nutritional requirements of head injured patients. J. Neurosurg., 64: 895–901, 1986.
8. Clifton, G. L., Robertson, C. S., and Contant, C. F. Enteral hyperalimentation in head injury. J. Neurosurg., 62: 186–193, 1985.
9. Clifton, G. L., Robertson, C. S., Hodge, S., et al. The metabolic response to severe head injury. J. Neurosurg., 60: 687–696, 1984.
10. Cooper, P. R., Moody, S., Clark, W. K., et al. Dexamethasone and severe head injury. A prospective double-blind study. J. Neurosurg., 51: 307–316, 1979.
11. Deitrick, J. E., Whedon, G. D., and Shorr, E. Effects of immobilization upon various metabolic and physiologic functions of normal men. Am. J. Med., 4: 3–36, 1948.
12. Demopoulos, H. B., Flamm, E. S., Seligman, M. L., et al. Further studies on free-radical pathology in major central nervous system disorders: Effect of very high doses of

methylprednisolone on the functional outcome, morphology, and chemistry of experimental spinal cord impact injury. Can. J. Physiol. Pharmacol., *60:* 1415–1424, 1982.

13. Deutschman, C. S., Konstantinides, F. N., Raup, S., *et al.* Physiological and metabolic response to isolated closed head injury. J. Neurosurg., *64:* 89–98, 1986.

14. Dick, A. R., McCallum, M. E., Maxwell, J. A., *et al.* Effect of dexamethasone on experimental brain edema in cats. J. Neurosurg., *45:* 141–147, 1976.

15. Duke, J. H., Jr., Jorgensen, S. D., and Broell, J. R. Contribution of protein to caloric expenditure following injury. Surgery, *68:* 168–174, 1970.

16. Elwyn, D. H. Nutritional requirements of adult surgical patients. Crit. Care Med., *8:* 9–20, 1980.

17. Faden, A. L., Jacobs, T. P., Patrick, D. H., *et al.* Megadose corticosteroid therapy following experimental spinal injury. J. Neurosurg., *60:* 712–717, 1984.

18. Fan, P. T., Yu, D. T. Y., Targoff, C., *et al.* Effects of corticosteroids on the human immune response. Suppression of mitogen-induced lymphocyte proliferation by "pulse" methylprednisolone. Transplantation, *26:* 266–267, 1978.

19. Faupel, G., Reulen, H. J., Mulr, D., *et al.* Double-blind study on the effects of steroids on severe closed head injury. In: *Dynamics of Brain Edema,* edited by H. M. Pappius and W. Feindel, pp. 337–343. Springer-Verlag, Berlin/New York, 1976.

20. French, E. A. The use of steroids in the treatment of cerebral edema. Bull. N.Y. Acad. Med., *42:* 301–311, 1966.

21. Gadisseux, P., Ward, J. D., Young, H. F., *et al.* Nutrition and the neurosurgical patient. J. Neurosurg., *60:* 219–232, 1984.

22. Giannotta, S. L., Weiss, M. H., Apuzzo, M. E. J., *et al.* High dose glucocorticoids in the management of severe head injury. Neurosurgery, *15:* 497–501, 1984.

23. Gobiet, W., Bock, W. J., Liesegan, J., *et al.* Treatment of acute cerebral edema with high dose of dexamethasone. In: *Intracranial Pressure III,* edited by J. W. E. Becks, D. A. Bosch, and M. Brock, pp. 231–235. Springer-Verlag, Berlin/Heidelberg/New York, 1976.

24. Gudeman, S. K., Miller, J. D., and Becker, D. P. Failure of high-dose steroid therapy to influence intracranial pressure in patients with severe head injury. J. Neurosurg., *51:* 301–306, 1979.

25. Haider, W., Lackner, F., Schlick, W., *et al.* Metabolic changes in the course of severe acute brain damage. Eur. J. Intens. Care Med., *1:* 19–26, 1975.

26. Hall, E. D. High-dose glucocorticoid treatment improves neurological recovery in head-injured mice. J. Neurosurg., *62:* 882–887, 1985.

27. Hall, E. D., and Braughler, J. M. Effects of intravenous methylprednisolone on spinal cord lipid peroxidation and $(Na^+ + K^+)$-ATPase activity. Dose-response analysis during 1st hour after contusion injury in the cat. J. Neurosurg., *57:* 247–258, 1982.

28. Hall, E. D., and Braughler, J. M. Effects of a single large dose of methylprednisolone sodium succinate on experimental posttraumatic spinal cord ischemia. Dose-response and time action analysis. J. Neurosurg., *61:* 124–130, 1984.

29. Kobrine, A. L., and Kempe, I. G. Studies in head injury. Part II. Effect of dexamethasone on traumatic brain swelling. Surg. Neurol., *1:* 38–42, 1973.

30. Long, C. L., Schaffel, N., and Geiger, J. W. Metabolic response to injury and protein needs from indirect calorimetry and nitrogen balance. J. Parenter Enter. Nutr., *3:* 452–456, 1979.

31. Marshall, L. F., King, J., and Langfitt, I. W. The complications of high-dose corticosteroid therapy in neurosurgical patients: A prospective study. Ann. Neurol., *1:* 201–203, 1977.

32. Marshall, L. F., Smith, R. W., and Shapiro, H. M. The outcome with aggressive treatment in severe head injuries. J. Neurosurg., *50:* 26–30, 1979.

33. Maxwell, R. E., Long, D. M., and French, L. A. The effects of glucocorticoids on cold-induced brain edema. J. Neurosurg., *34:* 477–487, 1971.
34. Michenfelder, J. D. The interdependency of cerebral functional and metabolic effects following massive doses of thiopental in the dog. Anesthesiology *41:* 231–236, 1974.
35. Miller, J. D., Becker, D. P., Ward, J. D., *et al.* Significance of intracranial hypertension in severe head injury. J. Neurosurg., *47:* 503–516, 1977.
36. Miller, J. D., and Leech, P. Effects of mannitol and steroid therapy on intracranial volume pressure relationships in patients. J. Neurosurg., *42:* 274–281, 1975.
37. Pitts, E. H., and Katkis, J. V. Effect of megadose steroids on ICP in traumatic coma. In: *Intracranial Pressure IV*, edited by K. Shulman, A. Marmarou, and A. Miller, pp. 638–642. Springer-Verlag, Berlin/Heidelberg/New York, 1980.
38. Ransohoff, J. The effects of steroids on brain edema in man. In: *Steroids and Brain Edema*, edited by H. J. Reulen and K. Schurmann, p. 211–217. Springer-Verlag, Berlin/Heidelberg/New York, 1972.
39. Rapp, R. P., Young, B., Twyman, D., *et al.* The favorable effect of early parenteral feeding on survival in head injured patients. J. Neurosurg., *58:* 906–912, 1983.
40. Rea, G. L., and Rockswold, G. L. Barbiturate therapy in uncontrolled intracranial hypertension. Neurosurgery, *12:* 401–404, 1983.
41. Robertson, C. S., Clifton, G. L., and Goodman, J. C. Steroid administration and nitrogen excretion in the head injured patient. J. Neurosurg., *63:* 714–718, 1985.
42. Robertson, C. S., Clifton, G. L., and Grossman, R. G. Oxygen utilization and cardiovascular function in head injured patients. Neurosurgery, *15:* 307–314, 1984.
43. Rockoff, M. A., Marshall, L. F., and Shapiro, H. M. High-dose barbiturate therapy in humans: A clinical review of 60 patients. Ann. Neurol., *6:* 194–199, 1979.
44. Saul, T. G., and Ducker, T. B. Effect of intracranial pressure monitoring and aggressive treatment on mortality in severe head injury. J. Neurosurg., *56:* 498–503, 1982.
45. Saul, T. G., Ducker, T. B., Saleman, M., *et al.* Steroids in severe head injury. A prospective randomized clinical trial. J. Neurosurg., *54:* 596–600, 1981.
46. Shapiro, H. M., Galindo, A., Wyte, S. R., *et al.* Rapid intraoperative reduction of intracranial pressure with thiopentone. Br. J. Anaesth., *45:* 1057–1062, 1973.
47. Shapiro, H. M., Wyte, S. R., and Loeser, J. Barbiturate-augmented hypothermia for reduction of persistent intracranial hypertension. J. Neurosurg., *40:* 90–100, 1974.
48. Sparacio, R. R., Lin, P. H., and Cook, A. W. Methylprednisolone sodium succinate in acute craniocerebral trauma. Surg. Gynecol. Obstet., *121:* 513–516, 1965.
49. Studley, H. O. Percentage of weight loss: A basic indicator of surgical risk in patients with chronic peptic ulcer. J.A.M.A., *106:* 458–460, 1936.
50. Tornheim, P. A., and McLaurin, R. L. Effect of dexamethasone on cerebral edema from cranial impact in the cat. J. Neurosurg., *48:* 220–227, 1978.
51. Ward, J. D., Becker, D. P., Miller, J. D., *et al.* Failure of prophylactic barbiturate coma in the treatment of severe head injury. J. Neurosurg., *62:* 383–388, 1985.
52. Waters, D. C., Hoff, J. T., and Black, K. L. Effect of parenteral nutrition on cold-induced vasogenic edema in cats. J. Neurosurg., *64:* 460–465, 1986.
53. Wilmore, D. W., Curreri, P. W., Spitzer, K. W., *et al.* Supranormal dietary intake in thermally injured hypermetabolic patients. Surg. Gynecol. Obstet., *132:* 881–886, 1971.
54. Young, B., Ott, L., Norton, J., *et al.* Metabolic and nutritional sequelae in the non-steroid treated head injury patient. Neurosurgery, *17:* 784–791, 1985.
55. Young, W., and Flamm, E. S. Effect of high-dose corticosteroid therapy on blood flow, evoked potentials, and extracellular calcium in experimental spinal injury. J. Neurosurg., *57:* 667–673, 1982.

29

Future Therapy of Head Injury

PAUL S. DWAN, M.D., DONALD P. BECKER, M.D., F.A.C.S.,
GEORGE GADE, M.D., and MARSHALL CHEUNG, PH.D.

INTRODUCTION

Trauma to the brain and spinal cord continues to challenge physicians at the patient's bedside as well as those in the research laboratory. Clinical trials, cooperative studies, and investigation into basic questions of pathophysiology and biochemistry have each contributed greatly to our understanding of nervous system trauma. The historically dismal outcome of patients with moderate-to-severe head injury has improved as a direct consequence of these efforts.

The Glasgow Coma Scale (GCS) and various numeric measures of outcome have aided our ability to compare groups of patients with respect to therapy and long-term return to function. Currently, those patients with severe head injuries (GCS < 7) experience an approximately 30–40% mortality rate (19, 25). An additional 50% recover full or partial function sufficient to live independently, while the remainder are left severely disabled or vegetative (24). This represents a considerable advance over similar patients treated during the first portion of this century but reflects a plateau in morbidity and mortality over the last decade. Improvement in the outcome of those with severe cerebral trauma remains elusive.

In those cases of head trauma associated with hematomas, early diagnosis, endotracheal intubation, surgical intervention, and maintenance of all metabolic parameters form the basis of therapy (2). Treatment of associated systemic injuries, electrolyte abnormalities, intracranial pressure elevations, and pulmonary insufficiency enhances the environment in which damaged but viable cerebral tissue may recover (6). Refinements in surgical technique will continue to play an important role in therapy of head injury, but an equal or greater contribution will be made by our understanding of basic mechanisms of cellular injury.

FUTURE THERAPY

Timely surgical decompression of posttraumatic cerebral mass lesions is the mainstay of the neurosurgical armamentarium (Figs. 29.1 and

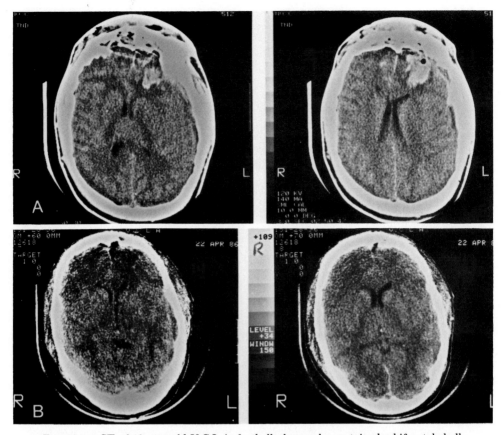

FIG. 29.1. CT of 19-year-old U.C.L.A. football player who sustained a bifrontal skull fracture and hemorrhagic contusion after a fall (A). Patient was confused with intermittent lethargy but without focal deficit. He underwent craniotomy with complete resection of hematoma and contused tissue. (B) Scan 5 days postoperatively shows mild edema but no evidence of hematoma or hemorrhagic tissue. Clinically, patient did well, returning to school 6 weeks after surgery. His only deficit was anosmia.

29.2). Focus on the direct compressive effects of subdural, epidural, and intraparenchymal hematomas neglects the impact of such space-occupying clots on distant tissues. Cerebral blood flow, and presumably metabolic rate, decline abruptly throughout the entire ipsilateral hemisphere in the presence of small contained basal ganglionic hematomas according to Mendelow and Bullock (7, 28). The same authors also studied the effects of uncontained (i.e., intraventricular, subarachnoid, and subdural) blood. Profound global reductions in cerebral blood flow were observed along with a significant ($p < 0.05$) rise in intracranial

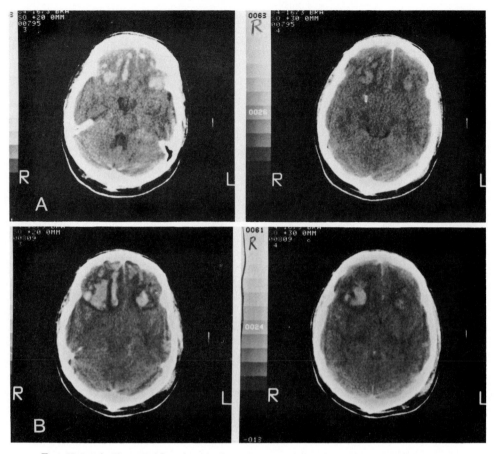

FIG. 29.2. A 23-year-old male struck in the occipital region with resultant bilateral contrecoup lesions (A). Upon presentation the patient was conversant but had deteriorated within 36 hours, becoming obtunded and posturing intermittently. CT showed consolidation and enlargement of hemorrhagic tissue (B). Management elsewhere included hyperventilation and steroids without surgery. Shortly after the second scan patient herniated and expired.

pressure to over six times those of control values. Mechanisms proposed to explain these effects are compromise of the microcirculation around the hematoma and the presence of vasoconstrictor substances released at the site of hemorrhage. By whatever means, the presence of basal cistern or intraventricular blood accelerates the cycle of cellular injury both through ischemia as well as unknown direct toxic effects. Recently, *in vitro* retina protein synthesis has been observed to decline in the presence of serum (M. Cheung, unpublished data, 1986). The removal of even small collections of blood may enhance recovery of tissue distant from the hemorrhage site by improvement in global and hemispheric blood flow and removal of toxic serum and red cell breakdown products. Safe and accurate means exist to stereotaxically evacuate small, deeply situated hematomas. The installation of hemolytic agents has also been advocated.

Hypertonic solutions such as urea, mannitol, and glycerol have been in use since the early 1950s and were arguably the first successful attempt to pharmacologically control increased intracranial pressure. Nevertheless, their chronic use may contribute to a reduction of cerebral blood flow and worsen cerebral perfusion. Therapy directed at increasing the cerebral perfusion pressure by manipulating systemic volume status rather than decreasing the intracranial pressure will enhance tissue oxygen and metabolite delivery. Moderate, induced hypertension combined with hypervolemic hemodilution with dextran-type polymers may play an increasing role in the management of severe head injuries.

The close similarity between the hypervolemic therapy proposed above and that currently in use for acute and chronic vasospasm seen after subarachnoid hemorrhage highlights the overlap between pathophysiology of cerebral injury from a wide variety of sources. Most reviews of the biochemistry of cerebral trauma emphasize the concurrent injury often seen as a result of cerebral hypoxia (29, 30).

In the absence of a decreased supply of oxygen and glucose in head injury what accounts for the decrease in adenosine triphosphate (ATP)? That such a decline in ATP even occurs in head trauma is still not established with certainty.

Using the rat acceleration concussion model Nilsson demonstrated in normoxic animals no depletion of energy stores in those undergoing a 7 m/s impact (31, 32). After a 9 m/s injury there was a significant fall in ATP limited to the pons. Lactate rose significantly in the brainstem but not cortex. By 15 minutes after trauma both ATP and lactate had nearly normalized. In those animals experiencing pulmonary edema and resultant hypoxia the energy stores were significantly lower both in brainstem and cortex. The implications according to the authors of these data are that an imbalance "between energy production and utilization" occurs, originating from an acutely increased metabolic activity. This excitation had abated in as little as 2 minutes following impact. Subsequent derangement in energy metabolism may occur because early vasospasm reduces the supply of substrates to the injured tissues (12). This vasospasm appears to be very short lived and may cause already damaged brain to be further compromised and rendered ischemic. Besides spasm another potential factor contributing to a decreased cerebral blood flow (CBF) is the global increase in intracranial pressure (ICP) (1–2 minutes) seen immediately after "uncontained" intraventricular or subarachnoid hemorrhage noted above.

The damaging effects of head trauma form a continuum which starts at the moment of impact and proceeds, unless corrected, for many days. The biomechanical nature of the injury, the presence or absence of immediate apnea, and systemic hypotension are key features to the clinician (26). Other phenomena such as acute vasospasm, depletion of energy stores, and lactate buildup may be quite short lived. The physician, of course, must initiate his therapy not at the moment of trauma but typically one-half to several hours later. Prompt surgical decompression, while a mainstay of treatment, addresses only the earliest factors in this "injury continuum." Beyond advances in surgical technique such as stereotaxic removal of deep hematomas, progress in the management of patients with moderate-to-severe cerebral injuries will largely depend on our improved understanding of the biochemical and structural bases of such injury.

The earliest effects of an acceleration-deceleration injury to the cranium are mechanical: distortion and stretching of axons, contusion, and vascular endothelial damage. These are followed shortly by a cascade of membrane-related biomechanical events which ultimately lead to ionic shifts, acidosis, cellular edema, further membrane dysfunction, and suppression of protein synthesis (Fig. 29.3). Therapy must be directed at halting or reversing the processes which damage tissue.

As reviewed above, the short-term imbalance between energy demanded by a hypermetabolic parenchyma and that supplied by a compromised vasculature leads inevitably to an ischemia-like state with loss of ATP available to the neurons and glia. Before examining the ionic changes which produce subsequent disruption, one must ask if the very early stimulation of metabolic demand occurring primarily in the brainstem might serve as a point of therapeutic intervention. Mechanical depolarization may explain a portion of initial excitation documented many years ago by continuous EEG monitoring during trauma (41). Evidence also is strong for a surge of catecholamines occurring centrally and peripherally which may play a role in early central nervous system (CNS) stimulation (18). The excitatory amino acids glutamate and aspartate are released in ischemic injury (11). CNS locations with high postischemic glutamate concentrations such as hippocampus may be susceptible to excitation and, as a result, outpace energy supplies. The presence of such an effect in cerebral trauma has been strongly considered but not yet demonstrated. A drug widely in use as a spasmolytic agent, baclofen, suppresses release of central stores of glutamate from presynaptic sources and thus may provide a means of preventing the early hypermetabolism which sets the stage for later depletion of ATP and electrolyte imbalances which occur in areas of trauma (20).

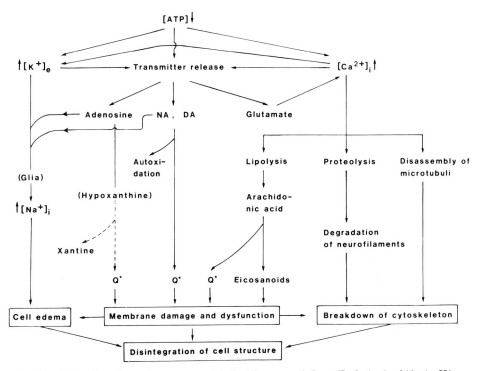

FIG. 29.3. Overview of events associated with energy failure. Early ionic shifts in K⁺ and Ca²⁺ trigger neurotransmitter release and subsequent cascades ultimately leading to irreversible structural and functional breakdown. See text for details. *NA*, noradrenaline; *DA*, dopamine. *Q*, free radical. (Reproduced with permission from Siesjo, B. K., and Weiloch, T. Cerebral metabolism in ischemia: Neurochemical basis for therapy. Br. J. Anaesth., *57:* 47–62, 1985. Copyright NINCDS.)

While the above effects are observed primarily at the site of impact there are a wide variety of cellular activities which are stimulated or suppressed ipsilateral to the injury or even globally. Dail found hemispheric reduction in α-glycerophosphate dehydrogenase (GPDH) following a highly focal lesion produced by undercutting a small portion of rat motor cortex (10). The activity of this enzyme reflects the rate of energy metabolism, and its suppression was observed solely in layers II and III. Within 9 days levels throughout the hemisphere had returned to preinjury values. Explanations for this or similar effects may aid our understanding of patients who suffer unexplained deteriorations despite near normal radiographic studies. Labeled energy intermediate compounds combined with positron emission tomography will allow future clinicians the ability to probe cerebral energy metabolism and design appropriate therapy, possibly by replacing depleted substrates. Intervention at the earliest stages in the development of cellular injury may demand that the focus of our therapy shift to the patient's first presentation in the Emergency Department or even to the scene of injury. As the complexity and urgency of therapy increases, the development of a local "neuro trauma" service consisting of field teams, emergency personnel, and neurosurgeons acting as a coordinated unit will enhance delivery of services to head injury victims. Just as the type and timing of surgery have become somewhat standardized within the past decade, so must protocols be organized to maximize cerebral recovery or, better yet, to prevent the cascades which promote CNS damage from occurring. Among the other early mechanical effects of trauma are vascular and cellular changes which promote shifts of water and various ions into and out of glia, neurons, and the interstitial space (42). Changes in vascular permeability will be addressed.

Fluid and solute movements occur as a consequence of early selective, and later generalized, changes in the blood-brain barrier (BBB) as suggested by Pardridge and others (33, 34). Dexamethasone may prove beneficial at these early stages of increased BBB permeability by blocking selective water transport (36). Beyond this particular use in "vasogenic" edema the role of steroids in head injury probably has no foundation in clinical or laboratory studies. The manipulation of two additional transport mechanisms may prove useful according to Pardridge, specifically, the polyamine and lactate systems. It is postulated that the basic amino acids arginine and ornithine provide substrates converted by CNS tissue into polyamines which themselves promote later changes in BBB permeability. These authors also suggest that enhancing lactate and ketone body transport across the BBB may provide a supplementary energy source inasmuch as brain can utilize these as well as glucose during times of increased metabolic demand.

The details of specific ionic movements following trauma are not precisely understood but these shifts, specifically of calcium (Ca^{2+}), appear to set the stage for a variety of secondary damaging effects. The accumulation of intraneuronal Ca^{2+} is likely a result of passive inflow from the extracellular environment driven by a 10,000-fold concentration gradient as well as its release from endoplasmic reticulum and mitochondria (41). Siesjo and Wieloch have suggested that failure of energy metabolism causes an outflow of intracellular potassium (K^+). As the extracellular K^+ exceeds about 10–15 μmol ml,$^{-1}$ voltage-dependent Ca^{2+} gates open allowing its pre- and postsynaptic entry (15). Presynaptic Ca^{2+} then triggers release of a variety of excitatory neurotransmitters (such as glutamate) which further enhances the inflow of postsynaptic Ca^{2+}. The considerable damage caused by this Ca^{2+} will be reviewed below, especially in relation to its effects on membranes.

The potential blockade of Ca^{2+} entry into neurons may be quite feasible with the newest generation of Ca^{2+} channel blocker, *e.g.*, diltiazem. In a primate model of induced ischemia the early data suggest that the severity of completed stroke as documented by brain mapping and neurological examination may be considerably less in the group treated with Ca^{2+} channel blockade. In such an experimental setting the biochemical manifestations of cerebral ischemia, notably, release of extracellular glutamate, appears to have been reduced (J. G. Frazee and P. S. Dwan, unpublished data, 1986). Glutamate and aspartate are also thought to act as agonists permitting the additional entry of Ca^{2+}. It is possible that the glutamate release blocker, baclofen, and the Ca^{2+} channel antagonist may act synergistically to reduce the Ca^{2+}-mediated cellular damage. Sequestered, mitochondrial Ca^{2+} already in the cell, of course, would not be reduced by the above means (38).

A wide variety of harmful intracellular events is triggered by the pathologic accumulation of Ca^{2+}. These include membrane phospholipid breakdown, inhibition of mitochondrial ATP production, destruction of the cytoskeleton, and protein phosphorylation.

The phospholipid constituents of cell membranes are in a dynamic process of reformation and dissolution. The entry of Ca^{2+} into cells activates phospholipases A and C which in turn promote membrane breakdown and ultimately prostaglandin synthesis and free oxygen radical formation (27, 43, 44). Ellis has demonstrated a rapid rise in brain prostaglandin following cerebral injury (13). These compounds have been shown to promote a variety of pathologic changes in cerebral vasculature, notably, long-term dilatation, and reduction of endothelial oxygen consumption (42). In experimental systems lithium has been shown to antagonize the Ca^{2+}-dependent activation of both phospholipases and may be of therapeutic benefit (Fig. 29.4) (16, 17). Free oxygen radical "scavengers" such as vitamin E may also prove useful at this early stage to help forestall membrane and vascular damage (23). As with the other therapies suggested above its early introduction systemically or locally within the subarachnoid space or ventricles would be necessary if its full benefits were to be realized.

Beyond the direct advantages to cerebral vasculature, the suppression of membrane breakdown would especially enhance the neurons' ability to maintain ionic gradients, and continue energy metabolism by mitochondria. The injured brain, however, shifts to anaerobic glycolysis in the absence of oxygen and glucose. An abrupt rise in the products of such glycolysis, including lactic acid, can be detected intercellularly and in the cerebrospinal fluid (CSF). Tissue acidosis is primarily due to this accumulation of lactate, although the influx of the hydrogen ion (H^+) also occurs after energy failure. The precise means by which lactate causes

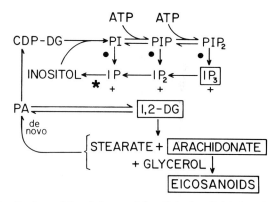

FIG. 29.4. Synthesis and breakdown of inositol. Agonist-induced calcium entry in trauma triggers activation of phospholipase A (●), and generation of second messengers (*enclosed in squares*). Lithium inhibits inositol-1-phosphate phosphatase which is responsible for resynthesis of inositol (★). Entry of inositol into CNS tissue is slow, and thus endogenous inositol formation is the rate-limiting step in subsequent synthesis of harmful second messengers which mobilize intracellullar Ca^{2+} stores. *Pl*, phosphatidylinositol; *PIP*, diphosphoinositide; *PIP₂*, phosphatidylinositol-4,5-biphosphate; *IP*, inositol-1-phosphate; *IP₂*, inositol-1,4-biphosphate; *IP₃*, inositol-1,4,5-triphosphate. CDP-DG, cytidine diphosphodiacyl glycerol. (Reproduced with permission from Hokin, L. E. Receptor and phosphoinositide generated second messengers. Annu. Rev. Biochem., *54:* 205–235, 1985. Copyright 1985 by Annual Reviews Inc.)

damage in injured or ischemic brain is unknown, but likely mechanisms include effects on mitochondrial function, cell volume control, postischemic blood flow, and free radical formation according to Rhencrona (37). Nevertheless, the severity of tissue acidosis has been correlated with poor outcome especially when tissue lactate exceeds 20 μmol/gm. Kalimo demonstrated that reperfusion caused lactate to be removed from brain and thus reversed the early histological effects of severe lactic acidosis (21).

Attempts to reverse lactic acidosis have recently focused on intra- and extracellular buffering agents especially tris hydroxymethyl aminomethane (THAM). This compound appears to be superior to other methods of correcting tissue acidosis such as hyperventilation, which produces secondary metabolic acidosis as compensation for the respiratory alkalosis. In a cat fluid percussion model the treatment group demonstrated a 60% survival rate compared with 20% in controls (1). In addition, ICP values were significantly ($p < 0.01$) less by 40%. Both experimentally and in initial clinical trials the ability to elevate arterial pH with THAM combined with mild hyperventilation proved greater than with hyperventilation alone. Clinical trials are underway to assess the role of reduction of tissue lactic acidosis in head injury.

Further reductions in cerebral lactic acidosis may be possible at present by simply controlling posttraumatic serum glucose. Animals made ischemic in the presence of hyperglycemia (glucose concentration of 28 μmol ml^{-1}) demonstrated a 4-fold increase in lactate over hypoglycemic animals (4.8 $vs.$ 20.7 μmol/gm) (38). The commonly observed steroid-induced hyperglycemia may well contribute to the persistence of damaging CNS acidosis. Serum and CSF electrolyte, glucose, pH, and pO_2, among other yet to be defined elements, constitutes the milieu in which potentially viable neurons and glia must attempt their recovery. Close attention to these systemic metabolic parameters may lessen secondary injury from edema and even enhance long-term structural recovery of axons.

Edema is both a consequence of the loss of cellular energy reserve seen in ischemia and trauma as well as a cause of subsequent cellular damage. Swelling occurs as Na^+ and Cl^- enter the astrocyte while entry of Ca^{2+} is largely confined to neurons (22). Siesjo, Cragoe, and others have suggested that two mechanisms produce this Na^+ entry (9, 38). The first is release by presynaptic endings of transmitters which stimulate membrane depolarization, and the second is tissue acidosis and resultant H^+ extrusion into the extracellular space, further driving Na^+ into glia. By employing agents which block the initial movement of Na^+ and H^+ across the glial membrane and by careful regulation of lactic acidosis as described above, one might halt the cascade of events which caused the formation of edema.

A wide variety of morphological changes has been observed following experimental head injury, mainly in the cat fluid percussion model (5). Neuronal and vascular alterations include dispersion of ribosomes and rough endoplasmic reticulum thinning (4). Of perhaps greater interest from a potential therapeutic viewpoint are the series of changes occurring in axons. These changes have been reviewed by Povlishock and others. Immediately after experimental injury no changes were seen in axons studied by electron microscopy (35). After 12–24 hours impairment of axoplasmic transport appeared along with clustering of organelles; however, the axon cylinders remained intact. Soon thereafter "axon ball" formation and gradual development of breaks in continuity are seen. This demonstrates that the initial blow does not tear or disrupt axons as had been earlier thought. Stretching appears to precipitate microscopic as well as functional changes (39). The more severe the stretch, the more likely one is to observe eventual axonal transection. Many regions of axon swelling give rise, within 2–3 weeks, to active sprouting which appears to be persistent. The fate of such newly generated sprouts is controversial, but the therapeutic implications are clear-cut. If a means can be found to induce such potential growth from damaged neuron processes, then potential repair may be possible. Recent evidence that stereotaxic implantation of fetal substantia nigra cells can lead to actual ingrowth, and incorporation of such cells raises the exciting possibility of implanting nerve growth trophic factors or even cultured neurons themselves into areas of damaged cortex. Even though highly speculative, such approaches clearly have a potential utility in lesions caused by processes other than trauma.

Beyond early surgical intervention and the future potential for therapy at the sites outlined above, attention must be focused on long-term consequences of head injury. The outcome of patients with head injury has been reviewed elsewhere (3). Intracranial mass lesions and increasing age correlate with poorer prognosis, and the majority of deaths occur within the first 48 hours (8). Good recovery or "moderate" disability will occur in 30–50% of patients, although the precise definition of either term varies among studies.

Deficits which develop as a result of focal cerebral damage such as epilepsy, paresis, dysphasia, and anosmia are more easily explained than disorders of intellect, behavior, and memory. Among survivors these latter deficits may impact heavily upon the ability to return to previous employment. Speculation on the cellular basis for these deficits might focus on long-term changes in synaptic activity and membrane permeability. Ca^{2+} is known to cause phosphorylation of a wide variety of proteins by activating protein kinases, an effect which persists long after the immediate ischemic episode has passed. Additionally, postsynaptic membranes in hippocampus may increase their affinity for glutamate by unmasking additional receptors as a further effect of Ca^{2+} according to Siesjo, Baudry, Lynch, and Halpain. The presence of increased sensitivity to an excitatory amino acid in temporal lobe structures has obvious implications for the promotion of seizures and possibly even personality disorders.

The proper function of both long- and short-term memory is disrupted to varying degrees, depending on the severity of head trauma. Ante- and retrograde amnesic effects are well known. Which processes are responsible for these lapses in memory? Recent evidence suggests that short-term memory (lasting hours) results from a covalent modification in intracellular proteins, while memory lasting days to months may require the induction of sequences of genes. Calcium plays a role in "intact" memory mechanisms by activating a series of proteases which leads to an increase in the number of glutamate receptors in the synaptic membranes thought to facilitate short- and long-term memory. Goelet, Castellucci, and others outline a series of events which results in the induction of specific messenger RNAs (mRNA), and ultimately new proteins (14, 40). Trauma has been shown to reduce protein synthesis by as much as 30% in rat cortex and brainstem (G. Gade, unpublished data, 1985). Future therapy may be directed at reversing or repairing many of these damaged protein synthetic functions.

CONCLUSIONS

Further advances in patient survival will arise from a better understanding of the mechanisms of cerebral injury. New means of surgical therapy may focus on the early evacuation of intracerebral hematomas, possibly by stereotaxic means. Future pharmacological intervention will be directed at preventing the various harmful "cascades" triggered by cerebral injury. Most of these are the result of early loss of energy stores, followed by ionic shifts (especially of Ca^{2+}), acidosis, changes in BBB permeability, cellular edema, membrane disruption, and effects on protein synthesis. Stimulation of normal reparative processes such as axonal sprouting may be a component of therapy in the future. Development of many of these treatments is currently feasible, but others will require major advances in all areas of neurobiology and will provide the clinician with an armamentarium of drugs which permits early and specific therapy.

REFERENCES

1. Becker, D. P. Acidosis in head injury. In: *Central Nervous System Trauma Status Report*, edited by D. P. Becker and J. T. Povlishock, Chap. 14. National Institutes of Health, National Institute of Neurological and Communicative Disorders and Stroke (NINCDS), Bethesda, Md., 1985.
2. Becker, D. P., and Miller, J. D. The outcome from severe head injury with early diagnosis and intensive management. J. Neurosurg., *47:* 491–502, 1977.
3. Becker, D. P., Miller, J. D., and Greenberg, R. P. Prognosis after head injury. In: *Neurological Surgery*, edited by J. A. Youmans, pp. 2137–2174. W. B. Saunders, Philadelphia, 1982.
4. Brown, L. J., Yoshida, N., Canty, T., *et al.* Experimental concussion: Ultrastructural and biochemical correlates. Am. J. Pathol., 67: 41–50, 1972.
5. Browning, M., Dunwiddie, T., Bennett, W., *et al.* Synaptic phosphoproteins: Specific changes after repetitive stimulation of the hippocampal slices. Science, *203:* 60–70, 1979.
6. Bruce, D. A., Langfitt, T. W., Miller, J. D., *et al.* Regional cerebral blood flow, intracranial pressure, and brain metabolism in comatose patients. J. Neurosurg., *38:* 131–144, 1973.
7. Bullock, R., Mendelow, A. D., Teasdale, G. M., *et al.* Intracranial hemorrhage induced at arterial pressure in the rat. Part 1. Neurol. Res., *6:* 184–188, 1984.
8. Carlsson, C. A., von Essen, C., Lofgren, J., *et al.* Factors affecting the clinical course of patients with severe head trauma. Part 1. Influence of biologic factors. Part 2. Significance of post traumatic coma. J. Neurosurg., *29:* 242–251, 1968.
9. Cragoe, E. T., Gould, N. D., Woltersdorf, O. W., *et al.* Agents for the treatment of brain injury. 1. (Aryloxy)alkanoic acids. J. Med. Chem., *25:* 567–574, 1981.
10. Dail, N. G., Feeney, P. M., Murray, H. M., *et al.* Responses to cortical injury. II. Widespread depression of the activity of an enzyme in cortex remote from a focal injury. Brain Res., *211:* 79–89, 1981.

11. Drejer, J., Beneviste, H., Diemer, N. H., *et al.* Cellular origin of ischemia induced glutamate released from brain tissue in vivo and in vitro. J. Neurochem., *45:* 145–151, 1985.
12. Ekelund, L., Nilsson, B., and Ponten, U. Carotid angiography after experimental head injury in the rat. Neuroradiology, *7:* 209–214, 1974.
13. Ellis, E. F., Wright, K. E., Wei, E. P., *et al.* Cyclooxygenase products of arachidonic acid metabolism in cat cerebral cortex after experimental brain injury. J. Neurochem., *37:* 892–896, 1981.
14. Goelet, P., Castellucci, V. F., Schacher, S., *et al.* The long and the short of long term memory—A molecular framework. Nature, *322:* 419–422, 1986.
15. Harris, R. J., Branston, N. M., Symon, L., *et al.* Changes in extracellular calcium activity in cerebral ischemia. J. Cereb. Blood Flow Metab., *1:* 203–210, 1981.
16. Hokin, L. E. Receptor and phosphoinositide generated second messengers. Annu. Rev. Biochem., *54:* 205–235, 1985.
17. Hubschman, O. R., and Nathanson, D. C. The role of calcium and cellular membrane dysfunction in experimental trauma and subarachnoid hemorrhage. J. Neurosurg., *62:* 698–703, 1985.
18. Huger, F., and Patrick, G. Effect of concussive head injury on central catecholamine levels and synthesis rates in rat brain regions. J. Neurochem., *33:* 89–95, 1979.
19. Jennett, B., and Teasdale, G. Prognosis of patients with severe head injury. Neurosurgery, *4:* 283–289, 1979.
20. Johnstone, G., Hailstone, M. H., and Freeman, C. Baclofen stereoselective inhibition of excitant amino acid release. J. Pharm. Pharmacol., *32:* 230–231, 1980.
21. Kalimo, H., Rhencrona, S., Soderfeldt, B., *et al.* Brain lactic acidosis and ischemic cell damage. 2. Histopathology. J. Cereb. Blood Flow Metab., *1:* 313–327, 1981.
22. Kimelberg, H. K., and Bourke, R. S. Mechanisms of astrocyte swelling. In: *Cerebral Ischemia*, edited by A. Bes, P. Braquet, R. Paoletti, and B. Siesjo, p. 131. Elsevier, Amsterdam, 1984.
23. Kontos, H. A., and Wei, E. P. Superoxide production in experimental brain injury. J. Neurosurg., *64:* 803–807, 1986.
24. Langfitt, N. Measuring the outcome from head injuries. J. Neurosurg., *48:* 673–678, 1978.
25. Levati, A., and Farina, M. Prognosis of severe head injuries. J. Neurosurg., *57:* 779–783, 1982.
26. Lillehei, K. O., and Hoff, J. T. Advances in the management of closed head injury. Ann. Emerg. Med., *14:* 789–795, 1977.
27. Meldrum, B., and Evans, T. Ischemic brain damage: The role of excitatory activity of calcium entry. Br. J. Anaesth., *57:* 44–46, 1985.
28. Mendelow, A. D., Bullock, R., *et al.* Intracranial haemorrhage induced at arterial pressure in the rat. Part 2. Neurol. Res., *6:* 189–193, 1984.
29. Miller, J. D. Head injury and brain ischemia. Br. J. Anaesth., *57:* 120–129, 1985.
30. Myers, R. E. A unitary theory of causation of anoxic and hypoxic brain pathology. Adv. Neurol., *26:* 195–217, 1979.
31. Nilsson, B., and Ponten, U. Experimental head injury in the rat. Part 2. Regional brain energy metabolism in concussive trauma. J. Neurosurg., *47:* 252–261, 1977.
32. Nilsson, B., and Ponten, U. Metabolism and neurophysiological function following head injury. In: *Central Nervous System Trauma Status Report*, edited by D. P. Becker and J. T. Povlishock, Chap. 28. National Institutes of Health, National Institute of Neurological and Communicative Disorders and Stroke (NINCDS), Bethesda, Md., 1985.

33. Pardridge, W. M. Brain metabolism: A perspective from the blood brain barrier. Physiol. Rev., *63:* 1481–1535, 1983.
34. Pardridge, W. M. Cerebral vascular permeability status in brain injury. In: *Central Nervous System Trauma Status Report*, edited by D. P. Becker and J. T. Povlishock, Chap. 36. National Institutes of Health, National Institute of Neurological and Communicative Disorders and Stroke (NINCDS), 1985.
35. Povlishock, J. T. The morphopathological responses to experimental head injuries of varying severity. In: *Central Nervous System Trauma Status Report*, edited by D. P. Becker and J. T. Povlishock, Chap. 30. National Institutes of Health, National Institute of Neurological and Communicative Disorders and Stroke (NINCDS), Bethesda, Md., 1985.
36. Reid, A. C., Teasdale, G. M., and McCulloch, J. The effects of dexamethasone administration and withdrawal on water permeability across the blood brain barrier. Ann. Neurol., *13:* 28–31, 1983.
37. Rhencrona, S. Brain acidosis. Ann. Emerg. Med., *14:* 770–776, 1985.
38. Siesjo, B. K., and Wieloch, T. Cerebral metabolism in ischemia: Neurochemical basis for therapy. Br. J. Anaesth., *57:* 47–62, 1985.
39. Thibault, L. E., and Gennarelli, T. A. Biomechanics and craniocerebral trauma. In: *Central Nervous System Trauma Status Report*, edited by D. P. Becker and J. T. Povlishock, Chap. 24. National Institutes of Health, National Institute of Neurological and Communicative Disorders and Stroke (NINCDS), Bethesda, Md., 1985.
40. Thompson, R. F. The neurobiology of learning and memory. Science, *233:* 941–947, 1985.
41. Walker, A. E., Kollros, J. J., and Case, T. J. The physiological basis of concussion. J. Neurosurg., *1:* 103–116, 1944.
42. Wei, E. P., Dietrich, W. D., and Povlishock, J. T. Functional, morphological, and metabolic abnormalities of the cerebral microcirculation after concussive brain injury in cats. Circ. Res., *46:* 37–47, 1980.
43. Wei, E. P., Lamb, R. G., and Kontos, H. A. Increased phospholipase C after experimental brain injury. Neurosurgery, *56:* 695–698, 1982.
44. Yoshida, S., Ikeda, M., Busto, R., *et al.* Cerebral phosphoinositide, triacylglycerol, and energy metabolism in reversible ischemia: Origin and rate of free fatty acids. J. Neurochem., *47:* 744–757, 1986.

The Neurosurgeon and Neurotrauma Care System Design

LAWRENCE H. PITTS, M.D.

Over 100,000 Americans die after trauma each year, and at least 25,000 or more are chronically institutionalized. Trauma accounts for more years of potential life lost than cancer and cardiovascular disease combined (Table 30.1) (13) because of its preponderance in the young (Table 30.2) (9). Head injury accounts for half or more of trauma deaths in most reported series, and for a majority of the disability incurred after injury. About 350–500 per 100,000 population are hospitalized each year after craniocerebral trauma (17). More people die from head injury than any other disorder treated by neurosurgeons, and trauma is second only to stroke as a cause of death from neurological diseases. In the aggregate, neurosurgeons spend almost 20% of their time treating patients with head and spinal cord injury (21).

Numerous authors have reported that the absence of regional trauma planning could result in as many as 20–30% more trauma deaths which might have been preventable (12, 28). Recent reports have noted significant improvement in trauma care where trauma centers existed (27) or after they were established (10, 11), including declines in preventable death rates (14% to 3%) and in suboptimally treated patients (32% to 4%) before and after institution of a regional trauma system (23). Such information has prompted many local, county, and State governments to begin design and enactment of trauma care systems. The necessary resources for optimal care of trauma patients have been specified by the American College of Surgeons Committee on Trauma (ACS-COT) (1, 4), and a number of hospitals are becoming trauma centers (15).

Central nervous system (CNS) damage is a major portion of serious trauma. However, there are far fewer neurosurgeons than other medical and surgical specialists who treat injury victims. In 1984, there were about 10 times as many Board-certified general surgeons and 6 times as many orthopaedists as the nearly 2800 neurosurgeons certified by the American Board of Neurological Surgery. Although not all general surgeons or orthopaedists treat trauma patients, neither do all neurosurgeons, making an even smaller group of surgeons treating CNS injuries.

TABLE 30.1

Potential Years of Life Lost before Age 65[a]

Trauma	41%
Cancer	18%
Heart disease	16%
All other	25%

[a] Modified from Center for Disease Control. Morb. Mort. Weekly Rep., *31:* 599, 1982.

TABLE 30.2

Percentage of Deaths from Various Causes[a]

Age	Injury	Cancer	Heart Disease	Other
1–4	46	7	4	43
5–14	55	14	3	28
15–24	79	5	3	13
25–34	62	10	6	22
35–44	31	21	20	28
45–64	7	32	36	25
65+	2	18	48	31

[a] Modified from Baker, S. P., O'Neill, B., and Karpf, R. *The Injury Fact Book.* Lexington Books, Lexington, Mass., 1984.

Since many hospitals are expanding their emergency medicine facilities as a source of new patients, and hospital staffs are asked to cover these emergency rooms (ER), the relative scarcity of neurosurgeons is even more noticeable. In some European countries, neurologists manage head injury patients not requiring surgery and, at times, they direct the postoperative care of patients with operated traumatic lesions. However, in agreement with the ACS-COT, neurosurgeons in the U.S. believe that "trauma is a surgical disease" and that neurotrauma is best treated by neurosurgeons.

Urgent or emergency treatment of traumatic injuries often disrupts the smooth pattern of routine medical care and elective surgery schedules during the day or, more commonly, preempts emergency medical and hospital resources and physician energies at night or on weekends (29), occurring at "unsocial hours" as noted by Bryan Jennett. For all of these reasons—the enormous impact of trauma on the public health particularly of the young, the prevalence of CNS injury in patients with severe trauma, the relatively small number of neurosurgeons available to treat trauma victims, and the strains placed on medical resources by the care of trauma and neurotrauma patients—it is imperative that trauma care planning in general and the neurosurgeon's role in particular be well defined in each locale to assure delivery of the quality of care that is now possible and that the public demands and deserves. Neurosurgeons must become involved in this planning process if their patients and their own needs and interests are to be met. The following elements should be considered during the planning process.

There have been explosive advances in the quality, diversity, and sophistication in emergency medical services (EMS) systems in the past decade which have had significant impact on a number of emergency medical problems (14). It is uncommon now for ambulance services to be staffed by firemen, policemen, or volunteers, although such staffing still may be found in rural areas. The overwhelming majority of EMSs are manned by highly trained professional paramedics or emergency medical technicians (EMTs) whose training programs include extensive exposure to didactic classroom presentations, practical clinical instruction, and on-the-job training in delivery of emergency medical care. These EMTs are all under a medical control structure which has ultimate responsibility for training and quality assurance, and it is this medical control structure through which EMTs must be coordinated with trauma-receiving facilities. There often is a fierce pride among paramedics and EMTs, and a careful balance must be struck between too lax and too tight a control on their activities. The former can lead to their making medical judgments too complex for their training, and the latter can preclude their exercising a good judgment under difficult circumstances in the field.

A number of important EMS issues must be addressed and settled during trauma system planning. Population density and distances to trauma facilities will dictate the style of initial EMS care. In urban environments, with designated trauma facilities nearby, a "scoop-and-run" technique will allow the most rapid delivery of critically injured patients to definitive care (18). In remote locations, more time probably should be spent "at the roadside" stabilizing the patient for a fairly long transport time by surface or air. An initial brief stop at a low level trauma facility may provide temporizing but lifesaving medical care such as placement of chest or endotracheal tubes, fracture splinting, or blood transfusions before transfer for definitive care. In suburban areas, careful guidelines must be established for EMS personnel, directing them to transport patients according to a defined local trauma care system, either to designated trauma hospitals or to nearby hospitals as best determined by the planning process.

An essential feature of an appropriate EMS response is patient evaluation and triage. Only some 8–10% of trauma patients require care at a Level 1 (1, 4) hospital (25). Inadequate triage either will send too many patients to Level 1 facilities with overutilization of costly resources when a lower level facility could deliver proper and more economical care; or it will send too few patients to Level 1 facilities, with some severely injured patients arriving at hospitals unable to manage them properly. Neurosurgeons, in their planning efforts, should define proper triage tools for neurological injuries and instruct EMS personnel in their use. It has been proposed, for example, that patients with a Glascow Coma Score (24) of less than 13 be taken to a Level 1 facility (2). Triage tools for trauma outside the nervous system also have been developed and should be considered by other surgeons in the trauma planning process (8).

In summary, neurosurgeons have a responsibility to develop and review EMS protocols regarding care of patients with neural trauma, and for EMS personnel training in evaluation and triage of neurologic injuries.

EMERGENCY ROOM ORGANIZATION

Since the founding of the American Board of Emergency Medicine in 1976, there has been a remarkable growth of the number of physicians who practice emergency medicine only. A number of emergency medicine residencies and fellowships have been developed nationwide, and research in delivery of emergency care has been conducted. These new emergency medical specialists have diverse training backgrounds, variously including general and thoracic surgery, medicine, pediatrics, or emergency medicine. Emergency resuscitation after major trauma is exacting and complex, and the spectrum of traumatic injuries demands considerable diagnostic skill. In the absence of a trauma surgeon, properly trained ER personnel, including emergency physicians, are required for optimum delivery of trauma care (26), and they are an invaluable resource in the immediate management of neurotrauma patients.

The ACS-COT Hospital Resources guidelines (1, 4), recognizing the prevalence and urgency of severe neurologic injury, require that a neurosurgeon be "in-house" in Level 1 and Level 2 facilities. Because it is impossible for fully trained neurosurgeons to be physically present in all of the trauma facilities across the country, provisions have been made to meet this in-house requirement by nonneurosurgeons who are approved by that hospital's Chief of Neurosurgery as being able to initiate immediate therapy and diagnostic procedures while the neurosurgeon is *en route* to the hospital after his presence is requested by ER personnel. In teaching hospitals, this function may be fulfilled by resident house staff or an in-house surgeon or emergency physician (Level 1 and 2 hospitals, respectively) who have been trained by the hospital's neurosurgeons to begin care of neurologic injury. It obviously is critical that the trauma facility's neurosurgical staff either provide neurosurgical coverage under their direct supervision, or train in-house trauma physicians to begin the therapy and diagnostic procedures most appropriate for the patient.

There is no question that outcome after severe head injury correlates adversely with shock and hypoxia (16, 22), and these secondary insults must be addressed aggressively in prehospital and emergency room neurotrauma care. Life-threatening hemorrhage or respiratory problems must be corrected immediately regardless of the neurologic status. Sequential neurologic evaluations carefully documented can be used to ascertain improvement or worsening and will dictate subsequent patient management.

Depending on the degree of neurologic abnormality or evidence of external injury, a number of diagnostic and/or therapeutic pathways may be taken. In patients who are either comatose or have significant mental status alterations, computed tomographic (CT) scanning is done routinely. If a patient rapidly becomes comatose or has signs of transtentorial herniation or brain stem compression with clear-cut evidence of trauma, diagnostic burr holes can be done without CT scanning and probably will reduce the time required to obtain brain decompression by craniotomy (6). Patients with altered mental status following a generalized seizure should improve within an hour of seizure, and patients who are intoxicated should improve over 2–3 hours of observation; their initial management may include serial observation. However, if they do not improve within these general time frames and there is evidence of head injury, CT scanning should be considered to rule out intracranial pathology requiring urgent attention. Specific protocols can be developed to determine those patients who routinely require admission and those who can be observed initially in the ER. It is incumbent upon neurosurgeons to help develop these protocols and, by instruction and monitoring of ER personnel, ensure that the protocols are followed. Since many patients with minor head injury can be treated appropriately without neurosurgery consultation, it is important that neurosurgeons help define who those patients are and encourage trauma physicians and ER physicians to treat them without consultation. Proper instruction of physicians who first see patients in the ER setting will reduce the number of unnecessary calls that neurosurgeons receive and more appropriately will allow their time to be spent on patients with significant head injuries best treated by neurosurgeons.

Thus, the neurosurgeon's role in the emergency management of patients with head injury is to help define appropriate patient categories and establish protocols for their diagnostic and therapeutic management, to instruct ER personnel in the use of their protocols and, finally, to monitor periodically the skill with which these protocols are carried out.

OPERATING ROOM ORGANIZATION

It is possible for the vast majority of hospitals in the U.S. to acquire necessary operating room (OR) equipment to manage even the most severe of traumatic injuries, including cardiac bypass capabilities. Proper neurosurgical equipment will be available in any OR where a full spectrum of elective neurosurgery cases are treated. Most neurotrauma cases do not require a microscope or microsurgical instruments, although they should be readily available if needed. Intraoperative ultrasound is being used more frequently for intracerebral hematomas or foreign bodies, and to insure adequate spinal canal decompression, and should be available if requested by the neurosurgeon. X-ray technicians and equipment should be available for intraoperative radiographs when requested.

Equipment generally is not a problem, but OR staffing certainly can be. For Level I and II trauma hospitals, an OR must be available *at all times* for emergency thoracotomy, laparotomy, or craniotomy, and appropriate anesthesia and nursing personnel must be available and in-house for such cases. It is unpopular, and certainly expensive, to commit resources in such a standby mode unless they are used frequently. Surgeons, particularly those with no interest in trauma care, seeking daytime elective OR time have little sympathy with the notion of an OR standing idle "waiting for a trauma case" when they could use it immediately if allowed to do so. Hospital administrators understandably would like to minimize salary costs for in-house anesthesia and nursing staff, but cannot reduce available personnel too much without losing the ability to initiate *immediate* surgery when needed. At least some minimal annual number of trauma cases is necessary for proper OR staffing to be cost-effective and to perform efficiently when emergency treatment is done. Neurosurgeons and their trauma colleagues must assure themselves of proper and timely hospital support for operative cases, or refuse to support trauma designation at that institution. Differences in institution commitment to OR, ER, and intensive care unit (ICU) staffing often will allow selection of the most appropriate institution for designation as a trauma-receiving facility, and neurosurgeons can best determine an institution's commitment to care of the neurotrauma patient.

NEUROTRAUMA INTENSIVE CARE

Intensive care management of trauma patients has changed dramatically in the past decade. Substantial numbers of intensive care unit (ICU) beds have been added in most acute care hospitals, having the effect of improving intensive management of critically ill patients but usually lowering the acuity of care of patients on general medical or surgical wards. Substantial technological advancements in physiologic monitoring and cardiopulmonary care have evolved in ICUs. Finally, with relatively large numbers of critically ill patients in ICUs, critical care specialists have arisen from a number of medical specialties, including neurosurgery, surgery, anesthesia, internal medicine, and pediatrics. In some institutions, neurological ICUs have remained under the direct control of neurologists and neurosurgeons, some of whom have had special fellowship training in intensive care. In other instances, local use of consultation from anesthesiologists, internists, and others has provided additional skills in appropriate cases.

As in other areas of planning for the care of the neurotrauma patient, individual neurosurgeons must assess their own skills and availability in deriving a plan for the optimum management of patients with neurotrauma.

No physician is better prepared than the neurosurgeon for the management of critically ill patients with nervous system injury. Assessment of patient status, particularly neurologic deterioration, should fall in his purview. Since the management of neurologic injury sometimes is at odds with the management of other problems, and since neurologic injury so commonly dictates eventual patient outcome, the neurosurgeon must maintain an important influence in patient management as long as the nervous system is physiologically unstable. For instance, in many cases of general trauma, fluid management can be quite liberal, and large fluid volumes commonly are used in resuscitation and in the acute phase of trauma management. However, when nervous system injury is present, overhydration in some patients can lead to increased cerebral swelling, particularly if serum sodium falls. The mild hypotension seen with many cervical spinal cord injuries is either best untreated or treated with low doses of vasopressor agents after possible internal hemorrhage has been excluded, instead of with infusion of large fluid volume so routinely used by trauma surgeons when hypotension is present. No other specialist will appreciate as well as the neurosurgeon some of these nuances of therapy and, thus, the neurosurgeon has an important role and obligation in the intensive management of patients with nervous system injuries.

Several different styles of organization can accomplish the above goal. When trauma is limited to nervous system injury, the neurosurgeon likely will be the patient's primary physician. By local agreement, in an ICU well staffed with specialists in intensive medicine, the neurotrauma patient may be managed jointly by the neurosurgeon and intensivist with each managing their areas of expertise. When such intensive care is not available or when the neurosurgeon has sufficient skills and is available, he may wish to manage the patient entirely without assistance from other specialists.

When multiple trauma is involved, the management scheme in the preceding paragraph may still pertain if the nervous system injury is the dominant injury. In this situation, the neurosurgeon still may be the primary or almost sole physician director, relying on other specialists in a relatively limited fashion. As the severity of injury to other organ systems increases, the neurosurgeon is progressively less likely to manage these non-CNS injuries by himself.

The ACS-COT guidelines (1, 4) require that a Trauma Service be an organizational unit of Level I and Level II trauma facilities. When such a service exists, multiple trauma victims often are managed by the "trauma team" (19) with essential input from other specialists such as neurosurgeons, urologists, and orthopaedic surgeons. Such an organization has been reported to reduce ICU mortality in severely injured patients (7). In many instances, as the various injuries become less acute, the patient eventually is transferred to the care of the specialist with the greatest expertise in caring for the most problematic residual injury, *e.g.*, an orthopaedist for the management of complex unstable fractures. Because of the prevalence in severity of injuries to the brain and spinal cord, often the patient is transferred to a neurosurgery service for management after the other organ injuries have become stable. This "trauma team" concept has been very successful in a large number of trauma centers. However, for it to work satisfactorily, there has to be a strong commitment by the hospital's surgical staff. In these instances, the trauma team becomes an important resource for managing patients with complex injuries. The neurosurgeon is an important member of this team whenever CNS injuries are present, and he or she can beneficially affect the management of the patient's neurologic injuries. If a well-developed trauma team does not exist in a given hospital, the neurosurgeon may need to become the trauma team leader and organize inputs from the various appropriate specialties in the management of a given patient. This is an arduous task in patients with multiple complex injuries that must fall to a surgeon skilled in the management of trauma who, in some institutions, will be the neurosurgeon.

Since the neurosurgeon will almost never be in the ICU on a full-time basis, he or she has an important additional role in planning ICU care in the form of nursing and staff education. The neurosurgeon should help develop charting and record-keeping in the ICU so that adverse changes in a patient's status can be appreciated using routine methods of neurologic status recording such as the Glasgow Coma Score and standardized muscle strength testing. Once appropriate scales have been incorporated into patient observation charts, the nursing staff must be instructed in their use. It is imperative that ICU physician and nursing staffs be able to evaluate neurosurgical patients adequately so that they can accurately detect patient deterioration and notify the neurosurgeon promptly. After the neurosurgeon has instituted appropriate instruction of the nursing staff in the proper use of neurological observation tools, he then should help monitor their use periodically to insure that their use is appropriate and adequate.

The neurosurgeon also needs to standardize management protocols insofar as possible. If intracranial pressure monitoring (ICP) is used in a given hospital, monitoring technique and ICP management protocols must be devised so that the nursing staff is competent in their use. Careful instruction of nurses to increase their skills and allay their fears will produce valuable allies for the neurosurgeon and his patients in the ICU.

RELATIONSHIPS AMONG HOSPITALS

Not all hospitals are able to or wish to participate in a region's trauma system. As noted above, there often will not be enough neurosurgeons in a given area to staff adequately all those hospitals which do seek trauma facility status. Finally, there will be instances when a trauma facility's neurosurgeon is unavoidably unavailable, such as with an ongoing trauma case, and adequate neurosurgical backup cannot be obtained. In all of these instances, it will be necessary to transfer patients with CNS trauma with or without other organ involvement to another facility inside or outside of that region for definitive neurosurgical care. Appropriate plans must be made in advance for orderly transfer of such patients under medical control to other facilities where prompt neurosurgical attention is available (5).

When a neurosurgeon who is responsible for trauma coverage at a given trauma receiving facility is unavailable, he should notify the hospital and try to work with them to secure adequate coverage until he is again available (3). In some cases, for limited periods of time one of the other neurosurgeons on the call schedule might be able to provide temporary coverage. If such coverage cannot be obtained, trauma cases involving the nervous system should be diverted to the nearest trauma receiving facility that does have coverage at that time. As soon as neurosurgical coverage is available at the first hospital, the diversion can be cancelled, and trauma patients can be received in the usual fashion. Emergency medical services should be notified when diversion is *temporarily in place* so that they can most expeditiously take a trauma victim to the appropriate facility without the potentially disastrous delay of taking a patient to a first facility only to find that adequate care cannot be delivered.

This sort of structure and written transfer agreements must be designed and implemented in advance, including appropriate financial agreements if a local or regional government is financially responsible for a patient's emergency medical care. Prearrangement will avoid potentially life-threatening delays which can occur shortly after injury. These matters cannot be dealt with smoothly at night or on weekends when most trauma occurs, and adequate planning is necessary for smooth transfers or diversions to occur.

CONCLUSIONS

For optimal care of neurotrauma, the neurosurgeon has an obligation to develop and implement schemes for emergency and urgent neurosurgical care. This must be done in advance of the need for such systems and further requires that a region's neurosurgeons and other trauma surgeons monitor the system that they have planned to assure its efficacy (18). The planning process requires that neurosurgeons assess their region's needs and their own ability to meet those needs. They must determine how many hospitals are required to provide appropriate trauma care availability and how they will staff those hospitals. This may exclude some facilities from providing trauma care for lack of adequate neurosurgical coverage. A designation of trauma facilities is a political process, and neurosurgeons should learn how to have their recommendations accepted and acted upon by regional and State trauma system directors. This obviously will be done best when neurosurgeons speak with a unified voice. It is in their and their patients' interest for neurosurgeons to agree to a single plan and then strive to have it accepted by other parts of the trauma care system.

The five particular areas which require neurosurgeons' involvement in planning include: (a) development and implementation of EMS protocols regarding neurotrauma; (b) ER management, including resuscitation and initiation of diagnostic procedures; (c) appropriate operating room organization that will allow immediate surgical care of appropriate patients; (d) Trauma Service and ICU organizational design to insure appropriate neurosurgical input in the care of the trauma victim; and (e) development of diversion and transfer plans when usual neurosurgical coverage at a trauma facility is unavoidably unavailable.

Trauma is a surgical disease, and neurotrauma should be treated preponderantly by neurosurgeons. Their involvement in neurotrauma care planning will best insure their appropriate dominance in this area and assure optimum care for their injured patients.

REFERENCES

1. American College of Surgeons Committee on Trauma. Hospital and prehospital resources for optimal care of the injured patient. Bull. Am. Coll. Surg., 71: 4–12, 1986.
2. American College of Surgeons Committee on Trauma. Hospital and prehospital resources for optimal care of the injured patient. Appendix F. Field categorization of trauma patients. Bull. Am. Coll. Surg., 71: 17–21, 1986.
3. American College of Surgeons Committee on Trauma. Hospital and prehospital resources for optimal care of the injured patient. Appendix I. Planning neurotrauma care. Bull. Am. Coll. Surg., 71: 22–23, 1986.
4. American College of Surgeons Committee on Trauma. *Hospital and prehospital resources for optimal care of the injured patient.* American College of Surgeons, Chicago, in press, 1987.
5. American College of Surgeons Committee on Trauma. Hospital and prehospital re-

sources for optimal care of the injured patient. Appendix C. Interhospital transfer of patients. American College of Surgeons, Chicago, 1987.

6. Andrews, B. T., Pitts, L. H., Lovely, M. P., et al. Is computed tomographic scanning necessary in patients with tentorial herniation? Results of immediate surgical exploration without computed tomography in 100 patients. Neurosurgery, 19: 408–414, 1986.

7. Baker, C. C., Degutes, L. D., DeSantis, J., et al. Impact of a trauma service on trauma care in a university hospital. Am. J. Surg., 149: 453–458, 1985.

8. Baker, S. P., and O'Neill, B. The injury severity score: An update. J. Trauma, 16: 882, 1976.

9. Baker, S. P., O'Neill, B., and Karpf, R. The Injury Fact Book. Lexington Books, Lexington, Ma., 1984.

10. Cales, R. H. Trauma mortality in Orange County: The effect of implementation of a regional trauma system. Ann. Emerg. Med., 13: 1–10, 1984.

11. Cales, R. H., Anderson, P. G., and Heilig, R. W. Utilization of medical care in Orange County: The effect of implementation of a regional trauma system. Ann. Emerg. Med., 14: 853–858, 1985.

12. Cales, R. H., and Trunkey, D. D. Preventable trauma deaths: A review of trauma care systems development. J.A.M.A., 254: 1059–1063, 1985.

13. Center for Disease Control. Morb. Mort. Weekly Rep., 31: 599, 1982.

14. Craren, E. J., Ornato, J. P., and Nelson, N. M. The investment. J. Emerg. Med. Serv., 5: 35–38, 1985.

15. Dunn, E. L., Berry, P. H., and Cross, R. E. Community hospital to trauma center. J. Trauma, 26: 733–737, 1986.

16. Eisenberg, H. M. Outcome after head injury: General considerations. In Central Nervous System Trauma Status Report 1985, edited by D. P. Becker and J. T. Povleshock. Prepared for the National Institute of Neurological and Communicative Disorders and Stroke, National Institutes of Health, pp. 271–280.

17. Frankowski, R. F., Annegers, J. F., and Whitman, S. Epidemiological and descriptive studies: The descriptive epidemiology of head trauma in the United States. In Central Nervous System Trauma Status Report 1985, edited by D. P. Becker and J. T. Povleshock. Prepared for the National Institute of Neurological and Communicative Disorders and Stroke, National Institutes of Health, pp. 33–43.

18. Lewis, F. R. Prehospital intravenous fluid therapy: Physiologic computer modelling. J. Trauma, 26: 804–811, 1986.

19. Maull, K. I., and Haynes, B. W. The integrated trauma service concept. J.A.C.E.P., 6: 497–499, 1977.

20. Maull, K. I., Schwab, C. W., McHenry, S. D., et al. Trauma center verification. J. Trauma, 26: 521–524, 1986.

21. Mendenhall, R. C., Watts, C., Radecki, S. E., et al. Neurosurgery in the United States: Log-diary study. Neurosurgery, 8: 267–276, 1981.

22. Miller, J. D., Sweet, R. C., Narayan, R., et al. Early insults to the injured brain. J.A.M.A., 240: 439–442, 1978.

23. Shackford, S. R., Hollingworth-Fridlund, P., Cooper, G. F., et al. The effect of regionalization upon the quality of trauma care as assessed by concurrent audit before and after institution of a trauma system: A preliminary report. J. Trauma, 26: 812–820, 1986.

24. Teasdale, G., and Jennett, B. Assessment of coma and impaired consciousness: A practical scale. Lancet, 2: 81–84, 1974.

25. Thompson, C. T. Trauma care: Commitment to excellence. Ann. Emerg. Med., 9: 538, 1980.

26. Thompson, C. T. The emergency physician, the trauma surgeon, and the trauma center. Ann. Emerg. Med., *12:* 235–237, 1983.
27. West, J. G., Cales, R. H., and Gazzaniga, A. B. Impact of regionalization: The Orange County experience. Arch. Surg., *118:* 740–744, 1983.
28. West, J. G., Trunkey, D. D., and Lim, R. C. Systems of trauma care—A study of two counties. Arch. Surg., *114:* 455, 1979.
29. Young, J. S., Burns, P. E., Bowen, A. M., *et al.* Spinal Cord Injury Statistics. Good Samaritan Medical Center, Phoenix, Ariz., 1982.

31

Nonoperative Management of Cervical Spine Injuries

VOLKER K.H. SONNTAG, M.D., F.A.C.S., and
MARK N. HADLEY, M.D.

INTRODUCTION

The incidence of spinal column trauma in the U.S. is approximately 5 per 100,000 of population. Many of these injuries involve the cervical spine and have a high associated incidence of paralysis and death. After cervical spine trauma, the neurological morbidity is between 45 and 60%; the mortality has been reported to be as high as 17% (5, 6, 28). Males are much more likely to sustain vertebral column trauma, particularly between the ages of 15 and 25 years. The most common causes of cervical spine injury are motor vehicle accidents, followed by falls and athletic-recreational accidents (5, 16, 18, 28, 37).

Nearly half of the patients who sustain cervical spine trauma will present without evidence of neurological injury (5, 28). That 10% of the patients in one review developed symptoms of cervical cord compression during evaluation in the emergency room or during some later phase of their hospitalization underscores the importance of proper cervical spine immobilization, careful and compulsive evaluation, and effective stabilization once the diagnosis is clear (29).

In this review we describe the common injuries of the cervical spinal column and outline which types of injuries may be managed optimally by nonoperative means. Treatment (nonsurgical *vs.* surgical) for a specific type of injury is often controversial and depends on the level and type of fracture, the presence of subluxation or instability, the patient's general physical condition, and his neurological status. These issues will be discussed later in this chapter.

EVALUATION

A high index of suspicion of spinal injury must be maintained until cervical fracture or instability can be ruled out by radiography. Immobilization of the head and neck with respect to the torso is essential during the initial resuscitation and evaluation of the patient. That 60% of patients with cervical fractures have other major organ system trauma highlights the importance of basic life support and resuscitation to avoid the potentially deleterious effects of hypoxia, hypovolemia, and hypotension on spinal cord function (28). Detailed serial neurological examinations document the patient's functional ability and serve as a reference for further determinations of recovery (or loss) of neurological function.

The radiographic evaluation of the cervical spine includes anteroposterior and lateral roentgenograms from the occiput through the first thoracic vertebra (34, 36). Open mouth or pillar views of the odontoid should be included. Areas of suspected pathology should be studied with thin-section, high-resolution computed tomography (CT) (1, 7, 8, 21). We obtain the CT evaluation before proceeding to dynamic flexion and extension radiographs (when indicated) and before obtaining myelographic, angiographic, or magnetic resonance studies (depending on individual patient pathology).

Every attempt should be made to achieve fracture-dislocation reduction with restoration of anatomic alignment early in the patient's hospital course (5, 10, 37). Traction with Gardner-Wells tongs (GWT) is usually effective for reduction but requires monitoring the patient closely. Immobilization of the head and neck with respect to the torso can be a problem despite GWT in the combative or uncooperative patient, partic-

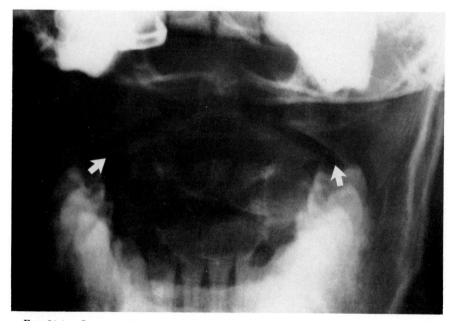

FIG. 31.1.   Open mouth x-ray of atlas-axis. The sum of the atlas-axis overlap (*arrows*) exceeds 7.0 mm.

ularly if a small amount of weight is required for reduction. We often place difficult patients with cervical spine instability in a rigid collar and sandbag both sides of the patient's head and neck (in addition to the GWT). These are the patients we attempt to immobilize with rigid external stabilization (halo vest) early in their hospital course to prevent subluxation and potential neurological injury (even if they are surgical candidates waiting for surgery). We treat patients with cervical spine injuries that require GWT in the intensive care unit (ICU) on a Stokes bed. The ICU setting also allows prompt treatment of spinal shock when present, promotes early prophylactic pulmonary-respiratory therapy, and facilitates treatment of other associated injuries. Of patients with a cervical spine fracture, 5–15% will have a second vertebral column fracture, an incidence that warrants a complete spinal column radiographic survey in suspected patients (11, 16, 28).

CERVICAL SPINE INJURIES

Atlas

Fractures of the atlas are uncommon and are rarely associated with neurological deficits (5, 32). The spinal cord injury service at our institution has treated 860 cervical spine fractures in the last 10 years

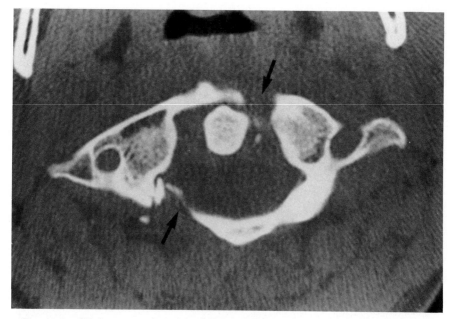

Fig. 31.2.   CT documentation of the Jefferson atlas fracture with multiple ring fractures (*arrows*).

(January 1976–January 1986), and only 42 (5%) were C1 fractures. Bursting fractures of the atlas were first reported by Jefferson (19). Other types of fractures, including unilateral arch fractures, have since been recognized (5, 19, 32, 35). Cadaver studies suggest that rupture of the transverse ligament causes instability at C1-C2 (35). If the lateral masses are spread by more than 7.0 mm (sum of the atlas-axis overlap on each side on the AP radiograph) (Figs. 31.1 and 31.2), the transverse ligament is no longer intact. Fractures with less lateral displacement are associated with less ligamentous disruption and may require less aggressive treatment (Figs. 31.3 and 31.4). The treatment of patients with atlas fractures with rotatory atlantoaxial dislocations, those with combinations C1 and C2 fractures, and those with persistent symptoms despite nonoperative therapy represent more complex management problems: Appropriate therapy must be individualized (5, 22, 26, 32, 35).

Axis

The unique anatomy and articulations of the axis predispose it to a variety of traumatic injuries (2). The second cervical vertebra is a common level of injury and represents 14–17.5% of all cervical fractures (2, 9, 16, 22). Axis fractures are known to occur in all age groups. We have reported the youngest patient—a 2 month old with a Hangman's

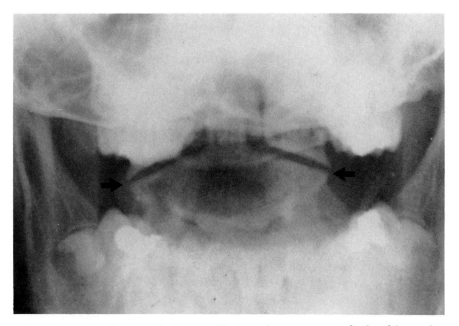

FIG. 31.3.   AP radiograph of atlas-axis. The lateral masses are not displaced (*arrows*).

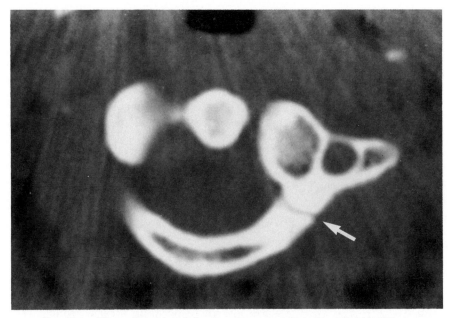

FIG. 31.4.   The unilateral arch fracture (*arrow*) of C1 is identified by CT.

fracture (16). Our oldest patient was a 94-year-old with an odontoid Type
II injury. Odontoid fractures are the most frequent type of C2 fracture
(2, 3, 9, 12, 16). In our series of 150 axis fractures, 86 were fractures of
the dens. Type II odontoid fractures were most common (67%) (Fig.
31.5), followed by Type III fractures (33%) (Fig. 31.6). We have not
encountered Type I odontoid fractures and we question whether they
exist (Table 31.1).

Miscellaneous fractures of the axis (non-odontoid, non-Hangman's
axis fractures) represent 22% of all C2 fractures. The most common
types are those involving the body and lateral mass (Figs. 31.7 and 31.8)
(15, 16). More force may be required to generate a body, pedicle, or
lateral mass axis fracture than that which results in an odontoid fracture.
In our series, miscellaneous fractures had 10 times the incidence of
associated neurological injury when compared to odontoid fractures
(Table 31.2).

Hangman's fractures, bilateral fractures through the pars interarticularis of the axis (Fig. 31.9), represented 21% of the 150 axis fractures we
reviewed. Neurological injury from a Hangman's fracture is rare because
the nature of the fracture essentially decompresses the spinal cord at the
C2 level (14, 16, 30, 31).

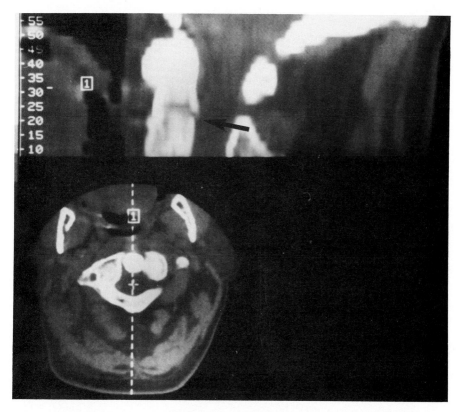

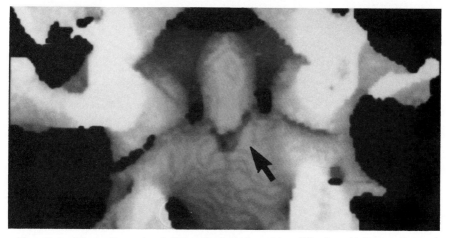

FIG. 31.6.   Three-dimensional CT study depicting a Type III odontoid fracture (*arrow*) (the fracture extends into the body of the axis).

TABLE 31.1

Cervical Fractures (N = 860) (January 1976–January 1986)

Level		No. of Patients	Percentage (%)
Axis		42	5.0
Atlas		150	17.5
Odontoid I	0		
Odontoid II	58		
Odontoid III	28		
Hangman's	31		
Miscellaneous	33		
C3-T1[a]		668	77.5

[a] Does not include isolated T1 fractures but includes fracture-dislocations at C7-T1.

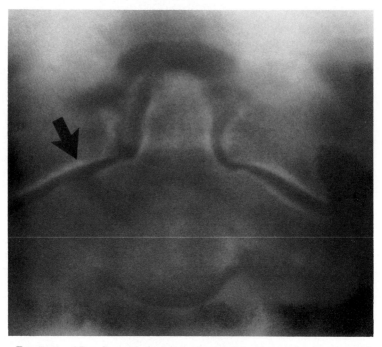

FIG. 31.7. AP radiograph depicting the axis lateral mass fracture (*arrow*).

Cervical Three through Thoracic One

A wide variety of fracture types occur between C3 and T1. Of the 300 acute cervical spine fractures reported by Bohlman, 76% were between these two levels (5, 6). This coincides with our experience, in which 77.5% of 860 cervical fractures were nonatlas, nonaxis injuries. The most common site of cervical vertebral body fracture is C5. The most common level of subluxation is at the C5-C6 interspace (37).

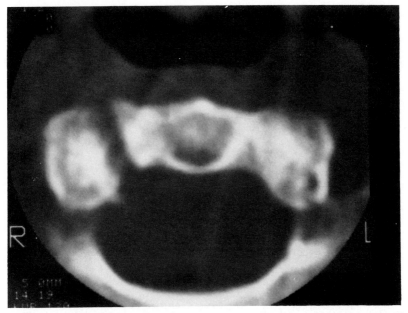

FIG. 31.8.   CT scan demonstrates the miscellaneous axis fracture (lateral mass) without dislocation or fragmentation.

TABLE 31.2

Neurological Injury—C2 Fractures

Odontoid fractures	1.2% (1/86)
Hangman's fractures	0% (0/31)
Miscellaneous fractures	12.0%[a] (4/33)

[a] Particularly with body, lateral mass fractures.

The incidence of neurological injury is considerably higher between C3 and T1 than it is for fractures at the two higher cervical levels (5, 6, 37). The most common injury patterns—in order of decreasing frequency— are fractures and/or subluxation of the articular processes (including unilateral and bilateral locked facets), fractures of a vertebral body, fractures of a lamina, spinous process fractures, and pedicle fractures (5). Subluxation complicating a vertebral column fracture increases both the likelihood and severity of the neurological injury (5, 6, 37). Subluxation involving the articular processes with facet dislocation and lock is particularly likely to be associated with neurological morbidity (33, 37). Of 31 patients in our series with bilateral locked facets, 1 was neurologically intact; 5 had incomplete myelopathies; and 25 had complete neurological injuries.

Few generalizations can be made regarding nonoperative *vs.* operative treatment of fractures and dislocations between C3 and T1. The specific

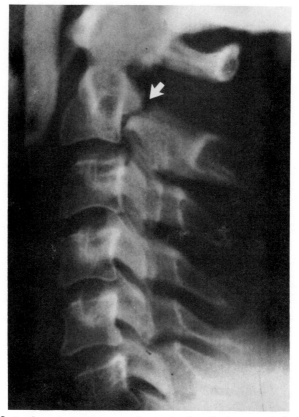

FIG. 31.9.   Lateral cervical spine x-ray demonstrating the hangman's fracture (*arrow*).

fracture type, the neurological condition of the patient, and the presence of associated traumatic injuries require individualization of treatment at each occurrence (5, 6, 10). Several guidelines, however, may assist the decision-making process. These will be outlined in the following section.

NONOPERATIVE THERAPY

Atlas fractures and dislocations are effectively treated with nonoperative external immobilization (Fig. 31.10). Rarely, severely comminuted fractures will fail to heal after a period of external immobilization, and surgical stabilization will be required (5, 26). A Philadelphia collar or another rigid neck brace is used for atlas fractures with less than 7.0 mm of lateral mass dislocation. Dislocations that measure greater than 7.0 mm are treated with the halo vest. The duration of therapy in the latter example is 10–12 weeks.

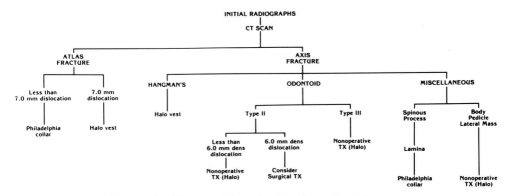

FIG. 31.10.   Treatment algorithm for atlas and axis fractures.

Several types of axis fractures are best treated by nonoperative means, including hangman's fractures, odontoid Type III fractures, and miscellaneous axis fractures (Fig. 31.10) (2, 14, 15, 16). All 31 patients with Hangman's fractures that we have treated had bony union and stability with external immobilization. We noted a shorter median duration of treatment with the halo vest (11 weeks) than with the SOMI (sternal occipital mandibular immobilizer) brace (14 weeks).

Odontoid Type III fractures rarely lead to nonunion or long-term instability if adequately immobilized with an external brace (16). Only 1 of 28 patients (3.5%) in our series required operative reduction and fusion. All others were treated effectively with external immobilization (26 halo, 1 SOMI) for 10–13 weeks duration.

We have treated 33 patients with miscellaneous fractures of the axis; 32 were stable with bony union after external immobilization. The majority of these fractures require treatment with a halo brace; however, treatment must be individualized according to the severity of the axis fracture. Obviously, an isolated lamina or spinous process fracture will not require the same type of immobilization or duration of therapy required to treat a lateral mass fracture with a 3-mm C2-C3 subluxation. One of the 33 patients we treated required late operation for nonunion after 15 weeks of halo vest immobilization. She had a C2 body fracture and a 4 mm C2-C3 subluxation.

The optimal treatment of odontoid Type II fractures has been the subject of considerable controversy. Patients' characteristics (age and neurological examination) and the degree and direction of the dens dislocation have been cited as criteria that help guide subsequent therapy (2, 3, 9, 12, 13, 16, 23). We discovered that the degree of dens dislocation was the single most important factor when considering the efficacy of nonsurgical therapy (Fig. 31.11) (16). Individuals with odontoid Type II

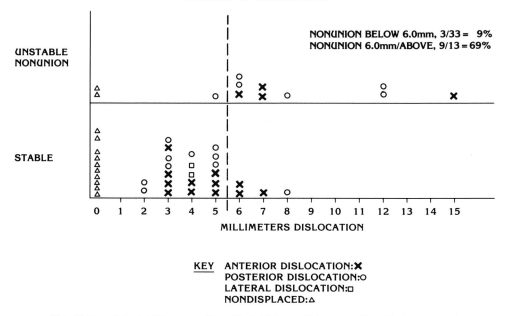

FIG. 31.11. Odontoid fractures, Type II: stability *vs.* dislocation. Graphic demonstration of the relationship between nonunion and the degree of dens dislocation for Type II fractures.

fractures with the dens dislocated less than 6.0 mm had only a 9% nonunion rate compared to a 69% nonunion rate for patients with a dens dislocation of 6.0 mm or greater, irrespective of the patient's neurological status or the direction of the dens dislocation ($p < 0.01$, chi square = 16.984). The age of the patient may be a factor when considering optimal therapy. Patients over 60 years of age in our series had a 38% incidence of nonunion (8 of 21 patients) compared to a 16% incidence for patients less than 60 years of age (4/25) (Fig. 31.12) ($p = 0.09$ chi square = 2.955). Patients 60 years of age and older had a slightly higher incidence of nonunion with a dens dislocation less than 6.0 mm (17%) compared to patients less than 60 years old (5%) ($p = 0.25$, chi square = 1.385). Both groups of patients had a statistically significant higher incidence of nonunion with a dens dislocation of 6.0 mm or more compared to the respective nonunion rates for a dens dislocation of less than 6.0 mm. (Age 60 and older: 17% *vs.* 67%, $p < 0.05$, chi square = 5.585. Less than age 60: 5% *vs.* 75%, $p < 0.01$, chi square = 10.470.) Research by other investigators supports these findings (9). We advocate 10–12 weeks of halo vest immobilization for these patients (less than 6.0 mm dens dislocation). Patients with Type II fractures with 6.0 mm (or greater)

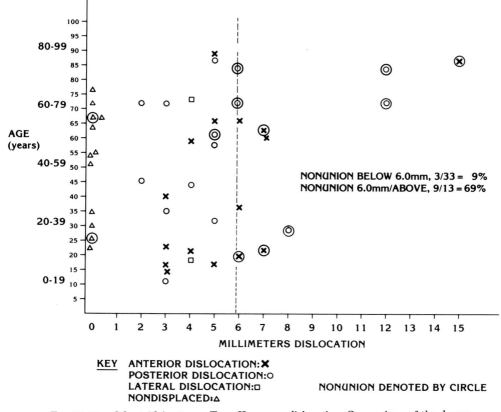

FIG. 31.12.   Odontoid fractures, Type II: age *vs.* dislocation. Comparison of the degree of dens dislocation and patient age with respect to nonunion for Type II odontoid fractures.

dens dislocation or those patients with traumatic injuries that preclude the application of the halo device should be offered early surgical therapy.

Acute cervical injuries between C3 and T1 require careful consideration and individualization of therapy (Fig. 31.13). One indication for nonsurgical management (*i.e.*, external immobilization) is a vertebral body fracture without cervical canal compromise (Fig. 31.14). Fractures of cervical vertebrae that remain in alignment or have been reduced to anatomical alignment heal well with rigid external immobilization (regardless of the neurological injury), unless there has been significant concomitant ligamentous disruption. A small percentage of patients with the latter condition will develop late cervical instability despite external immobilization and may require delayed surgical fusion. These patients are difficult to identify prior to initiating the primary therapy; therefore, serial follow-up examinations are necessary.

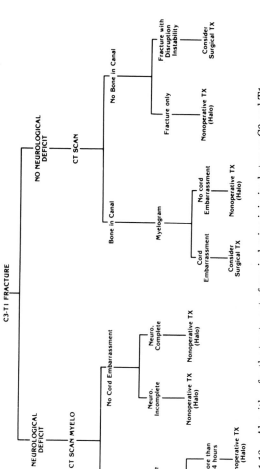

FIG. 31.13.   Algorithm for the treatment of cervical spine injuries between C3 and T1.

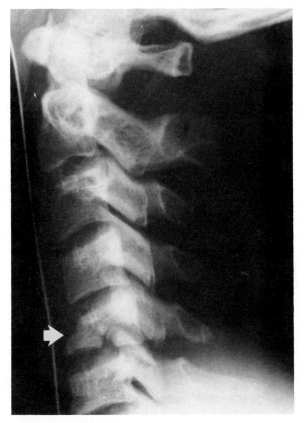

FIG. 31.14. Lateral radiograph of C5 vertebral body fracture (*arrow*).

Cervical fracture patterns that are controversial with respect to initial therapy (nonoperative *vs.* operative) include neurologically intact patients with compromise of the spinal canal. Equally controversial is the treatment of the neurologically injured patient who is improving despite bone or disc in the spinal canal. These patients are at risk for residual or delayed neurological sequelae, progressive kyphosis, premature cervical spinal stenosis, and radicular pain syndromes. While the incidence of these complications is not well known, their potential has been established (5, 27). Treatment must be individualized. But, in general, we advocate surgical decompression with fusion in patients with myelographic evidence of thecal sac embarrassment relatively early in their hospitalization (2–7 days postinjury) to remove the compressive pathology and to eliminate the potential for the aforementioned delayed complications.

The patient who has a complete neurological injury with bone in the spinal canal less than 24 hours after injury is also controversial with respect to initial therapy. The rare patient, described as complete pre-operatively, will have meaningful recovery of neurological function following emergent surgical decompression (1, 10). However, the vast majority of patients reported in the literature who have complete neurological injuries (in the absence of spinal shock) do not respond to any form of therapeutic intervention. We are aggressive with these patients with respect to early reduction of traumatic subluxation and have had functional motor and sensory recovery in one patient—a 16-year-old female who was complete 5 hours after injury from bilateral locked facets at C5-C6 (17). We have not seen significant recovery in any patient with a complete cervical neurological injury after operative intervention, regardless of the time of intervention.

Selected patients with locked facets (unilateral and bilateral) can be managed nonoperatively (Fig. 31.15) (4, 24, 33). Unilateral locked facets, particularly those with fracture fragments about the articular surfaces, can (once aligned) be treated effectively with halo vest immobilization. Bilateral locked facets are usually associated with major ligamentous disruption and instability (Fig. 31.16); however, those with fracture

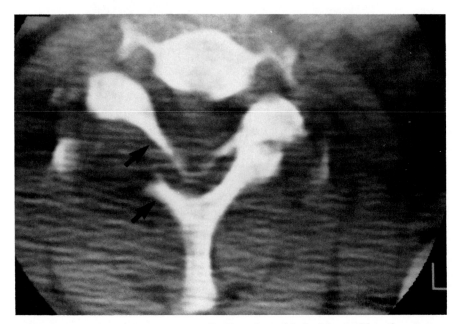

FIG. 31.15. CT scan of patient with C7-T1 unilateral locked facets. Note the rotatory subluxation (*arrows*).

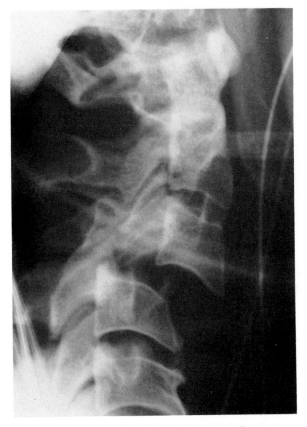

Fig. 31.16.   Lateral radiograph of patient with complete neurological deficit due to C3-C4 bilateral locked facets.

fragments (once aligned) will fuse with halo vest immobilization (24). Five of 6 patients we treated in this way were stable at last follow-up. The single patient who failed nonoperative management had repeated subluxation in her halo vest and required operative reduction and internal fixation.

The management of cervical spine injuries (traumatic subluxation) without evidence of fracture by CT or tomography is also controversial (Fig. 31.17). While most investigators advocate surgical treatment for ligamentous injuries (6, 10), we have managed 17 of these patients with halo vest immobilization for 12–16 weeks with good results (4). Fourteen patients were stable after therapy (82%), while 3 required later surgical reduction and fusion.

Indications for operative therapy include patients with a severely comminuted cervical vertebral body fracture and marked instability due

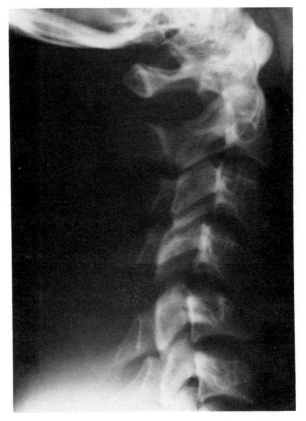

FIG. 31.17. Lateral x-ray of patient with spinal column instability at C4-C5 without evidence of fracture.

to posterior element disruption. These patients have a high likelihood of persistent instability and delayed kyphosis despite nonoperative immobilization (5, 6, 10). Finally, patients with an incomplete neurological injury with compromise of the spinal cord (bone, disc, blood, persistent subluxation) who either do not improve with nonoperative therapy or who demonstrate neurological deterioration *must* be treated surgically (5, 10). The latter example requires emergent operative decompression and stabilization.

Cervical Orthoses

Except for the most mild injuries (cervical sprain or isolated, stable spinous process fractures) foam collars should not be used as an orthotic device for the cervical spine. The Philadelphia collar, which provides

TABLE 31.3

Recipe for C-Spine Injury

ABCs-Immobilization in the field
  Resuscitation in ER with spine precautions
  Thorough neurological assessment
  Complete cervical spine radiographs, ± CT scan
  Stokes bed, early reduction with Gardner-Wells tongs
  Additional radiographic studies (myelo-angio-MRI) as needed
  Definitive therapy
    Nonoperative
    Operative
  Periodic follow-up

significantly better immobilization of the neck than the foam collar ($p <$ 0.001) (20, 38), has application in the treatment of minimally displaced atlas fractures and for several of the less severe miscellaneous axis fractures (15).

More significant fracture dislocations of the cervical spine require rigid immobilization of the head and neck with respect to the torso to maintain anatomic alignment and to insure bony union (20, 25, 38). Several cervicothoracic braces have been designed to serve this purpose. The SOMI brace provides fair immobilization with respect to flexion but allows considerable extension, rotation, and lateral bending of the cervical spine. The rigid cervicothoracic orthosis and the Yale brace were slightly better at head and spine immobilization than the SOMI; however, both allowed a significant range of neck flexion, rotation, and lateral bending compared to the halo immobilization brace. While not absolute in its ability to restrict head and neck movement, the halo ring attached to the plastic body vest represents the best form of external cervical spine immobilization currently available (15, 16, 20, 25, 38). We rely extensively on the halo vest immobilization device for nonoperative management of cervical spine fractures (C1 through T1) and have had good results with few complications. We use the rigid cervicothoracic brace as an alternative for patients who will not tolerate halo vest immobilization, particularly those with flexion injuries.

CONCLUSION

In summary, a wide variety of traumatic fractures and fracture-dislocations occur between the first cervical and the first thoracic vertebrae. Half of the patients who sustain cervical trauma will have significant neurological impairment. A measurable subpopulation of patients will either deteriorate neurologically or develop neurological symptoms only after arrival at the hospital, either during their evaluation or treatment.

The prompt resuscitation of traumatized patients and the early recognition and immobilization of cervical spine injuries will reduce these complications. Once the cervical spine injury has been characterized, early reduction and rigid immobilization are essential (Table 31.3). Many, if not the majority, of patients will be effectively treated nonoperatively.

REFERENCES

1. Allen, R. L., Perot, P. L., and Gudeman, S. K. Evaluation of acute nonpenetrating cervical spinal cord injuries with CT metrizamide myelography. J Neurosurg., *63:* 510–520, 1985.
2. Anderson, L. D. Fractures of the odontoid process of the axis. In: *The Cervical Spine*, edited by R. W. Bailey and H. H. Sherk, pp. 206–223. Lippincott, Philadelphia, 1983.
3. Apuzzo, M. L. J., Heiden, J. S., Weiss, M. H., *et al.* Acute fractures of the odontoid process: An analysis of 45 cases. J Neurosurg., *48:* 85–91, 1978.
4. Bloomfield, S. M., Browner, C. M., and Sonntag, V. K. H. Traumatic cervical spine subluxation without fracture: Review of 87 cases. Presented at the American Association of Neurological Surgeons and Congress of Neurological Surgeons, Joint Section on Spinal Disorders, San Diego, Calif., February 1985.
5. Bohlman, H. H. Acute fractures and dislocations of the cervical spine: An analysis of three hundred hospitalized patients and review of the literature. J. Bone Joint Surg., *61:* 1119–1142, 1979.
6. Bohlman, H. H., and Boada, E. Fractures and dislocations of the lower cervical spine. In: *The Cervical Spine*, edited by the Cervical Spine Research Society, pp. 232–267. Lippincott, Philadelphia, 1983.
7. Brant-Zawadski, M., Miller, E. M., and Federle, M. P. CT in the evaluation of spine trauma. AJR, *136:* 369–375, 1981.
8. Brown, B. M., Brant-Zawadski, M., and Cann, C. E. Dynamic CT scanning of spinal column trauma. AJR, *139:* 1177–1181, 1982.
9. Clark, C. R., White, A. A. III, and Cooper, P. Fractures of the dens: A multi-center study. Presented at the 35th Annual Meeting of Congress of Neurological Surgeons, Honolulu, Hawaii, September 1985.
10. Cooper, P. R., and Ransohoff, J. Surgical treatment. In: *The Cervical Spine*, edited by The Cervical Spine Research Society, pp. 305–317. Lippincott, Philadelphia, 1983.
11. Ducker, T. B. Comments. Neurosurgery, *18:* 330, 1986.
12. Dunn, M. E., and Seljeskog, E. L. Experience in the management of odontoid process injuries: An analysis of 128 cases. Neurosurgery, *18:* 306–310, 1986.
13. Ekong, C. E. U., Schwartz, M. L., Tator, C. H., *et al.* Odontoid fracture: Management with early mobilization using the halo device. Neurosurgery, *9:* 631–637, 1981.
14. Garfin, S. R., and Rothman, R. H. Traumatic spondylolisthesis of the axis (Hangman's fracture). In: *The Cervical Spine*, edited by The Cervical Spine Research Society, pp. 223–232. Lippincott, Philadelphia, 1983.
15. Hadley, M. N., Browner, C., and Sonntag, V. K. H. Miscellaneous fractures of the second cervical vertebra. Barrow Neurol. Inst. Q., *1:* 34–39, 1985.
16. Hadley, M. N., Browner, C., and Sonntag, V. K. H. Axis fractures: A comprehensive review of management and treatment in 107 cases. Neurosurgery, *17:* 281–290, 1985.
17. Hadley, M. N., Zabramski, J. M., Rekate, H. R., *et al.* Pediatric Spinal Trauma. Presented at the American Association of Neurological Surgeons and Congress of Neurological Surgeons, Joint Section on Spinal Disorders, San Diego, Calif., February 1986.

18. Heiden, J. S., Weiss, M. H., Rosenberg, A. W., et al. Management of cervical spinal cord trauma in Southern California. J Neurosurg., 43: 732–736, 1975.

19. Jefferson, G. Fracture of the atlas vertebra: Report of four cases and a review of those previously recorded. Br. J. Surg., 7: 407–422, 1920.

20. Johnson, R. M., Owen, J. R., Hart, D. L. H., et al. Cervical orthoses: A guide to their selection and use. Clin. Orthop. Related Res., 154: 34–45, 1981.

21. Keene, G. C. R., Hone, M. R., and Sage, M. R. Atlas fracture: Demonstration using computerized tomography. J. Bone Joint Surg. [Am.], 60A: 1106–1107, 1978.

22. Lipson, S. J. Fractures of the atlas associated with fractures of the odontoid process and transverse ligament ruptures. J. Bone Joint Surg. [Am.], 59: 940–943, 1977.

23. Maiman, D. J., and Larson, S. J. Management of odontoid fractures. Neurosurgery, 11: 471–476, 1982.

24. Marano, S. R., and Sonntag, V. K. H. Management of bilateral locked facets of the cervical spine. Presented at the American Association of Neurological Surgeons and Congress of Neurological Surgeons, First Meeting of the Joint Section on Spinal Disorders, San Diego, Calif., February 1985.

25. Morris, J. M. Spinal bracing. In: Neurosurgery, edited by R. H. Wilkins and S. S. Rengachary, pp. 2300–2305. McGraw-Hill, New York, 1985.

26. Pierce, D. S., and Barr, J. S., Jr. Fractures and dislocations at the base of the skull and upper cervical spine. In: The Cervical Spine, edited by The Cervical Spine Research Society, pp. 196–206. J. B. Lippincott, Philadelphia, 1983.

27. Ratcheson, R. A. Syllabus: Management of Acute Spinal Injuries: Late neurologic deterioration in spinal injury. Sponsored by the American Association of Neurological Surgeons; American Academy of Orthopaedic Surgeons; and Congress of Neurological Surgeons. Held in Scottsdale, Ariz., December 1985.

28. Reiss, S. J., Raque, G. H., Shields, C. B., et al. Cervical spine fractures with major associated trauma. Neurosurgery, 18: 327–330, 1986.

29. Rogers, W. A. Fractures and disolocations of the cervical spine: An end-result study. J. Bone Joint Surg. [Am.], 39: 341–376, 1957.

30. Schneider, R. C., Livingston, K. E., Cave, A. J. E., et al. "Hangman's fracture" of the cervical spine. J Neurosurg., 22: 141–145, 1965.

31. Seljeskog, E. L., and Chou, S. N. Spectrum of the hangman's fracture. J. Neurosurg., 45: 3–8, 1976.

32. Sherk, H. H., and Nicholson, J. T. Fractures of the atlas. J. Bone Joint Surg. [Br.], 52: 1017–1024, 1970.

33. Sonntag, V. K. H. Management of bilateral locked facets of the cervical spine. Neurosurgery, 150: 150–152, 1981.

34. Sonntag, V. K. H. The early management of cervical spine injuries. Ariz. Med., 10: 644–647, 1982.

35. Spence, K. F., Jr., Decker, S., and Sell, K. W. Bursting atlantal fracture associated with rupture of the transverse ligament. J Bone Joint Surg. [Am.], 52: 543–549, 1970.

36. Wales, L. R., Knopp, R. K., and Morishima, M. S. Recommendations for evaluation of the acutely injured cervical spine: A clinical radiologic algorithm. Ann. Emerg. Med., 9: 422–428, 1980.

37. Weiss, M. H. Mid- and lower cervical spine injuries. In: Neurosurgery, edited by R. H. Wilkins and S. S. Rengachary, Vol. 2, pp. 1708–1716. McGraw-Hill, New York, 1985.

38. Wolf, J. W., and Johnson, R. M. Cervical orthoses. In: The Cervical Spine, edited by The Cervical Spine Research Society, pp. 196–206. Lippincott, Philadelphia, 1983.

32

Operative Management of Cervical Spine Injuries

PAUL R. COOPER, M.D.

INTRODUCTION

There have been important recent advances which have increased our understanding of the biomechanics of spine injury and the relative importance of the various bony and ligamentous elements necessary for maintenance of spinal stability. As a result, there has been a more rational application of known techniques for spine stabilization as well as the development of new operative methods for more effective treatment of complex spine injuries.

There is a virtually unlimited combination of injuries which can affect the cervical spine, and delineation of the proper treatment of all of these would be impossible. In this chapter I shall review the most common injuries and synthesize the most recent information regarding the management of injuries to both the bony spine and its supporting ligamentous and cartilaginous structures. While the primary emphasis will be on the management of the *spine* injury, there will be both implicit and explicit consideration of the effect of operative treatment on the neural elements. The operative techniques described are not meant to be exhaustive, but using the principles for fixation described and understanding the nature of the injury, it is likely that one or a combination of operative approaches described will provide a solution for providing stability for most cervical spine injuries.

In another chapter in this volume the indications for nonoperative management of cervical spine injuries have been outlined. I shall therefore assume that the reader understands the principles and practice of closed (nonoperative) reduction and stabilization. Lesions such as spondylolisthesis of the axis (hangman's fracture), Jefferson fracture, and spinal cord contusion without fracture or subluxation rarely need operative management and will not be discussed.

RADIOGRAPHIC EVALUATION

A careful, logical radiographic evaluation of the patient with a cervical spine injury will enable the surgeon to define the specific anatomy of the injury and to choose the most appropriate operative approach. In essence, the surgeon must be aware of the site and extent of fractures and ligamentous injury, the presence of neural compression, and the likelihood that a lesion is stable or unstable.

Patients are evaluated with plain films, computed tomographic (CT) scan with bone windows, flexion-extension films, and CT/myelography. A modus operandi that we have found helpful is seen in the algorithm in Figure 32.1.

In essence, all patients with suspected cervical spine injuries are evaluated with plain films to define the general nature and the location of the injury. Plain film studies are followed by CT scanning with bone windows. The level of CT scanning is determined both by the patient's clinical signs and information provided by the plain films. It is tedious to scan the entire neck, and in general this is not done. However, at least 15% of patients will have a second, noncontiguous fracture (19), and a high index of suspicion is necessary lest such a lesion be missed. Before the advent and refinement of CT, polytomography was used for delineation of bony anatomy. While this remains an adequate diagnostic modality, we prefer CT scanning in our clinic because it gives a picture of the 3-dimensional cross-sectional anatomy of the spinal canal in a single scan and also provides information about injury to ligamentous or

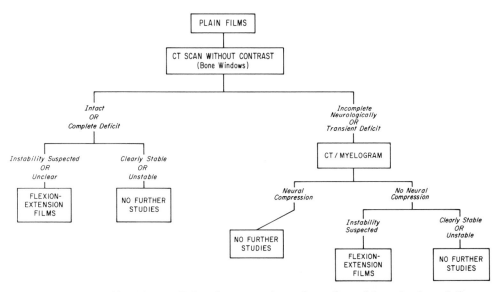

FIG. 32.1. Algorithm outlining the approach to the radiographic evaluation of the patient with a cervical spine injury. The studies performed and the order in which they are done depend on the patient's clinical status and information obtained from previous radiographic studies.

other soft tissue structures. Except for those patients who are experiencing neurological deterioration there is generally no urgency to performing a CT scan or any study other than plain films. In particular in patients with neurological deficit, immobilization and reduction of fractures and subluxations must take precedence over specialized diagnostic studies.

The choice of additional diagnostic tests depends on the patient's neurological function. All patients with incomplete or transient neurological deficit have CT scans after the subarachnoid introduction of a water-soluble contrast agent (iopamidol) to determine the presence of neural compression. The subsequent performance of flexion-extension films for the determination of stability will depend both on the presence or absence of neural compression seen on the CT/myelogram and on the likelihood of the existence of spinal instability as defined by plain films and the CT scan.

Ironically, further diagnostic evaluation in those patients who are (and have always been) neurologically intact and in those patients with a complete neurologic deficit is quite similar. We do not perform myelography in patients with complete functional spinal cord transection as we do not believe that decompression has any effect on their course. In patients who are intact, CT myelography is not performed as it is exceedingly unlikely that neural compression is present.

TIMING OF OPERATION

In patients with cervical spine injuries without neurologic deficit, operation is performed electively after medical problems have been resolved and fractures and subluxations have been reduced. The timing of operation is especially controversial in patients with neurologic deficit, either complete or partial, who have radiographic evidence of continued compression of neural structures.

At first glance it might seem self-evident that the sooner operation is performed and neural compression is relieved the more likely it would be that functional return would occur. Ducker et al. (9) are strong proponents of early operation in those patients seen within 6–12 hours of injury whose fracture/subluxations do not reduce readily and in those patients with persistent spinal cord compression demonstrated on myelography. Wagner (28) has also advocated operation in patients with neurologic deficit if reduction is not achieved within 1 hour of the institution of cervical traction. Yashon et al. (31) take a similar stand, and White et al. (30) state that decompression should be carried out "as soon as conditions permit."

In spite of these beliefs, there is no statistical evidence that early operation and decompression within the first hours after spinal cord injury result in any greater amelioration of neurologic deficit than operation performed days or weeks later. In particular, patients who have complete neurologic deficit on admission only rarely regain neurologic function. In these patients, when neurologic function returns it frequently does so without operative decompression. Thus, neurologic return after early operation cannot necessarily be ascribed to the salutary effects of decompression. Braakman (4) reported on 67 patients admitted within several hours of injury with complete neurologic deficit who did not undergo operation. At 6 hours five patients had regained some motor function, and by 24 hours an additional two had improved. No patient who had a complete neurologic deficit at 24 hours regained function other than minimal sensation.

Larson (15) examined the hypothesis that early operation could mitigate the effects of edema and presumably prevent neurologic deterioration. He remarked that deficit does not progress from edema, but rather from additional mechanical insult and that "the extent of recovery is independent of the interval between injury and operation." It seems most unlikely that early operation in patients who have complete or severe incomplete lesions will beneficially affect neurologic recovery; indeed, early operation in these patients may be associated with a much higher rate of complications. This has been noted by Braakman (4) and confirmed more recently by Marshall (20) in an analysis from a cooperative study of spinal cord-injured patients. It is my belief that the only absolute indication for early operation is neurologic deterioration in the presence of radiographic evidence of spinal cord compression by bone, soft tissue, or hematoma.

MANAGEMENT OF UPPER CERVICAL SPINE INJURIES

The overall goals of operative management are to prevent injury to neural structures; to ameliorate the effects of neural injury by decompressing the injured spinal cord or nerve roots; to produce mechanical stability of the cervical spine, permitting the earliest mobilization of patients both with and without neurologic deficit; and to prevent late spinal deformity.

For both conceptual and practical purposes it is convenient and appropriate to divide the discussion of operative management of cervical spine injuries into consideration of those which involve the upper cervical spine (C1 and C2) and those involving C3-C7. Hangman's fractures and Jefferson fractures rarely need operation; therefore, this discussion will be confined to management of fractures of the odontoid process.

Odontoid Fractures

Odontoid fractures comprise over 11% of all cervical spine fractures (16). Their management is controversial, and disagreement centers about the relative indications for operative and nonoperative treatment. Because odontoid fractures have a high rate of nonunion when they are treated nonoperatively with external immobilization some authorities (10, 18, 22, 25) advocate operative stabilization of most or all odontoid injuries. Others believe that halo or similar immobilization is generally satisfactory management (11). The literature on this fracture is extensive, and careful review shows that there are a number of clinical and radiographic criteria which may be used to predict the likelihood of fusion without operation: (a) age of the patient; (b) location of the fracture on the odontoid process; (c) direction of displacement of the fracture; (d) amount of subluxation; and (e) length of time from the injury to immobilization.

In general, the younger the patient the more likely it is that healing will take place without operative stabilization. The exact age after which patients should be considered operative candidates is unclear. The data of Dunn and Seljeskog (10) show that nonunion in Type II fractures increases from 22% in patients below the age of 50 to almost 60% in patients over this age. Apuzzo et al. (3) reported a similar relationship between the age of the patient and nonunion.

Fractures of the odontoid process have been divided by Anderson and D'Alonzo (2) into three types—those at the tip (Type I), those at the base (Type II), and those in which the fracture extends into the body of C2 (Type III) (Fig. 32.2). Type I fractures are rare and do not require operative stabilization. Type III fractures heal with external immobilization and rarely need operation. Type II fractures are the most common and have a significant incidence of nonunion which is related to several factors. Those fractures which remain anteriorly subluxed to a distance of 4 mm or greater have a high incidence of nonunion and should be treated primarily with operation (3, 11), although Dunn and Seljeskog (10) could find no relationship between the amount of anterior subluxation and the incidence of nonunion. On the other hand a posterior subluxation of greater than 2–3 mm is associated with a very high incidence of nonunion, and there is nearly universal agreement that these fractures should be fused primarily.

Lastly, the age of the fracture must be considered in deciding on therapy. Fractures which are months or years old with sclerosis around the fracture margins will not heal, even with extended immobilization, and should be fused. In general, fractures older than 2 weeks have a high rate of nonunion and should be fused as the primary treatment.

For individual patients the entire clinical and radiographic picture must be evaluated, and the chances of fusion with external immobilization should be discussed with the patient along with a description of the halo device and the limitations it may impose on activity and life-style.

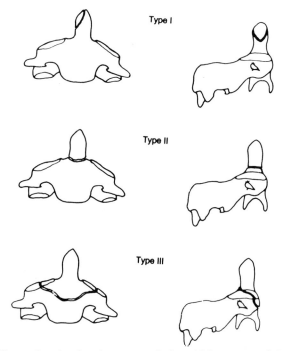

Type I

Type II

Type III

FIG. 32.2.   Illustration showing three types of odontoid fractures as defined by Anderson and D'Alonzo (2). (Reproduced with permission from Anderson, L. D., and D'Alonzo, R. T. Fractures of the odontoid process of the axis. J. Bone Joint Surg. [Am.], *56A:* 1663–1674, 1974.)

Some patients will prefer to have early definitive therapy with operation while others will be content to wear a halo for several months, knowing that there might be a 30 or 40% chance of nonunion even after several months of immobilization.

C1-C2 Ligamentous Instability

Ligamentous disruption between the odontoid process and C1 without fracture will also produce C1-C2 instability (Fig. 32.3). Purely ligamentous injuries will not heal spontaneously and all such patients must be fused.

Operative Approaches

ANTERIOR APPROACH

In almost all cases of odontoid fractures, stabilization is performed through a posterior approach. The anterior transoral approach (12) is used only for fractures which cannot be reduced and where there is persistent compression of the intradural contents by the fractured odon-

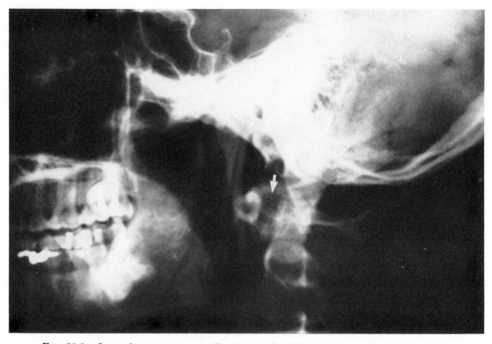

FIG. 32.3. Lateral roentgenogram illustrating C1-C2 ligamentous instability with forward subluxation of C1 on C2. *Arrow* delineates large space between anterior arch of C1 and the odontoid process.

toid process. This most commonly occurs in fractures which have not been recognized and which have healed in a subluxed state. Following removal of the odontoid process from an anterior approach, the majority of patients will be unstable at the C1-C2 level and must be fused. Although anterior C1-C2 fusion has been described, it provides little early stability after odontoidectomy, and patients are best served by posterior C1-C2 fusion (Fig. 32.4).

POSTERIOR APPROACH

A number of operations have been described for the stabilization of the C1-C2 complex, and a variety are effective. As a rule it is important that any operation provide immediate stability through the use of wire fixation and long-term stability with the use of bone grafts. Although fusions using acrylic (instead of bone) have been described (23), this substance is a foreign body and loses rather than gains strength with age as is the case with bone. Unless there are overriding considerations it is important that the fusion be limited to the C1-C2 posterior elements.

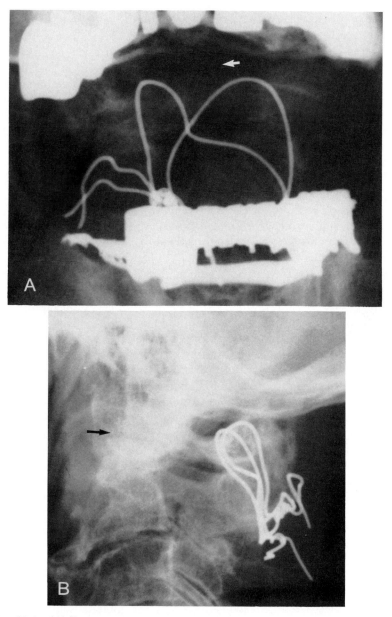

FIG. 32.4. (*A*) Postoperative roentgenogram in anteroposterior projection of patient
with myelopathy and irreducible C1-C2 subluxation. The odontoid process has been
removed (*arrow*) transorally and the posterior elements of C1 and C2 wired. (*B*) Lateral
roentgenogram of the same patient demonstrating absent odontoid process (*arrow*) and
bone and wire fusion posteriorly.

Extension of the fusion to the occiput should be performed only if there is also atlantooccipital instability; inclusion of the occiput in the fusion mass greatly decreases mobility of the neck and adds nothing to the strength of the C1-C2 fusion. Similarly, inclusion of C3 in the fusion does not improve the fusion and will also decrease mobility somewhat.

To achieve stabilization of C1-C2 we prefer to use the modification of the procedure described by Alexander et al. (1). Patients are brought to the operating room in cervical traction; intubation is carried out with the patient awake; and after intubation the patient is placed in a collar and turned to the prone position. For patients with anterior subluxation extension is the position of safety as the patient is being turned as well as intraoperatively. For the minority of patients with posterior odontoid subluxations, extension of the neck may exacerbate the subluxation and result in spinal cord compression; these patients should be turned while in a strictly neutral to very slightly flexed position and maintained in that position during operation.

All patients are placed prone on a horseshoe headrest in 5 lbs of traction. A lateral x-ray is taken, and the position of the neck is adjusted as appropriate. A midline incision is made from the suboccipital region to C3, and the paraspinous muscles are retracted laterally to expose the posterior ring of the foramen magnum and the posterior elements of C1 and C2. Using small curettes and dissecting instruments the ligaments are stripped off of the under (anterior) surface of the posterior elements of C1 and 2 to facilitate passage of sublaminar wires. Two strands of 1.0-mm in diameter stainless steel wire are passed beneath the posterior arch of C1 and are retracted to either side of the midline for later fixation of the bone graft. Two wires are also passed beneath the lamina of C2 in identical fashion also for graft fixation. A loop of 1.2-mm in diameter wire is then passed from inferiorly to superiorly beneath the arch of C1 in the midline; the loop is brought down inferiorly to catch the spinous process of C2, and the two free ends of the wire are tied below the spinous process of C2 and tightened by twisting firmly, binding the C1 and C2 posterior elements together. This central wire is most important as it provides immediate stability until the bone graft can fuse the C1 and C2 posterior elements. Nevertheless, the stainless steel wires may fatigue and break, and bone grafts are essential to provide long-term stability.

The bone graft is taken from the iliac crest and is split down the center so that two pieces of corticocancellous bone are created. These pieces are shaped, and the cancellous surface is placed on either side of the midline over the posterior elements of C1 and C2, which have previously been roughened with curettes or a high speed air drill. The four wires previously passed beneath C1 and C2 are tightened around these grafts, fixing them securely to the C1 and C2 posterior elements (Fig. 32.5). The wound

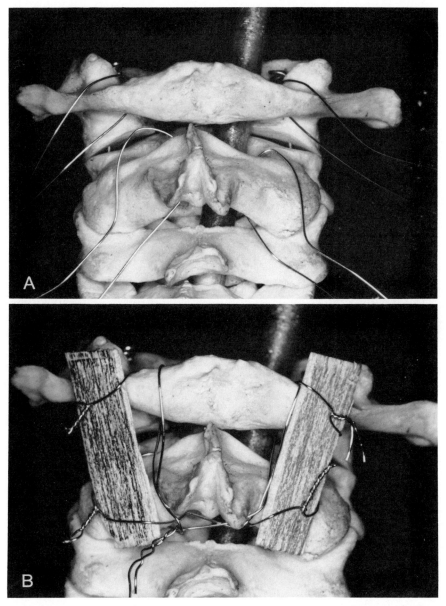

FIG. 32.5.   Technique for posterior wing of C1 to C2. (A) In this model wires have been passed beneath the posterior arch of C1 and lamina of C2. (B) A central wire has been passed beneath the arch of C1, looped around the spinous process of C2, and the ends twisted and tightened around the spinous process of C2. The grafts are secured in place by the previously placed lateral wires beneath the C1 and C2 posterior elements.

is closed routinely. Postoperatively patients should be immobilized in a Philadelphia or similar collar for 3 months.

The procedure is altered slightly for patients with posterior subluxation. In these patients, tightening of the central stabilizing wire can result in an increase in the posterior subluxation of the fractured odontoid process. To prevent this, a small block of bone is placed in the midline between the arch of C1 and the lamina of C2 before the midline stabilizing wire is tightened to prevent excessive posterior displacement of the arch of C1.

The process of posterior wiring and fusion of the C1-C2 complex is dependent on the integrity of the arch of C1 and the lamina of C2. If either of these has been fractured, then posterior wiring is not possible. In this case we have placed bone grafts over the posterior elements of C1 and C2 and have immobilized the patient in a halo vest for 3 months.

OPERATIVE MANAGEMENT OF MID AND LOWER CERVICAL SPINE FRACTURES

The goals of operative management of injuries to the mid and lower cervical spine are decompression of functional or potentially functional neural elements, establishment of stability, early mobilization of the injured patient, and prevention of future deformities of the spine when these aims cannot be achieved by nonoperative means.

Determination of Stability

White and Panjabi (29) have defined clinical stability as "the ability of the spine under physiologic loads to prevent initial or additional neurologic damage, severe intractable pain, or gross deformity." When the spine is subluxed it is obviously unstable (except in certain patients with locked facets). On initial radiographs, instability may be assumed if the anterior intervertebral body distance is greater than 3.5 mm or the intervertebral angulation is greater than 11° (29). In spines which do not appear subluxed on initial radiographic studies, stability may be ascertained by flexion-extension studies as outlined in a previous section of this chapter.

White *et al.* (30) have divided the elements which provide stability to the spine into anterior and posterior bony and ligamentous structures. They defined the anterior elements as the posterior longitudinal ligament and all structures anterior to it and the posterior elements as everything behind the posterior longitudinal ligament. They suggested that "any motion segment in which all the anterior elements or all the posterior elements are destroyed or are unable to function should be considered unstable (30)."

Choice of Operation

In another chapter in this volume, Sonntag has defined in detail which unstable injuries may be managed without operation and which may be successfully treated with external immobilization. As a general rule we utilize operative stabilization for all ligamentous disruption with minimal or no bony injury and in all other injuries with trauma to both anterior and posterior bony and ligamentous elements. Wherever possible our bias has been to stabilize fractures and subluxations through a posterior approach. We employ the anterior approach in those patients who have radiographic evidence of spinal cord compression from anteriorly and who also have some preservation of neurological function. We may also use the anterior approach for stabilizing the spine in those patients without neural compression who have such severe injury of the posterior elements that posterior stabilization cannot be performed.

Operative Technique

INTERSPINOUS WIRING

Subluxation of the vertebral bodies and facet joints with posterior ligamentous disruption occurs as a result of severe hyperflexion injury and is an indication for wiring and fusion of the posterior elements (26). When all of the ligamentous structures are disrupted, bilateral interfacet dislocation occurs so that the superior facets of the lower vertebra pass superiorly and posteriorly over the lower facet of the upper vertebra. Radiographically the anterior subluxation will be at least one-half of the anterior/posterior diameter of the vertebral body. Although it has been reported that 60% of bilateral facet dislocations without vertebral body compression fractures will heal with spontaneous intervertebral ankylosis (26), our experience has been that the vast majority of patients with this injury will need fusion (Fig. 32.6).

When there has been disruption of both facet joints and the posterior elements are intact, interspinous wiring with bony fusion provides both immediate and long-term stability. We position patients as previously described for posterior wiring of C1 to C2. If the patient has been in a halo vest, its attachment to the halo ring is loosened to permit adjustment and reduction of subluxations as well as approximation of the posterior elements when the posterior wires are tightened. X-rays are taken to confirm the maintenance of reduction in the prone position.

The muscles are stripped off of the posterior elements of the two vertebrae involved in the subluxation. Thus if there is a C5-C6 subluxation, the posterior elements of C5 and C6 are the ones that would be fused and are the only ones that will need to be exposed. If bilateral locked facets have not been reduced preoperatively or with traction after

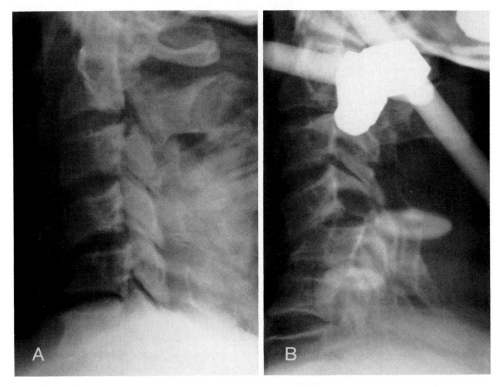

FIG. 32.6. (A) Lateral roentgenogram of a patient with bilateral facet disruption as well as anterior ligamentous instability after reduction. (B) Subluxation has recurred after attempted halo immobilization. Failure of the halo to immobilize this type of ligamentous injury is almost predictable, and such patients are best managed with posterior wiring and bony fusion.

the induction of anesthesia, an air drill may be used to remove the most superior portion of the superior facet, and an instrument can then be used to relocate the two vertebra. However, bilateral facet dislocation may be very resistant to relocation when more than 2 weeks have passed since injury.

A towel clip is used to make a hole as superiorly as possible in the upper posterior element where the spinous process joins the lamina. A wire 1.2 mm in diameter is passed through this hole, and both ends are then brought around the base of the lower spinous process to be fused. The ends are twisted together until no movement of the posterior elements can be appreciated. A bone graft is taken from the iliac crest and is split down the middle to give two pieces of corticocancellous bone. The laminae of the vertebra to be fused are abraded using a curette or preferably a small burr powered by a high speed air drill. It must be remembered that the laminae are mostly cortical bone and that any attempt at "decortication" of the laminae, as some authors propose, will result in significant loss of laminar strength. The bone graft (cancellous side of the graft against the lamina) bone is placed over the left and right hemilaminae of the two vertebrae which are to be fused. The length of each piece is adjusted to avoid fusion of more than two adjacent laminae. The grafts are held in place by the end of the twisted interlaminar wires (Fig. 32.7). If the muscle stripping is limited to the laminae to be fused, the tendency for the bone graft to settle inferiorly as the patient assumes the upright position, and to fuse additional (or wrong) levels is minimized.

Postoperatively patients may be immobilized in a Philadelphia or similar collar for a period of 3 months. However, in patients with severe ligamentous disruption, rigid external fixation in a halo vest may be necessary for successful immobilization and fusion (17). When instability exists at two levels and posterior elements are intact, the upper vertebra may be wired to the middle vertebra, which is then wired to the most inferior one. Although Maiman et al. (17) have combined posterior wiring with anterior fusion, we have not found this to be necessary.

The success of interspinous process wiring is absolutely dependent on the functional integrity of the laminae and spinous processes. If there are laminar, pedicular, or spinous process fractures, interspinous wiring will not provide sufficient stability. In this case the vertebra with the fractured posterior elements may be bypassed and a 3-level fusion carried out from the level above (Figs. 32.7B and C). However, it is important to note that the longer the fusion, the greater the forces at the site of the injury and the greater the chance of failure of bony fusion.

SUBLAMINAR WIRING

Sublaminar wiring in the cervical spine below the C1-C2 level is mentioned only to be condemned. At C1-C2, where the spinal canal is wide in relationship to the size of the spinal cord, sublaminar wiring is safe, and spinal cord injury from passage of the wires is unusual. In the middle and lower cervical spine, there is relatively little space between the bony canal and spinal cord; sublaminar passage of wires in this location is dangerous and should be avoided (26).

FACET TO SPINOUS PROCESS FUSION

Cahill et al. (6) believe that when one or both facets are fractured or disrupted, routine interspinous fusion is not adequate to maintain stability; further interspinous fusion above and below an injured posterior element may further compromise a damaged spine. In our own experience,

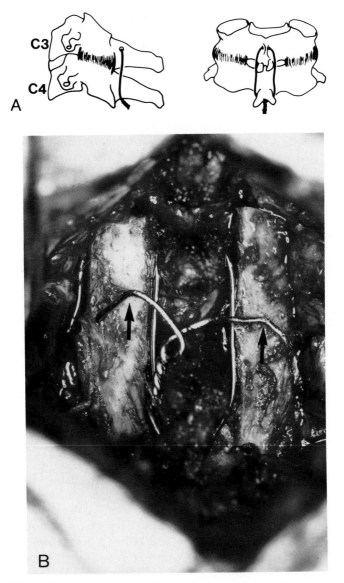

FIG. 32.7. (A) Illustration shows placement of wire for 2-level interspinous wiring and fusion. (Reproduced with permission from White, A. A., and Panjabi, M. M. *Clinical Biomechanics of the Spine.* Lippincott, Philadelphia, 1978.) (B) Operative photograph of C4-C6 wiring and fusion. Wire has been placed through the base of the spinous process of C4 and the ends twisted and tightened around the spinous process of C6. There were bilateral posterior element fractures of C5 precluding a fusion utilizing the spinous process of this vertebra. Note how the ends of the wires hold the bone grafts (*arrows*) in place. (C) Lateral roentgenogram showing placement of wires and bone graft (*arrow*).

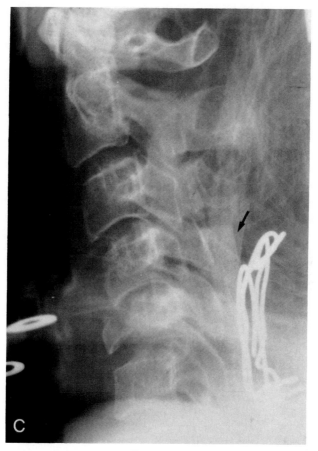

Fig. 32.7 C

posterior wiring as described in the previous section has provided adequate immobilization. Nevertheless, the facet to spinous process fusion will also provide very adequate stabilization in similar situations. This procedure is particularly useful when there is a unilateral jumped facet or there has been unilateral destruction of a facet joint. In this situation facet to spinous process fusion will prevent rotational subluxation. When the posterior elements are intact and there is severe facet injury, compromising a facet to spinous process wire loop, additional stability may be obtained by placing an interspinous wire.

The technique is simple and has been well described (6). After positioning of the patient and performing roentgenograms as outlined in previous sections of this chapter, the appropriate facet joints and spinous processes are exposed. If rotational deformity persists with a "locked" facet, an attempt is made to reduce the subluxation. The joint capsules are removed, and the articular cartilage is curetted. An air drill is used to make a hole in the upper facets at right angles to the articular surface. Double braided 22- or 24-gauge stainless steel wires are passed through the holes and looped around the lower spinous process and tightened. Bilateral wiring is performed even if the facet injury has been unilateral (Fig. 32.8). Corticocancellous bone is placed over the posterior elements for bony fusion. Postoperatively patients are placed in firm external immobilization for a period of 3 months.

POSTERIOR PLATES

The spine may be stabilized posteriorly with plates such as those described by Roy-Camille *et al.* (21). This form of stabilization is advantageous when there are spinous process or laminar fractures. Furthermore stabilization with Roy-Camille plates provides immediate immobilization at the lateral mass without the need for bony fusion. Most commonly

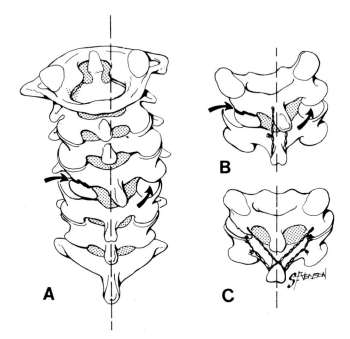

FIG. 32.8. (*A*) Illustration demonstrates rotational subluxation with unilateral facet fracture and bilateral facet joint disruption. (*B*) After interspinous wiring, rotational instability is not prevented. (*C*) Bilateral facet to spinous process wiring prevents rotational subluxation. (Reproduced with permission from Cahill, D. W., Bellegarrique, R., and Ducker, T. B. Bilateral facet to spinous process fusion: A new technique for posterior spinal fusion after trauma. Neurosurgery *13:* 1–4, 1983.)

the plates have two holes permitting fusion at one level (two vertebrae). But if there is instability at two adjacent levels, 3-hole plates allow stabilization at two levels (three vertebral bodies).

The plates work by stabilizing the articular masses and are placed bilaterally. Holes are drilled bilaterally in the articular masses of the vertebrae to be fused (Fig. 32.9A). The plates are placed so that their holes are directly over the holes drilled in the articular masses, after which screws (3.5 mm in diameter and 16 mm in length) are placed through the plate and into the drill holes at such an angle that both the roots and vertebral arteries are avoided (Fig. 32.9B). These plates provide immediate and permanent stability without the necessity for bone grafting, and patients need only a well-fitting cervical collar for three months postoperatively (Fig. 32.9C).

ANTERIOR CERVICAL FUSION

The indications for anterior cervical fusion for patients with spine trauma are few, in this author's opinion. As the sole means of operative stabilization anterior fusion is appropriate only for patients with: (a) some degree of neurologic preservation; (b) compression of the spinal cord from anteriorly; and (c) absence of posterior ligamentous instability.

Most of the techniques for anterior decompression of the spine were devised for removal of osteophytes or soft disc, and they must be modified when trauma has caused disruption to the vertebral body. We do not use the Cloward procedure (8) for trauma as the amount of bone removal is predetermined by the size of the drills, and the bone plug is round and cannot be readily adapted to the vertebrectomy that is so often needed with trauma. We employ a variation of the operation described by Smith and Robinson (24). We drill out the entire fractured body, adjacent discs, and cartilaginous end plates. The posterior longitudinal ligament must be removed and the dura identified to make absolutely certain that there are no hidden fragments of disc material compressing the dural tube posterior to the posterior longitudinal ligament. While the removal of the posterior longitudinal ligament has the disadvantage of decreasing stability (in what is often an already unstable situation), this is more than compensated for by the ability to visualize the dura and ascertain that there is no further disc material compressing the spinal cord.

Anterior cervical fusion is carried out using iliac crest bone graft. Both the bone graft and vertebra to be fused are notched or "keyholed" to decrease the chances of graft extrusion. If only anterior instability (as previously defined) exists, a well-fitting Philadelphia collar or similar orthosis may be sufficient to prevent graft extrusion.

More commonly there is coexisting posterior ligamentous instability, and removal of a destroyed vertebral body and posterior longitudinal

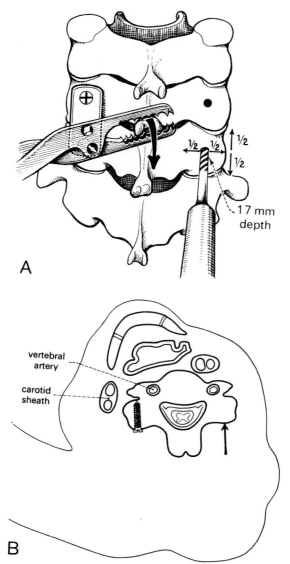

A

B

FIG. 32.9. (*A*) Illustration showing placement of screw holes in the exact center of the lateral mass for securing Roy-Camille plates. Instrument on spinous process demonstrates how subluxed posterior element may be rotated into proper position for plate fixation. (*B*) Illustration in axial plane showing how screw is placed lateral to vertebral artery. The screws are located midway between the upper and lower roots. (*C*) Operative photo showing position of plates after placement of screws. (Reproduced with permission Roy-Camille, R., Saillant, G., Berteaux, D. *et al.* Early management of spinal injuries. In: *Recent Advances in Orthopedics*, edited by B. McKibbon, pp. 57–87. Edinburgh, New York, London, Churchill Livingston, 1979.)

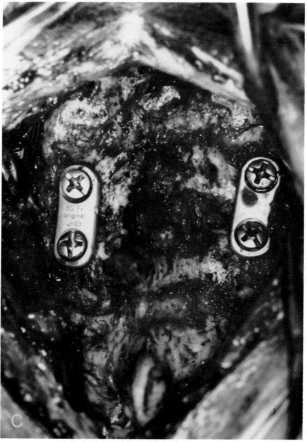

FIG. 32.9 C

ligament will, if anything, increase this instability. The placement of a bone graft (even one properly notched and fitted) will do little to establish immediate stability in this situation, and graft displacement is likely even if the patient is placed in a halo vest postoperatively (Fig. 32.10) (5, 7, 13, 27).

There are two potential solutions to this problem. In such patients one may first perform a posterior stabilization using interspinous wiring (or other posterior stabilizing techniques) and then proceed to anterior cervical decompression and fusion.

The other way of managing such patients is to perform a decompression and fusion in a standard fashion followed by anterior plating. One such technique has been detailed by Kaspar (14) and consists of fixation by screws of a plate to the vertebral bodies to be fused (Fig. 32.11). The tips of the screws must penetrate the posterior cortex of the vertebral body.

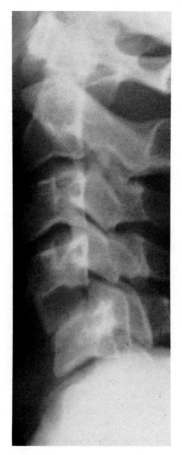

FIG. 32.10. Lateral roentgenogram demonstrates recurrent C4-C5 subluxation after anterior cervical fusion with an iliac crest bone graft in a patient with both anterior and posterior ligamentous instability.

If the screws are too short, they will not fix securely in the cancellous bone of the central portion of the vertebral body, and the screws will pull out, resulting in spinal instability and the possibility of esophageal penetration by the loosened screws (Fig. 32.12). Obviously excessive screw length with spinal cord compression or penetration is even more disastrous. Optimal screw length may be assured through the use of intraoperative fluoroscopic control. Postoperatively patients are provided with a well-fitting orthosis until the graft fuses.

CONCLUSION

The rational approach to the operative management of cervical spine trauma depends on a clear delineation of the radiographic anatomy of

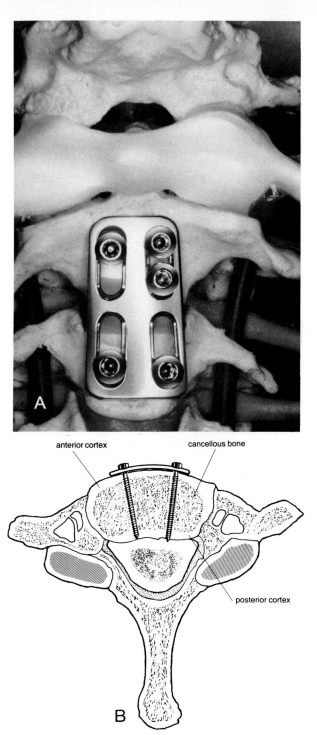

FIG. 32.11. (A) Model of cervical spine showing placement of Kaspar plate in adjacent cervical vertebrae. (B) Axial view shows placement of screws through posterior cortical bone. (Reproduced with permission from Kaspar, W. Anterior cervical fusion and interbody stabilization with the trapezial osteosynthetic plate technique. Aesculap Scientific Information, *12:* 1–36, 1985.)

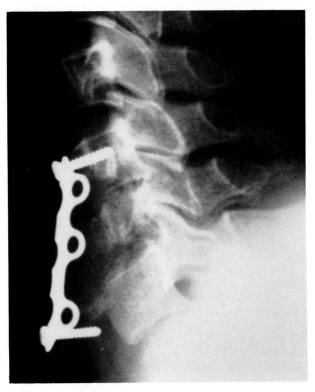

FIG. 32.12. Anterior cervical plate (not the Kaspar design) which pulled out as a result of screws which were too short to penetrate the posterior cortical bone.

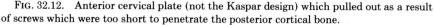

the injury. Specifically, radiographic assessment must define the sites of fractures and subluxations, the likelihood of stability and, in patients with residual neurologic function, the presence or absence of spinal cord compression.

Using information obtained from radiographic studies, the surgeon will be able to plan the most appropriate means of operative stabilization. In general we have preferred to stabilize most patients using a posterior approach as it will generally provide immediate stability without the necessity for any but the simplest of external stabilization devices in the postoperative period. The anterior approach is used in those patients with residual neurologic function who have evidence of persistent anterior spinal cord compression after reduction of subluxations. In this latter group of patients it may sometimes be necessary to stabilize the spine from both an anterior and posterior approach.

Whatever approach is used the goals of management remain: decompression of neural elements in patients with residual neurologic function and stabilization to prevent additional neural injury in the short term and progressive bony deformity in the long term.

REFERENCES

1. Alexander, E., Jr., Forsyth, H. F., Davis, C. H., Jr., et al. Dislocation of the atlas of the axis. The value of fusion of C1, C2, and C3. J. Neurosurg., 15: 353–371, 1958.
2. Anderson, L. D., and D'Alonzo, R. T. Fractures of the odontoid process of the axis. J. Bone Joint Surg. [Am.], 56A: 1663–1674, 1974.
3. Apuzzo, M. L. J., Heiden, J. S., Weiss, M. H., et al. Acute fractures of the odontoid process. An analysis of 45 cases. J. Neurosurg., 48: 85–91, 1978.
4. Braakman, R. Some neurological and neurosurgical aspects of injuries to the lower cervical spine. Acta Neurochir., 22: 245–260, 1970.
5. Bremer, A. M., and Nguyen, T. Q. Internal metal plate fixation combined with anterior interbody fusion in cases of cervical spine injury. Neurosurgery, 12: 649–653, 1983.
6. Cahill, D. W., Bellegarrigue, R., and Ducker, T. B. Bilateral facet to spinous process fusion: A new technique for posterior spinal fusion after trauma. Neurosurgery 13: 1–4, 1983.
7. Capen, D. A., Garland, D. E., and Waters, R. L. Surgical stabilization of the cervical spine. A comparative analysis of anterior and posterior spine fusions. Clin. Orthop., 196: 229–237, 1985.
8. Cloward, R. B. Anterior approach for removal of ruptured cervical discs. J. Neurosurg., 15: 602–617, 1958.
9. Ducker, T. B., Bellegarrigue, R., Salcman, M., et al. Timing of operative care in cervical spinal cord injury. Spine, 9: 525–531, 1984.
10. Dunn, M. E., and Seljeskog, E. L. Experience in the management of odontoid process injuries: An analysis of 128 cases. Neurosurgery, 18: 306–3110, 1986.
11. Ekong, C. E. O., Schwartz, M. L., Tator, C. H., et al. Odontoid fracture: Management with early management using the halo device. Neurosurgery, 9: 631–637, 1981.
12. Fang, H. S. Y., and Ong, G. B. Direct anterior approach to the upper cervical spine. J. Bone Joint Surg. [Am.], 44A: 588–1604, 1962.
13. Gassman, J., and Seligsen, D. The anterior cervical plate. Spine, 8: 700–706, 1983.
14. Kaspar, W. Anterior cervical fusion and interbody stabilization with the trapezial osteosynthetic plate technique. Aesculap Scientific Information, 12: 1–36, 1985.
15. Larson, S. J. Surgical treatment of cervical fractures. Contemp. Neurosurg., 6(8): 1–4, 1984.
16. Lipson, S. J. Fractures of the atlas associated with fractures of the odontoid process and transverse ligament ruptures. J. Bone Joint Surg. [Am.], 59A: 940–943, 1977.
17. Maiman, D. J., Banolat, G., and Larson, S. J. Management of bilateral locked facets of the cervical spine. Neurosurgery, 18: 542–547, 1986.
18. Maiman, D. J., and Larson, S. J. Management of odontoid fractures. Neurosurgery, 11: 471–476, 1982.
19. Maravilla, K. R., Cooper, P. R., and Sklar, F. H. The influence of thin section tomography in the treatment of cervical spine injuries. Radiology 126: 131–139, 1978.
20. Marshall, L., Knowlton, S., Garfin, S. R., et al. Deterioration following spinal cord injury. A multicenter study. J. Neurosurg., 66: 400–404, 1987.
21. Roy-Camille, R., Saillant, G., Berteaux, D., et al. Early management of spinal injuries. In: Recent Advances in Orthopedics, edited by B. McKibbon, pp. 57–87. Edinburgh, New York, London, Churchill Livingston, 1979.
22. Schiess, R. J., De Saussure, R. L., and Robertson, J. T.: Choice of treatment of odontoid fractures. J. Neurosurg., 57: 496–499, 1982.

23. Six, E., and Kelly, D. L., Jr. Technique for C-1, C-2 and C-3 fixation in cases of odontoid fracture. Neurosurgery, 8: 374–377, 1981.

24. Smith, G. W., and Robinson, R. A. Treatment of certain cervical spine disorders by anterior removal of the intervertebral disc and interbody fusion. J. Bone Joint Surg. [Am.], 40A: 607–623, 1958.

25. Southwick, W. O. Management of fractures of the dens (odontoid process). J. Bone Joint Surg. [Am.], 62A: 482–486, 1980.

26. Stauffer, E. S. Management of spine fractures C3-7. Orthop. Clin. North Am., 17: 45–53, 1986.

27. Stauffer, E. S., and Kelley, E. G. Fracture-dislocations of the cervical spine. Instability and recurrent deformity following treatment by anterior interbody fusion. J. Bone Joint Surg. [Am.], 59A: 45–48, 1977.

28. Wagner, F. C. Management of acute spinal cord injury. Surg. Neurol., 7: 346–350, 1977.

29. White, A. A., III, and Panjabi, M. The role of stabilization in the treatment of cervical spine injuries. Spine, 9: 512–522, 1984.

30. White, A. A., Southwick, W. O., and Panjabi, M. M. Clinical instability in the lower cervical spine. A review of past and current concepts. Spine, 1: 15–27, 1976.

31. Yashon, D., Tyson, G., and Vise, W. M. Rapid closed reduction of cervical fracture dislocations. Surg. Neurol., 4: 513–514, 1975.

33

Pharmacological Therapy of Acute Spinal Cord Injury: Studies of High Dose Methylprednisolone and Naloxone

WISE YOUNG, PH.D., M.D., VINCENT DeCRESCITO, PH.D.,
EUGENE S. FLAMM, M.D., ANDREW R. BLIGHT, PH.D., and
JOHN A. GRUNER, PH.D.

INTRODUCTION

Recent laboratory studies have suggested that some pharmacological treatments can improve functional recovery in experimental spinal-injured animals. In particular, naloxone (NLX), an opiate receptor antagonist, and methylprednisolone (MP), a synthetic glucocorticosteroid, were chosen to be subjects of a multicenter randomized clinical trial 2 years ago. Called the National Acute Spinal Cord Injury Study (NASCIS), this trial compares neurological recovery patterns of 300 patients treated with high dose MP (~30 mg/kg loading dose, and 50% of the loading dose IV per hour for 24 hours), NLX (~5.4 mg/kg loading dose, and 75% of the loading dose IV per hour for 24 hours), or placebo starting within 12 hours of injury. The trial is due to be completed next year.

Three observations influenced the protocols chosen in the NASCIS study. Although these findings have been pointed out in recent publications, they have received insufficient emphasis. First, laboratory studies suggest that very high doses of NLX and MP are required to produce an effect on functional recovery. The doses far exceed the levels of NLX and MP needed to block opiate receptors and produce glucocorticosteroid effects. Second, in these high doses, administration of both drugs together increased mortality in spinal-injured animals. Third, our studies did not find significant improvements in the histological appearance of the lesion site despite the enhancements in functional recovery after treatment with these agents.

We will describe here extended experimental studies carried out in our laboratory over the past 5 years, evaluating the effects of high dose NLX and MP administered 45 minutes after spinal cord injury in cats. Three doses of NLX (1, 3, and 10 mg/kg), a dose of MP (15 mg/kg), and a combination of NLX-MP (10 mg/kg + 15 mg/kg) were compared against placebo. Some of the naloxone findings have been published (41). The data here, however, represent the final results on extended groups. We will focus on the rationale for choosing NLX and MP treatments for spinal cord injury, seeking to look ahead to the challenges that lie in the post-NASCIS era. Whether the NASCIS trial shows positive or negative results, we still face the problem of optimizing the treatment or finding alternative therapeutic approaches with fewer side effects and greater potency.

METHODS

Surgical Procedures and Postoperative Care

We used exclusively female adult cats weighing 2.5–3.0 kg. After being anesthetized with pentobarbital (25 mg/kg I.V.), the T8-T9 spinal cords were exposed aseptically through a small laminectomy. The spinal cords were injured with a 20-gm weight dropped 20 cm onto the dorsal surface of the T8 thoracic spinal cord. The dura was not opened, and the spinal column was not stabilized. A Silastic sheet was placed over the laminectomy site to reduce adhesions. Muscle and skin were sutured together in layers over the laminectomy. The skin was then closed with stainless steel clips (removed at 10 days after surgery). The surgery and injury procedure usually took less than an hour.

The cats usually remained sedated for more than 24 hours after surgery. Because of the spinal cord injury, the cats were anesthetic below the lesion level. The cats reacted to firm squeezes of the forepaws but not to gentle manipulations of the wound site. The injured cats were cared for in boxes filled with 6 inches of absorbent pine shavings. The shavings effectively prevented decubiti and kept the skin dry. The cats received daily multiple bladder expressions and careful evaluations. When a cat appeared sick and failed to eat, our protocol was to rule out causes of illness and treat with antibiotics if necessary. Wound or bladder infections rarely occurred.

The 20 gm-20 cm Contusion Injury Model

The injury consisted of dropping a 20-gm weight 20 cm through a brass tube onto a thin (2-mm) cylindrical button with a diameter spanning the width of the spinal cord at T8 (5-mm). The cats were placed on a firm surface. The weight was released from a pin inserted through openings drilled into the tube. This relatively small impact typically compressed the spinal cord briefly and produced immediate losses of somatosensory evoked potentials (SEP) conducting from the hindlimb to the cortex. This is the spinal cord injury model in which we had carried out the earlier blood flow studies. This model of spinal cord contusion (1, 2) is probably the most widely used method of producing standardized injuries of the cat spinal cord. The outcome of this model has been found to be consistent as long as care is taken to maintain the injury conditions in detail (25, 67). The weight drop contusion produces a progressive central hemorrhagic necrosis at the lesion site (6, 7, 43). In our laboratory, the model consistently produces 85–90% incidence of long-term paraplegia in cats.

Treatment Protocols

All the treatments were given at 45 minutes after injury. Placebo controls (1 ml normal saline) were compared against three doses of NLX (1, 3, and 10 mg/kg), MP sodium succinate (15 mg/kg), and combined NLX and MP (10 mg/kg + 15 mg/kg). Table 33.1 summarizes the different treatment groups and the numbers of animals in each. All the animals received the treatments at 45 minutes after injury as an intravenous bolus without further maintenance doses. The rationale for this therapeutic approach is based on earlier studies showing that a single large early intravenous dose of NLX (10 mg/kg) or MP (15 mg/kg) was sufficient to prevent the typical posttraumatic white matter ischemia that occurs in the 20 gm-20 cm contusion model (85). The timing, 45 minutes, was chosen as a reasonable time at which drug treatment can be initiated in clinical spinal cord injury.

Assessment of Locomotor Recovery

The recovery of the cats from the spinal cord injury was judged from the locomotor and somatosensory evoked potential scores. At 6 and 12 weeks after injury, the locomotor ability of each cat was individually scored on a scale of 0–3 (0 = paralyzed hindlimbs, 1 = definite voluntary movements but inability to stand or walk, 2 = able to stand and walk unaided for short distances, 3 = able to walk across the room unaided). The scores were assigned by observers unaware of the treatments received by individual animals. Since supported animals even with transected spinal cords can exhibit spontaneous rhythmic motions related to locomotory generator sites in the lumbar spinal cord, we had to choose a behavior that required a substantial degree of descending control. Therefore, we emphasized *unaided* stance and locomotion in our scores. However, we felt that finer distinctions cannot be made through subjective observations of untrained animals.

Many investigators utilize modified Tarlov scales (76, 77) for scoring neurological recovery in animals. These scales typically required scoring of limbs independently for presence of spasticity and voluntary activity. Scores from individual limbs are summed. Such scales suffer from the weakness of substantial score overlap in animals that appear to function very differently. For example, an animal with normal scores on one hindlimb but totally paralyzed on the other may appear the same as an animal with low but present scores on both hindlimbs. Furthermore, the summed scores do not provide as much intuitive understanding of the recovery criteria as simple statements of the proportion of animals that recovered ability to walk unaided.

Somatosensory Evoked Potentials (SEPs)

SEPs were obtained at 6 weeks in all the cats. Activated by 2.3 Hz stimulation of the sciatic nerve with bipolar stainless steel needle electrodes, 200 responses were recorded and averaged from epidural electrodes contralateral to the stimulated side. The epidural electrodes were placed prior to injury and consist of small screws inserted into openings drilled in calvarium, one overlying the frontal midline and one overlying the somatosensory cortices on each side. The electrodes were held in place with dental acrylic. These screw electrodes provided a stable recording environment for the duration of the study.

The SEPs were graded on a scale of 0–3 (0 = absent response, 1 = trace, 2 = present but abnormal in latency or amplitude, 3 = normal). Three sets of SEP responses from each hindlimb were scored by three observers. To obtain a single score from two hindlimbs, we gave the animal an SEP score of 0 if both legs had no SEP responses or if one leg had a score of 1 and the other 0. If both hindlimbs had scores of 1 or one leg had 1 and the other 2, we gave the animal an overall SEP score of 1. If both legs had scores of 2 or one leg had 2 and the other 3, we gave the animal an overall SEP score of 2. Finally, if both legs had scores of 3, we gave an overall score of 3.

This SEP scoring approach was developed on pragmatic grounds. Although latencies and amplitudes of specific SEP components can be measured fairly reliably normally, spinal-injured animals and humans (84) have such abnormal and low amplitude SEP that specific components cannot be identified reliably. Furthermore, most of the SEP recordings showed no responses at all. The categories were chosen to minimize ambiguity and overlap. For example, the absence of responses can be readily assessed as no consistent response greater than background noise levels. Likewise, trace and abnormal responses can be distinguished easily from each other. However, because the greater source of disagreement between observers happened to be between the categories of 0 and 1, we tended to be more conservative in such situations.

Evaluation of Histological Appearance of the Lesion Site

At the end of 12 weeks, the cats were anesthetized with pentobarbital and perfused with formaldehyde fixatives. The spinal cords were removed, embedded in paraffin, and serially sectioned. The histological appearance of the spinal cords were assessed by ranking representative hematoxylin and eosin-stained coronal sections of the spinal cords in order of severity of damage. Severity of the lesion was subjectively judged on the basis of radial and longitudinal extent of the lesion site, as well as the amount of tissue surviving the lesion site. Three observers ranked coded coronal sections of the spinal cords.

Although quantitative morphometric assessments of injured spinal cords can be carried out (9–12) we chose not to do so in these experiments due to the large volume of histological material. The objective of the histological assessment was therefore limited to determining whether or not treatment differences can be detected on ranking of cord sections on the basis of light microscopic inspections. After rank ordering of the spinal cords, nonparametric statistical assessments of the treatment groups by the Wilcoxon test were carried out.

Statistical Analyses

The locomotor and SEP scores were assessed by the chi-square test. The ranking of the histological appearance of the lesion sites was then statistically assessed with the nonparametric Wilcoxon rank sum test. A p value of <0.05 served as criterion for statistical significance. To reduce observer bias, all scoring and rankings were done by observers unaware of the specific treatments received by individual animals. In most of the experiments, the treatments were randomized after injury.

Some animals were prospectively eliminated from the study. For example, cats that recovered SEP prior to the administration of treatments were excluded from the study. Mortality in the groups also posed a problem. Animals that died prior to the 6-week or 12-week assessment time points may have contributed to an inadvertent selection of the survivors with better functional recovery. To assess the magnitude of error contributed by mortality, we conducted a worst case analysis by assuming that all the animals that died would have remained paralyzed and would not have recovered SEP responses.

RESULTS

Table 33.1 lists the treatment groups and the numbers of animals studied in each group. Figures 33.1–33.4 summarize the locomotor, SEP, and mortality data in each treatment group at 6 weeks after injury. The control, NLX, MP, and combined NLX-MP results will be described separately below. The histological results will be presented last.

Control Untreated Group

A small number of cats died before the 6-week evaluation time. Of 20 cats in the control group, 3 died, representing a mortality rate of 15%.

TABLE 33.1
Treatment Groups

Name	Treatment	Dose (mg/kg)	No. of Animals
1. Control	Untreated		20
2. NLX1	Naloxone	1	7
3. NLX3	Naloxone	3	6
4. NLX10	Naloxone	10	28
5. MP	Methylprednisolone	15	14
6. NLX10 + MP15	Naloxone + Methylprednisolone	10 + 15	16
	Total no. of animals studied		91

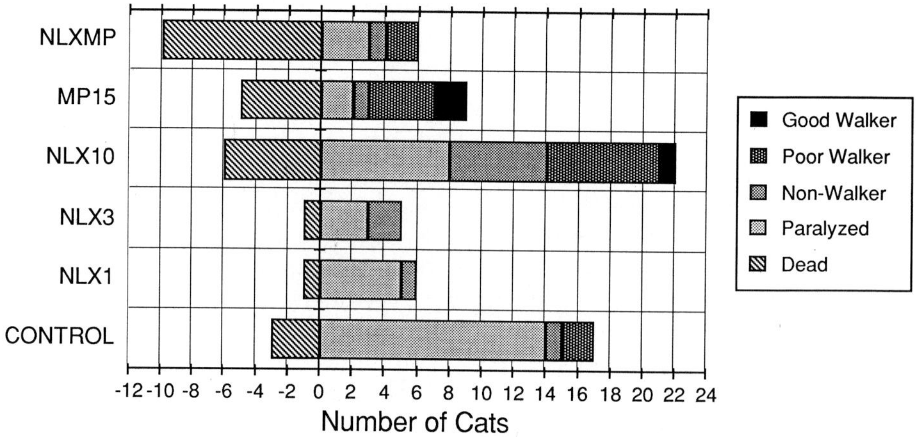

FIG. 33.1. Distribution of mortality and motor scores at 6 weeks. The numbers of animals that are *good walkers, poor walkers, non-walkers* (able to move but unable to stand and walk unaided), and *paralyzed* are plotted to the *right* of the ordinate. These are respectively equivalent to motor scores 3, 2, 1, and 0. The number of animals that died are shown on the *left* of the ordinate. The groups were given 10 mg/kg naloxone plus 15 mg/kg methyl-prednisolone (*NLXMP*), 15 mg/kg methylprednisolone (*MP15*), naloxone 10 mg/kg (*NLX10*), naloxone 3 mg/kg (*NLX3*), naloxone 1 mg/kg (*NLX1*), and controls (*CONTROL*).

All of the animals died more than 2 weeks after injury. None of the animals had frank infections of the surgery site or urological system. One cat had a pulmonary infection unresponsive to antibiotics and probably of viral origins. The other two simply were not feeding well and were losing weight. A mortality rate of 10–20% is consistent with previous studies in our laboratory.

A large majority of the untreated control cats did not recover motor function at 6 weeks after injury. Of the 17 cats in the group that survived

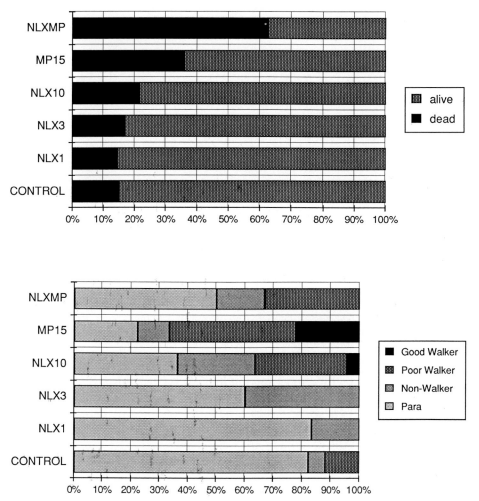

FIG. 33.3.   Percentage of cats in each motor score category. The percentage of animals is shown by motor categories respectively equivalent to the scores of 0, 1, 2, and 3. *Paralyzed* indicates lack of voluntary movements; *non-walker* indicates able to move voluntarily but unable to stand or walk unaided; *poor walker* indicates able to walk for a few steps unaided; and *good walker* indicates able to walk unaided. See Figure 33. 1 for explanation of groups.

to 6 weeks, 14 remained paralyzed; 1 showed some voluntary hindlimb movements but was unable to stand; 2 were able to stand and ambulate short distances unaided; and none were able to ambulate long distances. Thus, about 12% of the surviving controls recovered some locomotory ability; 6% had voluntary but nonfunctional hindlimb movements; and 82% were paralyzed. Figure 33.2 summarizes these results.

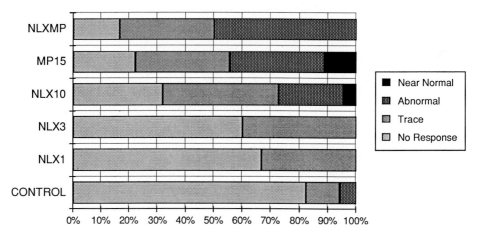

Figure 33.4. Percentage of cats in each SEP score category. The percentage of animals is shown by categories respectively equivalent to somatosensory scores of 0, 1, 2, and 3. *No response* indicates no consistent cortical somatosensory evoked potential waveform discernible within the first 50 msec in either hindlimb or very small response in only one hindlimb; *trace* response indicates a small but definite response in at least two limbs; *abnormal* indicates a robust response that is abnormal in latency and amplitude in at least both limbs; *near normal* indicates strong responses present in both limbs and responses close to normal in one or both limbs. See Figure 33.1 for explanation of groups.

SEP recovery reflected the locomotor scores. One of the two cats that recovered some ambulatory function had a trace response (SEP = 1) and the other present but abnormal (SEP = 1.5). One cat had trace SEP responses on one leg (SEP = 0.5). The remainder had no detectable SEP responses on either leg (SEP = 0). Thus, 14 of 17 animals or 82% of the surviving cats in the group had no detectable cortical SEP elicitable from either hindlimb. Only 1 cat or 6% of the surviving controls had more than trace SEP responses.

Naloxone Groups

Mortality rates in the NLX-treated groups were slightly higher than those of the controls. In the 1 mg/kg, 3 mg/kg, and 10 mg/kg groups, 1 of 7, 1 of 6, and 6 of 28 cats died before 6 weeks, respectively, 14%, 17%, and 21%, respectively. This suggests a trend of increasing mortality with the 10 mg/kg dosage of NLX administered at 45 minutes after spinal cord injury. Statistical analysis, however, indicated that the mortality rate of the 10 mg/kg-treated cats was not significantly (Chi-square value of 0.316, 1 *df*, *p* > 0.25) higher than that of the controls.

The low dose NLX-treated groups (1 and 3 mg/kg) did not show significant motor recovery at 6 weeks. None of six cats treated with 1 mg/kg and none of the five cats treated with 3 mg/kg recovered motor scores to 2 or more. Only 1 of the 6 (17%) cats treated with 1 mg/kg and 2 of the 5 (40%) cats treated with 3 mg/kg NLX showed any evidence of voluntary activity in the hindlimbs. The SEP scores in these two groups similarly support the lack of a beneficial effect of NLX at 1 mg/kg and 3 mg/kg doses. One of 6 cats (17%) in the 1 mg/kg group had trace responses on both hindlimbs, and another (17%) had trace SEP responses in one hindlimb. Two of 5 cats (40%) of the 3 mg/kg group had trace responses in one or both hindlimbs. None had SEP scores above 1 on any limb.

The high dose NLX-treated group (10 mg/kg) showed greater recovery than controls at 6 weeks. Of the 22 cats surviving to 6 weeks, 8 or 37% achieved motor scores of 2 or higher; 14 or 64% had motor scores of 1 or greater. The motor scores in the 10 mg/kg NLX-treated group were significantly greater than those of controls on statistical analysis (Chi-square value 8.147, 3 df, $p < 0.05$). SEP scores also were significantly higher in the 10 mg/kg NLX-treated group compared to those of the 1 mg/kg and 3 mg/kg groups. Approximately 51% of the 10 mg/kg NLX-treated group had SEP responses with scores of 1 or greater on both legs, compared to 12% in the controls (Chi-square value 6.309, 1 df, $p < 0.05$).

Methylprednisolone Group

High doses of MP (15 mg/kg) increased mortality rates. Of 14 cats studied, 5 or 36% died within 6 weeks after injury. Although this increase appears to be not statistically significant, the trend approaches significance (Chi-square value of 4.706, 1 df, $0.05 < p < 0.1$). Of the 9 surviving cats treated with 15 mg/kg methylprednisolone, 6 (66%) achieved motor scores of 2 or better. This is significantly different from the scores of the controls (Chi-square value of 8.327, 1 df, $p < 0.05$). This salutary effect of MP on the motor scores continued to be significant even when we did the worst case analysis by assuming that all the cats that died would not have recovered motor scores of >1 (Chi-square value of 4.894, 1 df, $p < 0.05$).

The SEP scores supported the results of the motor evaluation. Of the 9 cats treated with 15 mg/kg MP and evaluated at 6 weeks, 6 had SEP scores of 1 or greater in both hindlimbs (Chi-square value of 8.327, 1 df, $p < 0.001$). Even if we assumed that all the cats that died prior to the 6-week evaluation would not have recovered SEP, the results would still be statistically significant (Chi-square value of 4.894, 1 df, $p < 0.05$).

Combination Naloxone-Methylprednisolone Group

Combining NLX and MP greatly increased postoperative mortality. By 6 weeks after injury, 63% of the animals had to be sacrificed due to failure to thrive despite intensive care. This is statistically significant from control (Chi-square value of 8.693, 1 df, $p < 0.001$). Of the 6 surviving cats treated with combined NLX and MP, 4 had SEP scores of 1 or greater in both hindlimbs (Chi-square value of 6.933, 1 df, $p < 0.01$). However, worst case analysis suggests that recovery results in the group given combined NLX and MP may not be significant. If we assume that all the cats that died prior to evaluation would not have had SEP, the difference between their recovery results and those of the controls was no longer statistically significant (Chi-square value of 2.148, 1 df, $0.20 < p < 0.1$).

Histological Evaluation of the Lesion Site

Based on the locomotory and SEP recovery of the different groups, we expected the histological appearance of the lesion site to reflect the extent of function recovery observed. Three independent observers ranking hematoxylin and eosin-stained sections of the lesion site could not distinguish in that respect between the groups. The Wilcoxon ranked sum test suggested that none of the treated groups could be distinguished from each other on the basis of their ranks at a confidence level of $p < 0.05$.

DISCUSSION

We will first review some of the literature on the use of NLX and MP in spinal cord injury and then focus on three issues: the high doses of NLX and MP required to achieve functional effects, the potential deleterious effects of combined MP and NLX, and our failure to detect any significant difference in the histological appearance of the lesion site in the different treatment groups.

NLX Treatment of Spinal Cord Injury

NLX belongs to a class of morphine analogues in which the methyl group on the N carbon is replaced by a larger alkene chain. These drugs specifically bind opiate receptors, displacing other opiate compounds from the receptors with variable efficiency. Many of these drugs themselves activate opiate receptors and thus produce so-called agonist action, in addition to antagonizing the existing opiates. NLX has the least agonist activity of this class of substances and is one of the most potent, reversing exogenous opiates in doses of 0.01–0.10 mg/kg. It, however, is metabolized rapidly and has a half-life of about 30 minutes (39).

Faden and Holaday (32, 33) first reported a beneficial effect of NLX on posttraumatic hypotension and neurological recovery of cats subjected to experiment cervical spinal contusion. These experiments stemmed from earlier observations (31) that NLX improves blood pressure in hemorrhagic and endotoxic models of hypotensive shock. Thus, when they found that 2 mg/kg/hour of NLX given intravenously not only prevented the hypotension but improved neurological recovery of the cats, they suggested that the posttraumatic hypotension is caused by endogenous opiates and that NLX improved spinal cord blood flow by increasing blood pressure (36).

We (85) subsequently assessed the effect of NLX on spinal cord white matter blood flow and found that a 10 mg/kg bolus dose prevented the typical posttraumatic spinal white matter hypoperfusion. The spinal cord blood flow improvement, however, did not correlate with higher systemic pressures in individual animals. Furthermore, by the time blood flow began to fall at 2–3 hours after injury, blood pressure was typically beginning to normalize. White matter blood flow usually did not differ significantly from preinjury levels and was even slightly higher during the first hour after injury (83, 85–88). We concluded that NLX probably alters blood flow directly in the spinal cord through a mechanism other than systemic pressure. This conclusion has found support in studies suggesting that naloxone causes cerebral arterial vasodilatation (78).

The mechanism of the NLX effect in spinal cord injury is still not well understood. The cause-effect relationship between the NLX-induced improvement in blood flow and functional recovery has not been established. Naltrexone, an opiate receptor blocker closely related to naloxone, increases central nervous system (CNS) tissue metabolic activity (44). The posttraumatic decline in spinal blood flow, however, may be a manifestation rather than a cause of tissue damage (83). In fact, the site of action of NLX in spinal cord injury is not known, *i.e.*, whether NLX acts directly on the spinal cord or through some indirect systemic effect. Although NLX has been reported to be beneficial in cerebral and spinal cord ischemia (55, 64), the findings have not been reproducible by all of the laboratories studying the phenomenon and remain controversial (54, 57, 69).

Current research on the subject has focused on other opiate receptor blockers. Soon after their initial studies on NLX, Faden and Holaday (30, 34, 37, 38) reported that thyrotropin-releasing hormone (TRH) had effects on spinal cord injury similar to those of NLX. TRH is not even a direct opiate receptor antagonist but has indirect affects on opiate receptors other than the μ class of receptors. NLX antagonizes most classes of opiate receptors but shows the greatest affinity for the μ class of receptors. Consequently, Faden *et al.* (30) have proposed that the effect of NLX is mediated by the κ class of opiate receptors (58).

MP Treatment of Spinal Cord Injury

A large body of literature suggests that corticosteroids exert beneficial effects in spinal cord injury. The effects of steroid administration on functional recovery and histological appearance of the lesion site have been studied by Campbell *et al.* (22), Black and Markowitz (8), Eidelberg *et al.* (27), Green *et al.* (45), Means and Anderson *et al.* (3, 65), Pappius (69), and many others (26, 35, 38, 50, 51, 59, 61, 65, 72). These studies have relied on several animal species and injury models, a variety of steroids, widely different dosages, and many methods of evaluating injury outcome. More recent studies have focused on the biochemical and physiological effects of high dose MP, usually 15–30 mg/kg (15–21, 46–49, 73, 88), reporting that very high doses are required to reduce lipid peroxidation. Given the variety of methods and models, it is not surprising that workers in the field have not been unanimous in their reports of steroid treatment effects. Although a majority of investigators using high doses of steroids have reported morphological, biochemical, physiological, or functional improvements in spinal injury models, some did not (8, 35, 38, 51).

Classically, corticosteroids are believed to act as hormones with marked effects on protein metabolism leading to negative protein balance. They increase gluconeogenesis, lipid metabolism, Na retention, K excretion, glandular secretions, and CNS excitability. In addition, in large doses, they "stabilize" cell membranes, prevent formation of vasoactive kinins, and alter a multitude of other biological processes, possibly through indirect mechanisms (53, 62, 82). In doses higher than endogenous levels, corticosteroids have been shown to inhibit inflammation and immune responses. Thus, corticosteroids have proven indispensable for therapy of hypersensitivity reactions, rheumatoid diseases, ulcerative colitis, dermatitis, and other conditions.

However, in spinal cord injury, the mechanism of action may involve none of these hormonally mediated effects of corticosteroids. MP belongs to a class of synthetic steroids of greater (4×) glycosteroid potency than cortisone but of less than dexamethasone (25×). For beneficial effects to be seen in spinal cord injury, most recent studies suggest that at least 15 mg/kg of MP must be given. This is more than 1000 times the level needed to activate glucocorticosteroid receptors in the body. Some workers have consequently focused on a direct chemical effect of the steroid unrelated to its hormonal action. Demopoulos *et al.* (24), for example, theorized that steroids play an important role in stabilizing membranes by inhibiting free radical reactions set into motion by trauma. This theory has been supported recently by work from Braughler and Hall (15–20), who showed that large doses of MP (30 mg/kg) will reduce lipid peroxidation in injured spinal cords. They also showed that high dose steroids will protect membrane-bound enzymes, such as ATPase, and intracellular substances, such as neurofilaments, as well as reverse pathological lactic acid accumulation at the lesion site.

In recent studies, we found that 15 mg/kg MP had a significant but delayed effect on blood flow and ionic changes. These blood flow increases were maximally produced at dosages of 30 mg/kg. Hall and Braughler (18–20, 47) showed a clear dose-response relationship between MP dosage and the attenuation of lactoacidosis, neurofilamentous degradation, and ATPase activity loss in injured spinal cords. The dosage window appears to be very narrow. At 60–90 mg/kg, according to Hall and Braughler, MP actually worsened all the parameters studied.

The High Doses of MP and NLX Required to Produce Functional Recovery

Our data presented above suggest strongly that very high doses of NLX are required to improve functional recovery of spinal-injured cats. Cats treated with 1 mg/kg and 3 mg/kg of NLX did not differ from controls. Note the trend for better SEP and motor recovery with increasing NLX dose, suggesting that >3 mg/kg of NLX is required to produce significant functional recovery from spinal cord injury and that 3 mg/kg may represent the threshold of drug effect. Faden and Holaday had found 2 mg/kg/hour of NLX to be efficacious (32, 33, 36, 38). The discrepancy between their experimental results and ours may stem from the injury models used and the drug administration protocol. Their model consisted of a contusion of the cervical spinal cord, which allowed some neurological recovery in a majority of untreated cats at 6 weeks after injury whereas only 15% of untreated cats subjected to our model recovered. Our protocol also differed in that NLX was given as a bolus injection at 45 minutes whereas they gave a continuous infusions of 2 mg/kg/hour.

In humans, 0.4–1.0 mg of NLX given to a 70-kg person will reverse narcotic overdoses, 3 orders of magnitudes less than the 10 mg/kg dose that we used in this study. Likewise, the recommended dosage for the hormonal effects of MP is about 50–500 μg/kg per day to an average-sized human. The dose of 15 mg/kg we gave in this study represents 30–300 times the dose required to produce glucocorticoid effects. Clearly, a strong likelihood exists that neither of the drugs may be acting via their normally accepted mechanism of action as an opiate receptor blocker or a glucocorticosteroid. Although it is possible that naloxone may be acting on κ-receptor sites which would require higher doses, we still lack an explanation of what κ-receptors have to do with spinal cord injury. The role of κ-receptors in mammalian CNS is still controversial (52). Likewise, although it is possible that the MP is mediated by one of its many hormonal effects which simply requires total saturation of all the steroid receptors, it is unclear what effect this might be and how it can act so rapidly as to produce a change in spinal cord blood flow within minutes after a 30 mg/kg dose of MP has been given.

Neither drug, especially NLX, had been given to spinal-injured patients at such high doses. We therefore embarked on a Phase I clinical trial to ascertain the feasibility of giving such high doses of these two drugs to spinal-injured patients. A total of 60 patients with spinal cord injury were treated with either MP or NLX within 24 hours after injury. Due to the extensive clinical experience with giving 1 gm of MP to patients with spinal cord injury (15 mg/kg), we went to 30 mg/kg MP loading dose followed by 50% of that dose every hour for 24 hours. In the case of NLX, 29 patients were given doses of NLX ranging from 0.14 to 5.4 mg/kg. The first 3 patients were started on 0.14 mg/kg loading dose, followed by 20% of the loading dose per hour for 48 hours. The dose was doubled every 3–5 patients when no side effects were noted. The last 9 patients received 2.7–5.4 mg/kg loading dose, followed by 75% of that dose per hour for 24 hours. The results of this clinical trial have been published (41).

This Phase I trial served to allay three concerns. First, our worry that NLX, being an opiate receptor blocker, may enhance pain in patients who had just recently suffered trauma turned out to be immaterial. Although 4 of 29 patients experienced pain, only one had to be withdrawn from the study because of pain. A large majority tolerated the high doses with no major side effects. The four patients who experienced pain all had some preserved sensations below the lesion level and had a reason for pain. The one patient that was withdrawn had a fractured hip. Because of the naloxone, opiate analgesics cannot be used. Second, in the previous NASCIS trial involving 1 gm of MP given for 10 days, there was a trend towards increasing morbidity (13, 14). Although not statistically significant, we were concerned that the higher 30 mg/kg dose of MP might have greater adverse side effects. This did not turn out to be the case. The incidence of infection, pulmonary complications, and upper gastrointestinal tract hemorrhage did not increase in the patients treated with 30 mg/kg MP, followed by maintenance dosages of 15 mg/kg/hour for 24 hours. Some previous studies suggested that naloxone can produce cardiorespiratory complications (4, 5, 40, 63, 66, 75) and psychological changes (23). Third, the mortality rates of both the MP- and NLX-treated patients were not significantly different from historical untreated controls.

Possible Deleterious Effects of High Dose MP and NLX

High dose MP (30 mg/kg) and NLX (10 mg/kg) produced a higher mortality rate in our animal studies. Although, when judged by strict statistical criterion of $p < 0.05$, the mortality of neither group was significantly different from that of controls, it is important to apply a less conservative criterion to avoid a Type II statistical error. Thus, we decided to use a $p < 0.25$ for the test of significance. By this criterion, the mortality rate of the groups treated with 15 mg/kg MP, however, appeared to be of borderline significance ($0.05 < p < 0.1$). The mortality rates of the 1 mg/kg, 3 mg/kg, and 10 mg/kg NLX-treated cats was not significantly different from those of untreated control ($p > 0.25$). There were no doubts, however, about the statistical significance of the mortality rate in the combined NLX-MP-treated group ($p < 0.001$), wherein 10 of 16 cats died within 6 weeks after spinal cord injury.

Most of the NLX-MP treated cats died at about a week after injury, sometimes without obvious cause, and despite intense care. Some had evidence of pulmonary edema and right heart failure, but this was not a consistent finding. There was no evidence of frank infections of the lungs, urinary tract, or central nervous system. Because we had not expected this high a mortality rate from the studies using only NLX or MP, we had not prepared for more detailed investigations of the cats. For example, the immunological status of the animals was not assessed. Nevertheless, the high mortality rate in this group of cats led us to recommend strongly to the NASCIS committee to take as much precaution as possible to exclude patients receiving either drug in high doses prior to admission to the protocol. The Phase I trial was likewise carried out with the same precautions.

High doses of NLX (4 mg/kg) have been reported to produce temporary decreases in memory performance and mood changes in normal human volunteers. In addition, there are several reported cases of adverse effects of small doses of naloxone in patients, usually in the setting of general anesthesia. For example, hypertension, pulmonary edema, ventricular arrhythmias, and cardiac arrests (4, 5, 40, 66, 75) have been observed with 0.2–0.8 mg of naloxone. In most of these cases, factors in addition to the naloxone administration may have contributed to the complications. None of our NLX-MP-treated animals died acutely during the surgery or injury procedures when they were anesthetized.

Recently, Sapolsky and Pulsinelli (74) reported that glucocorticosteroids increased the extent of neuronal death in a model of transient cortical ischemia in rats. It is unclear whether this finding is relevant to the NASCIS study for the following reasons. First, they used adrenalectomy to test the role of glucocorticosteroids. Their study failed to consider the possibility that adrenalectomy may have altered blood levels of catecholamines and other substances which may be a contributing factor to the ischemic lesion. Second, the reported deleterious effect occurred in hippocampal neurons that are known to be susceptible to transient ischemia and also have the highest concentration of glucocorticoid hormonal receptors in the CNS. Third, MP has also been used in large numbers of patients with CNS tumors and inflammatory diseases with no report of neurological problems. Fourth, a recent study by Braughler and Lainer (21) showed that very high doses of MP (60 mg/kg) improved the mortality and functional recovery of gerbils subjected to bilateral carotid occlusions. Similar protective effects on glucocorticoids have been reported in other models of neuronal injury (60, 62, 68, 70, 71, 79). Finally, a deleterious effect of MP on the injured spinal cord is inconsistent with our data so far on recovery of function in spinal cord injury.

We, however, must not become complacent about the use of such high doses of MP or NLX. The beneficial effects of MP appear to be restricted to a dosage range of 15–30 mg/kg, a very narrow therapeutic window. Braughler and Hall have shown that MP doses exceeding 60 mg/kg can aggravate the injury process in injured cat spinal cords, including enhanced lactoacidosis and lipid peroxidation. This is one of the major limitations of high dose MP treatments. Due to variables such as blood flow, drug delivery to the nervous system may conceivably produce spinal cord MP concentrations wider than a two-fold concentration range. Therefore, both beneficial and deleterious effects may be produced by high dose MP treatments, and the latter may be masked by the former. The NLX therapeutic dosage range similarly may be narrow although, to our knowledge, there are no studies that have systematically investigated naloxone effects on injured spinal cords at doses greater than 10–20 mg/kg.

Histological Appearance of the Lesion Site and Functional Recovery

The histological appearance of the lesion sites did not correlate significantly with functional recovery. Despite the significant differences between the treated and untreated groups behaviorally, we were unable to find consistent differences in the qualitative light microscopic appearance of the treated and untreated spinal cords. The lack of correlation between the morphological appearance of the spinal cords and the extent of functional recovery raises a critical question. How can the animals recover so strikingly without improvement in the morphological appearance of the lesion site?

Quantitative morphometric analysis of injured spinal cords (9–12) suggested that the difference in the numbers of axons that can support locomotor function may be too small to be detected by subjective assessments of the spinal cord. Normal cats have approximately 500,000 axons countable on light microscopy in the T9 thoracic spinal cord. In our 20 gm-20 cm contusion model of spinal cord injury, an average of 17,000 axons ± 20,000 survive at 3–4 months after injury or <5%. In cats with locomotor scores of 2 or greater, axon counts ranged from 25,000 to >100,000. In several studies carried out in the past 3 years in our laboratory, total axon counts were compared with walking ability. No cat that had less than 20,000 axons was able to walk unassisted.

While very low axon counts can rule out recovery, high axon counts do not necessarily predict locomotory ability. For example, some cats with >50,000 axons were unable to walk. *In vitro* recordings suggest that the lack of recovery is attributable in part to demyelination (9, 10). Note that 50,000 axons represent only 10% of the normal axon count. Thus, approximately 20,000–30,000 axons are necessary and sometimes sufficient to support functional locomotion in cats. These findings support the observations of Windle *et al.* (80, 81) that section of as much as 90% of a cat spinal cord will still allow recovery of locomotory function. Likewise, Eidelberg *et al.* (28, 29) found that relatively few axons can support locomotor function in cats.

These findings may explain our inability to detect a difference in the histological appearance of the lesion site. A discrepancy of several thousand or even tens of thousands of axons, *i.e.*, 1–2% of the spinal white matter, is not easily detectable by means other than quantitative axon counts. That argues for the necessity for quantitative axon counts in experimental spinal cord injury studies. Potentially misleading conclusions can arise from relying on the histological appearance of the spinal cord or even mapping the size of the lesion site.

Beyond NASCIS

Spinal cord injury, by necessity, involves mechanical damage to axons. A large proportion of the axons at the lesion site must die or become disconnected as a direct result of mechanical damage, no matter how attractive the theories concerning secondary nonmechanical injuries to axons may sound. The number of axons that can be salvaged by any pharmacological treatment must be limited in cases of severe spinal cord injury. The finding of walking animals with <10% of spinal axons imparts a breath of optimism in this otherwise dismal picture. It suggests that saving or regeneration of as little as 5–10% of axons in the spinal cord may restore some function in spine-injured animals.

Our findings suggest that treatments that can prevent 5–10% of nondisrupted axons at the lesion site from dying may restore some motor and sensory function. There are likely to be a large number of pharmacological approaches to this goal. Neither NLX or MP are optimal therapies. Both were discovered serendipitously to have beneficial effects on spinal cord injury, at dosages that essentially preclude their normal mechanisms of action as opiate receptor blockers or steroid hormones. They both have undesirable side effects which, although sufficiently tolerable at present to be tested in a clinical trial, may lead to problems when either are used clinically in large populations. The results of our animal study suggest a trend for both NLX and MP to increase mortality rates, albeit not statistically significantly. There are approximately 10,000 cases of acute spinal cord injury in the U.S. yearly. Even a 2–3% increase in mortality rates, not detectable with our small trials, would be unacceptable, especially if the clinically significant gain in function occurs only in a small fraction of treated patients.

Whether or not the current NASCIS trial demonstrates beneficial effects of NLX or MP, further laboratory research must be carried out. If the trial indicates that neither are effective, we must not only identify new treatments but also explain why the clinical results do not correlate with laboratory findings. Many questions will need answers. Should the treatment be given earlier, for longer periods of time, or directly to the spinal cord? Should the treatment be restricted only to certain types of spinal cord lesions? Are the animal models that we devote so much effort to representative of the human condition?

The mechanisms of action of MP and NLX must be elucidated. It is likely that the effects of both of these drugs on injured spinal cords are unanticipated drug effects unrelated to their classic receptor activities. More specific and potent drugs can probably be found. Without understanding their mechanisms, better drugs with more focused activities and fewer side effects will be difficult to find. Empirical trial-and-error approaches to drug discovery are hopelessly inefficient. Therein lies the challenge of the post-NASCIS era.

ACKNOWLEDGMENTS

This work is supported in part by NIH Grants NS 10164, NS 15990, and NS17267. We are grateful to Fred Holmes, Ben Ayala, and James Sinaly for excellent technical assistance.

REFERENCES

1. Allen, A. R. Surgery of experimental lesion of spinal cord equivalent to crush injury of fracture dislocation. J. A. M. A., *50:* 941–952, 1911.
2. Allen, A. R. Remarks on histopathological changes in spinal cord due to impact: An experimental study. J. Nerv. Ment. Dis., *41:* 141–147, 1914.
3. Anderson, D. K., Means, E. D., Waters, T. R., *et al.* Microvascular perfusion and metabolism in injured spinal cord after methylprednisolone treatment. J. Neurosurg., *56:* 106–113, 1983.
4. Andree, R. A. Sudden death following naloxone administration. Anesth. Analg. (Cleve.), *59:* 782–784, 1980.
5. Azar, I., and Turndoff, H. Severe hypertension and multiple atrial premature contractions following naloxone administration. Anesth. Analg. (Cleve.), *59:* 524–525, 1979.

6. Balentine, J. D. Pathology of experimental spinal cord trauma. I. The necrotic lesion as a function of vascular injury. Lab. Invest., *39:* 236–253, 1978.

7. Balentine, J. D. Pathology of experimental spinal cord trauma. II. Ultrastructure of axons and myelin. Lab. Invest., *39:* 254–255, 1978.

8. Black, P., and Markowitz, R. S. Experimental spinal cord injury in monkeys: Comparison of steroids and local hypothermia. Surg. Forum, *22:* 409–411, 1971.

9. Blight, A. R. Cellular morphology of chronic spinal cord injury in the cat: Analysis of myelinated axons by line sampling. Neuroscience, *10:* 521–543, 1983.

10. Blight, A. R. Axonal physiology of chronic spinal cord injury in the cat: intracellular recording in vitro. Neuroscience *10:* 1471–1486, 1983.

11. Blight, A. R. Delayed demyelination and macrophage invasion: A candidate for "secondary" cell damage in spinal cord injury. CNS Trauma, *2:* 299–315, 1985.

12. Blight, A. R., and DeCrescito, V. Morphometric analysis of experimental spinal cord injury in the cat: The relation of injury intensity to survival of myelinated axons. Neuroscience, *19:* 321–341, 1986.

13. Bracken, M. B., Collins, W. F., Freeman, D. F., *et al.* Efficacy of methylprednisolone in acute spinal cord injury. J. A. M. A., *251:* 45–52, 1984.

14. Bracken, M. B., Shepard, M. J., Hellenbrand, K. G., *et al.* Methylprednisolone and neurological function 1 year after spinal cord injury. J. Neurosurg., *63:* 704–713, 1985.

15. Braughler, J. M., and Hall, E. D. Acute enhancement of spinal cord synaptosomal (Na^+-K^+)-ATPase activity in cats following intravenous methylprednisolone. Brain Res., *219:* 464–469, 1981.

16. Braughler, J. M., and Hall, E. D. Correlation of methylprednisolone pharmacokinetics in cat spinal cord with its effect on (Na^+-K^+)-ATPase, lipid peroxidation and motor neuron function. J. Neurosurg., *56:* 838–844, 1982.

17. Braughler, J. M., and Hall, E. D. The uptake and elimination of methylprednisolone from the contused cat spinal cord following an intravenous injection of the sodium succinate ester. J. Neurosurg., *58:* 538–542, 1983.

18. Braughler, J. M., and Hall, E. D. Lactate and pyruvate metabolism in the injured cat spinal cord before and after a single large intravenous dose of methylprednisolone. J. Neurosurg., *59:* 256–261, 1983.

19. Braughler, J. M., and Hall, E. D. Pharmacokinetics of methylprednisolone in cat plasma and spinal cord following a single intravenous dose of sodium succinate ester. Drug Metab. Dispos., *10:* 551–552, 1983.

20. Braughler, J. M., and Hall, E. D. Effects of multi-dose methylprednisolone sodium succinate administration on injured cat spinal cord neurofilament degradation and energy metabolism. J. Neurosurg., *61:* 290–295.

21. Braughler, J. M., and Lainer, M. J. The effects of large doses of methylprednisolone on neurologic recovery and survival in the Mongolian gerbil following three hours of unilateral carotid occlusion. CNS Trauma, *3:* 153–161, 1986.

22. Campbell, J. B., DeCrescito, V., Tomasula, J. J., *et al.* Effect of antifibrinolytic and steroid therapy on contused cords of cats. J. Neurosurg., *55:* 726–733, 1974.

23. Cohen, M. R., Cohen, R. M., Pickar, D., *et al.* High-dose naloxone infusions in normals. Dose-dependent behavioral, hormonal, and physiological responses. Arch. Gen. Psychiatry, *40:* 613–619, 1983.

24. Demopoulos, H. B., Flamm, E. S., Pietrenigro, D. D., *et al.* The free radical pathology and the microcirculation in the major central nervous system disorders. Acta Physiol. Scand. Suppl., *492:* 91–119, 1980.

25. Dohrmann, G. J., and Panjabi, M. M. "Standardized" spinal cord trauma: biomechanical parameters and lesion volume. Surg. Neurol., *6:* 263–267, 1976.

26. Ducker, T. B. and Hamit, H. F. Experimental treatments of acute spinal cord injury. J. Neurosurg., *30:* 693–697, 1969.

27. Eidelberg, E., Staten, E., Watkins, L. J., *et al.* Treatment of experimental spinal cord injury in ferrets. Surg. Neurol., *6:* 243–246, 1976.

28. Eidelberg, E., Story, J. L., Walden, J. G., *et al.* Anatomical correlates of return of locomotor function after partial spinal cord lesions in cats. Exp. Brain Res., *42:* 81–88, 1981.

29. Eidelberg, E., Straehley, D., and Erspamer, R. Relationship between residual hindlimb assisted locomotion and surviving axons after incomplete spinal cord injuries. Exp. Neurol., *56:* 312–322, 1977.

30. Faden, A. I. Opiate antagonists and thyrotropin-releasing hormone. II. Potential role in the treatment of central nervous system injury. J. A. M. A., *252:* 1452–1454, 1984.

31. Faden, A. I., and Holaday, J. W. Opiate antagonists: A role in treatment of hypovolemic shock. Science, *205:* 317–318, 1979.

32. Faden, A. I., Jacobs, T. P., and Holaday, J. W. Opiate receptor antagonist improves neurologic recovery after spinal injury. Science, *211:* 493–494, 1981.

33. Faden, A. I., Jacobs, T. P., and Holaday, J. W. Comparison of early and late naloxone treatment in experimental spinal injury. Neurology, *32:* 677–681, 1982.

34. Faden, A. I., Jacobs, T. P., and Holaday, J. W. Thyrotropin-releasing hormone improves neurologic recovery after spinal trauma in cats. N. Engl. J. Med., *305:* 1063–1067, 1981.

35. Faden, A. I., Jacobs, T. P., Patrick, D. H., *et al.* Megadose corticosteroid therapy following experimental traumatic spinal injury. J. Neurosurg., *60:* 712–717, 1984.

36. Faden, A. I., Jacobs, T. P., Mougey, E., *et al.* Endorphins in experimental spinal injury: Therapeutic effect of naloxone. Ann. Neurol., *10:* 326–332, 1981.

37. Faden, A. I., Jacobs, T. P., and Smith, M. T. Thyrotropin-releasing hormone in experimental spinal injury: Dose response and late treatment. Neurology, *34:* 1280–1284, 1984.

38. Faden, A. I., Jacobs, T. P., Smith, M. T., *et al.* Comparison of thyrotropin-releasing hormone (TRH), naloxone, and dexamethasone treatments in experimental spinal injury. Neurology, *33:* 673–678, 1983.

39. Fishman, J., Hahn, E. F., and Norton, B. I. Comparative *in vivo* distribution of opiate agonists and antagonists by means of double isotope techniques. Life Sci., *17:* 1119–1126, 1975.

40. Flacke, J. W., Flacke, W. E., and Williams, G. D. Acute pulmonary edema following naloxone reversal of high-dose morphine anesthesia. Anesthesiology, *47:* 376–378, 1977.

41. Flamm, E. S., Young W., Demopoulos H. B., *et al.* Experimental spinal cord injury: Treatment with naloxone. Neurosurgery, *10:* 227–231, 1982.

42. Flamm, E. S., Young, W., Collins, W. F., *et al.* A Phase I trial of naloxone treatment in acute spinal cord injury. J. Neurosurg., *63:* 390–397, 1985.

43. Goodkin, R., and Campbell, J. B. Sequential pathological changes in spinal cord injury. Surg. Forum, *20:* 430–432, 1969.

44. Grandison, L., Buchweitz, E., and Weiss, H. R. Effect of naltrexone on regional brain oxygen consumption in the cat. Brain Res., *233:* 367–379, 1982.

45. Green, B. A., Kahn, T., and Klose, K. J. A comparative study of steroid therapy in acute experimental spinal cord injury. Surg. Neurol., *13:* 91–97, 1980.

46. Hall, E. D., and Braughler, J. M. Acute effects of intravenous glucocorticoid pretreatment on the *in vitro* peroxidation of cat spinal cord tissue. Exp. Neurol., *72:* 321–324, 1981.

47. Hall, E. D., and Braughler, J. M. Effects of methylprednisolone on spinal cord lipid peroxidation and (Na⁺-K⁺)-ATPase activity: Dose response analysis during the first hour after contusion injury in the cat. J. Neurosurg., *57:* 247–253, 1982.

48. Hall, E. D., and Braughler, J. M. Glucocorticoid mechanisms in acute spinal injury: A review and therapeutic rationale. Surg. Neurol., *18:* 320–327, 1982.

49. Hall, E. D., Wolf, D. L., and Braughler, J. M. Effects of a single large dose of methylprednisolone sodium succinate on experimental posttraumatic spinal cord ischemia. J. Neurosurg., *61:* 124–130, 1984.

50. Hansebout, R. R. A comprehensive review of methods of improving cord recovery after acute spinal cord injury. In: *Early Management of Acute Cervical Spinal Cord Injury*, edited by C. H. Tator, pp. 181–196. Raven Press, New York, 1982.

51. Hedeman, L. S., and Sil, R. Studies in experimental spinal cord trauma. Part 2. Comparison of treatment with steroids, low-molecular weight dextran and catecholamine blockade. J. Neurosurg., *40:* 44–51, 1974.

52. Hiller, J. M., and Simon, E. J. Specific, high affinity [³H]ethylketocyclazocine binding in rat central nervous system: Lack of evidence for κ receptors. J. Pharmacol. Exp. Ther., *214:* 516–519, 1980.

53. Hirata, F., Schiffman, E., Venkatasubramanian, K., *et al.* A phospholipase A₂ inhibitory protein in rabbit neutropils induced by glucocorticoids. Proc. Natl. Acad. Sci. U.S.A., *77:* 2533–2536, 1980.

54. Holaday, J. W., and D'Amato, R. J. Naloxone or TRH fails to improve neurological deficits in gerbil models of "stroke." Life Sci., *31:* 385–392, 1982.

55. Hosobuchi, Y., Baskin, O. S., and Woo, S. K. Reversal of induced ischemic neurologic deficit in gerbils by the opiate antagonist naloxone. Science, *215:* 69–71, 1982.

56. Jarrott, D. M., and Domer, F. R. A gerbil model of cerebral ischemia suitable for drug evaluation. Stroke, *11:* 203–209, 1980.

57. Kastin, A. J., Nissen, C., and Olson, R. D. Failure of MIF-1 or naloxone to reverse ischemia-induced neurological deficits in gerbils. Pharmacol. Biochem. Behav., 17: 1083–1085, 1982.

58. Kosterlitz, H. W., and Leslie, F. M. Comparison of the receptor binding characteristics of opiate antagonists interacting with μ- or κ-receptors. Br. J. Pharmacol., *64:* 607–614, 1978.

59. Kuchner, E. F., and Hansebout, R. R. Combined steroid and hypothermia treatment of experimental spinal cord injury. Surg. Neurol., *6:* 371–376, 1976.

60. Laha, R. K., Dujovny, M., Barrionvevo, P. F., *et al.* Protective effects of methylprednisolone and dimethylsulfoxide in experimental middle cerebral artery embolectomy. J. Neurosurg., *49:* 508–516, 1978.

61. Lewin, M. G., Hansebout, R. R., and Pappius, H. M. Chemical characteristics of traumatic spinal cord edema in cats. Effects of steroids on potassium depletion. J. Neurosurg., *56:* 106–113, 1974.

62. Lombard, J. H., Loegering, D. J., and Stekiel, W. J. Prevention by methylprednisolone of norepinephrine depletion in vascular tissue during severe hemorrhage in dogs. Blood Vessels, *17:* 276–280, 1980.

63. Martin, W. R., Eades, C. G., Thompson, J. A., *et al.* The effects of morphine and nalorphine like drugs in the nondependent and morphine dependent chronic spinal dog. J. Pharmacol. Exp. Ther., *197:* 517–532, 1976.

64. McNicholas, L. F., and Martin, W. R. New and experimental therapeutic roles for naloxone and related opioid antagonists. Drugs, *27:* 81–93, 1984.

65. Means, E. D., Anderson, D. K., Waters, T. R., *et al.* Effect of methylprednisolone in compression trauma to the feline spinal cord. J. Neurosurg., *55:* 200–208, 1981.

66. Michaelis, L. L., Hickey, P. R., Clark, T. A., et al. Ventricular irritability associated with the use of naloxone hydrochloride. Two case reports and laboratory assessment of the effect of the drug on cardiac excitability. Ann. Thorac. Surg., 28: 608–614, 1974.
67. Molt, J. T., Nelson, L. R., Poulos, D. A., et al. Analysis and measurement of some sources of variability in spinal cord trauma. J. Neurosurg., 50: 784–791, 1979.
68. Palmer, G. C., Taylor, M. D., and Callahan, A. S. Therapeutic protection of adenylate cyclase systems following bilateral stroke in gerbils. Fed. Proc., 42: 1367, 1983.
69. Pappius, H. M. The therapeutic effects of drugs in injured central nervous system. CNS Trauma, 2: 93–98, 1985.
70. Pappius, H. M. Dexamethasone and local cerebral glucose utilization in freeze-traumatized rat brain. Ann. Neurol., 12: 157–162, 1982.
71. Pappius, H. M. Effect of drugs on local cerebral glucose utilization in traumatized brain: Mechanisms of action of steroids revisited. In: Recent Progress in the Study and Therapy of Brain Edema, edited by K. G. Go and A. Baethmann, pp. 11–26. Plenum, New York, 1984.
72. Parker, A. J., and Smith, C. W. Functional recovery from spinal cord trauma following dexamethazone and chlorpromazine therapy in dogs. Res. Vet. Sci., 21: 246–247, 1976.
73. Pietrenegro, D. D., DeCrescito, V., Tomasula, J. J., et al. Ascorbic acid: A putative biochemical marker of irreversible neurologic functional loss following spinal cord injury. CNS Trauma, 2: 85–92, 1985.
74. Sapolsky, R. M., and Pulsinelli, W. A. Glucocorticoids potentiate ischemic injury to neurons: Therapeutic implications. Science, 229: 1397–1400, 1985.
75. Taff, R. H. Pulmonary edema following naloxone administration in a patient without heart disease. Anesthesiology, 59: 576–577, 1983.
76. Tarlov, I. M. Spinal Cord Compression, Mechanisms of Paralysis and Treatment. Charles C Thomas, Springfield, Ill., 1957.
77. Tarlov, I. M., and Klinger, H. Spinal cord compression studies. II. Time limits of recovery after acute compression in dogs. Arch. Neurol. Psychiatry, 71: 271–290, 1954.
78. Turner, D. M., Kassell, N. F., Sasaki, T., et al. High dose naloxone produces cerebral vasodilation. Neurosurgery, 15: 192–197, 1984.
79. Tornheim, P. A., and McLaurin, R. L. Effect of dexamethasone on cerebral edema from cranial impact in the cat. J. Neurosurg., 48: 220–227, 1978.
80. Windle, W. F., Smart, J. O., and Beers, J. J. Residual function after subtotal spinal cord transection in adult cats. Neurology, 8: 518–521, 1958.
81. Windle, W. F. Concussion, contusion, and severance of the spinal cord. In: The Spinal Cord and Its Reactions to Traumatic Injury, edited by W. F. Windle. Marcel Dekker, New York, 1980.
82. Woodbury, D. M., and Vernadkis, A. Effects of steroids on the central nervous system. Methods Horm. Res., 5: 1–56, 1966.
83. Young, W. Blood flow, metabolic and neurophysiological mechanisms in spinal cord injury. In: Central Nervous System Trauma Status Report—1985, edited by D. P. Becker and J. T. Povlishock. pp. 463–473. National Institutes of Health, NINCDS, Bethesda, Md., 1985.
84. Young, W. Correlation of somatosensory evoked potentials and neurological findings in clinical spinal cord injury. In: Management of Acute Cervical Spinal Injury, edited C. H. Tator, pp. 153–166. Raven Press, New York, 1981.
85. Young, W., Flamm, E. S., Demopoulos, H. B., et al. Effect of naloxone on posttraumatic

ischemia in experimental spinal contusion. J. Neurosurg., *55:* 209–219, 1981.

86. Young, W., Yen, V., and Blight, A. Extracellular calcium activity in experimental spinal cord contusion. Brain Res., *253:* 105–113, 1982.

87. Young, W., Koreh, I., Yen, V., *et al.* Effect of sympathectomy on extracellular potassium activity and blood flow in experimental spinal cord contusion. Brain Res., *253:* 115–125, 1982.

88. Young, W., and Flamm, E. S. Effect of high dose corticosteroid therapy on blood flow, evoked potentials, and extracellular calcium in experimental spinal cord injury. J. Neurosurg., *57:* 557–673, 1982.

Index

Page numbers in *italics* denote figures; those followed by *t* denote tables

699